# Hearing Loss

Covering all aspects of the anatomy, physiology, diagnosis, and treatment of hearing loss, this is an accessible and comprehensive text for all clinicians interested in expanding their knowledge of hearing loss.

There have been many exciting developments in the nearly two decades since the fourth edition was published. This revised edition includes new material on cochlear biology, synaptopathy, regenerative therapy for sensorineural hearing loss, systemic causes of hearing loss such as autoimmune inner ear disease, advances in audiometry and aural rehabilitation, and many other topics. In addition, it contains expanded chapters on tinnitus, dizziness, and facial paralysis, as well as updated material on otoacoustic emissions, sudden hearing loss, hearing protection devices, temporal bone tumors, nutraceutical research and hearing in dogs. The book is extensively augmented with case reports that illustrate important principles.

The book is of value to otolaryngologists, general practitioners, pediatricians, residents, medical students, audiologists, nurses, audiometric technicians, attorneys, and other professionals with an interest in the ear and hearing.

# Hearing Loss

## Fifth Edition

Robert Thayer Sataloff, MD, DMA, FACS
Professor and Chair, Department of Otolaryngology—Head and Neck Surgery
Senior Associate Dean for Clinical Academic Specialties
Drexel University College of Medicine
Adjunct Professor, Department of Otolaryngology—Head and Neck Surgery
Sidney Kimmel Medical College, Thomas Jefferson University
Chair, American Institute for Voice and Ear Research
Philadelphia, Pennsylvania, USA

Pamela C. Roehm, MD, PhD
Professor and Vice Chair, Department of Otolaryngology—Head and Neck Surgery
Drexel University College of Medicine
St. Christopher's Hospital for Children
Philadelphia, Pennsylvania, USA

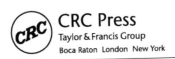

CRC Press
Taylor & Francis Group
Boca Raton London New York

CRC Press is an imprint of the
Taylor & Francis Group, an **informa** business

Designed cover image: Authors' own image

Fifth edition published 2025
by CRC Press
2385 NW Executive Center Drive, Suite 320, Boca Raton, FL 33431

and by CRC Press
4 Park Square, Milton Park, Abingdon, Oxon, OX14 4RN

CRC Press is an imprint of Taylor & Francis Group, LLC

© 2025 Robert Thayer Sataloff and Pamela C. Roehm

Fourth edition published by CRC Press 2005

ISBN: 9781032568669 (hbk)
ISBN: 9781032567594 (pbk)
ISBN: 9781003437444 (ebk)

DOI: 10.1201/b23379

Typeset in Minion
by KnowledgeWorks Global Ltd.

**DEDICATION**

*To our families
and to
Joseph Sataloff, MD, DSc,
one of the founders of the subspecialty of
Otology and author of the first
edition of* Hearing Loss *(1966)*

# Contents

## Appendices

# Preface to the Fifth Edition

As noted in the prefaces to the first (1966), second (1980), third (1993), and fourth (2006) editions of *Hearing Loss,* this work is written for a broad audience. It includes introductory and more advanced reference materials of value to otolaryngologists, general practitioners, pediatricians, residents, medical students, audiologists, nurses, audiometric technicians, attorneys, and other professionals with an interest in the ear and hearing. Although it incorporates a great deal of information, an effort has been made to continue the tradition of the first four editions by keeping the language "readable" not only for physicians, but also for those without an extensive medical vocabulary. There have been many exciting developments in the nearly two decades since the fourth edition was published. This revised edition includes new material on cochlear biology, synaptopathy, regenerative therapy for sensorineural hearing loss, systemic causes of hearing loss such as autoimmune inner ear disease, advances in audiometry and aural rehabilitation, and many other topics. In addition, it contains expanded chapters on tinnitus, dizziness, and facial paralysis, as well as updated material on otoacoustic emissions, sudden hearing loss, hearing protection devices, temporal bone tumors, nutraceutical research and hearing in dogs. The book is extensively augmented with case reports that illustrate important principles.

Chapter 1 provides a succinct overview of hearing loss, emphasizing both medical and societal considerations. Chapter 2 is an accessible review of aspects of the physics of sound pertinent to clinical measurement of hearing and noise. It provides the reader with an understanding of the decibel, hertz, weighting networks, and techniques for calculating the effect of multiple noise sources. Chapter 3 introduces the anatomy and physiology of hearing, and a basic classification of hearing loss. Chapter 4 introduces

clinical elements of the history and physical examination for patients with otologic complaints. The fifth edition also includes an expanded list of Essential Questions to be asked when taking a history.

Chapter 5 reviews the principles and techniques for measuring hearing loss, and it includes a discussion of who should do audiometry. It also includes suggested subjects to be covered in training programs for audiometric technicians and hearing conservationists. In addition, it provides updated information on computerized audiometry. Chapter 6 explains the audiogram and its interpretation, including basic information about masking. This is followed in Chapter 7 by a discussion of special hearing tests, which includes material updated from the third edition. Chapter 8 includes information on auditory-evoked response testing, one of the newer techniques for hearing assessment. Chapter 9 offers an in-depth overview of causes of conductive hearing loss and their management. Before providing a similar overview of over 100 pages for sensorineural hearing loss, Chapter 10 includes a summary of the latest concepts in cochlear biology essential for understanding sensorineural hearing loss. Chapter 11 is a particularly important new addition to the book. In this chapter, the principles and appropriate applications of synaptopathy are summarized definitively by Dr. Charles Liberman whose research identified and characterized this important new topic. In Chapter 12, Dr. Samuel Gubbels provides fascinating insights into research in regenerative therapy for sensorineural hearing loss in another classic new chapter. Chapter 13 discusses the complex and controversial problem of sudden sensorineural hearing loss and its treatment, including the most current concepts (as with all chapters). Chapter 14 presents the problems of mixed, central, and functional hearing loss, including information on auditory processing disorders.

Chapter 15 provides updates to the unique chapter on systemic causes of hearing loss. This chapter summarizes not only the most common and important hereditary causes of hearing loss, but also many of the systemic causes of sensorineural hearing loss, including hypertension, diabetes, syphilis, autoimmune inner ear disease, COVID-19 and many other conditions. Chapter 16 discusses many important common causes of hearing problems in children, the special consequences of hearing impairment in pediatric patients, and important research considerations. Chapter 17 reviews the difficulties and complexities associated with establishing an accurate diagnosis of occupational hearing loss. It summarizes pertinent literature on this subject and includes a review of the criteria established by the American Occupational Medicine Association. It also includes information on many cofactors associated with occupational hearing loss, as well as non-occupational factors that may affect or be confused with occupational hearing impairment.

Chapter 18 has been revised substantially, particularly regarding hearing aids. Information about the latest concepts in amplification has been included, as well as information about cochlear implants. Chapter 19 discusses hearing protection devices for industry, and for special applications such as use by musicians, and has been updated to provide the most current information on the subject. Chapter 20 reviews the problems of tinnitus, a condition often associated with hearing loss. Chapter 21, a newly expanded chapter, provides a comprehensive treatment of the problems associated with balance disorders, as well as a review of modern techniques of evaluation, including videonystagmography, computerized dynamic posturography, rotary chair testing, and other modalities. Chapter 22 covers the problem of facial paralysis. This condition may accompany sensorineural hearing loss, especially following trauma or tumor. Neoplasms of the ear and related structures are among the more serious causes of hearing loss. In the first two editions, only acoustic neuromas were discussed in any detail. Chapters 23 and 24 have been added to provide the reader with overviews of our current understanding of squamous cell carcinoma (Chapter 23) and sarcoma (Chapter 24) of the temporal bone. Both chapters have been updated extensively for this edition. Chapter 25

is presented for general information and fascination, as well as for reference for people working in industries or avocations in which dogs may be employed as guards or to perform work in noisy areas, or in which they may be exposed to noise for other reasons. It describes what is known about hearing in dogs. This information is included in the book not only because of its intrinsic interest, but also because understanding the species differences described so beautifully in this updated chapter, all of us must give considerable thought to how we interpret research data based upon experimentation in animals, many of which are even further distant from humans than are canines. Chapter 26 has been revised extensively and discusses research on nutraceutical modulation of Glutathione, which affects the Cytokine system (among other things), and on other substances that may play a role in future hearing research and care. Chapter 27 is composed of tables summarizing the differential diagnosis of hearing conditions and is especially valuable for quick review. The book also contains four appendices. They provide outline summaries of more detailed information about anatomy of the ear; pathology of the ear; otosclerosis, Paget's disease, and osteogenesis imperfecta; and neurofibromatosis. They are intended to provide in "easy reference" fashion, more detailed information on these subjects than was considered appropriate for the body of the text. We hope that they will prove particularly useful for students and residents.

This book is associated with another work by the same authors: *Occupational Hearing Loss*, Fourth Edition. Some of the chapters in *Hearing Loss*, Fifth Edition also appear in *Occupational Hearing Loss*, Fourth Edition.

We are deeply indebted to Mary Hawkshaw, R.N., B.S.N, our indefatigable editorial assistant; our audiologists; and Debbie Westergon and Melanie Culhane for their expert and tireless efforts in preparation of the manuscript.

We also are indebted deeply to the late Dr. Joseph Sataloff whose pioneering contributions helped establish the fields of Otology and of Occupational Hearing Loss. Many of the chapters in this book retain wisdom that he contributed.

**Robert Thayer Sataloff**
**Pamela C. Roehm**

# Authors

**Robert Thayer Sataloff**, MD, DMA, FACS, is Professor and Chair, Department of Otolaryngology—Head and Neck Surgery and Senior Associate Dean for Clinical Academic Specialties, Drexel University College of Medicine. Dr. Sataloff holds Adjunct Professorships in the Departments of Otolaryngology—Head and Neck Surgery at Thomas Jefferson University and the Philadelphia College of Osteopathic Medicine, and he is on the faculty of the Academy of Vocal Arts. He serves as Conductor of the Thomas Jefferson University Choir. Dr. Sataloff is also a professional singer and singing teacher. He holds an undergraduate degree from Haverford College in Music Theory and Composition; graduated from Jefferson Medical College, Thomas Jefferson University; received a Doctor of Musical Arts in Voice Performance from Combs College of Music. He completed a Residency in Otolaryngology—Head and Neck Surgery and a Fellowship in Otology, Neurotology and Skull Base Surgery at the University of Michigan. Dr. Sataloff is Chair of the Boards of Directors of the Voice Foundation and of the American Institute for Voice and Ear Research. He also has served as Chair of the Board of Governors of Graduate Hospital, President of the American Laryngological Association, the International Association of Phonosurgery, the Pennsylvania Academy of Otolaryngology—Head and Neck Surgery, and the American Society of Geriatric Otolaryngology; and in numerous other leadership positions. Dr. Sataloff is Editor-in-Chief of the *Journal of Voice*; Editor Emeritus of the *Ear, Nose and Throat Journal*; Associate Editor of the *Journal of Singing*; on the Editorial Board of *Medical Problems of Performing Artists*; and is an editorial reviewer for numerous otolaryngology journals. He is a member of the Editorial Panel of the AMA Guides to the Evaluation of Permanent Impairment. Dr. Sataloff has written over 1000 publications including 76 books, and he has been awarded more than $5 million in research funding. His *h*-index is 47 (as of March 2024). He has invented more than 75 laryngeal microsurgical instruments distributed currently by Integra Medical, ossicular replacement prostheses produced by Grace Medical, and a novel laryngeal prosthesis (patent pending). He holds a patent on a unique thyroplasty implant. His medical practice is limited to care of the professional voice and to Otology/Neurotology/Skull base surgery. Dr. Sataloff has developed numerous novel surgical procedures including total temporal bone resection for formerly untreatable skull base malignancy, laryngeal microflap and mini-microflap procedures, vocal fold lipoinjection, and vocal fold lipoimplantation. Dr. Sataloff is recognized as one of the founders of the field of voice, having written the first modern comprehensive article on care of singers, and the first chapter and book on care of the professional voice, as well as having influenced the evolution of the field through his own efforts and through the Voice Foundation for over four decades. Dr. Sataloff has been recognized by Best Doctors in America (Woodward White Athens) every year since 1992, *Philadelphia Magazine* since 1997, and Castle Connolly's "America's Top Doctors" since 2002.

**Pamela C. Roehm**, MD, PhD, is a graduate from Johns Hopkins School of Medicine. She completed a Residency in Otolaryngology at the University of Pittsburgh and Fellowship in Neurotology and Skull Base Surgery at the University of Iowa. She is board certified in Otolaryngology by the American Academy of Otolaryngology— Head and Neck Surgery and holds a Certificate of Added Qualification in Neuro-Otology. Her subspecialty areas of expertise include all diseases of the ear including hearing loss, cochlear implantation, ear infections, cholesteatoma, and ear tumors. She previously worked at New York University, where she was the Associate Program Director for Otolaryngology and Neurotology Fellowship Site Director at Bellevue Hospital and the Veterans Administration Hospital in Manhattan. She then relocated to Temple, where she was promoted to Professor and served as the Division Director of Otology and Neurotology and Director of the Medical Student Rotation in Otolaryngology. She joined the St. Christopher's Otolaryngology Division in June 2020. She also works with the Specialty Physicians Associates Otolaryngology group in Bethlehem, PA, and is the Founding Residency Director for the St. Luke's University Otolaryngology Residency. Dr. Roehm is Professor and Vice Chair in the Department of Otolaryngology—Head and Neck Surgery at Drexel University College of Medicine.

# Contributors

**Arianne Abreu**
Philadelphia College of Osteopathic Medicine
Philadelphia, Pennsylvania, USA

**Mark T. Agrama**
South Florida ENT Associates
Jupiter, Florida, USA

**Alexander J. Barna**
Drexel University College of Medicine
Philadelphia, Pennsylvania, USA

**Hye Rhee Chi**
Philadelphia College of Osteopathic Medicine
Philadelphia, Pennsylvania, USA

**Cynthia L. Chow**
Consulting Audiology Associates, LLC
Chicago, Illinois, USA

**D. Caroline Coile**
Suwannee River Station
Live Oak, Florida, USA

**Skylar Drexel**
AUD Specialty Physicians Associates
Bethlehem, Pennsylvania, USA

**Daniel Eichorn**
Philadelphia College of Osteopathic
   Medicine
Philadelphia, Pennsylvania, USA

**Samuel P. Gubbels**
University of Colorado Anschutz Medical
   Campus
Aurora, Colorado, USA

**Mary J. Hawkshaw**
Drexel University College of Medicine
and
American Institute for Voice and Ear Research
Philadelphia, Pennsylvania, USA

**Thomas A. Kwyer** (Deceased)
Private Practice
Toledo, Ohio, USA

**Kevin L. Li**
Temple University Hospital
Philadelphia, Pennsylvania, USA

**M. Charles Liberman**
Eaton Peabody Laboratories
Boston, Massachusetts, USA

**Camryn Marshall**
Charles E. Schmidt College of Medicine
Florida Atlantic University
Boca Raton, Florida, USA

**Brian McGovern**
Cooper University Health Care
Camden, New Jersey, USA
and
Drexel University College of Medicine
Philadelphia, Pennsylvania, USA

**Katherine Mullen**
Geisinger Commonwealth School
   of Medicine
Scranton, Pennsylvania, USA
and
Graduate School of Biomedical Sciences &
   Professional Studies
Drexel University College of Medicine
Philadelphia, Pennsylvania, USA

**Brian A. Neff**
Department of Otorhinolaryngology
Mayo Clinic
Rochester, Minnesota, USA

**Kerrin E. Richard**
Oticon, Inc.
Somerset, New Jersey, USA

**Pamela C. Roehm**
Department of Otolaryngology—Head and Neck
 Surgery
Drexel University College of Medicine
Saint Luke's Hospital—Bethlehem Campus
and
St. Christopher's Hospital for Children
Philadelphia, Pennsylvania, USA

**Joseph Sataloff** (Deceased)
Thomas Jefferson University
Philadelphia, Pennsylvania, USA

**Robert Thayer Sataloff**
Drexel University College of Medicine
American Institute for Voice and Ear Research
and
Thomas Jefferson University
Philadelphia, Pennsylvania, USA

**Leona J. Tu**
Drexel University College of Medicine
Philadelphia, Pennsylvania, USA

**Danielle L. Walter**
St. Christopher's Hospital for Children
Philadelphia, Pennsylvania, USA

**Thomas O. Willcox Jr.**
Thomas Jefferson University
Philadelphia, Pennsylvania, USA

# Hearing loss: An overview

ROBERT THAYER SATALOFF AND PAMELA C. ROEHM

Although the importance of good hearing can hardly be overestimated, it has not been appreciated by the public, or even by the medical community. Over 40 million Americans have hearing loss, and there is still a stigma attached to deafness. Little has changed from the days when society had to be admonished: "Thou shall not curse the deaf." Although hearing loss may not be regarded widely as a punishment from God, it is seen still as an embarrassing infirmity, or a sign of aging and senility, and it is associated with a loss of sexual attractiveness. Too often patients do not seek medical attention of their own accord. Many deny and tolerate hearing loss for a considerable period of time before being coerced by a family member to seek medical care. Patients accept the need for eyeglasses, but it is unusual to tell someone that he/she needs a hearing aid without causing distress. This is as common in 70-year-old patients as it is in teenagers.

When hearing loss occurs early in childhood, its devastating consequences are more obvious than when it occurs insidiously in adult life. Normal psychological maturation involves progression from oneness with a child's mother to self-image definition. In this process, the child develops patterns of human interrelationship and modes of emotional expression. A substantial hearing deficit in infancy interferes with this process. It delays self-image development, impairs the child's expression of needs, and often results in alienation from the child's family, sometimes to a permanent deficit in his or her ability to establish relationships. Severe hearing loss makes learning a mammoth task for the child, and he/she frequently reacts with frustration or isolation. The personality distortion that results from this sequence affects the person and his or her family throughout their lives.

Even more mild forms of hearing loss early in life can cause great difficulty. We frequently see a child who developed within normal limits but is not doing well in school, is inattentive, and is frequently considered "not too bright." It is not uncommon to discover a moderate hearing loss in such a child. When the hearing loss is corrected, the parents invariably report that the child is "like a different person." Fortunately, many of the hearing impairments that lead to these and other consequences are preventable or readily treatable.

When hearing loss occurs in an adult, more subtle manifestations of many of the same problems may be found. Most people with age- or noise-induced hearing loss lose hearing in the high frequencies first, making it difficult for them to distinguish consonants, especially s, f, t, and z. This makes a person strain to understand what is being said in everyday conversation. The person knows that there is speech because he/she can hear the vowels, but he/she cannot easily distinguish the difference between "yes" and "get." This makes talking to one's spouse, going to the movies, going to church, and other pleasures that most of us take for granted stressful chores. It is also the unrecognized source of considerable marital discord. For example, a man who has worked hard for many years in a noisy environment like a factory will often have a substantial hearing loss, especially if he has not worn ear protection. When he comes home and sits down to read a newspaper,

DOI: 10.1201/b23379-1

if his wife starts talking to him from another room (especially if there is competing noise such as running water or air conditioners), he will be able to hear her talking but not understand her words. Before long, it becomes so difficult to say "what" all the time that he stops listening. Soon she thinks he does not pay any attention to her or love her anymore, and neither of them realizes that he has a hearing loss underlying their friction. Otologists see this scenario daily in the office. Although each of these patients can be helped through counseling and rehabilitation, we still have no cure for many cases of sensorineural deafness. Despite that, there is relatively little support for research. We undergo a constant barrage of requests for funds for sight, cancer, muscular dystrophy, multiple sclerosis, and numerous other entities, but it is hard to remember the last call for help for the deaf.

Although otologic advances have made almost all forms of conductive hearing loss surgically curable, the inner ear function in patients with sensorineural hearing loss can be restored in only a few conditions (syphilis, cytomegalovirus, hypothyroidism, and a few others). Despite advances in our understanding of hearing loss and in hearing aid and cochlear implant technology, which make it possible to improve the lives of almost every patient with hearing loss, deafness prevention is still our best cure. A thorough understanding of the function of the ear and related structures reveals many possibilities for prevention of injury and restoration of function. Avoidance of damaging noise, ototoxic drugs, and adequate treatment of diseases such as syphilis and other measures often prevent hearing loss. Even when sensorineural hearing loss occurs, systematic, comprehensive assessment may reveal a treatable underlying cause. Fortunately, this is true in an increasing number of patients, as medical knowledge increases.

Today, although not all hearing loss can be cured, virtually every patient with hearing impairment can be helped through accurate diagnosis, understanding, education, medication, aural rehabilitation, amplification, and/or cochlear implantation. Major advances have been made in the last few decades, and even more may be anticipated as exploration continues into the mysteries of the inner ear and ear–brain interface.

# The physics of sound

ROBERT THAYER SATALOFF AND PAMELA C. ROEHM

A fundamental understanding of the nature of sound and terms used to describe it is essential to comprehend the language of otologists, occupational health physicians, audiologists, and industrial engineers. Moreover, studying basic physics of sound helps one recognize complexities and potential pitfalls in measuring and describing sound and helps clarify the special difficulties encountered in trying to modify sources of noise.

## SOUND

Sound is a form of motion. Consequently, the laws of physics that govern actions of all moving bodies apply to sound. Sound measurement is not particularly simple. The study of physics helps us to understand many practical aspects of our daily encounters with sound. For example, why does an audiologist or otologist use a different baseline for decibels (dBs) in their office from that used by an engineer or occupational health physician who measures noise in a factory? Why is it that when hearing at high frequencies is tested, a patient may hear nothing and then suddenly hear a loud tone? Yet, all the examiner did was move the earphone a fraction of an inch. Why is it when two machines are placed close together, each making

60 dB of noise, the total noise is not 120 dB? Everyone concerned with noise or hearing loss should have sufficient familiarity with the physics of sound to understand the answers to these basic questions.

## SOUND WAVES

Sound is the propagation of pressure waves radiating from a vibrating body through an elastic medium. A *vibrating body* is essential to cause particle displacement in the propagating medium. An *elastic medium* is any substance whose particles return to their point of origin as soon as possible after they have been displaced. *Propagation* occurs because displaced particles in the medium displace neighboring particles. Through this mechanism, sound energy travels forward in space. *Pressure waves* are composed of areas with slightly greater than ambient air pressure (compression) and slightly less than ambient air pressure (rarefaction). These are associated with the bunching together or spreading apart of the particles in the propagating medium. The pressure wave makes receiving structures such as the eardrum move back and forth with the alternating pressure. For example, when a sound wave is generated by striking a tuning fork, by speaking, or by others means, the vibrating object moves molecules of the air, causing them alternately to be compressed and rarefied in a rhythmical pattern. This sets up a chain reaction with adjacent air molecules and spreads at a rate of ~1100 ft/s (the speed of sound). This is *propagation* of the pressure waves.

Sound requires energy. Energy is used to set a body into vibration. The energy is imparted to particles in the propagating medium and then is distributed over the surface of the receiver (eardrum or microphone) in the form of sound pressure.

Energy is equal to the square of pressure ($E = P^2$). However, we are unable to measure sound energy directly. Only the pressure exerted on the surface of a microphone can be quantified by sound-measuring equipment.

## CHARACTERISTICS OF SOUND WAVES

Sound waves travel in straight lines in all directions from the source, decreasing in intensity at a rate inversely proportional to the square of the distance from their source. This is called the inverse-square law. This means that if a person shortens his/her distance from the source of a sound and moves from a position 4 ft away to only 2 ft from the source, the sound will be four times as intense rather than merely twice as intense. In practical application, this inverse-square law applies only in instances in which there are no walls or ceiling. This relationship does not always hold true in a room where sound waves encounter obstruction or reflection, which can amplify the intensity of the sound. Thus, increasing the distance of a whisper or a ticking watch from the subject rarely can provide an accurate or reliable assessment of hearing.

Sound waves travel through air more rapidly than through water. They are conducted by solids at different speeds. An ear placed close to the iron rail of a train track will detect the approach of the train before the airborne sounds can reach the observer. Thus, sounds travel through different media at different speeds; the speed also varies when the medium is not uniform. However, sound waves are not transmitted through a vacuum.

This can be demonstrated by the classic experiment of placing a ringing alarm clock inside a bell jar and then removing the air. The ringing will no longer be heard when the air is exhausted, but it will be heard again immediately when air is readmitted. This experiment emphasizes the importance of the medium through which sound waves travel.

The bones of the head also conduct sounds, but ordinarily the ear is much more sensitive to sounds that are airborne. Under certain abnormal conditions, as in cases of conductive hearing loss, a patient may hear better by bone conduction than by air conduction. Such an individual can hear the vibrations of a tuning fork much better when it is held directly touching the skull than when it is held next to the ear but without touching the head.

Distortion of sound waves by wind is common. The effect varies according to whether the wind blows faster near the ground or above it. When sound travels through air and encounters an obstruction such as a wall, the sound waves can bend around the obstacle similar to water passing around a rock in a stream. The behavior of sound waves striking an object depends upon several factors, including wavelength. Sound waves may pass unaffected through an object, be reflected off the object, or may be partially reflected and partially passed through or around the object (shadow effect). Low-frequency sounds of long wavelength tend to bend (diffraction) when encountering objects. Diffraction is less prominent with sounds >2000 Hz. The behavior of sound waves encountering an object also depends upon the nature of the object. The resistance of an object or system to the transmission of sound is called impedance. This depends upon a variety of factors such as mass reactants, stiffness reactants, and friction. The ability of an object to allow transmission of sound is called its admittance, which may be thought of as the opposite of impedance.

### Components of sound

A simple type of sound wave, called a *pure tone*, is pictured in **Figure 2.1**. This is a graphic representation of one and one-half complete vibrations or cycles, or periods, with the area of compression represented by the top curve and the area of rarefaction by the bottom curve. Although pure tones do not occur in nature, the more complicated sounds that we encounter in daily life are composed of combinations of pure tones. Understanding the makeup of this relatively simple sound helps us analyze more complex sounds. Fourier analysis is used to separate complex signals into their simple tonal components.

A pure tone has several important characteristics: One complete vibration consists of one compression and one rarefaction (**Figure 2.2**). The number of times such a cycle occurs in a given period of time (usually 1 second) is called *frequency*. Frequency is usually recorded in cycles per second or hertz (Hz). The psychological correlate of frequency is *pitch*. In general, the greater the frequency, the higher the pitch, and the greater the intensity, the louder the sound. However, there is a difference between actual physical phenomena (such as frequency or intensity) and people's perceptions of them (pitch and loudness). A tuning fork is constructed so that it vibrates at a fixed frequency no matter how hard it is struck. However, although it will vibrate the same number of times per second, the prongs of the tuning fork will cover a greater distance when the fork is struck hard than when it is struck softly. This increased *intensity* we perceive as increased *loudness*. In the sine wave diagram of a pure tone, a more intense sound will have a higher peak and lower valley than a softer sound. Greater intensity also means that the particles in the propagating medium are more compressed. The height or depth of the sine wave is called its amplitude. Amplitude is measured in dBs. It reflects the amount of pressure (or energy) existing in the sound wave.

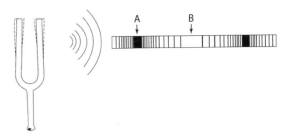

Figure 2.2 Areas of compression (A) and rarefaction (B) produced by a vibrating tuning fork.

*Wavelength* is the linear distance between any point in one cycle and the same point on the next cycle (peak-to-peak, for example). It may be calculated as the speed of sound divided by the frequency. This is also one *period*. Wavelength is symbolized by the Greek letter lambda ($\lambda$) and is inversely proportional to frequency (**Figure 2.3**). This is easy to understand. Since sound waves travel at ~1100 ft/s, simple division shows us that a 1000-Hz frequency has a wavelength of 1.1 ft/cycle and a 2000-Hz tone has a wavelength of ~6.5 in. Similarly, a 100-Hz tone has a wavelength of ~11 ft. The wavelength of a frequency of 8000 Hz would be 1100 divided by 8000 or 0.013 ft (~1 in.). Wavelength has a great deal to do with sound penetration. For example, if someone is playing a stereo too loudly several rooms away, the bass notes will be heard clearly, but the high notes of violins or trumpets will be attenuated by the intervening walls. Low-frequency sounds (long wavelengths) are extremely difficult to attenuate or to absorb, and they require very different acoustic treatment from high-frequency sounds of short wavelengths. Fortunately, they are also less damaging to hearing.

Any point along the cycle of the wave is its *phase*. Because a sine wave is a cyclical event, it can be described in degrees like a circle. The halfway point of the sine wave is the 180° phase point. The first peak occurs at 90°, etc. The interaction of two pure tones depends on their phase relationship. For example, if the two sound sources are identical and are perfectly in phase, the resulting sound will be considerably more intense than either one alone (constructive interference). If they are 180° out of phase, they will nullify each other and no sound will be heard (destructive interference) (**Figure 2.4**). Interaction of sound forces also depends upon other factors such as resonance which is affected by the environment and the characteristics of the receiver (such as the ear canal and ear).

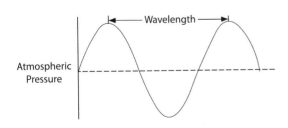

Figure 2.1 Diagram of a pure tone (sine wave).

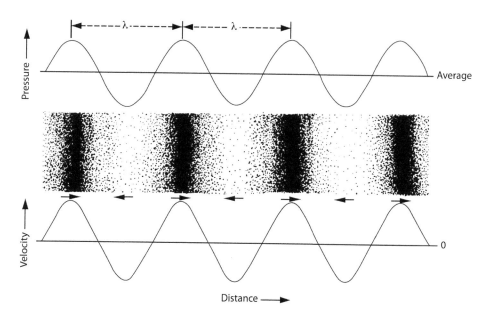

Figure 2.3 Diagram showing wavelength in relation to other components of a sound wave. (Adapted from Van Bergeijk et al. [1].)

Speech, music, and noise are *complex sounds* rather than pure tones. Most sounds are very complex with many different wave forms superimposed on each other. Musical tones usually are related to one another and show a regular pattern (complex periodic sound), whereas street noise shows a random pattern (complex aperiodic sound) (**Figure 2.5**).

It is somewhat difficult to define noise accurately because so much of its meaning depends on its effect at any specific time and place rather than on its physical characteristics. Sound can in one instance or by one individual be considered as very annoying noise, whereas on another occasion or to another observer, the same sound may seem pleasant and undeserving of being designated "noise." For the purpose of this book, the term *noise* is used broadly to designate any unwanted sound.

An interesting aspect of sound waves related to hearing testing is a phenomenon called the *standing wave*. Under certain circumstances, two wave trains of equal amplitude and frequency traveling in opposite directions can cancel out at certain points called "nodes." **Figure 2.6** is a diagram of such a situation. It will be noted that when a violin string is plucked in a certain manner, at point "n" (node) there is no displacement. If this point falls at the eardrum, the listener will not be aware of

any sound because the point has no amplitude and cannot excite the ear. This phenomenon occasionally occurs in hearing tests, particularly in testing at ≥ 8000 Hz. These higher frequencies are likely to be involved because the ear canal is ~2.5 cm long, and the wavelength of sound at such high frequencies is of a similar length. The point of maximum displacement is called antinode.

Furthermore, when sound waves are produced within small enclosures, as when an earphone is placed over the ear, the sound waves encounter many reflections, and much of the sound at high frequencies is likely to be in the form of standing waves. Such waves often do not serve as stimuli to the inner ear, and no sensation of hearing is produced because of the absence of transmission of sound energy.

Sometimes, by simply holding the earphone a little more tightly or loosely to the ear in testing the higher frequencies, suddenly no sound may be produced at all when it should be loud, or a loud sound may be heard when a moment before there seemed to be no sound. This phenomenon occurs because of the presence of standing waves. During hearing testing, one often uses modulated or "warbled" tones to help eliminate standing wave problems that might result in misleading test results.

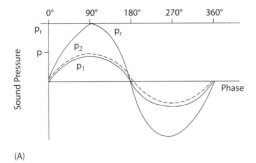

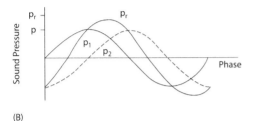

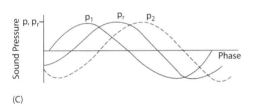

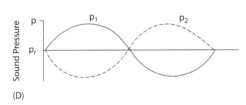

Figure 2.4 Combination of two pure tone noises ($p_1$ and $p_2$) with various phase differences. (A) 0° phase difference: $p_r = 2p$ ($p_r = p + 6$ dB). (B) 90° phase difference: $p_r = 1.4p$ ($p_r = p + 3$ dB). (C) 120° phase difference: $p_r = p$ ($p_r = p + 0$ dB). (D) 180° phase difference: $p_r = 0$.

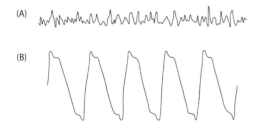

Figure 2.5 (A) Typical street noise and (B) "C" on a piano.

In addition, resonant characteristics of the ear canal play a role in audition. Just like organ pipes, the ear may be thought of as a pipe. It is closed at one end and has a length of ~2.5 cm. Its calculated resonant frequency is ~3400 Hz (actually 3430 Hz if the length is exactly 2.5 cm, and if the ear were really a straight pipe). At such a resonant frequency, a node occurs at the external auditory meatus, and an antinode is present at the tympanic membrane, resulting in sound pressure amplification at the closed end of the pipe (eardrum). This phenomenon can cause sound amplification of up to 20 dB between 2000 and 5000 Hz. The resonance characteristics of the ear canal change if the open end is occluded, such as with an ear bud insert or headphone used for hearing testing. These factors must be taken into account during equipment design and calibration, and when interpreting hearing tests.

The form of a complex sound is determined by the interaction of each of its pure tones at a particular time. This aspect of a sound is called *complexity*, and the psychological counterpart is *timbre*. This is the quality of sound that allows us to distinguish among a piano, oboe, violin, or voice all producing a middle "C" (256 Hz). These sound sources combine frequencies differently and consequently have different qualities.

## MEASURING SOUND

The principal components of sound that we need to measure are frequency and intensity. Both are measured with a technique called scaling. The frequency scale is generally familiar because it is based on the musical scale or *octave*. This is a logarithmic scale with a base of 2. This means that each octave increase corresponds to a doubling of

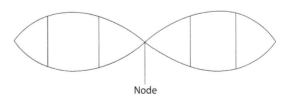

Figure 2.6 Diagram of a standing wave, showing the nodal point at which there is no amplitude.

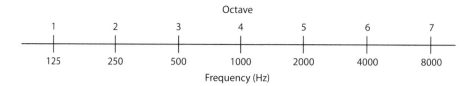

Figure 2.7 Scaling for octave notation of frequency levels.

frequency (**Figure 2.7**). Linear increases (octaves) correspond with progressively increasing frequency units. For example, the octave between 4000 and 8000 Hz contains 4000 frequency units, but the same octave space between 125 and 250 Hz contains only 125 frequency units. This makes it much easier to deal with progressively larger numbers and helps show relationships that might not be obvious if absolute numbers were used (**Figure 2.8**).

Another reason for using octave scaling was pointed out in the 19th century by psychophysicist Gustav Fechner. He noted that sensation increases as the log of the stimulus. This means that ever-increasing amounts of sound pressure are needed to produce equal increments in sensation. For example, loudness is measured in units called SONES. Other psychoacoustic measures include the PHON scale of loudness level and the MEL scale for pitch. The sone scale was developed by asking trained listeners to judge when a sound level had doubled in loudness relative to a 1000-Hz reference at 40 dB. Each doubling was defined as one sone. (This is similar to doubling in pitch being referred to as one octave.) One-sone increments correspond to ~10-dB increases in sound pressure or about a 10-fold energy increase. So, in addition to being arithmetically convenient, logarithmic scaling helps describe sound more as we hear it.

In the kind of noise measurement done in industry, the chief concern is with very intense noise. In the testing of hearing, the primary concern is with very weak sounds because the purpose is to determine the individual's thresholds of hearing. Accurate intensity measurement and a scale that covers a very large range are necessary to measure and compare the many intensities with which we have to work.

The weakest sound pressure that the sensitive, young human ear can detect under very quiet conditions is ~0.0002 µbar, and this very small amount of pressure is used as the basis or the reference level for sound measurements. This base usually is determined by using a 1000 Hz tone (a frequency in the range of the maximum sensitivity of the ear) and reducing the pressure to the weakest measurable sound pressure to which the young ear will respond. In some instances, the keen ear under ideal conditions will respond to a pressure even weaker that 0.0002 µbar, but it is the 0.0002-µbar pressure that is used as a base.

Of course, sound pressures can be increased tremendously above the weakest tone. The usual range of audible sound pressures extends upward to ~2000 µbar, a point at which the pressure causes discomfort and pain in the ears. Higher pressures can damage or even destroy the inner ear. Because this range (0.0002–2000 µbar) is so great, the use of the microbar as a measurement of sound is too cumbersome.

## INTENSITY

Measuring intensity or amplitude is considerably more complex than measuring frequency. Intensity is also measured on a logarithmic ratio scale. All such scales require an arbitrarily established zero

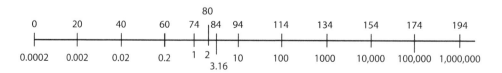

Figure 2.8 Decibel scaling (sound pressure level [SPL]). Measurements in dB SPL are written over the line, and sound intensities in µbar are written beneath the line. (After Lipscomb [2].)

point and a statement of the phenomenon being measured. Usually, sound is measured in dBs. However, many other phenomena (such as heat and light) also are measured in dBs.

## DECIBEL

The term "decibel" has been borrowed from the field of communication engineering, and it is this term that most generally is used to describe sound intensity. The detailed manner in which this unit was derived and the manner in which it is converted to other units is somewhat complicated and not within the scope of this book. However, a very clear understanding of the nature of the dB and the proper use of the term is most valuable in understanding how hearing is tested and sound is measured.

## A unit of comparison

The dB is simply a unit of comparison, a ratio, between two sound pressures. In general, it is not a unit of measurement with an absolute value, such as an inch or a pound. The concept of the dB is based on the pressure of one sound or reference level, with which the pressure of another sound is compared. Thus, a sound of 60 dB is a sound that is 60 dB more intense than a sound that has been standardized as the reference level. The reference level must be either implied or specifically stated in all sound measurement, for without the reference level, the expression of intensity in terms of dBs is meaningless. It would be the same as saying that something is "twice," without either implying or referring specifically to the other object with which it is being compared.

## Two reference levels

For the purpose of this book, two important reference levels are used. In making physical sound measurements, as in a noisy industry, the base used is the sound pressure of 0.0002 µbar (one millionth of one barometric pressure or of one atmosphere), which is known as *acoustical zero* dBs. Sound-measuring instruments such as sound-level meters and noise analyzers are calibrated with this reference level. Several other terms have been used to describe acoustical zero. They include 0.0002 dyne/cm², 20 µN/m², and 20 µPa. Now, 0.0002 µbar

has been accepted. When a reading is made in a room and the meter reads so many dBs, the reading means than the sound pressure level (SPL) in that room is so many dBs greater than acoustical zero. The designation SPL means that the measurement is SPL relative to 0.0002 µbar. When SPL is written, it tells us both the reference level and the phenomenon being measured.

The other important reference level is used in audiometry and is known as *zero decibels* (0 dB) *of hearing loss or average normal hearing*. This level is not the same as that used as a base for noise measurement. Rather, it is known as hearing threshold level or HTL. In the middle-frequency range (~3000 Hz), it is 10 dB above the reference level known as acoustical zero. In testing hearing with an audiometer, 40-dB loss in hearing on the audiogram means that the individual requires 40 dB more sound pressure than the average normal person to be able to hear the tone presented.

As the baseline or reference level is different for the audiometer than it is for noise-measuring devices, it should be clear now that a noise of, say, 60 dB in a room is not the same intensity as the 60-dB tone on the audiometer. The noise will sound less loud because it is measured from a weaker reference level.

## Formula for the decibel

With these reference levels established, the formula for the dB is worked out. To compare the two pressures, we have designated them as Pressure 1 ($P_1$) and Pressure 2 ($P_2$), with $P_2$ being the reference level. The ratio can be expressed as $P_1/P_2$.

Another factor that must be taken into account is that in computing this ratio in terms of dBs, the computation must be logarithmic. A logarithm is the exponent or the power to which a fixed number or base (usually 10) must be raised in order to produce a given number. For instance, if the base is 10, the log of 100 is 2, because $10 \times 10 = 100$. In such a case, 10 is written with the exponent 2 as $10^2$. Similarly, if 10 is raised to the fourth power and written as $10^4$, the result is $10 \times 10 \times 10 \times 10$, or 10,000; the logarithm of 10,000 is, therefore, 4. If only this logarithmic function is considered, the formula has evolved as far as dB = log $P_1/P_2$. But it is not yet complete.

When the dB was borrowed from the engineering field, it was a comparison of sound powers and not pressures, and it was expressed in bels and not dBs. The dB is 1/10 of a bel, and the sound pressure is proportional to the square root of the corresponding sound power. It is necessary, therefore, to multiply the logarithm of the ratio of pressures by 2 (for the square root relationship) and by 10 (for the bel–dB relationship). When this is done, the dB formula is complete, and the dB in terms of SPLs is defined thus:

$$dB = \frac{20\log P_1}{P_2}$$

For instance, if the pressure designated as $P_1$ is 100× greater than the reference level of $P_2$, substitution in the formula gives dB = 20 × log 100/1. As it is known that the log of 100 is 2 (as $10^2 = 100$), it can be seen that the formula reduces to dB = 20 × 2 or 40 dB. Therefore, whenever the pressure of one sound is 100× greater than that of the reference level, the first sound can be referred to as 40 dB. Likewise, if $P_1$ is 1000× greater, then the number of dBs would be 60, and if it is 10,000× greater, the number of dBs is 80. A few other relationships are convenient to remember. If sound intensity is multiplied by 2, sound pressure increases by 6 dB. If intensity is multiplied by 3.16 (the square root of 10), sound pressure increases by 10 dB. When intensity is multiplied by 10, sound pressure increases by 20 dB. These relationships can be seen clearly in **Figure 2.8**.

In actual sound measurement, if $P_1$ is 1 μbar—being a pressure of 1 dyne/cm²—then the ratio is 1/0.0002 or 5000. By the use of a logarithmic table or a special table prepared to convert pressure ratios to dBs, the pressure level in such a case is found to be 74 dB, based on a reference level of 0.0002 μbar (**Figure 2.8**). **Figure 2.9** shows where a number of common sounds fall on this dB scale in relation to a 0.0002-μbar reference level. This base level is used for calibrating standard sound-measuring instruments.

In *audiometric testing*, which uses a higher reference level than that for sound measurement, the tester does not need to be concerned with additional mathematical formulas because the audiometer used in testing is calibrated to take into account the increase above acoustical zero to provide the necessary reference level for audiometry of average normal hearing (0 dB of hearing loss) at each frequency tested.

## Important points

The important thing to remember is that the dB is a logarithmic ratio. It is convenient unit because 1 dB approaches the smallest change in intensity between two sounds that the human ear can distinguish.

An important aspect of the logarithmic ratio is that as the ratio of the pressures becomes larger, because the sound becomes more intense, the rate of increase in dBs becomes smaller. Even if the ratio of the pressures is enormous, such as one pressure being 10,000,000× that of another, the number of dBs by which this ratio is expressed does not become inordinately large, being only 140 dB SPL. This is the principal reason for using the dB scale. From the psychoacoustic perspective, it takes comparatively little increase in sound pressure to go from 0 to 1 dB, and the normal ear can detect this. However, when an attempt is made to increase the sound pressure from 140 to 141 dB—also an increase of 1 dB, which the ear can barely detect—it takes an increase of ~10,000,000× as much in absolute pressure.

A point to be remembered is that the effect of adding dBs together is quite different from that of adding ordinary numbers. For example, if one machine whose noise has been measured as 70 dB is turned on next to another machine producing 70 dB, the resulting level is 73 dB and not 140 dB. This is obtained as follows: When combining dBs, it is necessary to use an equation that takes into account the energy or power exerted by the sound sources rather than the sound pressure exerted by this energy. The equation is as follows:

$$dB_{power} = 10\log_{10}\frac{E_1}{E_0}$$

where $E_1$ is a known power (energy) and $E_0$ is the reference quantity.

$$dB = 10\log_{10}\frac{2}{1}$$

(there were two machines operating rather than one, resulting in a 2:1 ratio)

$$= (10)(0.3010) \quad \text{(the logarithm of 2 is 0.3010)}$$
$$= 3.01$$

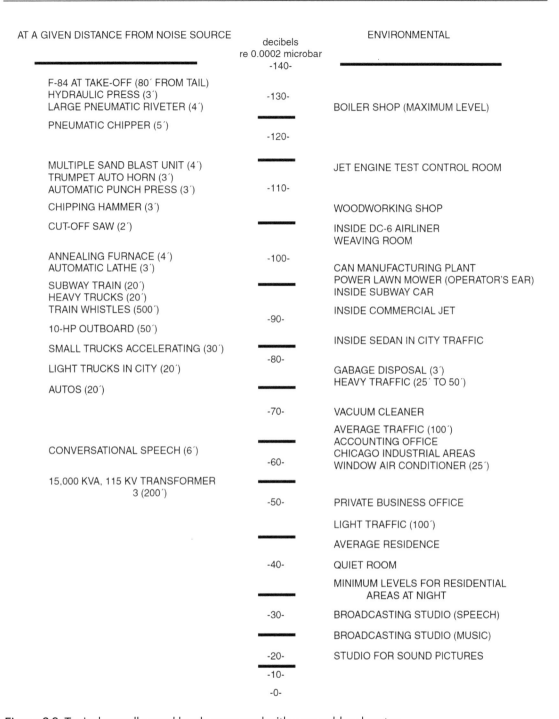

AT A GIVEN DISTANCE FROM NOISE SOURCE

decibels
re 0.0002 microbar
-140-

ENVIRONMENTAL

F-84 AT TAKE-OFF (80′ FROM TAIL)
HYDRAULIC PRESS (3′)                   -130-
LARGE PNEUMATIC RIVETER (4′)                    BOILER SHOP (MAXIMUM LEVEL)

PNEUMATIC CHIPPER (5′)
                                       -120-

MULTIPLE SAND BLAST UNIT (4′)                   JET ENGINE TEST CONTROL ROOM
TRUMPET AUTO HORN (3′)
AUTOMATIC PUNCH PRESS (3′)              -110-

CHIPPING HAMMER (3′)                            WOODWORKING SHOP

CUT-OFF SAW (2′)                                INSIDE DC-6 AIRLINER
                                               WEAVING ROOM

ANNEALING FURNACE (4′)                  -100-
AUTOMATIC LATHE (3′)                            CAN MANUFACTURING PLANT
                                               POWER LAWN MOWER (OPERATOR'S EAR)
SUBWAY TRAIN (20′)                              INSIDE SUBWAY CAR
HEAVY TRUCKS (20′)
TRAIN WHISTLES (500′)                           INSIDE COMMERCIAL JET
                                       -90-
10-HP OUTBOARD (50′)

SMALL TRUCKS ACCELERATING (30′)                 INSIDE SEDAN IN CITY TRAFFIC
                                       -80-
LIGHT TRUCKS IN CITY (20′)                      GABAGE DISPOSAL (3′)
                                               HEAVY TRAFFIC (25′ TO 50′)
AUTOS (20′)

                                       -70-    VACUUM CLEANER

                                               AVERAGE TRAFFIC (100′)
                                               ACCOUNTING OFFICE
CONVERSATIONAL SPEECH (6′)                      CHICAGO INDUSTRIAL AREAS
                                       -60-    WINDOW AIR CONDITIONER (25′)

15,000 KVA, 115 KV TRANSFORMER
          3 (200′)
                                       -50-    PRIVATE BUSINESS OFFICE

                                               LIGHT TRAFFIC (100′)

                                               AVERAGE RESIDENCE

                                       -40-    QUIET ROOM

                                               MINIMUM LEVELS FOR RESIDENTIAL
                                                    AREAS AT NIGHT

                                       -30-    BROADCASTING STUDIO (SPEECH)

                                               BROADCASTING STUDIO (MUSIC)

                                       -20-    STUDIO FOR SOUND PICTURES
                                       -10-
                                       -0-

Figure 2.9 Typical overall sound levels measured with a sound-level meter.

**Figure 2.10** is a chart showing the results obtained from adding noise levels. It may be used instead of the formulas. On this chart, it will be seen that if 70 and 76 dB are being added, the difference of 6 dB is located on the graph, and this difference is found to produce an increase of 1 dB, which is added to the higher number. Therefore, the combined level of noise produced by the two machines is 77 dB above the reference level.

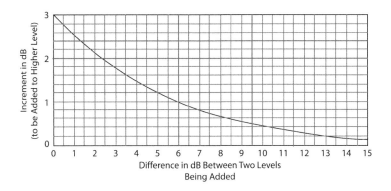

Figure 2.10 Results obtained from adding noise levels.

## dBA MEASUREMENT

Most sound level meters that are used to measure noise levels do not simply record SPL relative to 0.0002 μbar (dB SPL). Rather, they are generally equipped with three filtering networks: A, B, and C. Use of these filters allows one to approximate the frequency distribution of a given noise over the audible spectrum (**Figures 2.11** and **2.12**). In practice, the frequency distribution of a noise can be approximated by comparing the levels measured with each of the frequency ratings. For example, if the noise level is measured with the A and C networks and they are almost equal, then most of the noise energy is > 1000 Hz because this is the only portion of the spectrum where the networks are similar. If there is a large difference between A and C measurements, most of the energy is likely to be < 1000 Hz. The use

of these filters and other capabilities of sound level meters are discussed in Chapter 14.

The A network is used when measuring sound to estimate the risk of noise-induced hearing loss because it represents more accurately the ear's response to loud noise. It is not possible to describe a noise's damaging effect on hearing simply by stating its intensity. For instance, if one noise has a spectrum similar to that shown in curve A in **Figure 2.11**, with most of its energy in the low frequencies, it may have little or no effect on hearing. Another noise of the same overall intensity, having most of its sound energy in the higher frequencies (curve C), could produce substantial hearing damage after years of exposure. Examples of low-frequency noises are motors, fans, and trains. High-frequency noises are produced by sheet metal work and air pressure hoses. Although the human ear is more sensitive in the frequency range 1000–3000 Hz than it is

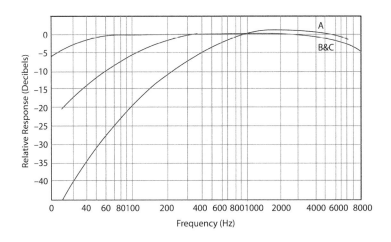

Figure 2.11 Frequency–response characteristics of a sound level meter with A, B, and C weighting. *Abbreviation*: SPL, sound pressure level.

| Center Frequency (Hz) | A-Weighting Adjustment (dB) | Center Frequency (Hz) | A-Weighting Adjustment (dB) |
|---|---|---|---|
| 10 | −70.4 | 500 | −3.2 |
| 12.5 | −63.4 | 630 | −1.9 |
| 16 | −56.7 | 800 | −0.8 |
| 20 | −50.5 | 1000 | 0.0 |
| 25 | −44.7 | 1250 | +0.6 |
| 31.5 | −39.4 | 1600 | +1.0 |
| 40 | −34.6 | 2000 | +1.2 |
| 50 | −30.2 | 2500 | +1.3 |
| 63 | −26.2 | 3150 | +1.2 |
| 80 | −22.5 | 4000 | +1.0 |
| 100 | −19.1 | 5000 | +0.5 |
| 125 | −16.1 | 6300 | −0.1 |
| 160 | −13.4 | 8000 | −1.1 |
| 200 | −10.9 | 10000 | −2.5 |
| 250 | −8.6 | 12500 | −4.3 |
| 315 | −6.6 | 16000 | −6.6 |
| 400 | −4.8 | 20000 | −9.3 |

Figure 2.12 Adjustments by frequency for A-weighting scale.

in the range < 500 and > 4000 Hz (**Figure 2.13**), this frequency-specific differential sensitivity does not explain fully the ear's vulnerability to high-frequency sounds. Although various explanations have been proposed involving everything from teleology to redundancy of low-frequency loci on the cochlea to cochlear shearing mechanics, the phenomenon is not completely understood. Mechanisms of noise-induced hearing loss are discussed in Chapter 14.

There are other important and interesting aspects of the physics of sound that might be discussed; the subject is a complex and fascinating one. The average physician concerned with the problems of hearing loss will find that a reasonable comprehension of the material thus far presented will be helpful—especially the fact that the term "decibel" expresses a *logarithmic ratio to an established reference level.*

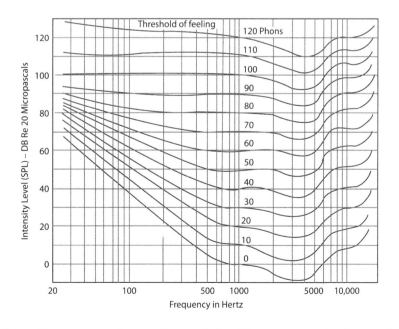

Figure 2.13 Fletcher–Munson curves showing the sensitivity of the ear to sounds of various frequencies.

Understanding the basic physics of sound is invaluable in medical and legal interactions involving hearing loss. Deeper knowledge is required in many instances, and the consultation services of good physicists and engineers with practical understanding of the problems of medicine and industry are indispensable.

## REFERENCES

1. Van Bergeijk WA, Pierce JR, David EE. Waves and the Ears. New York: Doubleday and Co., 1960:44.
2. Lipscomb DM. Noise and occupational hearing impairment. Ear Nose Throat 1980; 59:13–23.

# 3

# The nature of hearing loss

ROBERT THAYER SATALOFF AND PAMELA C. ROEHM

Hearing loss is one of the most challenging problems confronting medicine, not only because there are some 40 million Americans with hearing loss but also especially because it can affect personality so adversely. A mild hearing loss sometimes may produce more psychological disturbance than a greater hearing deficit in conditions such as Ménière's disease. It is this effect of hearing loss on the patient's emotions, rather than the actual deafness, that may persuade the patient to seek the help of a physician. The hearing loss often bothers the people around him/her more than it does the patient. Deafness is a rather strange symptom, for it is not accompanied by pain, discomfort, itch, or fear, as is true of cancer and other diseases that compel patients to seek medical aid. Hearing loss is really a symptom rather than a disease.

Consider, for a moment, what motivates a patient to visit a doctor and complain of problems with hearing. Perhaps a number of embarrassing situations begin to occur with greater frequency in everyday life. For example, it may be a failure to hear or to understand an employer when given directions, especially in noisy conditions. An assistant may fail to take dictation correctly, and the resulting mistakes may cause a great deal of tension in the office. A young woman may try to hide from herself and her friends that her hearing is impaired, but when she goes out on a date, she repeatedly gives the wrong answers, especially when it is dark in the car, and she is unable to read the lips of her companion. A husband may sit and read his newspaper and fail to understand what his wife is saying while she is running water in the kitchen; this may lead to constant friction between husband and wife, with complete lack of communication and, eventually, serious martial stress.

These situations are typical of the embarrassing circumstances that produce feelings of inadequacy and insecurity. Yet the patient is unable to face this problem and seek the help of a physician. When he/she does visit a physician to complain of deafness, it is rarely of his/her own free will. The patient usually is nagged into going by a spouse, friend, or boss, who have been trying for years to get the person to do something about his/her hearing difficulty.

Not infrequently, when a husband and a wife walk into the otologist's office, the dialogue follows a familiar pattern. The physician asks the man what his difficulty is, and before he has a chance to answer, his wife blurts out that he is deaf and

DOI: 10.1201/b23379-3

does not pay attention to her. The husband generally looks meek and bewildered, as if he is not sure what is going on, but he certainly does not want to assume the blame for all of his difficulty. It soon becomes apparent that arguments are his key problems and that they were brought on by his hearing loss. One of the most heartbreaking episodes the authors have encountered in otologic practice occurred with a 21-year-old man who pleaded from some cure for his bilateral nerve deafness secondary to meningitis contracted 6 years earlier. The patient offered to turn over all of the money he had in the bank if he could be given even a moderate cure for his hearing loss. When asked what prompted him to seek help now, 6 years after the onset of deafness, he replied tearfully that it was important to hear his new baby when she cried during the night.

## EARLY STAGES OF A HEARING LOSS

People do not really notice any hearing deficit until their hearing level has dropped rather markedly or suddenly. In the early stages of a high-frequency hearing loss, for example, there actually are no symptoms, except that the patient may say he/she cannot hear their phone in one ear as well as in the other. If the patient notices this, he/she may seek help early, but most people are not this fortunate. Often, the hearing loss is usually rather substantial before one seeks medical attention.

## EVERY PATIENT CAN BE HELPED

Because hearing deficiency can cause emotional trauma, it can be stated categorically that every patient with a hearing loss who visits a physician can be helped in some way. It may not always be possible to restore hearing to normal capacity or to improve it to a no handicapping level, but it is always possible to mitigate the psychological impact of a hearing loss on the patient. He/she can be taught to hear better with the hearing that is left and correct the pessimistic and antagonistic attitude toward the hearing problem, and he/she can be helped to communicate better. It is the physician's responsibility to improve the patient's quality of life.

## REFERRAL OF PATIENTS BY VARIOUS SPECIALISTS

Interestingly, many patients are referred to an otolaryngologist not by a general practitioner, internist, or pediatrician but by a surprising variety of other physicians such as obstetricians, dermatologists, psychiatrists, and even proctologists. Patients seem to have a strange inclination to reveal their hearing loss symptoms under the most unusual circumstances. For example, astute obstetricians have referred to us many patients who complained of buzzing in their ears during the last month of pregnancy or early postpartum. The usual finding in these cases is otosclerosis, which accounts for the buzzing tinnitus. Obstetricians should be alert for a family history of hearing loss because this is associated with otosclerosis, a condition that is often aggravated by pregnancy and may present initially after delivery.

Hearing loss commonly is reported in dermatologists' offices by patients whose ear canals repeatedly collect debris from an exfoliative dermatitis. Unless the debris is removed carefully, the canal walls can be injured, and the dermatitis can be aggravated. Psychiatrists should be cognizant of the relationship between hearing loss and emotional disturbance. Hard-of-hearing patients often have been under a psychiatrist's care for a long time before being referred to an otologist for a hearing evaluation. Many psychological and emotional disturbances can be corrected or mitigated by early attention to the patient's hearing. Lamentably, some deaf but otherwise normal children have been found in mental institutions.

Curiously, some patients are most disturbed by their hearing loss when they fail to hear the little sounds, such as the passing of urine or flatus, that eventually may cause them serious embarrassment. Several patients have been referred to us by proctologists and urologists for complaints that the patients never had discussed with their general practitioners.

With the advent of the Occupational Safety and Health Act (OSHA) and routine audiometry in industry, occupational physicians and nurses have become chief sources of referral of large numbers of employees for otologic examination and diagnosis. This is important not only to detect noise-induced hearing loss but also to find patients with correctable or serious causes of hearing impairment.

Industry is in a unique position to help improve the hearing health of the working force.

When hard-of-hearing patients are not under a physician's responsible guidance, they may go directly to hearing aid dealers without a diagnosis or even a medical examination. Although many "hearing centers" and hearing aid websites are operated in an ethical manner, there are some that will sell any patient a hearing aid without investigating whether the deafness could have been cured. Some people use their hearing aids incorrectly because they fail to receive proper instruction at the time of purchase.

In many types of hearing loss, a hearing aid provides the only possible improvement. It is necessary for the patient to realize that no hearing aid can overcome the distortion produced by sensorineural deafness and that his/her hearing never will be "normal." Nevertheless, it is painful for a patient to accept these disagreeable facts. It takes skill to select the right hearing aid and time to learn to use it. Often, the patient's only chance to receive a clear explanation of the hearing trouble—what he/she has to look forward to and what can be done about it—is to go to a physician and audiologist who can communicate the facts and advise him/her properly.

The patient's personality and financial need to hear, as well as his/her willingness to wear a hearing aid and perhaps to take up lip reading, also enter into the way he/she adapts to a hearing impairment. A person who must earn a living may put up with these inconveniences more readily than an elderly person who may be more willing to retire into the comfortable silence of a restricted existence. The popularity of ear-level devices for hearing electronic devices has made it more acceptable for younger people to wear hearing aids.

## THE VALUE OF UNDERSTANDING AND CONDUCTING HEARING TESTS

Detecting hearing loss is often such a simple procedure that physicians of every specialty should have some understanding of hearing tests and be able to perform basic screening in their offices whenever the need arises. When talking with patients, one of the most effective screening tools used in determining whether or not a patient has a hearing loss is simply asking him/her, "Do you feel that you have a hearing loss?" Additionally, a simple test can be done with a 512 Hz tuning fork. This instrument can prove to be invaluable and very reliable in discovering substantial hearing impairment. It is used to help determine whether a hearing loss is caused by damage to the outer and middle ear or to the sensorineural mechanism. However, a tuning fork (even tuning forks of different frequencies) may not supply sufficient information in cases involving minimal high-frequency losses >1000–2000 Hz and other mild hearing deficiencies. Because the tuning fork will not provide a quantitative determination of hearing loss, it is necessary to use an audiometer, particularly in cases in which the loss is limited to the high-frequency range.

A good audiometer is well worth the price and effort needed to acquire skill in its use. The audiometer should be equipped to do air conduction and bone conduction tests with masking. Directions for using an audiometer and for avoiding some of the pitfalls in its use are discussed in Chapter 5.

Every community should have facilities to test hearing. An otolaryngologist can supply such services. In small communities, the pediatrician, general practitioner, or school nurse may be doing hearing tests. Many industries and small hospitals throughout the country have established hearing centers directed by well-trained audiologists and technicians. It is advisable for all physicians to have a clear understanding of audiometrics, so they may interpret the reports sent to them from the ear specialist. For these reasons, a basic discussion of audiometry is included in this book, and the results of various types of hearing tests are interpreted.

## ANATOMY AND PHYSIOLOGY OF THE HUMAN EAR

The ear is divided into three major anatomical divisions: (a) the outer ear, (b) the middle ear, and (c) the inner ear (**Figure 3.1**).

The outer ear has two parts: (a) the "trumpet-shaped" apparatus on the side of the head called the auricle or pinna and (b) the tube leading from the auricle into the temporal bone called the external auditory canal. The opening through the auricle into the external auditory canal is called the meatus.

The tympanic membrane, or "eardrum," stretches across the inner end of the external ear canal separating the outer ear from the middle ear.

The middle ear is a tiny cavity in the temporal bone. The three auditory ossicles, malleus (hammer), incus (anvil), and stapes (stirrup), form a bony bridge from the external ear to the inner ear. The bony bridge is held in place by muscles and ligaments. The middle ear chamber is filled with air and opens into the throat through the eustachian tube. The eustachian tube helps to equalize pressure on both sides of the eardrum.

The inner ear is a fluid-filled chamber divided into two parts: (a) the vestibular labyrinth, which functions as part of the body's balance mechanism, and (b) the cochlea, which contains the hearing–sensing nerve. Within the cochlea is the organ of Corti, which contains thousands of minute, sensory, hairlike cells (**Figure 3.2**). The organ of Corti functions as the switchboard of the auditory system. The eighth cranial or acoustic nerve leads from the inner ear to the brain, serving as the pathway for the impulses the brain will interpret as sound. Additional information on ear anatomy may be found in Appendix I and in Chapter 10.

Sound creates vibrations in the air somewhat similar to the "waves" created when a stone is thrown into a pond. The outer ear "trumpet" collects these sound waves, and they are funneled down the external ear canal to the eardrum. As the sound waves strike the eardrum, they cause it to vibrate. The vibrations are transmitted by mechanical action through the middle ear over the bony bridge (ossicular chain) formed by the malleus, incus, and stapes. These vibrations, in turn, cause the membranes over the openings to the inner ear to vibrate, causing the fluid in the inner ear to be set in motion. The motion of the fluid in the inner ear excited the nerve cells in the organ of Corti, producing electrochemical impulses that are gathered together and transmitted to the brain along the acoustic nerve. As the impulses reach the brain, we experience the sensation of hearing.

The sensitivity of the hearing mechanism is extraordinary. Near threshold, the eardrum only moves approximately one 1,000,000th of an inch. Our intensity range spans extremes from the softest sounds to sounds of jet engine intensity, covering an intensity range of ~100,000,000–1. Over this range, we are able to detect tiny changes in intensity and in frequency. Young, healthy humans can hear frequencies from ~20 to 20,000 Hz and can detect frequency differences as small as 0.2%. That is, we can tell the difference between a sound of 1000 Hz and 1002 Hz. Consequently, it is no

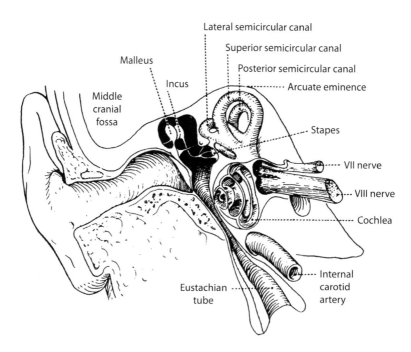

Figure 3.1 Diagrammatic cross-section of the ear. The semicircular canals are connected with maintaining balance.

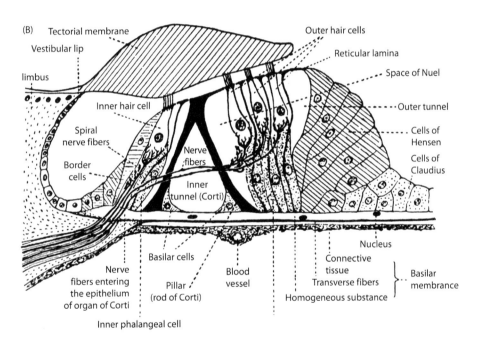

(A)

Spiral artery

Spiral ganglion

Capsule of ganglion cell

Myelin sheath

Scala vestibuli

Vestibular membrane (Reissner)

Limbus spiralis

Internal spiral sulnus

Basilar membrane

Scala tympani

Secreting epithelium

Area vascularis

Ductus cochlearis

Tectorial membrane

Crista basilaris

Spiral organ (Corti)

External spiral sulcus

Spiral ligament

(B)

Tectorial membrane

Vestibular lip

limbus

Inner hair cell

Spiral nerve fibers

Border cells

Nerve fibers

Inner tunnel (Corti)

Nerve fibers entering the epithelium of organ of Corti

Basilar cells

Pillar (rod of Corti)

Blood vessel

Inner phalangeal cell

Outer hair cells

Reticular lamina

Space of Nuel

Outer tunnel

Cells of Hensen

Cells of Claudius

Nucleus

Connective tissue

Transverse fibers

Homogeneous substance

Basilar membrance

Figure 3.2 A cross-section of the organ of Corti. (A) Low magnification. (B) Higher magnification. (After Rasmussen [1].)

surprise that such a remarkable complex system can be damaged by various illnesses and injuries.

## Causes of hearing loss

There are two basic types of hearing loss: *conductive* and *sensorineural*. They are discussed in detail throughout this book.

## ESTABLISHING THE SITE OF DAMAGE IN THE AUDITORY SYSTEM

The cause of a hearing loss, like that of any other medical condition, is determined by carefully obtaining a meaningful history, performing a physical examination, and obtaining certain tests. In otology, hearing tests parallel the function of clinical laboratory tests in general medicine.

Despite recent advances in otology, we still lack certain information about the ear and, as a result, cannot always determine the cause of hearing impairment. Fortunately, if the site of damage in the auditory system can be established, it is possible to decide on the best available treatment and the prognosis. When a hearing loss is classified, the point at which the auditory pathway has broken down is localized, and it is determined whether the patient's hearing loss is conductive, sensorineural, central, functional, or a combination of these.

*Conductive hearing loss* is due to any condition that interferes with the transmission of sound through the external and middle to the inner ear. If it is in the middle ear, the damage may involve the footplate of the stapes, as in otosclerosis, or the mobility of the drum and ossicles caused by fluid. Conductive hearing losses generally are correctable.

In *sensorineural hearing loss*, the damage lies medial to the stapedial footplate—in the inner ear, the auditory nerve, or both. Many physicians call this condition "nerve deafness." In the majority of cases, it is not curable. The cochlea has ~30,000 hair cells that connect with nerve endings. Those hair cells in the large end of the cochlea respond to very high-pitched sounds, and those in the small end respond to low-pitched sounds. These hair cells, and the nerve that connects them to the brain, are susceptible to damage from a variety of causes.

In *central hearing loss*, the damage is situated in the central nervous system at some point from the auditory nuclei (which are located in the medulla oblongata) to the auditory cortex. Knowledge about the subject still is limited.

In *functional hearing loss*, there is no detectable organic damage to the auditory pathways, and some underlying psychological or emotional problem is at fault.

Frequently, a patient experiences two or more types of hearing impairment, a problem called *mixed hearing loss*. However, for practical purposes, this term is used only when both conductive and sensorineural hearing losses are present in the same ear.

Each type of hearing loss has specific, distinctive characteristics, which make it possible to classify the vast majority of cases seen in clinical practice. When certain basic features are found, the classification usually can be made with confidence.

## CONDUCTIVE HEARING LOSS

In cases of conductive hearing loss, sound waves are not transmitted effectively to the inner ear because of some interference in the external ear canal, the eardrum, the ossicular chain, the middle ear cavity, the oval window, the round window, or the eustachian tube. For example, damage to either the middle ear, which transmits sound energy efficiently, or the eustachian tube, which maintains equal air pressure between the middle ear cavity and the external canal, could result in a mechanical defect in sound transmission. In pure conductive hearing loss, there is no damage to the inner ear or the auditory neural pathways.

Patients diagnosed as having conductive hearing loss have a better prognosis than those with sensorineural loss because modern techniques make it possible to cure or at least improve the vast majority of cases in which the damage occurs in the outer or middle ear. Even if they are not improved medically or surgically, these patients benefit greatly from a hearing aid because what they need most is amplification. They are not bothered by distortion and other hearing abnormalities that often occur in sensorineural loss.

## SENSORINEURAL HEARING LOSS

The word "sensorineural" was introduced to replace the ambiguous terms "perceptive deafness" and "nerve deafness." It is a more descriptive and more accurate anatomical term. Its dual character suggests that two separate areas may be affected, and actually, this is the case. The term "sensory" hearing loss is applied when the damage is localized in the inner ear. Useful synonyms are "cochlear" or "inner ear" hearing loss. "Neural" hearing loss is the correct term to use when the damage is in the auditory nerve, anywhere between its fibers at the base of the hair cells and the auditory nuclei. This area includes the bipolar ganglion of the eighth cranial nerve. Other common names for this type of loss are "nerve deafness" and "retrocochlear hearing loss." These names are useful if applied appropriately and meaningfully, but too often they are used improperly.

Although at present it is common practice to group together both sensory and neural components, it has become possible in many cases to attribute a predominant part of the damage, if not all of it, to either the inner ear or the nerve. Because of some success in this area and the likelihood that ongoing research will allow us to differentiate between even more cases of sensory and neural hearing loss, we shall divide the terms and describe the distinctive features of each type. This separation is advisable because the prognosis and the treatment of the two kinds of impairment differ. For example, in all cases of unilateral sensorineural hearing loss, it is important to distinguish between a sensory and neural hearing impairment because the neural type may be due to an acoustic neuroma which could be serious or even life-threatening. Those cases which we cannot identify as either sensory or neural and those cases in which there is damage in both regions we shall classify as sensorineural.

There are various and complex causes of sensorineural hearing loss, but certain features are characteristic and basic to all of them. Because the histories obtained from patients are so diverse, they may contribute more insight into the etiology than into the classification of a case.

Sensorineural hearing loss is one of the most challenging problems in medicine. A large variety of hearing impairments fall under this category. The prognosis for restoring an ear with sensorineural hearing loss to normal function with presently available therapy is poor in most cases. Although some spontaneous remissions and hearing improvements have occurred with therapy, particularly in cases involving sensory loss, there is still a need for further research.

## MIXED HEARING LOSS

In this book, the term "mixed hearing loss" will be used to indicate a conductive hearing loss accompanied by a sensory or a neural (or a sensorineural) loss in the same ear. However, the emphasis is on the conductive hearing loss because available therapy is so much more effective for this group. Consequently, the otologic surgeon has a special interest in cases of mixed hearing loss in which there is primarily a conductive loss complicated by some sensorineural damage.

## FUNCTIONAL HEARING LOSS

Functional hearing loss occurs in clinical practice more frequently than many physicians realize. This is the type of condition in which the patient does not seem to hear or respond to certain sounds: yet the handicap may be caused not by any organic pathology in the peripheral or the central auditory pathways but rather by psychological factors.

The hearing difficulty may have an entirely emotional or psychological etiology, or it may be superimposed on some mild organic hearing loss, in which case it is called a functional or a psychogenic overlay. Often, the patient really has normal hearing underlying the functional hearing loss. A carefully recorded history may reveal some hearing impairment in the patient's family or some reference to deafness which served as the nucleus for the patient's functional hearing loss. Rarely, patients who have secondary gain issues may have no hearing loss or may have a mild hearing loss and yet will demonstrate severe hearing loss on some tests of hearing. Reasons can include trying to elicit sympathy from romantic partners, potential financial gain associated with injury, and other causes that lead people to feign hearing loss. This type of functional hearing loss is called malingering.

The most important challenge in such a case is to classify the condition properly. It may be quite difficult to determine the underlying cause, but if the classification is made accurately, the proper therapy can be instituted. Too often, the emotional origin of a functional hearing loss is not recognized, and patients receive useless otologic treatments for prolonged periods. In turn, this process may aggravate the emotional element and cause the condition to become more resistant. Therefore, early and accurate classification is imperative.

## CENTRAL HEARING LOSS (CENTRAL DYSACUSIS)

Although information about central hearing loss is accumulating, it remains a mystery in otology. Physicians know that some patients cannot interpret or understand what is being said and that the cause of the difficulty is not in the peripheral mechanism but somewhere in the central nervous system. In central hearing loss, the problem is not a lowered pure-tone threshold but rather the patient's ability to interpret what he/she hears. Obviously, it is a more complex task to interpret speech than to respond to a pure-tone threshold; consequently, the tests necessary to diagnose central hearing impairment must be designed to assess a patient's ability to handle complex information. Most of the tests now available were not created specifically for this purpose, and so, it still requires a very experienced audiologist and almost intuitive judgment on the physician's part to make an accurate diagnosis. (Although aphasia sometimes is considered to be related to central hearing loss, it is outside the realm of otology.)

Central auditory processing disorders of lesser severity actually are much more common than recognized previously. Patients with this problem have difficulty filtering out competing auditory signals. Typically, they have trouble "hearing" in crowds, concentrating or reading with a radio on, and having conversations in noisy restaurants. The cause is often unknown, but the condition can result from head trauma. Thresholds often are normal, but impaired thresholds and increasing age may aggravate the symptoms.

## REFERENCE

1. Rasmussen AT. Outlines of Neuro-Anatomy. Dubuque, IA: WC Brown, 1947.

# 4

# The otologic history and physical examination

ROBERT THAYER SATALOFF AND PAMELA C. ROEHM

The first concern of a physician who is consulted by a patient with a hearing problem should be to put him/her at ease. The patient is likely to be anxious because he/she already has suffered much embarrassment from failure to understand other people, who have not always been patient with his/her handicap. The first step is to face the patient and to speak in a distinct and moderate tone. If the patient is wearing a hearing aid, there usually is no need to use a loud voice, but it helps to speak slowly and distinctly.

A hearing difficulty is quite different from the usual complaints presented to a physician. Other patients may be concerned about discomfort, itching, or pain. Perhaps they are worried that they have cancer. In comparison, the patient with a hearing loss is likely to be in good health.

A person who experiences a hearing loss usually sees a physician because of an inability to communicate successfully in social and vocational situations. The hearing loss itself is not the main issue. Therefore, when he/she first tells the doctor about the hearing trouble, the patient probably will have a great deal to unburden about psychological, social, and business problems.

Otolaryngologists (ear, nose, and throat doctors) are specialists in ear problems, among other things. Otology is a subspecialty of otolaryngology, practiced by physicians with special interests and knowledge of ear problems. Neurotology is a subspecialty of otolaryngology, and really a subspecialty of otology. Although the field is over 40 years old, there are still few practitioners who have the experience or fellowship training beyond otolaryngology residency to qualify them as neurotologists. Otolaryngologists subspecializing in this area are specially trained in the diseases of the ear and ear–brain interface and in skull base surgery for problems such as acoustic neuroma, glomus jugulare, intractable vertigo, total deafness, and traditionally "unresectable" neoplasms. They are distinct from otoneurologists, whose background is in neurology but who have special interest in disorders afflicting the hearing and balance system. Consultation with an otologist or neurotologist often is advisable during evaluation of ear and hearing problems which are often more complex than they appear to be at first.

DOI: 10.1201/b23379-4

## ESSENTIAL QUESTIONS

The physician often can save much time and be more helpful to the patient by asking certain meaningful questions that have a direct bearing on the nature of the patient's problem. The answers to these questions may help to establish a differential diagnosis of the hearing impairment.

These are among the helpful questions:

1. In which ear do you think you have hearing loss?
2. How long have you had a hearing loss?
3. If you first noticed it in relation to a head injury, exactly when did you become aware of it?
4. Who noticed it: You, family members, or others?
5. Did your hearing decrease slowly, rapidly, or suddenly?
6. Is your hearing now stable?
7. Does your hearing fluctuate?
8. Do you have distortion of pitch?
9. Do you have distortion of loudness (bothered by loud noises)?
10. Can you use both ears on the telephone?
11. Do you have a feeling of fullness in your ears?
12. Are you aware of anything (foods, weather, and sounds) that makes your hearing loss better or worse?
13. Does your hearing change with straining, bending, nose blowing, or lifting?
14. Did you have ear problems as a child?
15. Have you ever had ear drainage?
16. Have you had recent or frequent ear infections?
17. Have you ever had ear surgery?
18. Have you ever had ear surgery recommended, but not performed?
19. Have you ever had a direct injury to your ears?
20. Have you ever had problems similar to your current complaints prior to your current injury?
21. Do you have ear pain?
22. Have you had recent dental work?
23. Do you have any medical problems (diabetes, blood pressure, and others)?
24. Have you ever had syphilis or gonorrhea? Do you have AIDS?
25. Does anyone in your family have a hearing loss?
26. Has anyone in your family undergone surgery for hearing?
27. Do you have parents, brothers, or sisters with syphilis?
28. Have you ever worked at a job noisy enough to require you to speak loudly in order to be heard?
29. Do your ears ring or have other noises?
30. Do you have temporary hearing loss when you leave your work environment?
31. Do you have any noisy recreational activities, such as rifle shooting, listening to rock and roll music, snowmobiling, motor cycling, and wood working?
32. Do you wear ear protectors when exposed to loud noise?
33. Do you frequently scuba dive?
34. Do you fly private aircraft or skydive?
35. Do you have dizziness?

When the patient is a child, parents should be asked to supply information about any possible difficulties at birth and early childhood problems such as anoxia, severe jaundice, blood dyscrasias, or a hemorrhagic tendency. They should also be asked to provide information regarding any history and causes of seizures and high fevers.

## THE IMPORTANCE OF GETTING ACCURATE ANSWERS

The patient often, inadvertently, gives inaccurate answers to some of the questions in the history. This is particularly true when he/she is asked to specify how long he/she has had hearing loss. Usually, the patient underestimates the duration of the impairment.

It is an advantage to have the patient's husband or wife present at the taking of the history because he or she often supplies more accurate information. Many hearing losses develop insidiously, and the patient may not be aware of any trouble until long after the problem has become obvious to everyone else. Some patients refuse to recognize or to admit that their hearing is defective, even though others have suggested the possibility to them. This common observation illustrates the psychological overtones that frequently complicate certain forms of hearing impairment.

The exact time of onset of hearing loss may be crucial, particularly when it is sudden. Hearing may be lost instantly when a patient puts a finger in his/her ear and thereby blocks the ear canal with a plug of wax. Sudden onset may be caused by Ménière's disease, mumps, viruses, exposure to sudden very loud noises (like bombs), rupture of the round window membrane or a blood vessel, or by other causes including acoustic neuroma. In practically all such cases, only one of the ears is involved. Both ears may be affected as a result of meningitis, autoimmune inner ear disorders, or a severe head injury. Most frequently, hearing loss develops slowly over many years, especially in presbycusis, otosclerosis, deafness following exposure to intense noise, and hereditary nerve deafness.

Because otosclerosis, presbycusis, and hereditary nerve deafness are determined genetically, or at least have a tendency to recur in families, the question of familial occurrence is of some importance. Frequently, the patient is certain there is no history of deafness in the family, and yet, when the studies are completed, the diagnosis may point to a hereditary or familial condition. After further questioning, the patient sometimes recalls that one or several members of his/her family were afflicted with a hearing impairment. More often the patient insists that there has been no deafness in the family. This statement can be true, for in many cases of hereditary deafness, the hearing loss may not manifest itself for many generations, may be recessive, or the patient may be the first person in the family with a hereditary condition. In otosclerosis, for example, there may be no recent evidence of deafness in any living member of the family, and yet it is known that otosclerosis tends to be inherited.

## PROGNOSIS AND DIAGNOSIS

A vital question in the minds of both the physician and the patient is: "Will the hearing loss get worse?" The answer depends on the diagnosis. For example, some cases of hereditary nerve deafness are likely to get worse and may become quite profound. Otosclerosis may progress initially but level off and

not become very severe. Some otosclerotics, however, tend to develop sensorineural loss and suffer hearing deterioration early in life. Congenital hearing loss progresses infrequently.

The patient often can help the otologist arrive at a more definite diagnosis, even on the first visit, by indicating with some certainty whether the hearing loss has remained constant or has been getting worse over a period of months or years. It helps the otologist to distinguish between deafness caused by noise and that caused by hereditary or advancing age. A diagnosis that reveals an inherently nonprogressive condition is a source of great comfort and satisfaction to both the otologist and the patient.

## DIFFERENTIATING SYMPTOMS

## SENSORINEURAL OR CONDUCTIVE HEARING LOSS

Asking a patient whether he/she hears better in a quiet or a noisy environment usually provokes an expression of bewilderment. "I wonder what that means?" seems to be written on the patient's face. Actually, the answer to this question provides a valuable preliminary clue as to whether the patient has a sensorineural or a conductive hearing loss. In many cases of conductive hearing loss, especially in otosclerosis, there is a tendency to hear better in noisy places, whereas in sensorineural hearing loss, there often is a tendency to hear much more poorly in a noisy environment. The ability to hear better in the presence of noise is called paracusis of Willis, or paracusis Willisii, and is named after Thomas Willis, the physician who first described this phenomenon.

## TINNITUS

One of the least understood and therefore most frustrating conditions encountered by the otologist is tinnitus or "ear noises." Because various types of tinnitus are associated so often with specific types of hearing impairment, a complaint of tinnitus and a description of its characteristics can be helpful. This subject is discussed throughout this book and especially in Chapter 18.

## VERTIGO

Vertigo is also a frequent companion of hearing loss. Because the hearing and the balance mechanisms are related so intimately and bathed in the same labyrinthine fluid, vertigo often accompanies hearing difficulties. Some disturbances in the labyrinthine fluid such as Ménière's syndrome produce not only hearing loss but also interference with balance. To the otologist, vertigo does not mean light-headedness, fainting, or seeing spots before the eyes. It does not mean merely a slight sensation of loss of balance. Rather, it conveys a sensation of movement, a feeling that the room or the patient is revolving or being pushed or pulled. A sick feeling in the stomach, or nausea, often accompanies the sensation of rotary vertigo, which is similar to that felt by an inexperienced sailor on a storm-tossed ship. Labyrinthine vertigo can cause a loss of balance during walking; the patient may find it difficult to walk in a straight line because of a sensation of swaying from side to side. Full discussions of tinnitus and vertigo are found in Chapters 18 and 19.

## FLUCTUATION IN HEARING

Almost all people with hearing trouble are aware of fluctuation in their hearing. Many patients seem to hear better in the morning than at night. Some claim they hear better after they inflate their ears (by pinching the nose, closing the lips, and blowing—the so-called Valsalva maneuver). Several factors are involved in a fluctuating hearing level. For example, most people seem to hear much better when they are rested and relaxed than when they are tired and upset, as at the end of a hard day. Alertness may sharpen, whereas inattention may dull auditory efficiency. Sharp fluctuations in hearing are inherent in some types of hearing loss, such as Ménière's disease.

## SELF-INFLATION

Although it is true that some people actually can improve their hearing temporarily by inflating their ears, the vast majority experience only a clear feeling in their ears, which leads them to feel subjectively better without really hearing better. This subjective improvement usually is short-lived and provides little benefit. Moreover, indiscreet self-inflation can lead to ear infections and abnormal eardrums.

## FACTS IN THE HISTORY THAT MAY BE IMPORTANT

## OTOTOXIC DRUGS

Hearing loss can be caused by taking large doses of certain drugs such as gentamycin, neomycin, kanamycin, aspirin, and many others. The physician should learn whether the patient has used any of these drugs extensively because the information may have an important bearing on the diagnosis. Knowledge of previous ear or systemic infections also may yield important clues.

## SPEECH DEFECT

Because the development of speech depends on hearing, deafness or defective hearing in infancy or early childhood can result in speech problems. This is the reason that for centuries people who were deaf from birth also were considered to be mentally impaired since they could neither hear nor speak. One of the important clues the otologist uses in diagnosis is the patient's speech. Features such as loudness, strain, and poor articulation all help to indicate the type of hearing loss and its prognosis.

For example, a hard-of-hearing patient who speaks in a loud and strained voice probably has a sensorineural type of hearing loss. If his/her voice is unusually soft, the loss probably is conductive. If a child has a speech deficit, particularly involving consonants, she/he most likely have a high-frequency sensorineural defect.

## NOISE-INDUCED LOSS

Questions that determine the patient's line of work help to establish whether he/she has been exposed to very intense noise. A history of military service or other exposure to gunfire also is important. The large number of people who lose their hearing because of exposure to intense industrial noise is a subject of serious concern.

The importance of the patient's history cannot be emphasized enough. Often it suggests a diagnosis that then may require only a few special tests for confirmation. In such instances, many needless studies can be eliminated, and much time and energy can be saved.

## PREVIOUS EAR SURGERY

At one time it could be established readily that the patient had had ear surgery by looking for the postauricular mastoidectomy scar. Today, modern otologic surgery leaves little or no scarring. Surgery for correction of otosclerosis and ossicular defects leaves no detectable scar. Even the most observant otologist cannot know whether a patient has had previous surgery, in many cases. Not uncommonly, a patient who has had stapes surgery is embarrassed or unwilling to admit that he/she is undergoing a revision rather than an initial procedure. Therefore, it is always important to ask directly whether a patient has had any surgery to correct deafness.

Every patient who complains of a hearing loss, tinnitus, vertigo, or any other aural symptom requires a complete examination of the head and the neck. It is not sufficient to examine only the ears because the source of some otologic symptoms lies in the nasopharynx, the posterior choanal region, the temporomandibular joint, or even the throat. Ear pain, for example, may be a presenting symptom of cancer of the larynx.

## A STANDARD PATTERN FOR A COMPLETE EXAMINATION

It is advisable to develop a standard pattern for a complete examination so that nothing is overlooked. If this pattern is followed consistently, it becomes routine to examine the opposite ear and the nasopharynx even when the presumptive cause of the patient's symptoms is located immediately and cleared up, as in the case of removing impacted cerumen from one ear.

Physical examination of the patient with otological complaints should begin with a general assessment as the patient enters the physician's office. While physical examination outside the head and neck is deferred to other specialists,

initial observations of skin color and turgor, gait, affect, and other characteristics frequently provide valuable information that may trigger the appropriate referral.

Some physicians begin their examinations by first inspecting the ear about which the patient complained. The authors prefer to examine first the nose, then the neck and the throat, then the presumably normal ear, and finally the so-called bad ear. We suggest this sequence because it is possible to overlook the opposite ear, nasopharynx, and other structures while concentrating on the symptomatic ear. Occasionally, the patient asks pointedly, "Doctor, aren't you going to look at my other ear or my throat?"—but we should not have to be reminded.

## ENDOSCOPIC EXAMINATION OF THE NOSE AND NASOPHARYNX

The time required to perform a complete examination can be shortened by first inspecting the nose with a nasal speculum and at the same time spraying the nasal cavities with a vasoconstrictor and 1% cocaine or Pontocaine to prepare them to receive the nasal endoscope or nasopharyngoscope.

It is important to check the condition of the turbinates and osteomeatal complex and also look for possible discharge and obstruction caused by polyps. If pus is found in the nose, its source should be identified. Does it originate in the middle meatus or further back toward the nasopharynx? Any discharge should be evacuated with a fine nasal suction before passing the nasopharyngoscope. The appearance and consistency of the mucosa over the turbinates also should be noted. Is it pale and boggy, or is it red and tense? Does it shrink markedly after the cocaine is applied? What about the nasal airway? Is it adequate before shrinkage? What happens after shrinking?

The authors avoid passing the nasopharyngoscope until the last part of the nasal examination. A small amount of 4% cocaine should be applied to the floor of the nose with a fine probe tipped with cotton. In only a few minutes, the medication anesthetizes the floor sufficiently to pass the nasopharyngoscope. Many patients tolerate this procedure well even without topical anesthesia. Extreme gentleness should be practiced when passing probes, especially a nasopharyngoscope, into the nasal passage. If a direct passage still is not clearly visible after shrinking the mucosa, use the other naris. In many cases, it is also possible to visualize the nasopharynx by placing a small mirror at the back of the patient's throat (**Figure 4.1**). Whichever method is used, it is important to obtain a good view. The nasopharyngeal examination enables the physician to see the roof of the nose and the posterior aspects of the turbinates. Finally, the nasopharynx, eustachian tube, and fossae of Rosenmüller are scrutinized carefully on both sides.

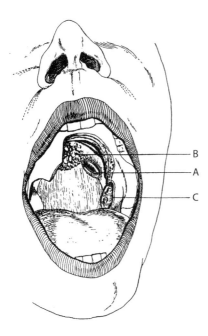

**Figure 4.1** (A) The eustachian tube opening in the back of the throat behind the soft palate that has been partially removed. (B) Adenoids. (C) Tonsils.

## THE EUSTACHIAN TUBE

The functional efficiency of the eustachian tube can be estimated in part by looking at the prominent cartilaginous lips (tori) of the tubal orifice through the nasopharyngoscope while the patient swallows. The tori should move freely. If a bubble covers the tubal orifice and the tube is normal, the bubble should break during swallowing. It is most important to look for thick bands of adhesions or growths of adenoid tissue in Rosenmüller's fossae behind the tubal opening. Sometimes these can be seen best by placing a moderate-sized (1 cm) mirror on the depressed tongue and looking up into the nasopharynx.

## THE MOUTH AND THROAT

The oral cavity should be examined carefully with attention not only to all mucosal surfaces but also to the teeth and gingiva. Wear facets on teeth and malocclusion may indicate that temporomandibular joint problems are causing ear pain. Palpation is an essential part of oral cavity examination because the examining finger can detect early tumors in the oral cavity, the base of the tongue, and the nasopharynx. The physician should always look specifically for a submucous cleft palate, which may be associated with ear disease. This is particularly important if a bifid uvula is found.

Examination of the larynx with a mirror should provide a good view of the epiglottis, true and false vocal cords, pyriform sinuses, and the base of the tongue at rest and during phonation. Better visualization can be obtained with a nasopharyngoscope or through strobovideolaryngoscopy.

Systematic examination of the neck includes bimanual palpation of the temporomandibular joints and parotid and submandibular glands. In addition, various triangles of the neck, the thyroid gland, and the carotid arteries must be palpated. Auscultation of the carotids for bruits should be routine, especially when the patient complains of dizziness or pulsatile tinnitus. A test for laryngeal crepitus also should be performed because absence of crepitus may be the only clue to a postcricoid cancer.

A basic neurological examination with special attention to the cranial nerves also is a routine part of a good otologic assessment and is especially important in the evaluation of unilateral or asymmetrical hearing loss, where neurological findings may lead to the diagnosis of acoustic neuroma, multiple sclerosis, or other important health problems.

## EARS

A head mirror, rather than an otoscope, provides a better view of the auricle and the entrance to the external canal. The shape of the external ear and its position on the head should be noted. The examiner also must look behind the ear for scars, cysts, or other abnormalities. Sometimes a small cyst or furuncle situated just at the entrance to the canal may be overlooked and cause pain when the otoscope is inserted. Choose an otoscope with as large a tip as will fit comfortably. A large tip affords broader vision and fits more snugly in the canal so that alternative positive and negative pressure can be applied to the eardrum with a small rubber bulb to test the mobility of the eardrum. This procedure is useful also in determining whether there is a perforation in the eardrum. Some patients may experience dizziness and eye movement as a result of this test if the eardrum is perforated. If there is an eardrum perforation or a mastoid cavity, this is called a positive fistula test and may signify an erosion of a semicircular canal. If the eardrum is intact, it is a positive Hennebert's sign which may suggest Ménière's syndrome or a perilymph fistula. Actually, a positive fistula test requires conjugate deviation of the eyes, but in practice, subjective dizziness is accepted as a positive fistula test or Hennebert's test.

# EARDRUM

## Removal of wax or debris

If wax or debris is present, it should be removed carefully so that the entire drum can be seen. Whenever possible, the wax should be picked out gently with a dull ear curette or an alligator forceps. Irrigation should be reserved for those cases in which there is no likelihood of a perforation, and the wax is impacted and difficult to pick or wipe out. When the drum has a perforation, irrigation may result in middle ear infection. Any debris, such as that caused by external otitis or otitis media, should be wiped out carefully with a thin cotton-tipped applicator or removed with a fine suction tip. Generally, a culture should be obtained if infection is suspected. If the physician notes bony protrusions (exostoses) in the canal, he/she should be especially gentle because injury to the thin skin covering them could result in bleeding and infection. If a large tip on the otoscope makes it difficult to see the drum, a smaller tip is used; care should be taken when inserting it deeply in order to avoid pain or injury. Findings can be documented easily using a videootoscope.

## Cone of light

We can derive much information from scrutiny of the eardrum. In a normal eardrum, a cone of light is seen coming from the end of the umbo or handle of the malleus because of the way in which the sloping drum reflects the otoscopic light. In some eardrums, the cone of light may not be seen, but this does not necessarily mean that an important abnormality exists. Absence of the cone of light may be due to abnormal slope of the drum or the angle of the external canal, a thickening of the eardrum, or changes due to aging that do not allow the light to be reflected. It also may be caused by middle ear effusion and other abnormalities.

## Intact or perforated eardrum

It is essential to find out whether the drum is intact. Most of the time a hole (perforation) in the eardrum is readily visible (**Figure 4.2**). Sometimes, however, it is difficult to see a perforation (**Figure 4.3**), and occasionally what appears to be one really is an old perforation that has healed over completely with a thin, transparent film of epithelium. If a patient has a discharge that does not come from the external canal, or if the discharge is mucoid, the physician always must look carefully for the perforation through which the discharge issues. A pinpoint perforation should be suspected when a patient complains that air whistles through the ear whenever he/she blows his/her nose or sneeze.

There are several ways to detect a perforation in the eardrum. One method is to move the drum back and forth with air pressure in the external canal (pneumatic otoscopy). This is done with a special otoscope or the rubber bulb attached to some otoscopes. If the drum moves back and forth freely, it probably is intact. If it does not move or moves only slightly, the perforation may become visible because the perforated area moves more sluggishly than the rest of the drum. Decreased eardrum mobility also may be caused by middle-ear fluid or adhesions. If a perforation is high in the area of Shrapnell's membrane, the eardrum still may move fairly well. Another technique (politzerization) to detect a perforation is to have the patient swallow while a camphorated mist is forced into one nostril and the other nostril is pinched shut. If the eustachian tube is patent and there is a perforation in the eardrum, the examiner, looking into the external auditory canal, will see the mist coming out through the small perforation. Sometimes spraying a film of powder, such as boric acid powder, on the drum delineates the edges of the perforation. This can also be done with the patient lying down, with the eardrum covered with water or a clear eardrop. When air passes through the eustachian tube, the examiner sees bubbles at the site of the perforation. All these procedures can be used also to see whether there is a transparent film over a healed perforation; gentleness and care are essential to avoid breaking the film.

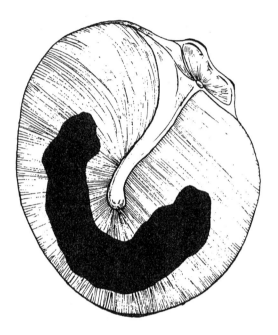

Figure 4.2 Tympanic membrane with large central perforation.

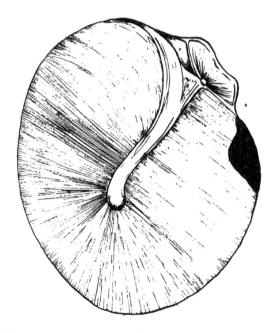

Figure 4.3 Tympanic membrane with small marginal perforation.

The use of an otologic microscope enhances accurate assessment of the eardrum and middle ear.

## Shadow formations

It is important to look for shadow formations behind the drum, particularly those caused by fluid in the middle ear. To accomplish this, the otologist should try to look through the drum rather than merely at it. In this way, what seemed to be a simple surface becomes a map with a dark shadow for the round window niche, a lighter area for the promontory, a pink area for the incus, and many other features.

## Fluid in the middle ear

Fluid in the middle ear often eludes detection, even though it causes hearing loss. Failure to discover the fluid could result in a wrong diagnosis. For example, a patient may have a 30 dB conductive hearing loss with an eardrum that appears to be practically normal. The diagnosis naturally would be otosclerosis, and stapes surgery would be indicated. When the eardrum is reflected during surgery, however, a thick mucoid, gelatinous mass is found, especially around the oval and the round windows, and the correct diagnosis is not otosclerosis but secretory otitis media. The fluid was simply not detected preoperatively.

A diligent search should be made for fluid in the middle ear if bone conduction is reduced slightly in an otherwise classic picture of conductive hearing loss. There are several ways to detect fluid in the middle ear. If a well-defined fluid level is seen through the eardrum, the diagnosis is simple. It should be borne in mind, however, that strands of scar tissue in the drum and bands in the middle ear can stimulate a fluid level. It helps to see whether the apparent fluid level stays in position while the patient's head is bent forward and backward. With air pressure in the external canal, it is difficult to get free to-and-fro motion of the drum if there is much fluid behind it in the middle ear. In contrast, a normal drum moves easily. Occasionally, bubbles can be seen in the fluid confirming the diagnosis. Impedance audiometry is useful in patients who might have an abnormality in the eardrum and middle ear, and computerized tomography (CT) scans can help to clarify the status of the middle ear in selected patients.

*Politzerization* is of great help in detecting fluid but should not be performed in the presence of an upper respiratory infection, particularly one affecting the nose. During politzerization, the fluid and the bubbles can be seen briefly through the drum; then they usually disappear. The patient may profess to suddenly hear better. Politzerization also should be avoided in patients who have undergone stapedectomy.

Whenever there is any suspicion of the pressure of middle ear fluid, a *myringotomy* should be performed for diagnostic and therapeutic reasons. In an adult, this can be done without local or general anesthesia by using a sharp knife to puncture the inferior portion of the drum. If fluid is present, some usually will ooze out spontaneously, or it can be forced out by politzerization or suction through the myringotomy. A ventilation tube can be placed, if appropriate.

## Scars and plaques, color, and tumors

The eardrum may reveal still other findings such as scars and plaques. These reflect previous infections and tissue changes in the eardrum. They rarely in themselves cause any significant degree of hearing loss. Occasionally, an eardrum appears to be blue or purple. This may be due to a blockage in the middle ear or to entrapped fluid, or it may be merely a peculiar type of retracted eardrum. A reddish color sometimes is caused by a tumor (glomus jugulare) extending into the middle ear. If there is any possibility of the presence of such a tumor, manipulation should be avoided until further studies have clarified the diagnosis.

## Retracted eardrum

This is another abnormal finding. It is easy to understand why one physician will look at a drum and consider it to be normal, whereas another will say it is retracted. Eardrums vary in their appearance, and the concept of retraction is subject to comparable variations. Even a moderate amount of retraction *per se* may not cause any significant hearing loss. Only when the drum is retracted markedly, and especially when it is pulled onto the promontory, is there a correlation between retraction and hearing. In such instances, politzerization can restore hearing by returning the drum to its original position. Occasionally, the drum is overdistended during politzerization, and then it appears to be flaccid and relaxed. It recovers spontaneously in most cases, often after a swallow or two.

In all cases of retracted eardrum (especially unilateral), the cause should be sought in the nasopharynx, the sinuses, and the eustachian tube. Allergies and enlarged adenoids are the most common causes, but neoplasms also must be ruled out, especially in unilateral cases. Aerotitis media may be another cause of a retracted eardrum. In some patients, politzerization is not possible, and a small eustachian catheter has to be introduced gently into the mouth of the eustachian tube, generally guided by a nasopharyngoscope positioned through the other naris. The air can be forced in carefully until the tube is opened. By placing one end of a listening tube (Toynbee tube) in the patient's ear and the other end in the physician's ear, the sound of air can be heard as it enters the middle ear.

## Erosion, previous surgery, and drainage

Perhaps the most confusing otologic picture presents itself when the eardrum is largely eroded and the middle ear is discharging; a similar problem arises when some kind of mastoid surgery has deformed the normal landmarks. In such cases, it is necessary to appraise the condition of the middle ear in order to decide on the proper treatment and to evaluate the chances of restoring hearing. In view of the extensive amount of otologic surgery that has been performed in recent years, it is always wise to look at scars of previous operations, both postauricular and endaural, the latter being situated just above the tragus. A postauricular scar usually indicates mastoid surgery. If the eardrum is practically normal, most likely a simple mastoidectomy or tympanomastoidectomy was done, and the hearing may be within normal limits. If the eardrum is gone and the malleus and the incus also are absent, the operation may have been a radical mastoidectomy, and the conductive hearing loss should be ~50–60 dB. Intermediate between the simple and the radical mastoidectomies are various surgical procedures aimed at both preserving as much hearing as possible and eradicating the infection or cholesteatoma. These procedures usually are called modified radical tympanomastoidectomies. Most of the time, the eardrum or part of it is visible, and some form of ossicular chain is present. In modern techniques, a prosthesis may have been inserted to restore ossicular continuity; also, a graft may have been applied to replace the eardrum that had been removed or damaged previously. The endaural scar also could indicate a fenestration operation; an eardrum will be visible, but it will seem to be out of place, and at least some part of the mastoid bone will have been exenterated. Quite often these cavities are covered with debris and require gentle cleaning to permit a clear view. Caution is necessary in cleaning such a cavity around the fenestrated area to avoid inducing vertigo and nystagmus.

Many stapes operations are performed. Because this procedure rarely leaves an evident scar, previous stapes surgery must be uncovered in the history. In stapes surgery, the incision is made inside the external auditory canal on its posterior wall, and the eardrum is reflected forward upon itself so that the surgeon can work in the middle ear. Healing is almost free of visible scars in the canal although absence of bone along the posterior scutum may be noted after this surgery.

It is becoming much more common to see eardrums of a very peculiar appearance in which infection has played no part. In most cases, the unusual features are the result of myringoplasties (surgical repair of the eardrum) with skin, fascia, or other grafts. The drum may appear to be thick and flaccid or whitish, and it may show few landmarks. Ideally, the patient or previous medical records can supply the pertinent information in such instances. Sometimes one will see an eardrum with something that looks like a small tube sticking out of it. A tiny piece of polyethylene, silastic, metal, or Teflon tubing has been inserted through a small perforation to prevent closure and to allow ventilation of the middle ear. This usually is done in cases of persistent secretory otitis media.

## NEUROTOLOGICAL EXAMINATION

In addition to complete otoscopic examination, a pneumatic otoscope is used to move each eardrum to determine whether this maneuver causes dizziness and/or nystagmus. If there is a hole in the eardrum, this is called a fistula test. If the eardrum is intact, it is called Hennebert's test. Although technically conjugate deviation of the eyes is required for the test to be positive, in general practice a clear subjective response of dizziness is considered a positive test, especially if nystagmus is present. A positive Hennebert's test may occur with endolymphatic hydrops or a fistula. Hitselberger's sign is sought by testing sensation of the lateral posterior/superior aspect of the external auditory canal. This is the area that receives sensory supply from the facial nerve. Lesions putting pressure on the nerve such as acoustic neuromas or anterior/inferior cerebellar auditory vascular loops often cause a sensory deficit in this area or a positive Hitselberger's sign. Prior ear surgery may also cause decreased sensation in this area. The eyes are examined for extraocular muscle function and spontaneous nystagmus. This examination is aided by Frenzel glasses which prevent visual fixation. It is important to note that the examiner's eye is an order of magnitude more sensitive in detecting nystagmus than an electronystagmography (EMG). Videonystagmography (VNG) is more sensitive than EMG, but certain eye movements will not be analyzed correctly by algorithms used to automatically analyze the test. For instance, only 3D VNG will correctly detect torsional eye movements using these examinations.[1] However, VNG records these eye movements and the resulting video can be reviewed frame by frame to reveal these otherwise overlooked abnormalities. So, direct observation of the eyes during physical examination (and review of videos) should not be omitted. Other cranial nerves should be examined, as well. The olfactory nerve may be tested by asking the patient to inhale vapors from a collection of different scents. The optic nerve is tested at least by visual confrontation, if not by referral to an ophthalmologist. Fundoscopic examination is added in some cases, especially if increased intracranial pressure or significant microvascular disease is suspected.

Trigeminal nerve sensation is tested by assessing sensation in all three divisions on both sides. The trigeminal nerve also supplies motor fibers to muscles of mastication which can be evaluated by assessing jaw movement and muscle strength. In addition to Hitselberger's sign, the facial nerve is assessed through observations of facial movement and tone. Tear flow, stapedius muscle reflex, salivary flow, and taste can also be tested as part of a facial nerve evaluation. The glossopharyngeal nerve is evaluated by testing gag reflex in the posterior third of the tongue or oropharynx, and sensation along the posterior portion of the palate, uvula, and tonsil oropharyngeal sensory function also can be tested and quantified using functional endoscopic sensory testing with air pulses that trigger the laryngeal reflex. Abnormal vocal fold or palatal motion is often the most obvious sign of tenth nerve dysfunction. Eleventh cranial nerve abnormality is diagnosed in the presence of sterno-cleidomastoid or trapezius muscle weakness, and 12th nerve dysfunction causes unilateral tongue paralysis. Examination of the nose and oral cavity is performed routinely. Special attention is paid to nasal obstruction when taste and smell disorders have been identified and to clear rhinorrhea which may indicate a cerebrospinal fluid leak following head injury. Examination of the larynx should include special attention to symmetry of vocal fold motion and to any signs of direct laryngeal trauma. In addition, hoarseness or any other voice change should be noted and investigated with strobo-videolaryngoscopy, objective voice measures, and other state-of-the-art evaluations. Examination of the neck includes palpation not only of the anterior neck but also of the posterior aspect looking for muscle spasm and tenderness of the cervical vertebrae. These findings are associated often with limitation of motion, especially in patients who have dizziness associated with changes in head and neck position. Attention should be paid to the regions of C1 and C2, especially in patients with posttraumatic dizziness. Neck examination should also include auscultation of the carotid arteries and palpation of the superficial temporal arteries. If there is any question of vascular insufficiency, ultrasound of the carotid and vertebral arteries, MR angiography (MRA), MR venography (MRV), or arteriography should be considered. In addition, Romberg testing, gait assessment, cerebellar function testing, and other neurologic evaluation should be carried out.

## OTHER CONDITIONS TO CONSIDER

In addition to asking questions directed specifically to otologic problems, the physician must obtain a complete general medical history. Many systemic conditions are associated with otologic symptoms such as hearing loss, tinnitus, and dizziness. Such conditions include diabetes, hypoglycemia, thyroid dysfunction, cardiac arrythmia, hypertension, hypotension, renal disease, collagen vascular disease, previous meningitis, multiple sclerosis, herpes infection,

previous syphilis infection (even from decades ago), glaucoma, seizure disorders, and many other conditions. Psychiatric conditions also are relevant because many of the medications used to treat them and to treat various systemic diseases may cause otologic symptoms as side effects. Otologic symptoms can also be caused by a variety of antibiotics and toxic chemicals, such as lead and mercury. Previous radiation treatment to the head and neck may result in microvascular changes that cause hearing loss, tinnitus, or dizziness. Even excess consumption of alcohol or caffeine may produce symptoms that could be confused with other etiologies. Chickenpox occasionally leaves a small pockmark on the eardrum that may persist for many years and be confused with a clinically relevant problem. Blood in the middle ear following head injury generally indicates a fracture in the temporal bone and may result in eardrum scar or hearing loss. Hearing tests help to determine the extent of involvement, especially if the inner ear is damaged. Whenever there is a possibility of an acoustic neuroma, additional tests including magnetic resonance imaging (MRI) and a neurological evaluation are indicated. The interpretation of many of these tests is not included in this book.

Objective tinnitus is a noise that can be heard by the examiner as well as the patient. To detect these cases, the physician should put his/her ear to the patient's ear or use a listening tube (Toynbee tube) or stethoscope to find out whether there is a bruit indicating a vascular disorder. Another cause of objective tinnitus is an intermittent spasm of the soft palate that produces a clicking sensation heard in the ear, and this also may be heard with a Toynbee tube or stethoscope. There are also many other conditions that should be considered in otologic patients. In addition to those discussed later in this book, a great many more may be reviewed in medical textbooks of otology/neurotology.

## TESTS

## TESTS OF HEARING AND BALANCE

Testing of hearing and balance function is fundamental in patients with otological complaints. Specific appropriate tests will be discussed in detail in subsequent chapters.

## METABOLIC TESTS

Metabolic tests must be selected on the basis of clinical need in each individual case. However, certain conditions have such profound importance in otologic symptoms that they are sought with nearly routine frequency. Most of these conditions are discussed in greater detail in later chapters.

Luetic labyrinthitis is a highly specific syphilis infection of the inner ear. Luetic labyrinthitis can cause hearing loss, tinnitus, and vertigo. Untreated, it may eventually cause total deafness. Routine serologic testing (RPR and VDRL) is normal. In order to detect luetic labyrinthitis, an FTA absorption test, MHA-TP, or other sophisticated syphilis antibody test must be obtained.

Similarly, Lyme disease, which is caused by infection with Borrelia bacteria, can lead to sensorineural hearing loss, tinnitus, balance, and facial nerve dysfunction. Treatment for Lyme disease can limit hearing loss and reverse tinnitus, imbalance, and facial paralysis. To detect Lyme disease, a Lyme panel (antibody testing followed by confirmatory Western blot) should be ordered.

Diabetes and especially reactive hypoglycemia may produce symptoms of dizziness. In some cases, hypoglycemia may provoke symptoms similar to endolymphatic hydrops (Ménière's syndrome). A 5-hour glucose tolerance test is often necessary in dizzy patients to rule out hypoglycemia, although other tests are available to detect diabetes.

Even mild hyperthyroidism may produce fluctuating hearing loss, tinnitus, and disequilibrium in some patients. It is frequently necessary to obtain T3, T4, and TSH to establish this diagnosis.

Hyperlipoproteinemia has been associated with sensorineural hearing loss, as well. When sensorineural hearing loss of unknown etiology is under investigation, measurement of cholesterol and triglyceride levels may be helpful.

Diabetes mellitus and collagen vascular disease produce vascular changes which compromise perfusion and may cause otologic symptoms. In addition to routine screening for diabetes, tests for collagen vascular disease including rheumatoid factor, antinuclear antibody, and sedimentation rate may be indicated.

Autoimmune inner ear pathology has been well documented. When suspected, a variety of tests of immune function is required, as discussed later in this book.

In at least a small number of patients, allergies may cause otologic symptoms. In the authors' experience, this association is less common than some literature would suggest. However, in the appropriate clinical setting, allergy evaluation and treatment may be required for otologic symptoms including dizziness, tinnitus, and hearing loss.

A great many other tests may be appropriate depending upon clinical presentation. Many viruses, sickle cell disease, and numerous other problems may cause neurotologic symptoms that may be difficult to differentiate from symptoms caused by noise or other etiologies without appropriate studies.

## RADIOLOGIC TESTS

Neurotologic diagnosis has been revolutionized by modern radiologic technology. In many patients with otologic symptoms, radiologic investigation is essential.

## MAGNETIC RESONANCE IMAGING

MRI is the mainstay of radiologic evaluation of the neurotologic patient. MRI of the brain and internal auditory canals is required for complete assessment. In the neurotologic patient, it is essential to rule out demyelinating disease, neoplasms, subdural hematomas, and other conditions that may be responsible for the patient's neurotologic complaints. High-resolution gadolinium-enhanced MRI of the internal auditory canal is required to rule out acoustic neuroma. Very high-quality studies are necessary, and MRI should be performed on a magnet of at least 1.5 Tesla strength.

## COMPUTERIZED TOMOGRAPHY

CT scan has been performed much less frequently in the recent years because of improvements in MRI. However, CT testing may still be extremely valuable. MRI does not show bony detail. A high-resolution CT of the ears may show birth defects or even hairline fractures or other bony abnormalities of great clinical importance that may not be invisible on MRI. One should not hesitate to order both studies if indicated by history or physical examination findings.

## AIR-CONTRAST CT

Air-contrast CT involves infusion of 3–5 cc of air through a lumbar puncture. The procedure should be performed with a small gauge spinal needle and is done routinely on an out-patient basis. Air is allowed to rise into the cerebellopontine angle (CPA), and the internal auditory canal and neurovascular bundle can be visualized well. This test was standard for detection of small acoustic neuromas before MRI was developed. Now it is performed infrequently, but it still has use particularly in people who cannot undergo MRI when there is a high suspicion of a small tumor. It shows the region much more clearly than MRI and often allows detection of abnormalities such as anterior inferior cerebellar artery loop compression of the eighth cranial nerve with arachnoid response at the contact point, a condition that cannot be assessed definitively by MRI.

## ULTRASOUND AND ARTERIOGRAPHY

When there is a question regarding the adequacy of carotid or vertebral blood flow, ultrasound provides a noninvasive, painless, expeditious method for assessing blood flow. In patients with positional vertigo, vertebral ultrasound with the neck in neutral, flexed, extended, and turned positions may reveal intermittent vertebrobasilar artery system occlusion. If the results are equivocal, if significant vascular compromise is identified, or if there is very strong clinical suspicion of vascular occlusion despite an unimpressive ultrasound, arteriography may be required. While this test is more definitive, it may be associated with serious complications and is ordered only when truly necessary. MRA is less invasive and may provide the needed information in many cases. Angiography also provides information about intracranial vascular anatomy. In some cases, additional information about intracranial vascular flow may be necessary, and new techniques of intracranial doppler study are available for this purpose.

## DYNAMIC IMAGING

Single-photon emission computed tomography (SPECT) or positron emission tomography (PET) also have been used for neurotologic evaluation. In some patients, they may show blood flow abnormalities in the microcirculation of the auditory structures that may be the only objective abnormalities identified for some patients.[2,3] However, it is not used commonly in the evaluation of patients with hearing loss.

## REFERENCES

1. Gananca MM, Caovilla HH, Gananca FF. Electronystagmography versus videonystagmography. Braz J Otorhinolaryngol, 2010;76(3):399–403.
2. Sataloff RT, Mandel S, Muscal E, Park CH, Rosen DC, Kim SM, Spiegel JR. Single-photon-emission computed tomography (SPECT) in neurotologic assessment: A preliminary report. AJO, 1996;17(6):909–916.
3. Joglekar SS, Bell JR, Caroline M, Chase PJ, Domesek J, Patel PS, Sataloff RT. Evaluating the role of single photon emission computed tomography (SPECT) in the assessment of neurotologic assessment. Ear Nose Throat J, 2014;93(4–5):168–171.

# 5

# Classification and measurement of hearing loss

ROBERT THAYER SATALOFF AND PAMELA C. ROEHM

## HEARING TESTS WITH THE TUNING FORK

Two basic types of testing are done with a tuning fork routinely: air conduction and bone conduction. The best all-purpose tuning fork to use is a 512 Hz steel tuning fork. Tuning forks of lower frequencies produce a greater tactile sensation that is felt rather than heard or that can be felt before the tone is heard. However, tuning forks of various frequencies from 125 to 8000 Hz may be useful in some situations. Although forks of frequencies higher than 512 Hz are attenuated quickly, they can supply useful information. With the 512 Hz tuning fork, it is possible for the examiner to obtain a rough estimate of the extent of the hearing loss and to speculate whether the cause is conductive or sensorineural. In some cases, it is even possible to establish whether the damage is in the inner ear or in the nerve.

A tuning fork should not be struck very hard; a blow that is too forceful produces overtones that might give false information. Furthermore, a very loud tone may startle some patients who are especially sensitive to noise because of hyperrecruitment, a condition often present in Ménière's disease. Tuning forks should be struck on something that is firm but not too hard. The knuckle, the elbow, and the neurological rubber hammer are all satisfactory for this purpose. Tabletops and wooden chairs generally should not be used to activate tuning forks.

In testing for air conduction, the tuning fork should be held close to, but should not touch, the ear, and the broad side of one of the prongs must face the ear (**Figure 5.1**). It is wrong to hold the two prongs parallel to the side of the ear. Such an application often produces a dead spot, and, consequently, the listener may hear no tones, even though his/her hearing may be normal. To verify this fact, the examiner should place the tuning fork to his/her own ear and rotate it. The tone will appear to go off and on as the fork turns.

Air conduction measures the ability of airborne sound waves to be transmitted to the inner ear along the external auditory canal, the eardrum, and the ossicular chain. This is done by holding the vibrating tuning fork near, but not touching, the external auditory canal. Bone conduction measures, to some

DOI: 10.1201/b23379-5

degree, the ability of the inner ear and the nerve to receive and to utilize sound stimuli. In this test, the external auditory canal and the middle ear are bypassed. The base or the handle of the vibrating tuning fork is held directly on the skull so that the vibrations can reach the inner ear directly (**Figure 5.2**). The fork may be held on the mastoid bone, the forehead, the nasal dorsum, the closed mandible, or the upper teeth. Gentle application to the upper incisors or even to dentures provides the best clinical measurement of bone conduction. This effect can be produced more sterilely by first having the patient bite down on a tongue depressor and then pressing the handle of the vibrating fork onto the portion of the tongue depressor which projects out from the mouth. These sites are preferable to the mastoid area or forehead with regard to sensitivity.

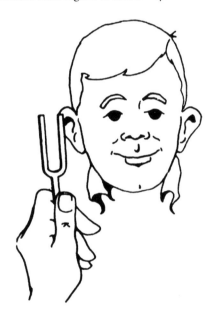

Figure 5.1 Position of the tuning fork for air conduction testing.

## FACTORS IN EVALUATION

## APPROXIMATE RESULTS WITH THE TUNING FORK

Despite efforts, no reliable method to calibrate tuning forks quantitatively has been found. Therefore, the tuning fork makes it possible to obtain only a rough approximation of a patient's ability to hear. For example, the physician can strike the fork gently, apply it successively to the left and to the right ear, and ask the patient to specify in which ear the tone sounds louder, or the examiner can compare the patient's ability to hear a tuning fork with his/her own, presumably normal (or, at least, known) hearing. However, because it is not possible to express the results of tuning fork tests in quantitative terms such as decibels, the use of an audiometer is required.

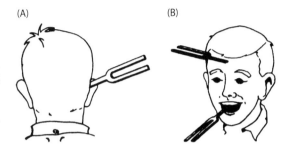

(A)            (B)

Figure 5.2 Placement of the handle of the fork on the mastoid (A) and on the forehead and the upper incisors (B) for bone conduction testing.

## TRANSMISSION OF SOUND TO THE OPPOSITE EAR

When testing hearing with a tuning fork or an audiometer by either air or bone conduction, it is important to remember that sounds of sufficient intensity, when applied to or held near one ear, are transmitted around the head or through the bones of the skull and are heard by the opposite ear.

In air conduction testing, the tone near one ear has to be quite loud to be carried around the head and heard by the opposite ear. There is roughly a 40-dB attenuation between the ears; in other words, if a tone near one ear is 40 dB or louder, it can be heard by the opposite ear. In bone conduction testing, the problem is far more complex because there is little or no attenuation by the skull of low-frequency bone conducted sound. Although the examiner thinks he/she is testing the *left* ear when he/she holds a tuning fork to the *left* mastoid bone, he/she actually is testing *both* ears because the right ear receives the sound at almost the same intensity as the left ear.

## MASKING THE OPPOSITE EAR

For these reasons, it is necessary, especially in bone conduction testing, to mask the opposite ear hearing so that responses only from the ear being tested are received. This also applies to air conduction testing, particularly when there is a difference of ~40 dB or more in hearing acuity between the two ears.

It might seem that the opposite ear could be masked by inserting a plug or covering it with the patient's hand. Actually, these measures would not only fail to mask the ear but also they would cause the tuning fork to sound even louder. To prove this, you need to merely strike a tuning fork and hold the handle to your upper incisors. Generally, if your hearing is normal, the fork will be heard throughout the head. Plugging an ear with a finger does not mask it; instead, it produces a conductive hearing loss and misleading results. When testing one ear with a tuning fork, a good way to mask the opposite ear is to have an assistant or the patient rub a page of stiff writing paper over the opposite ear. The noise made by this paper occupies the nerve pathway of that ear, and then you can be sure of getting a response only from the ear to which you apply the tuning fork. The air-pressure hose that is used to spray noses also can serve as a masking device. It should be used cautiously in order to avoid injuring the eardrum. The air nozzle should be applied somewhat sideways in the ear so that the noise goes into the canal without too much air pressure. A special noisemaker called a Bárány noise apparatus also is available. This device is very inexpensive and small; it is activated by winding it up and pressing a button, and it can help mask hearing in the contralateral ear.

## USING THE TUNING FORK IN DIAGNOSIS

Now that we know the basics of tuning fork testing, let us proceed to use the fork in helping to make a diagnosis in routine office practice. Bear in mind that if only a mild hearing loss is present (i.e., < 25 dB for the frequency being tested by the fork), the tuning fork may not provide accurate information. It is reliable only when the hearing loss is ≥ 25 dB.

## SYSTEMATIC EVALUATION

Let us suppose a patient complains of hearing trouble in his/her left ear, and the otoscopic examination shows normal external canals and eardrums in both ears. What steps are taken to find exactly where in the auditory pathways the damage has occurred, and what is the most likely cause? First, it is necessary to determine whether there really is a hearing loss in the patient's left ear. To do this, strike the tuning fork gently, hold it to your own normal ear until the tone gets weak, then quickly put the fork near the patient's left ear and ask if he/she hears it. If not, put it to the right and presumably normal ear to be sure the fork is still vibrating. Finally, put it back to your own ear to be certain the tone is still present.

Obviously, if the fork is heard either in your ear or in the patient's good right ear but not in the left, or bad, ear, he/she probably have some hearing loss in the left one. Then, by striking the tuning fork a little harder each time and listening with your own normal ear before and after you place it to the patient's left ear, you can determine how loud the fork's vibrations must be for the patient to hear them. In this way, a rough idea of the degree of his/her hearing loss can be gained.

Converting this finding to decibels by an "educated guess" is surprisingly difficult. It should not be attempted even by so-called experts. If the patient seems to hear what you believe to be an extremely weak tone (almost as weak as you can hear), his/her hearing loss, if it exists, probably is too mild to be studied with a tuning fork, or perhaps it is present only in the higher frequencies. In either case, audiometric studies are required.

## RINNE TEST

Now let us presume that the patient does have a moderate hearing loss in the left ear and does not respond to a vibrating tuning fork that you hear. The next step is to determine whether the damage is in the conductive area (the outer or the middle ear) or in the sensorineural pathways (the inner ear or the auditory nerve). The patient now is asked to tell you whether the vibrating tuning fork seems to sound louder when it is held beside the left ear (by air) or behind the left ear directly on the mastoid bone (by bone). The tuning fork is struck hard enough so that the patient should be able to hear it fairly well, and it is held beside the left ear for about a second. Then, it is quickly moved until its handle touches the left mastoid bone, where it is held for another second. Move the fork back and forth between these two points, striking the fork again, if necessary, until the patient can tell whether it is louder by air or behind the ear. This is called the Rinne test. Applying the handle to the upper incisors is another good method of testing and will detect smaller air–bone gaps (20–25 dB) than will mastoid testing (30–35 dB).

If the fork is louder behind the ear on the patient's mastoid bone or on the teeth, bone conduction is considered to be better than air conduction, and therefore, he/she has a conductive hearing loss. In other words, the sensorineural pathway is working, but something is blocking the sound waves from reaching the inner ear.

Furthermore, because the outer ear had been examined and was found to be normal, the probable diagnosis is some defect in the ossicular chain, such as otosclerosis.

## WEBER TEST

To confirm these findings, the tuning fork now is struck again, and the handle is placed on the patient's forehead nasal dorsum, gently touching his/her upper incisor teeth, or on a tongue depressor bitten between the patient's teeth. The patient is then asked to indicate in which ear the fork sounds louder (the Weber test). In a conductive hearing loss, the tone will sound louder in the bad ear, the left one in this case. Something like this happens when you plug your own ear while the fork is on your teeth; you probably will be surprised that it sounds louder in the plugged ear. Plugging the ear produces a conductive hearing loss just as otosclerosis does. In sensorineural hearing loss, the tuning fork sounds louder in the good ear.

## SCHWABACH TEST

Occasionally, a patient will find it difficult to lateralize the fork to either ear, that is, to tell in which ear the fork sounds louder. This reaction does not rule out conductive deafness but, rather, suggests the need for further studies, particularly with an audiometer. To complete the tuning fork tests on this particular patient, who has a presumptive diagnosis of otosclerosis, strike the fork gently, press it against the patient's left mastoid area until he/she barely hear it, and then move the instrument quickly to your own mastoid (the

Schwabach test). The patient will hear the tuning fork much better and longer by bone conduction on his/her mastoid than even you yourself can hear it. This is called prolonged bone conduction and substantiates a diagnosis of conductive hearing loss.

## FURTHER TESTS

Now let us examine a different patient with normal otoscopic findings who also is complaining of left-sided hearing loss. When we compare his/her ability to hear by air and bone conduction (Rinne test), we find he/she hears much better by air conduction than by bone, in contrast to the previous patient. Furthermore, when we put the tuning fork to his/her teeth, it sounds louder in his/her good ear than in his/her bad ear (Weber test). It is important in this last test to mask the good ear with noise so that the sound of the fork pressed against the mastoid of the bad ear may not be heard in the good ear. The site of damage in this patient is not in his/her middle or outer ear, as in the previous case, but in his/her inner ear or auditory nerve. The patient has sensorineural hearing loss, and the most likely cause will have to be determined by exploring the history and performing many more tests, some of which require special equipment. Chapter 10 includes an explanation of how it is possible with a tuning fork to decide in some patients whether the damage is located specifically in the inner ear proper or auditory nerve by testing for diplacusis (pitch distortion) or recruitment (loudness distortion).

## DIFFICULT CASES

The two patients mentioned earlier were comparatively easy to classify. Actually, most patients are just as easy to test, but, occasionally, more difficult cases are encountered, as when the same patient has a severe or even total loss of hearing in one ear and a partial conductive hearing loss in the other. A great deal of masking and careful interpretation of hearing tests are necessary in such cases; yet the tuning fork can provide the essential information, and each ear often can be classified properly.

Determining the site of damage usually can be done readily with a tuning fork. In some instances, however, this may become difficult, and it may be especially hard to decide which of many possible causes applies. More sophisticated tests with an audiometer and other equipment are helpful in such cases, but the tuning fork should be used routinely to confirm or to challenge the results obtained with the more discriminating and complex equipment.

## THE AUDIOMETER AND THE TUNING FORK

Few general practitioners have audiometers today, but it might be rewarding to purchase one and learn to perform audiometric hearing tests. It would enable them to render better service to some of their patients, just as electrocardiography refines their service to others. The technique for performing good audiometry and the pitfalls to be avoided are described later in this chapter. If a practitioner prefers not to use an audiometer and refers his/her patients to a local otolaryngologist, audiologist, or hearing center, he/she should make it a routine policy to confirm all studies done by consultants with his/her own tuning fork tests. Although a consultant may have more elaborate equipment and testing experience, the general practitioner should not underestimate the importance of the simple tuning fork in the diagnosis of hearing loss or the possibility for errors in audiometric test results. Boothless audiometry measurement computer application can make these services more affordable. These programs must be calibrated to ambient noise and are inherently less sensitive and reliable than audiometers. However, they are significantly less costly and take up substantially less space. Hearing tests from boothless audiometry computer programs would require confirmation to ensure accuracy, and they do not meet Occupational Safety and Health Act (OSHA) requirements for use in industry.

## ASPECTS OF TESTING

## COOPERATION OF THE PATIENT

At present, physicians have at their disposal only a few reliable *objective* methods of measuring hearing (Chapter 7). In routine testing, some voluntary response of the patient is necessary as an indication that he/she hears the sound used to test hearing. The sound may be a word, a sentence, a pure tone, a noise, or even the blast of a loud horn. The patient's response may consist of raising his/her finger or hand, pressing a button, answering a question, repeating a sentence, turning in the direction of the sound, or merely blinking his/her eyes. The test sound is reduced in intensity until the patient hears it ~50% of the times it is presented. In such an instance, the intensity level at which the patient just hears the sound is called the *threshold of hearing*. Speech may be used at a reasonably loud level, and the patient is asked to repeat words or combinations of words to determine how well he/she distinguishes certain speech sounds. This is called *discrimination testing*.

## DEVELOPMENT OF THE AUDIOMETER

The ideal method of testing hearing would be to measure and to control everyday speech accurately and to present it to the patient in such a manner that, without requiring any voluntary response from the patient, the physician could determine whether the patient had received and understood it clearly through both ears and with the participation of his/her brain. Unfortunately, many unsolved complex problems have prevented the development of such a method. Even the very first step of controlling and measuring the intensity of speech itself has not yet been perfected.

The old method of testing hearing—one that some physicians still use—is to stand 15 ft away and to whisper a number of words to the patient, who is plugging his/her distal ear with a finger. The examiner gradually comes closer until the patient just begins to repeat the whispered words correctly. If the patient responds correctly to every word at 15 ft, the examiner gives him/her a score of 15/15, or normal hearing, but if the physician must approach to within 5 ft to obtain a correct response, the patient receives a 5/15 score for his/her hearing impairment. Then, the patient faces the opposite way, with a finger plugging the other ear, and the procedure is repeated.

It is extremely difficult to duplicate this test under identical conditions. Furthermore, it is virtually impossible to compare the results of different patients or to maintain an accurate sound-intensity level. Factors such as the acoustics of the test room, the choice of words, the examiner's accent, enunciation, and ability to control and to project his/her voice as well as the degree of hearing loss in either or both of the patient's ears render this testing procedure highly inaccurate.

## THE PURE-TONE AUDIOMETER

These shortcomings and the impossibility of controlling and reproducing speech sounds accurately with the early forms of electronic equipment led to the development of the pure-tone audiometer. Its designers recognized that their chief objective was to determine to what degree speech must be amplified to be just heard by the patient. They therefore analyzed speech and found that it encompassed frequencies from ~128 to 8192 Hz.

At that time, electronic equipment was readily available to measure pure tones with a great deal of accuracy, though no equipment was available to measure speech. Because it was not practical to test all frequencies from 128 to 8192 Hz, the developers of the audiometer decided to sample certain pure-tone frequencies within the speech range. They selected a series of doubles: 128, 256, 512, and so on to 8192. Frequencies bearing this double relationship to each other represent octaves on the musical scale.

## FREQUENCY RANGE

Later, the numbers were rounded off so that today audiometers are calibrated for frequencies 250, 500, 1000, 2000, 3000, 4000, 6000, and 8000 Hz. This frequency range does not cover the entire gamut of normal hearing; it covers only the speech range. The young human ear is sensitive to sound waves from frequencies as low as 16 Hz to as high as 20,000 Hz. Its most sensitive area is in the range between 1000 and 3000 Hz because of ear canal resonance, as discussed in Chapter 2. In this so-called middle-frequency range, it takes less sound energy to reach the threshold of hearing than it does for tones > 3000 and < 1000 Hz. **Figure 5.3** shows that the ear is more sensitive at the middle frequencies than at the higher and lower frequencies, and so, it is necessary to make higher and lower tones louder to permit the normal ear to hear them.

Because the audiogram has a 0-dB reference level for normal hearing, which is depicted as a straight line across the audiogram, it was necessary to introduce a *correction factor* to the lower and the higher frequencies to adjust the reference level to a straight, rather than a curved, line. The straight-line reference level makes it easier to read and to interpret an audiogram.

Above the range of normal human hearing is the ultrasonic domain. Dogs and bats can hear those high frequencies that are inaudible to the human ear. Bats have such sensitive ears that they use these frequencies to guide their flight in a manner that parallels closely the principle of the modern sonar system. Because the human ear is not sensitive to these frequencies, it does not suffer damage from ultrasonics, even at reasonably high intensities.

## REFERENCE HEARING THRESHOLD LEVELS

The American Standards Association (ASA) 1951 reference level of 0 dB was derived from studying "normal" individuals in a national hearing survey. A large number of hearing tests were performed on young people with presumably normal hearing to find the intensity that could be considered normal at each frequency. Because this was an average value, some subjects had better-than-average normal hearing, causing some otologists to complain that it was awkward to express the results of a hearing test on a person with above-normal hearing in minus figures (e.g., as −5 dB). It also was cumbersome to have to speak in terms of "hearing loss" rather than "residual hearing." Because the reference hearing level used in some European countries was lower, or better, than that of the ASA, the International Standards Organization (ISO), of which the American National Standards Institute (ANSI) is the United States' member body, changed the standard to conform to the European standard. The ISO updates its standards periodically (1), and audiometers must be calibrated to specific standards (2).

**Table 5.1** shows the difference in decibel readings between the ASA and ISO/ANSI standards.

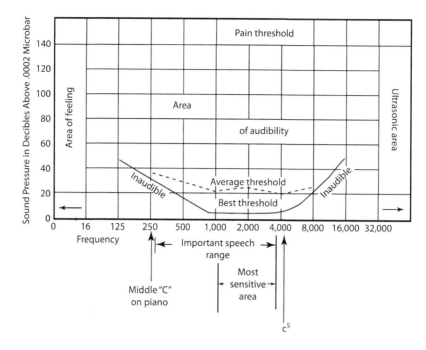

Figure 5.3 Graph showing area of audibility and sensitivity of the human ear, known as the minimum audibility curve. The best threshold (solid line) separates the audible from the inaudible sounds. This level generally is the reference level for sound-level meters. The average threshold of hearing (dashed line) lies considerably above the best threshold and is the reference level used in audiometers. The ear is most sensitive between 1000 and 3000 Hz. The sound pressures are measured in the ear under the receiver of an audiometer. (Modified from Davis and Silverman [3].)

## THE NEED FOR EXAMINERS WITH SPECIALIZED TRAINING

Presently the most reliable and accepted way to test hearing is to use a standard pure-tone audiometer. The ability to use this instrument satisfactorily requires specialized training because the testing requires the voluntary cooperation of the subject.

One of the most important functions of every training program is to teach the tester how to make the responses of the subject a reliable indication of whether or not he/she is hearing the test tone. This can be accomplished best by following these principles: (a) The method of testing should be explained to the listener in a simple and positive manner, and a practical demonstration should be given if the person ever had a hearing test before. (b) The method of response should be as simple as possible—for example, raising a finger or a hand, or pressing a button is simpler than writing down an answer. (c) The subject should be conditioned to give a positive response and encouraged to give

Table 5.1 A Comparison of ASA-1951 and ISO-1963/ANSI-1969 Reference Hearing Threshold Levels

| Frequency (Hz) | Reference threshold level (dB) | | |
|---|---|---|---|
| | ASA-1951[a] | ISO/ANSI[b] | Difference |
| 125 | 54.5 | 45.5 | 9.0 |
| 250 | 39.5 | 24.5 | 15.0 |
| 500 | 25.0 | 11.0 | 14.0 |
| 1000 | 16.5 | 6.5 | 10.0 |
| 1500 | (16.5) | 6.5 | 10.0 |
| 2000 | 17.0 | 8.5 | 8.5 |
| 3000 | (16.0) | 7.5 | 8.5 |
| 4000 | 15.0 | 9.0 | 6.0 |
| 6000 | (17.5) | 8.0 | 9.5 |
| 8000 | 21.0 | 9.5 | 11.5 |

Abbreviations: ANSI, American National Standards Institute; ASA, American Standards Association; ISO, International Standards Organization.
[a] The figures in parentheses are interpolations.
[b] It is common practice to add 10 dB at 500, 1000, and 2000 Hz when converting hearing thresholds from ASA to ANSI. ISO/ANSI values are from W.E. 705A earphone data.

reliable answers quickly and concisely. (d) The subject should be given just enough time to respond after the presentation of each sound signal.

One of the responsibilities of a trained tester is *to be certain* that the responses obtained are reliable and are an accurate indication of the subject's hearing. Frequently, the experienced tester develops an intuitive feeling as to the reliability of the test and can change the technique when there is any question about the cooperation of the subject. For example, if a tester notes that the subject seems to be indecisive and does not give precise answers, he/she may ask the subject to raise his/her entire hand or to say "yes" instead of using the finger response.

## ANSWERS TO QUESTIONS

Why is special training necessary to perform hearing tests? Why cannot one become proficient just by following the directions supplied with the audiometer or be trained by the salesman who sells the audiometer? The answers already were suggested in part when it was emphasized that audiometry is a subjective test and that subjects are not always anxious or able to give reliable responses. Accurate audiometry requires a very carefully trained tester to determine when these instances occur.

Experience has shown that though they have performed several hundreds or even thousands of audiograms and consider themselves to be authorities on audiometry, testers without adequate audiometric training do in fact make serious mistakes of which they are unaware and thus produce hearing tests that are neither reliable nor valid. This kind of circumstance has been verified in every phase of audiometry in otologic practice, industry, and school systems. It was demonstrated dramatically in a report by a subcommittee of the ASA in which only a few hundred audiograms were found to be reliable out of several thousand performed in industry by presumably trained people.

To perform satisfactory audiometry, a tester must be trained thoroughly to understand the importance of his/her responsibility and to take pride and interest in his/her work. Without this training, unsatisfactory test results may be obtained that may prove to be more a liability than an asset. Such training in hearing testing is available in numerous institutions throughout the country, or it can be supplied by well-trained audiologists and otologists.

## WHO SHOULD PERFORM AUDIOMETRY?

Ideally, the physician should do his/her own audiometry because in this way he/she can make a good appraisal of the hearing level of his/her patient. Unfortunately, this is not usually possible because of the time factor in the busy schedule of the otologist, general practitioner, pediatrician, industrial physician, or the school physician. Partly as a consequence, the profession of audiology has developed. Audiologists are trained professionals, usually with a master's degree, AuD or PhD, and with certification. They are generally the most fully trained personnel at performing routine and specialized hearing tests. However, it is neither necessary nor practical to use a fully trained audiologist for screening audiometry in every noisy workplace, school, or clinical setting. Nurses, medical assistants, and other personnel available in industry can be trained to perform excellent audiometry. The training may take several days or weeks, depending on individual aptitude and the manner in which the program is organized. The principal purposes of the training program are to teach the tester to utilize the best available technique, to be completely aware of the potential pitfalls in hearing testing, to understand the limitations of his/her training and the situations in which testing should be referred to a certified audiologist, and to understand the serious consequences of an incorrect report. The responsibility of the tester, unless he/she is a physician, is not to interpret results but, rather, to produce valid, reliable test results. People trained to do hearing tests must also have a firm basic understanding of the hearing mechanism.

## TRAINING OF AUDIOMETRIC TECHNICIANS

Audiometric technicians are used commonly in industry and in some physicians' offices. No certifying agency has been accepted universally, although there are now two recognized organizations supervising technician training (one for offices practice and one for industry), as discussed below. So, many such technicians have no certification credential as audiometric technicians or occupational hearing conservationists. Consequently, the content and quality of training programs for technicians are not consistently good. While this problem is being addressed, a few principles should be kept in mind. Any training course should consider the following objectives:

1. Introduction to basic anatomy and physiology of the ear.
2. Introduction to basic physics of sound and hearing.
3. Understanding of the types of hearing loss, audiometric patterns, and variations.
4. Basic understanding of audiometric techniques and the ability to perform basic audiometry, for example, pure-tone air and bone conduction and speech audiometry, and tympanometry.
5. Awareness of other audiometric techniques, such as evoked response, electro-cochleography (ECoG), and central testing.
6. Basic examination of the external ear, including evaluation for impacted cerumen, and the use of tuning forks.
7. Basic introduction to causes of hearing loss and audiometric patterns.
8. Recognition of the limits of knowledge and understanding the need for supervision by a physician or audiologist. Understanding of the need for diagnosis by a physician.

The following course outline details the kind of information the authors feel would be necessary and useful for fully trained audiometric technicians. A few of the subjects listed are omitted routinely in training programs specifically designed for hearing conservationists whose practice is limited to the industrial setting.

Programs such as the one outlined here should include ample "hands-on training" under supervision. This kind of training program is useful for audiometric technicians who will be working in a physician's office, preferably under the supervision of an otologist and audiologist. It is especially important that such technicians understand the great difference between their training and that of a certified audiologist. Technicians should have specific guidelines regarding appropriate patients to test, those who require a referral, and exactly which patients they are qualified to test with masking. The American Academy of Otolaryngology—Head and Neck Surgery has established a certificate program

recently (but not a certification program). It is excellent and includes the important features listed above.

1. Basic Science of the Ear
   a. Anatomy
   b. Physiology
   c. Examination
   d. Hearing loss
      i. Types
      ii. Causes

2. Basic Physics of Sound
   a. Sound waves
   b. Measurement of sound
   c. The decibel
   d. Frequency and pitch
   e. Intensity and loudness
   f. Complex sounds and speech

   *Laboratory*

   a. Study of ear models
   b. Physics of sound
   c. Physical examination of ear
   d. View relevant video or films

   *Audiometry*

   Equipment

   a. Development and history
   b. Types of audiometers
      i. Manual
      ii. Self-recording
      iii. Computerized
   c. Terminology
   d. Reference hearing thresholds
   e. Audiometer performance check
   f. Calibration
   g. Record keeping
   h. Testing environment
   i. Ambient noise levels

3. The Audiogram
   a. Definition and terms
   b. Reference hearing levels
   c. Calibration
   d. Graphic representation and symbols
   e. Numerical representation
   f. Audiometric forms

4. Audiometric Technique
   a. Basic concepts
   b. Subject instructions

c. Demonstration of test procedures
d. Routine audiometry
e. Special situations
f. Screening audiometry
g. Errors of audiometry
h. Pure-tone air conduction
i. Pure-tone bone conduction
j. Basic concepts of masking
k. Speech reception threshold
l. Speech discrimination

5. Impedance Technique
   a. Impedance audiometry
   b. Tympanometry
   c. Compliance
   d. Acoustic reflex
   e. Demonstration of test procedure

*Laboratory*

Practicum

a. Pure-tone air and bone
b. Speech reception threshold
c. Speech discrimination
d. Impedance and tympanometry
e. Acoustic reflex
f. Equipment check

*Audiometric Interpretation*

Interpretation

a. Sensorineural hearing loss
b. Conductive hearing loss
c. Mixed hearing loss
d. Differential diagnosis
e. Functional vs. malingering
f. Inability to diagnose from audiogram alone
g. Technician's responsibilities and limitations
h. Need for physician's diagnosis

*Special Hearing Tests*

a. Recruitment
b. Short-Increment Sensitivity Index (SISI)
c. Békésy
d. Alternate binaural loudness balance
e. Tone decay testing
f. Central auditory testing
g. Pseudo-hypoacusis tests ("functional" hearing loss)
h. ECoG

i. Evoked response audiometry
j. Acoustic emissions

*Hearing Aids and Devices*

Evaluation

a. Candidates
b. Types of aids available
c. Making an earmold
d. Auditory rehabilitation
e. Auditory devices
f. Cochlear and hearing aid implantation
g. Hearing protectors

*Other Considerations*

Diagnostic Problems

a. Tinnitus
b. Vertigo
c. Conductive hearing loss
d. Sensorineural hearing loss
e. Anatomical problems
   i. Ventilation tubes
   ii. Collapsing canals
   iii. Draining ears
   iv. Others
f. Uncooperative patient

6. Hearing Conservation Programs
   a. Federal regulations
   b. State and local regulations
   c. Worker's compensation
   d. Impairment versus disability
   e. Reporting and record keeping

7. Limitations of Training
   a. Masking
   b. Problem patients
   c. Unusual patterns of audiograms
   d. Referrals necessary
   e. Interpretation of results
   f. Hearing aids
   g. Special tests

Training for occupational hearing conservationists whose duties are limited to the industrial setting can be slightly different. Industrial audiometric technicians and hearing conservationists must acquire considerable knowledge in order to generate reliable, valid results and participate in an effective hearing conservation program. The required information can usually be obtained during a 2- or 3-day course, supplemented with reading materials. The most widely accepted certification is a 20-hour course that leads to designation as certified Occupational Hearing Conservationist (COHC) by the Council for Accreditation in Occupational Hearing Conservation (CAOHC). If CAOHC training is not available, a similar curriculum should be utilized.

At present, as a minimum we recommend the following training curriculum for hearing conservationists:

| Training program for occupational hearing conservationists | |
|---|---|
| **Day 1** | |
| 8:00 | Introduction: Hearing Conservation in Noise |
| 9:00 | Physics of Hearing |
| 9:15 | The Audiometer and Audiometry—OSHA Requirements |
| 10:30 | Supervised Audiometric Testing |
| 12:15 | Review of Technique and Pitfalls |
| 12:45 | Supervised Audiometric Testing |
| 1:45 | Record Keeping and OSHA Requirements |
| 3:00 | Physics of Sound/Noise Analysis |
| 4:00 | Review—Questions and Answers |
| **Day 2** | |
| 8:00 | Physiology and Pathology of the Ear |
| 9:00 | The Audiometer/Calibration of OSHA Requirements |
| 10:15 | Audiogram Review |
| 10:45 | Supervised Audiometric Testing |
| 12:30 | Hearing Protection and OSHA Requirements |
| 1:30 | Use of Tuning Fork and Otoscope, Fitting of Hearing Protection |
| 2:15 | Federal and State Noise Regulations Worker's Compensation |
| 3:15 | Review—Questions and Answers |
| **Day 3** | |
| 8:00 | Self-Recorders, Microprocessors |
| 9:00 | Noise Analysis Continued |
| 9:45 | Written Examination |
| 11:00 | Review of Written Examination |
| 11:30 | Summary of Hearing Conservation Program Adjourn |

*Abbreviations:* OSHA, Occupational Safety and Health Act.

## METHODS OF TESTING HEARING

There are several methods of using pure tones to test hearing. The best technique and the one that we recommend for all physicians is the procedure for performing an individual audiogram described in Chapter 6. Some other methods also are useful, as discussed subsequently.

## SCREENING METHOD

If a large number of people, such as in the armed forces and school systems, have to be tested in a short time and routine threshold audiometry would be too time-consuming and impractical, it may be necessary to use a screening method. In a screening test, the intensity of each frequency is set at a specific level, for example, 20 dB, and the individual is asked whether he/she hears each tone—yes or no. If the tones are heard, the test is passed; if not, the person may be scheduled for threshold testing. Such screening audiometry, using above-threshold levels, does not meet the proper requirements of medical practice or industrial medicine, nor do testing environments with excessive ambient noise that may alter test results.

## GROUP PURE-TONE TESTING

Another method of testing hearing is group pure-tone testing, in which many subjects are given the same tones at the same time through multiple earphones; then the subjects are asked to fill out certain coded forms establishing whether or not they hear the levels tested. Although this method may have some usefulness in the military and in certain school systems, it is recommended that all personnel tested in this manner be rechecked by threshold audiometry when the opportunity arises.

## SELF-RECORDING AUDIOMETRY

Self-recording audiometry with either individual pure tones or continuously changing tones is a modification of the standard manual technique. Self-recording audiometers are being used in increasing numbers, and often a hearing tester is not required to be in constant attendance. The sounds are presented to the subject in a standardized manner using computerized controls, and the subject records a written record of his/her auditory acuity by recording their perception of the presence or absence of the tone. In industries where compensation is an issue, the tester should be in attendance during most of the test to be certain the responses are accurate.

## HOW TO SELECT THE TEST ENVIRONMENT

## CRITERIA

Because it is difficult to hear very soft sounds in a noisy room and audiometers are calibrated on subjects tested in a quiet room, all testing of hearing should be done in a quiet room. If there is excessive ambient noise in the test room when hearing tests are done, the subject invariably has difficulty hearing the weaker threshold tones and gives invalid responses. Prefabricated "soundproof" rooms are

desirable but expensive and generally are not purchased by general practitioners or even by all otologists. Some schools and industries have purchased such rooms, but often efforts are made to find a satisfactory test room without spending a great deal of money.

When selecting the location for testing hearing, the physician should bear in mind that the room should be close to his/her regular examining office. The test room should be as far as possible from ringing telephones, elevators, air-conditioning systems, air ducts, water pipes, drainpipes, and other sources of disturbing and extraneous noise. The ceiling should not transmit the noise of people walking on the floor above. The room should have as few windows as possible and only one door. In spite of these apparent limitations, a satisfactory test room can be found in almost every physician's office. If a physician does a great amount of hearing testing and is interested in optimal results, he/she should purchase a prefabricated hearing test booth.

## TESTS FOR AMBIENT NOISE

### Sound-level meter

Several methods can be used to determine whether or not a room is satisfactory for testing hearing. One of the best methods is to use a sound-level meter/octave band analyzer. The physician can obtain the services of a local engineer, particularly if there are large industries in the area, to do the measurements for him/her. Most major industries have properly trained personnel and equipment and are glad to cooperate with physicians. If the sound study shows that the ambient noise falls at or below the levels in **Table 5.2**, the room can be considered satisfactory for the test frequencies listed and for using earphones to test hearing.

Table 5.2 Maximum allowable sound pressure levels—ANSI S3.1, 1977 and 1991

| Test tone frequency (Hz) | 500 | 1000 | 2000 | 3000 | 4000 | 6000 | 8000 |
|---|---|---|---|---|---|---|---|
| Octave band level | 21.5 | 29.5 | 34.5 | 39.0 | 42.0 | 41.0 | 45.0 |
| One-third octave band level | 16.5 | 24.5 | 29.5 | 34.5 | 37.0 | 36.0 | 40.0 |

The readings on the sound-level meter should be taken several times during the day, especially when the outside environment is noisiest. In this way, the physician can determine what is probably the best time to do hearing tests.

## A comparison of hearing tests

If a sound-level meter is not available, another good method can be used. In a very quiet test room, perhaps available at a local institution or university, the examiner should use his/her audiometer to test several subjects who have already been found to possess normal hearing ability. These same subjects should then be retested by the examiner in the room that he/she wants to use for hearing tests. If it can be determined that the hearing of these individuals is similar in both rooms, it may be assumed that the physician's room is suitable for obtaining satisfactory audiograms.

## REDUCING AMBIENT NOISE

If there is a significant difference between the thresholds of the tests performed in the room in question and those in the very quiet room, and if other variables have been ruled out, the ambient noise level of the test room is probably *too high*. Some measures have to be taken to reduce it. Most of the time, the interference occurs in the low frequencies at 250 and 500 Hz. When comparing the thresholds, the physician should keep in mind that a 5-dB difference is within expected variation in audiograms and is not caused necessarily by the masking effect of the ambient noise. However, if it is > 5 dB, something will have to be done to quiet the room before it can be used. The following steps can be taken. Make sure there is a tight-fitting, solid door or, better yet, a double door at the entrance to the room. Put a soft rug on the floor and perhaps acoustic tile on the ceiling and walls. Hang drapes on the windows. Signs reading "Quiet, please" also should be posted.

## FURNITURE AND REGULATIONS

The test room should be furnished as simply as possible with a table, a chair, and lighting fixtures that do not produce a loud hum. If air-conditioning units, electric fans, or telephones are in the room, shutoff switches should be easily accessible so that they may be silenced during the testing period.

## THE AUDIOMETRIC BOOTH

All audiometric testing in industry should be done in an audiometric booth that meets standards specified in the OSHA Hearing Conservation Amendment. (These levels are less restrictive than those shown in **Table 5.2**.)

There are several good commercially manufactured booths available. Major differences between them include the placement of the doors, viewports, ventilation systems, and, of course, sound reduction capabilities.

They should be noiseproof enough to bring the ambient noise down to acceptable testing levels in accordance with OSHA specifications.

Windows and earphone jack plugs are situated so that the instrument can be placed, and the tester can be seated so as to see the patient being tested without the patient being able to see the operation of the audiometer.

The patient should not be required to sit in the closed booth any longer than necessary to minimize claustrophobia. Showing the subject how to open the door from the inside should help to ease apprehension. Instructions should be given to the seated subject with the door wide open. Only when the actual testing is under way should the door be closed.

If it becomes necessary to interrupt the test or leave in the middle of a test to attend to a more urgent matter, open the door, remove the earphones, and invite the subject to leave the booth until you are able to give him/her your attention again.

Although the use of a booth may be unfamiliar, usually the patient will not become nervous unless he/she senses insecurity or hesitancy on the part of the tester. Practice is necessary to ensure confidence of the patient and accuracy of the procedure.

Loud sounds and talking in the immediate area of the booth will disturb the subject. Stop the test during any such disturbance. Sometimes low-flying aircraft or street traffic causes this problem, and the examiner should be familiar with the attenuation qualities of the booth.

## SUMMARY

1. Booths should be used in all industrial audiometric testing.
2. The booth must lessen ambient noise but does not completely deaden the spoken voice or factory rumble.
3. Once inside the booth, the patient's test should proceed as efficiently as possible.
4. Practice and familiarity of the instrument and booth will result in very accurate test results.
5. Noise levels inside the booth should be within ANSI specifications.
6. Periodic checks on booth noise levels should be made, especially if repair work has been done on the booth (leaky seals), or if production noise levels increase near the test area.
7. All locations will prepare a designated area to conduct audiometric tests that must meet prevailing standards. If existing facilities with or without modifications are not available, an approved sound booth must be installed.

## THE KIND OF AUDIOMETER TO PURCHASE

An audiometer is a precision instrument that produces pure tones of known intensity. The instrument is very delicate and must be handled carefully, with particular attention to the earphones. Although standard specifications for approved audiometers are established by ANSI, audiometers differ in many features. These differences help to determine which audiometer is best suited for a particular use. For the general practitioner, the pediatrician, or the director of a school testing program, it is advisable that the audiometer be as simple as possible, as it is likely that only air and perhaps bone conduction tests are to be done. If bone conduction audiometry is to be performed, it is essential that masking of known intensity be available. In industry, bone conduction rarely is done, and only air conduction aspects of the audiometer are of importance. Most commercial audiometers are now of reasonably high quality. Certain features are essential to all audiometers:

1. They should meet ANSI S3.6–2018 (R2023) standards.
2. They should be easy to operate and should have as few complicating and intricate extras as possible.
3. They should be able to test at least the following frequencies: 500, 1000, 2000, 3000, 4000, 6000, and 8000 Hz.
4. Unless the physician intends to use more complicated tests, accessories such as speech testing apparatus, dual channels, and various others should not influence the purchase of the equipment.
5. The tone presenter switch should not click when it is operated.
6. The audiometer should be purchased from a supplier who will guarantee prompt attention in case of malfunction and supply a substitute calibrated audiometer if the instrument has to be removed for repairs. This last feature is of utmost importance; otherwise a physician or facility may be without an audiometer for long periods of time.

## THE MANUAL AUDIOMETER

A manual audiometer has a series of switches and controls to direct its operation (**Figure 5.4**). The on–off switch controls the power on the audiometer. This should be turned on at least 15 minutes before use, especially in older audiometers, and, if possible, it should be left on all day rather than turned on and off as the need dictates. A frequency selector dial designates the tone that is produced in the earphones.

The attenuator determines the intensity of the tone produced. Attenuators usually are calibrated in 5-dB steps from 0 to 110 dB, with the exception of the very low and high frequencies, for which the maximum usually is ~90 dB. Readings should not be made between the 5-dB steps. As the maximum output at 250 and 8000 Hz generally is not >90 dB, one should bear in mind while testing that exceeding 90 dB on the dial does not increase the intensity of the tone produced. The tone presenter switch is used to turn the tone on and off. The tone always should be off, unless the tester wishes to turn it on for testing purposes.

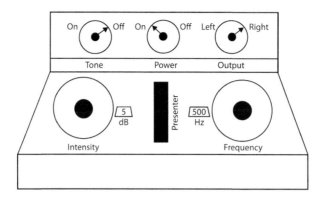

Figure 5.4 Main switches and dials of a typical clinical screening audiometer. Included are the frequency dial, which controls the tonal output, in this case set at 500 Hz; the attenuator, which controls the volume output in decibels, here set at 5 dB; the earphone selector switch; and the tone presenter, which turns the signal on and off. The presenter is left in the "off" position and pressed to the "on" position when the tone is to be presented. Modern sophisticated diagnostic audiometers have many additional switches, functions, and designs, but the basic principles remain unchanged.

Two wires leading from the audiometer are attached to earphones connected by a spring headband. The earphones should be handled with extreme caution because they are very delicate and can easily be thrown out of adjustment. They are part of a mechanism that converts electric current into sound. The earphones are equipped with a rubber cushion that is of considerable importance. It must be of a specified size so that the volume of air it encloses is precisely the same as that provided when the instrument was calibrated (~6 cc). The cushion cannot be replaced by a larger or smaller one for reasons of comfort without disturbing the calibration of the instrument. If a type of cushion is purchased to provide better attenuation, the audiometer then must be calibrated with the cushion in place.

Some audiometers are accompanied by a push-button cord that allows the patient to signal his response by pressing the button. When the subject hears the tone, he/she presses the button, causing a light to appear on the instrument panelboard. This is one way of getting a response from the subject. Many experienced testers prefer to have the patient raise a finger or a hand.

## THE MICROPROCESSOR AUDIOMETER

The millions of audiograms being performed in industry because of OSHA and worker's compensation stimulated development to make audiometry more reliable and data handling more efficient. Noteworthy is the microprocessor audiometer, which was useful especially for larger plants and corporations.

The instrument was extremely helpful for plants performing large numbers of audiograms. It is also an efficient way of obtaining audiometric data and otologic histories and sending them in print or on a disk to a consultant otologist for diagnosis.

The audiogram can be performed manually, semiautomatically, or automatically. Information questions can be inserted, deleted, or modified. Automatic calculation of standard or significant threshold shift with or without age correction can be programmed along with any other useful information. Calibration is performed readily and documented. Automatic validity tests are generally standard in each testing sequence. In the best instruments, the computer can be used for other purposes when it is not used for hearing testing. Additional copies of printed data can be reprinted from stored data. The data can also be transferred to a central computer or an attached microcomputer. **Figure 5.5** shows a sample printout.

The efficiency of data management depends on the software. Many of the most commonly used instruments employ a software program developed by HCNC (Hearing Conservation Noise Control, Inc.) in conjunction with the E. I. DuPont de Nemours & Company, Inc., whose hearing conservation program has been in operation for > 50 years. The HCNC Computerized Audiometric Testing

Program is a combined data storage and evaluation program. This program interfaces with many audiometers and has been modified, updated, and renamed. These programs provide a printed copy of the audiogram for permanent records.

```
      TRACOR INSTRUMENTS
         AUSTIN, TEXAS
   DATE   00 00 00
   TIME      00:00

   SUBJECT:

   X................

   SS#/ID#    000000000
   JOB#    000000000000
   NOISE EXP.    000000
   TEST TYPE    0
   TYPE PROTECTOR    0
   BIRTH DATE 00 00 00
   SEX    F

   CURRENT AUDIOGRAM
   FREQ.    L/DB   R/DB
   1KHZ TEST 50    50
    500HZ     60    50
   1000HZ     50    50
   2000HZ     30    30
   3000HZ     30    30
   4000HZ     50    30
   6000HZ     30    30
   8000HZ     30    30
   AV 234     36    30

   MODE       PULSED

   RA400   SER#.
   VERSION    3.4
   CAL. ANSI 1969 STD

   CAL. DATE   00/00
   EXAMINER ID#
   000000000

   X................

   LOCATION CODE
   000000
```

Figure 5.5 Typical computerized audiogram.

An immediate evaluation of the hearing test for the occurrence of OSHA Standard Threshold Shift (STS) should be performed and documented.

Data storage of employee information, hearing thresholds, and otoscopic/otologic examination histories should be performed and documented.

## CALIBRATION PROCEDURE

If a change in an audiometer's operating characteristics is sudden and extensive, it is obvious that the instrument should be serviced. However, a slow change may not be obvious. If changes in instrument accuracy go undetected, poor measurements may be made over many weeks or months before a calibration check discloses the inaccuracy. Wasted measurements can be prevented by simple daily checks designed to detect changes in an instrument's operating characteristics and potential trouble spots.

The following tests and inspections should be made by the technician at the beginning of each day:

1. All control knobs on the audiometer should be checked to be sure that they are tight on their shafts and not misaligned.
2. Earphone cords should be straightened so that there are no sharp bends or knots. If the cords are worn or cracked, they should be replaced. A recalibration is not necessary when earphone cords are replaced.
3. Earphone cushions should be replaced if they are not resilient or if cracks, bubbles, or crevices develop. A recalibration should not be necessary when earphone cushions are replaced.
4. The audiometer calibration should be checked by measuring the hearing threshold at each test frequency of a person who has normal hearing and whose hearing levels are well known (biological calibration). If a persistent change of > 10 dB occurs from day to day in this person's hearing threshold at any test frequency, and it cannot be explained by temporary threshold shifts caused by colds, noise exposure, or other factors, an instrument recalibration is indicated. A technician who has normal hearing may serve as the test subject. At the beginning and end of each day of testing, these threshold levels should be

recorded serially in ink, with no erasures, if the records are to have legal significance. Any mistakes made in these record entries should be crossed once with ink, initialed, and dated.

5. The linearity of the hearing level control should be checked, with the tone control set on 2000 Hz, by listening to the earphones while slowly increasing the hearing level from threshold. Each 5-dB step should produce a small, but noticeable increase in level without changes in tone quality or audible extraneous noise.

6. Test the earphone cords electrically, with the dials set at 2000 Hz and 60 dB, by listening to the earphones while bending the cords along their length. Any scratching noise, intermittency, or change in test tone indicates a need for new cords.

7. Test the operation of the tone presented, with dials set at 2000 Hz and 60 dB, by listening to the earphones and operating the presenter several times. Neither audible noise, such as clicks or scratches, nor changes in test tone quality should be heard when the tone presenter is used.

8. Check extraneous noises from the case and the earphone not in use, with the hearing level control set at 60 dB and the test earphone jack disconnected from the amplifier. No audible noise should be heard while wearing the earphones when the tone control is switched to each test tone.

9. Check the headband tension by observing the distance between the inner surfaces of the earphone cushions when the headset is held in a free, unmounted condition. At the center of its adjustment range, the distance between cushions should be ~0.5 in. The band may be bent to reach this adjustment.

When a tester observes that audiograms indicate a persistent, unexplainable hearing impairment at either all or specific frequencies, he/she should stop testing patients and test several ears known to be normal, in order to confirm that the instrument is calibrated properly.

After testing for the day has been completed, testers should recheck the instrument on themselves and on several normal ears and then record all results. This final check is necessary because the tester may not be aware that at some time during

the day the audiometer had gone out of adjustment. By establishing the calibration of the audiometer at the end of the day, the tester will know whether there is a need to retest any subjects, and he/she also will have an important confirmation for medicolegal purposes if ever required.

When a tester uses his/her own or other normal ears to verify the calibration of an audiometer, he/she is testing only the calibration at threshold and also is assuming that the attenuator is working properly and producing accurate readings at above-threshold levels. Electronic instruments are necessary to perform above-threshold and other calibration measurements.

When an instrument's accuracy is suspect, the possibility that the tester may not be using the instrument properly should not be overlooked. For this reason, it is always wise to discuss the problem with some person who is very familiar with the operation of the instrument to determine whether a simple solution is available.

## RECORD OF CALIBRATION TESTING

It is important for testers to keep a daily record of their biological calibration testing, indicating the exact time and manner in which the audiometer in use was checked for calibration. Electronic calibration records also should be maintained. This is an important precaution, particularly in medicolegal cases.

## AUDIOMETER REPAIRS

When an audiometer's accuracy is suspect, it should be serviced and calibrated by a qualified laboratory.

It can be difficult to find competent audiometer calibrator services. Even the audiometer distributor may not be competent in repair or calibration procedures. When a calibration service is located, some understanding should be reached about the kind of calibration to be performed. Determine that hearing level accuracy will be checked for each test tone at each 5-dB interval throughout the operating range. For industrial applications, the range should cover hearing levels from 10 to 70 dB with reference to ANSI S.6–2018 (R2023) and at least test tones of 500, 1000, 2000, 3000,

4000, 6000, and 8000 Hz. Calibration specifications include tolerance limits on attenuator linearity, test tone accuracy and purity, tone presenter operation, masking noise, and the effects of power supply variations. It is always good practice to require a written report that includes all measurement data. A simple statement that the audiometer meets ANSI specifications should not be accepted without some evidence that all tests have been made. Electronic-acoustical calibration should be conducted routinely on an annual basis.

Rarely, the instrument must be shipped away for service or calibration. At those times, it may be advisable to have another instrument on hand. Another solution may be to borrow an instrument during the repair period. If a second instrument is used, its calibration must be established carefully, and a note must be made on each audiogram stating the change of instruments.

Accuracy of the instrument should not be taken for granted following a factory adjustment, particularly after shipment. The instrument always should be checked subjectively as described earlier.

## REFERENCES

1. International Organization for Standardization ISO 7029:2017. Acoustics-Statistical Distribution of Hearing Thresholds Related to Age and Gender. Reviewed and confirmed in 2023.
2. Acoustical Society of America. Specification for Audiometers ASA/ANSI s3.62018(R2023). American National Standard, March 23, 2023.
3. Davis H, Silverman SR, eds. Hearing and Deafness, revised edition. New York, NY: Holt, 1960.

# 6

# The audiogram

ROBERT THAYER SATALOFF, DANIELLE L. WALTER, AND PAMELA C. ROEHM

A more detailed discussion of audiometry can be found in this chapter; the basic information needed to interpret an audiogram will be presented here. We will cover the following questions: What do the numbers mean? What is 0 dB, or normal, hearing, and what is a –5 dB hearing level? What is a high-tone or a low-tone loss?

## DEFINITION

An audiogram is a written record of a person's hearing level measured with specific pure tones. The pure tones generally used are the frequencies 250, 500, 1000, 2000, 3000, 4000, 6000, and 8000 Hz; these tones are generated electronically by the audiometer. This frequency range includes the pitches of sound included in our speech.

## TERMS

If 0 dB represents ideal normal hearing, a 60 dB hearing threshold level also can be called a 60-dB "hearing loss." Although both terms describe the same condition, the term "hearing level" is currently more popular in otology because it emphasizes the hearing that the patient still has rather than the hearing that he/she has lost. Also, because a –5-dB level is a gain rather than a loss among

DOI: 10.1201/b23379-6

persons with normal hearing, the "level" avoids the confusion of "negative losses" and contributes to a more positive approach in helping patients with deficient hearing.

However, because the term "hearing loss" still is in common use and this book is concerned with the diagnosis of hearing loss, the words "loss" and "level" will be used interchangeably to indicate the threshold of a person's hearing.

## REFERENCE HEARING LEVEL

The original American Standards Association (ASA 1951) 0-dB reference level was established from data obtained between 1935 and 1936. Newer data obtained some 30 years later indicated that the human ear was ~10 dB more sensitive. This information led to the International Standards Organization (ISO 1964) reference level, which was later adopted by the American National Standards Institute (formerly ASA) now known as ANSI 1989. The actual differences are shown in Chapter 5. Because many otologists may still be using ASA-calibrated audiometers and thousands of old audiograms are based on the old reference level, graphic audiograms throughout this book will show both references—ASA on the left and ANSI on the right. Most hearing levels recorded in numerals and serial form will be on the ANSI reference level.

## HORIZONTAL AND VERTICAL VARIABLES IN A GRAPHIC AUDIOGRAM

Ideally, one should measure a patient's ability to hear speech, but because of several difficulties, pure tones are still used. For simplicity, only specific frequencies were selected for routine use. They are called *octave frequencies* because each successive tone is an octave above the one immediately below it, and the number of cycles per second from one tone to the next is doubled. Octave frequencies constitute the horizontal variable in an audiogram: How well the patient hears at each frequency. Does he/she hear the tone as well as a person with normal hearing, or does it have

to be made louder to be heard and, if so, how much louder? To make this comparison, one must have a normal baseline for each frequency. There are certain shortcomings inherent in any system that relies on sampling of this sort. In order to improve audiologic tests, frequencies between the usual octaves are also often tested, particularly 3000 and 6000 Hz. Frequencies above the usual test range may also be useful, including 10,000, 12,000 Hz, and sometimes higher frequencies. High-frequency testing is particularly useful when assessing noise exposure in a subject.

## WHAT IS NORMAL HEARING?

The threshold at the various frequencies of a person with normal hearing ability originally was obtained by testing a large number of young people between the ages of 20 and 29 and determining the intensities of the thresholds at the various frequencies. It was found that the thresholds fluctuated over an ~25-dB range even in subjects with assumably normal hearing. An average was reached at each frequency tested and defined as 0 dB of hearing. Some subjects heard better than 0; many of them heard tones as weak as −10; others did not hear a sound until it was amplified to a level between 0 and 15 dB. This variation indicated that the range between −10 and +15 dB could be considered normal for the average young person (ASA). The range for the ANSI scale is 0–25 dB. In clinical practice, however, a patient with a 15 dB hearing level in most frequencies may be considered to having a hearing loss.

Average normal hearing, or 0 dB, is the reference level on the audiometer. A hearing loss at some specific frequency is expressed and recorded as the number of decibels by which a tone must be amplified for a patient to hear it.

## WHAT THE AUDIOMETER MEASURES

Commercial audiometers are calibrated and recording methods are standardized in such a way that what is recorded is not a patient's ability to hear but, rather, his/her hearing *loss* in the frequencies tested. If he/she can hear 0 dB, he/she has no hearing loss, but if he/she cannot hear until the tone is 30 dB louder than 0 dB, he/she has a hearing loss of 30 dB. The pure-tone audiometer offers the best means yet devised for routine hearing measurement.

## FORMS OF THE AUDIOGRAM

The audiogram, which shows a patient's hearing threshold for the standard range of frequencies, can be recorded in several ways. The most common is a *graph* on which the frequencies are marked off from left to right, and the tone intensities range up and down. A statement that **O** is for the right ear and **X** for the left should appear at the bottom of each graph. **Figure 6.1** shows such a graph and indicates the conventional marks by which the curve for the left ear can be distinguished from that for the right ear. A series of **X** marks connected by a dashed line denotes the left; circles connected by a solid line represent the right ear. The short arrows found on some audiograms hereafter indicate that there was no response to the test tone at the output limits of the audiometer.

One of the chief disadvantages of using this type of graph in industry and otology is that if 8 or 10 audiograms are done in a year on a certain subject, the record becomes bulky, and it becomes difficult to compare one curve with another performed on a different date.

**Figure 6.2** shows another form of recording these thresholds in which the intensities are recorded numerically and serially instead of being plotted. This form, which is more acceptable and practical, is recommended for industry, schools, and otologic practice. It is called a serial form. The authors routinely use this form in their practice, but because the graph form may be familiar to some readers, it is used often in this book. In a serial audiogram, instead of using a symbol for the right and left ears, the number of decibels designating the threshold is recorded at each frequency. The notation NR on the serial form denotes that there was "no response" to the test tone at the output limits of the audiometer.

The letters WN indicate that "white noise" was used for masking. Furthermore, a place for comments and a brief history is available on this type of serial audiogram.

Serial audiograms make it easier to record all thresholds obtained independently. For example, in the routine retesting of 1000 Hz, both thresholds, even if alike, should be recorded in the space provided. In legal situations, these multiple numbers will confirm that the threshold was rechecked several times. It is necessary to record *every* threshold that is derived independently, even if there is marked variation, for this may have considerable significance. It is important that every serial audiogram include the date and the signature of the tester as well as other information that can be placed under Comments.

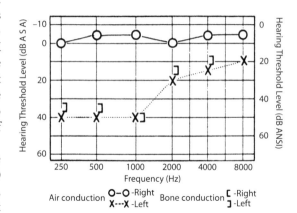

Figure 6.1 Audiometric findings: Right ear thresholds for air and bone conduction pure tones are normal. Left ear has reduced air and bone thresholds of about the same magnitude (no air–bone gap). The right ear was masked during all testing of the left ear. Speech reception threshold: right, 5 dB; left, 45 dB. Discrimination score: right, 98%; left, 62%. Tuning fork lateralizes to right ear. Tuning fork on left shows air is better than bone conduction (A > B), and bone conduction is reduced on the left mastoid. In general, brackets ([ and ]) are used to indicate masked bone conduction. Unmasked right ear is symbolized with an O, unmasked left ear with an **X**. *Abbreviations*: ANSI, American National Standards Institute; ASA, American Standards Association.

JOSEPH SATALOFF, M.D.
ROBERT THAYER SATALOFF, M.D.
1721 PINE STREET    PHILADELPHIA, PA 19103

**HEARING RECORD**

JOSEPH SATALOFF, M.D.
ROBERT THAYER SATALOFF, M.D.
1721 PINE STREET    PHILADELPHIA, PA 19103

NAME _____    AGE _____

### AIR CONDUCTION

| | | | RIGHT | | | | | | | | LEFT | | | | | |
|---|---|---|---|---|---|---|---|---|---|---|---|---|---|---|---|---|
| DATE | Exam | LEFT MASK | 250 | 500 | 1000 | 2000 | 4000 | 8000 | RIGHT MASK | 250 | 500 | 1000 | 2000 | 4000 | 8000 | AUD |
| ANSI | | | 10 | 5 | 5 | 10 | 5 | 5 | | 50 | 50 | 50 | 30 | 25 | 20 | |
| | | | | | | | | | | | | | | | | |
| | | | | | | | | | | | | | | | | |
| | | | | | | | | | | | | | | | | |
| | | | | | | | | | | | | | | | | |
| | | | | | | | | | | | | | | | | |
| | | | | | | | | | | | | | | | | |

### BONE CONDUCTION

| | | | RIGHT | | | | | | | LEFT | | | | | |
|---|---|---|---|---|---|---|---|---|---|---|---|---|---|---|---|
| DATE | Exam | LEFT MASK | 250 | 500 | 1000 | 2000 | 4000 | RIGHT MASK | 250 | 500 | 1000 | 2000 | 4000 | | AUD |
| | | | | | | | | | 45 | 45 | 50 | 25 | 20 | | |
| | | | | | | | | | | | | | | | |
| | | | | | | | | | | | | | | | |
| | | | | | | | | | | | | | | | |

### SPEECH RECEPTION

| DATE | RIGHT | LEFT MASK | LEFT | RIGHT MASK | FREE FIELD | MIC. |
|---|---|---|---|---|---|---|
| ANSI | 15 | | 55 | | | |
| | | | | | | |
| | | | | | | |

### DISCRIMINATION

| | | | RIGHT | | | | LEFT | | |
|---|---|---|---|---|---|---|---|---|---|
| DATE | % SCORE | TEST LEVEL | LIST | LEFT MASK | % SCORE | TEST LEVEL | LIST | RIGHT MASK | EXAM. |
| | 98 | | | | 62 | | | | |
| | | | | | | | | | |
| | | | | | | | | | |

### HIGH FREQUENCY THRESHOLDS

| | RIGHT | | | | | | | LEFT | | | | |
|---|---|---|---|---|---|---|---|---|---|---|---|---|
| DATE | 4000 | 8000 | 10000 | 12000 | 14000 | LEFT MASK | RIGHT MASK | 4000 | 8000 | 10000 | 12000 | 14000 |
| | | | | | | | | | | | | |
| | | | | | | | | | | | | |

| RIGHT | | WEBER | LEFT | | HEARING AID | | |
|---|---|---|---|---|---|---|---|
| RINNE | SCHWABACH | ← | RINNE | SCHWABACH | DATE | MAKE | MODEL |
| | | | A > B | RED. | RECEIVER | GAIN | EXAM |
| | | | | | EAR | DISCRIM. | COUNC |

REMARKS

Figure 6.2 Serial form used in clinical practice.

## INTERPRETING THE TYPICAL AUDIOGRAM

Now let us look at a typical audiogram and interpret it.

In **Figure 6.1**, the left ear (**X**s connected with dashed lines) shows a level of ~40 dB (ASA) up to 1000 Hz; then the curve approaches more normal hearing (the 0 line on the graph). We would say, then, that this patient hears high tones better than low tones. This is an ascending curve, and the patient is said to have a low-tone or low-frequency hearing loss. Hearing in the right ear is normal.

## SOME BASIC CONCEPTS

The reader is referred to Chapter 7 for information on special studies, including bone conduction, adaptation, recruitment, and speech discrimination. However, because these concepts are discussed in the earlier chapters on classification of hearing loss, it is necessary to define them briefly here.

## AIR CONDUCTION

This denotes the ability of the ear to receive and conduct sound waves entering the external ear canal. Normally, these waves cause the eardrum to vibrate, and the vibrations are transmitted through the chain of ossicles to the oval window. When air conduction is impaired as a result of damage to the outer or middle ear and the sensorineural mechanism of the inner ear is intact, the maximum difference between air and bone conduction thresholds is ~60–70 dB. This is so because when the sound is > 60–70 dB, it will be conducted by the bones of the skull directly to the cochlea.

## BONE CONDUCTION

To some extent, this is a measure of the patient's ability to hear sound vibrations that are transmitted directly to the cochlea through the bones of the skull, bypassing the outer and the middle ear. Bone conduction is unimpaired in simple conductive hearing loss. Thus, conductive hearing loss can be distinguished from sensorineural hearing loss by tuning forks or bone conduction audiometry.

Tuning fork tests, reviewed in Chapter 5, always should be performed to confirm the audiometric findings. When inconsistencies occur, the tuning-fork test often turns out to be correct.

Although sounds up to ~50 dB directed to one ear by air conduction through an earphone usually are heard by the ear alone, this is not the case with bone conduction. Bone conducted sounds are heard almost equally well by both ears no matter where the vibrations are impressed upon the skull. This holds true of both the tuning fork and the audiometer vibrator. The proper way to minimize confusion is to mask the opposite ear by introducing enough neutral sound into it to occupy its auditory pathway and prevent the test from reaching it.

A common method of recording bone conduction by a graph type of audiogram is shown in **Figure 6.1**. The open cusps, or brackets, are used to symbolize the ear as it faces the examiner. A caricature of a face showing that "]" is the left ear and "[" the right should clarify this concept (**Figure 6.3**). Bone conduction also can be recorded numerically, as in the serial type of audiogram (**Figure 6.2**).

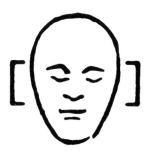

Figure 6.3 Brackets are used in graphic audiograms to indicate left and right ears. The correct side may be remembered if they are thought of as earmuffs.

When the bone conduction and the air conduction curves or levels are of the same magnitude, there is *no air–bone gap*. But if the bone conduction level is better (i.e., shows less hearing loss and is closer to the normal hearing level), an *air–bone gap* is said to exist.

## SPEECH RECEPTION THRESHOLD

This is a measure of a person's ability to hear speech, not pure tones, using a speech audiometer that controls the intensity of the speech output. One can test the speech reception threshold (SRT) by means of simple two-syllable words or sentences to determine the weakest intensity at which the subject can hear well enough to repeat the spoken words or the sentences. A person who hears normally can hear and repeat these words at a level of 0–15 dB. For hard-of-hearing individuals, the SRT is higher (i.e., the speech must be louder to enable them to repeat it). The higher the number of decibels, the greater the hearing loss.

## DISCRIMINATION SCORE

This does not measure the weakest intensity at which the patient hears speech sounds but, rather, how well he/she can correctly repeat certain representative words delivered to the ear at ~30 or 40 dB above the individual's SRT. The person with normal hearing discriminates between 90% and 100% of the words. Patients with sensorineural losses may have moderate and sometimes severe discrimination losses, although they also may be normal.

## RECRUITMENT

To a patient with recruitment, compared with someone without it, a tone that sounds soft becomes loud more suddenly and rapidly when its intensity is increased. This abnormally great and abrupt increase in the sensation of loudness, especially marked in patients with sensory hearing loss, generally is absent in patients with conductive hearing loss.

## ABNORMAL TONE DECAY OR PATHOLOGICAL ADAPTATION

This finding occurs predominantly in neural hearing loss. A patient who exhibits abnormal tone decay is unable to continue hearing a tone at threshold when it is prolonged at a uniform level of intensity; his/her hearing fatigues rapidly. The phenomenon is called pathological fatigue or abnormal tone decay.

Someone who has normal hearing continues to hear a very weak threshold tone for several minutes, but an individual with abnormal tone decay may hear the sound only for several seconds. Then, the sound is made louder. When this is done, the patient will hear the sound again for a few seconds, only to lose it again quickly and request that the volume be increased and so on.

## HOW TO PERFORM A ROUTINE AUDIOGRAM

It has been demonstrated repeatedly that though hearing testers without adequate training may have performed many hundreds of audiograms and may consider themselves to be experts, many of them are making mistakes of which they are unaware, and they are producing test results that often are inaccurate.

Although audiometric testing may appear to be disarmingly simple, by no means is it easy to obtain accurate thresholds consistently. Because reliable and valid audiograms are of such great diagnostic importance, such valuable guides to therapy, and so decisive in medicolegal cases, it is essential that they be performed well. This chapter provides an outline of basic technique, with emphasis on the essential features of good audiometry. This presentation is followed by a discussion of the more common pitfalls that beset routine audiometry.

## PREPARING THE SUBJECT

Before starting the audiogram, the tester should consider the following preliminary steps:

1. Seating the subject.
2. Instructing the subject.
3. Placing the earphones on the subject.

## SEATING THE SUBJECT

If the tester and the subject are in the same room, the subject should be seated in a comfortable, squeakless chair so that his/her hands can rest on the arms of the chair or on the far end of the tester's table. The subject's profile should be turned toward the tester because the tester must be able to observe the subject's hands, face, and head, but the subject must not be able to observe the tester's hands and arms or the control panel of the audiometer.

Having the subject close his/her eyes while listening may help the patient to concentrate more on threshold sounds and prevents him/her from receiving visual clues from the examiner's movements.

Although some technicians advocate seating the subject with his/her back to the tester, the authors feel this is unsatisfactory, even if the push button is used to register the response. This arrangement hinders the tester from numerous indications that help establish an opinion as to the validity of the thresholds and the cooperation of the subject including the subject's possible malingering.

## INSTRUCTING THE SUBJECT

Proper, concise instructions directed to the subject are critical for obtaining reliable responses. A successful method of instruction is as follows:

Have you had your hearing checked before?

Yes.

That's fine—let me remind you of what we're going to do. You will be listening for some tones. Each time you hear a tone, raise your finger. [*Demonstrate how you want this done.*] When the tone goes away, lower your finger. [*Demonstrate how you want this done.*] No matter how faint the tone, raise your finger when you hear it. [*Demonstrate how you want this done.*] And lower it when the tone goes away. [*Demonstrate how you want this done.*] Do you hear better in one ear than the other?

No.

Then we will check your right ear first. [*If there is a difference in hearing, check the better ear first in case of the need to introduce masking to eliminate the cross-over effect.*]

## PLACING THE EARPHONES ON THE SUBJECT

It is very important to place the receivers snugly on the subject's ears so that no leakage exists between them and the sides of the head. The headband should be adjusted to the subject's head size so that the phones are comfortable. The tester should ask the subject to remove earrings and push away hair covering the ears. Items such as glasses, hearing aids, and earrings also should be removed because they can prevent the receiver from fitting snugly or can block out the test tones. The phone should not bend the ear over; the center of the phone should be directly aligned with the opening of the ear canal.

Insert earphones are another popular option as they yield low test–retest variability for high frequencies without the need to remove glasses or earrings. This is particularly beneficial when monitoring noise-induced threshold changes because noise exposure changes often occur in high frequencies. When placing inserts, the tester should place the foam insert plug deeply into the subject's ear canal to avoid the leakage of sound.

Audiometric testing performed in non-sound-treated rooms should take into special consideration background noise. To overcome ambient noise, the tester should use insert earphones to provide low-frequency attenuation of ambient noise which may mask the test tone.

The tester should make sure that the cord leading from the earphones is not draped over the front of the subject; otherwise, the subject's movements could rub the cord and introduce distracting noises into the earphones.

When the tester places the earphones on the subject, the red phone or insert must be placed on the right ear and the blue phone or insert must be placed on the left ear.

The earphones should not be placed on the subject until directions have been given and the tester is ready to proceed with the production of the audiogram. Also, it is preferable to remove eyeglasses and hearing aids after the instructions have been given. When the earphones are in place, the tester should start the test immediately. The tester should not make the subject wait while you fill in the date, signature, serial number, and other information.

## THE AUDIOGRAM

The tester should determine the subject's threshold at the specific frequencies in the following order: 1000, 2000, 3000, 4000, 6000, 8000, 1000 (repeat), 500, and 250 Hz. The 1000-Hz tone is tested first because usually this is the easiest one for which to establish a definitive threshold. The threshold at 1000 Hz is confirmed by repeating it, to help confirm test accuracy, and because the subject who has not previously had an audiogram may not have recognized the tone as such the first time. Both readings are recorded on the form. Tests at higher frequencies such as 10,000, 12,000, and 14,000 Hz may also be performed. Findings at these frequencies may be helpful in differentiating occupational hearing loss from presbycusis and in early damage detection from ototoxic drugs.

With the earphone selector switch properly set and the frequency dial at 1000 Hz, turn on the tone with the tone presenter beginning at 30 dB HL. If the subject does not respond, it will be necessary for the tester to increase the dial in 20-dB increments until the subject responds. Stop the tone, allowing the subject to lower his/her finger. Present the tone once again at this response level to confirm the initial response. If the patient responds, turn off the tone and *decrease* the intensity by 10 dB. Present the tone. There should be no response to this 10-dB reduction in intensity. If there is no response, turn the tone off, *increase* intensity 5 dB, and then present the tone. If there is a response to this 5-dB increase, turn off the tone and decrease by 5 dB. Present the tone. If no response occurs, turn the tone off, *increase* by 5 dB, and present to tone. If there is a response, this is the threshold; record the number of the last response. The objective is to get at least two ascending "yes" responses.

Most young subjects will have extremely good hearing and will respond to the tone while the hearing level dial is still at 0 dB. It is good practice to obtain at least two or three "yes" responses to ascertain the threshold. Do not neglect to get a confirmation of the initial response, which was obtained during the rollup of the volume control dial.

If there is no confirmation of the initial response, turn on the tone again and continue to roll the volume control dial up in 20-dB increments until there is a response and a confirmation. Then, make the 10-dB reduction and proceed from that point. A "yes" response requires the tone to be made softer until the subject stops responding.

All tones presented to the subject should be brief bursts of sound and should be held for no longer than 1 or 2 seconds.

When the threshold for 1000 Hz has been determined and recorded, the threshold for each succeeding frequency is determined in the same manner. After rechecking 1000 Hz, test 500 Hz and then 250 Hz. For good test–retest reliability at 1000 Hz, the threshold should not deviate more than (plus or minus) 10 dB when rechecked. However, a (plus or minus) 10-dB difference indicates to the technician that the first threshold may be invalid, and the same may be true for the other thresholds. When this difference is noted, several of the succeeding frequencies should be rechecked until reliability is obtained. Then, recheck and record the 1000-Hz threshold before testing 500 Hz.

When the tester has completed the recording of thresholds for one ear, the earphone selector is then switched to the opposite ear, and the identical procedure is repeated, except that it is not necessary to retest 1000 Hz on the second ear. Recheck the thresholds for those frequencies indicating a loss >25 dB. The tester always should record all independently obtained thresholds on the audiogram.

## ORDER OF TESTING

*First ear*: 1000, 2000, 3000, 4000, 6000, 8000, 1000, 500, and 250 Hz.

*Second ear*: 1000, 2000, 3000, 4000, 6000, 8000, 500, and 250 Hz. Interoctave intervals such as 750 and 1500 Hz should be tested when there is a 20-dB threshold difference in adjacent octaves.

## RECORDING AUDIOGRAMS

The relative merits of *graph* and *serial* audiograms were discussed earlier. For industrial applications, we strongly recommend the use of serial audiograms.

## SECURING OBJECTIVITY

Because of the possibility that the tester, in an attempt to complete the test quickly, may be influenced by a previously obtained threshold, it is advisable to avoid looking at the preceding audiogram on the serial chart. For this reason, it is helpful to have an assistant record while the tester calls off the threshold obtained at each frequency. If a tester cannot find a satisfactory assistant for this purpose, he/she should place a card over every previously obtained audiogram so that he/she is not influenced in any way. A special mask that allows only the blank spaces on the audiogram to be seen can also be prepared. This type of self-restriction will assure the tester that he/she is performing as objective a test as possible.

## PRESERVING RECORDS

Original audiograms should not be destroyed, even if they are transcribed from one form to another. They are important written records of a subject's hearing. Thresholds should not be erased when a repeat check finds the original threshold to differ from the most recent one. Instead, all thresholds should be recorded. The difference may be significant, and this may have an important bearing on the interpretation of any hearing loss.

## AVOIDING ERRORS IN AUDIOMETRY (PITFALLS)

In the performance of audiometry, it is important to avoid certain errors and pitfalls encountered by testers who are not adequately acquainted with the limitations of this testing procedure.

1. When depressing the tone presenter switch, the tone should not be presented for > 1–3 seconds. The tones should be *short bursts* rather than prolonged. Each tone should be presented for about the same length of time, except in situations where the tester may want to check the subject's response to the cessation as well as the onset of the tone.
2. Every audiogram should be done as *rapidly as possible* without sacrificing the reliability and the validity of the threshold testing. Taking too long to do an audiogram will fatigue the subject and result in inaccurate responses.
3. However, rushing through the test is as bad as wasting time. The tester should appreciate that some subjects take longer to respond than others. It is essential that the tester *allows sufficient time for the response*. Faster and more definitive responses often can be obtained from the subject if he/she is given concise and explicit directions prior to testing.
4. The tester should *always be certain that the subject is not directly or indirectly watching* the control panel of the audiometer and/or the tester.
5. Some testers tend to present the signal and then look up at the subject as if to ask if he/she has heard the tone; others may move a hand away from the audiometer after a dial change. Both actions constitute visual, rather than aural, clues and can elicit false-positive responses. *It is poor audiometric testing technique to signal your move.*

6. Another possible error is to place the wrong phone on the ear. Repeated checks should be made to see that the *phones are placed on the proper ear*, that they correspond with the switch on the control panel, and that the threshold is recorded for the ear being tested. Red corresponds to the right ear, and blue corresponds to the left ear.
7. The tester should remember to recheck the threshold at 1000 Hz after the ear is tested for other frequencies, as the initial determination may not have been completely accurate.
8. If, during the testing of many subjects, significant hearing losses are found repeatedly in the same frequencies, it is wise for the tester to *recheck the earphones* on himself/herself to be sure that nothing has gone wrong during the testing procedures. Conversely, if all subjects seem to have normal hearing, the audiometer may be generating tones louder than the hearing level dial indicates.
9. At all times, the tester must *avoid rhythmical presentation* of the signals.
10. Some subjects will complain, particularly after listening to very loud tones, that the tones continue to linger even after the signal itself has stopped. This so-called *aftertone* happens occasionally in certain ears and *must be taken into consideration*. More time and more careful determination of threshold are indicated for such subjects.
11. Occasionally, a tester will encounter a subject who has tinnitus such as a ringing noise in his/her ears. When the threshold of certain frequencies is being obtained, such a subject may state that the "head noise" is confusing his/her responses. If a *threshold cannot be determined in a routine manner to the tester's satisfaction, several other methods are available*. One of these is to use several short, interrupted bursts of tone two or three times instead of a single tone or to use a frequency-modulated pulsed tone that can be produced by same audiometers. Sometimes this will enable a subject to respond more accurately because they are able to distinguish the pure tone from the tinnitus. This change in technique and the fact that the subject complains of tinnitus should be noted on his/her record.

12. Sometimes a tester may encounter a subject whose responses are so varied that an accurate threshold cannot be obtained at that time. In this case, the test should be terminated and repeated on another day. It is *unsatisfactory for a tester to report vague general thresholds* on such a subject, especially because accurate responses may be attainable. The reliability of the subject's responses should be documented in the patient's record.

13. When recording the hearing losses at 250 and 8000 Hz, *one should not record higher levels than the maximum output of the audiometer.* The tester should be familiar with the limitations of the audiometer. These output limits are generally printed on the frequency dial.

14. When depressing the *tone presenter switch*, the tester must be particularly *careful not to press it down too hard or let it spring back too quickly*; otherwise, it will make a click and may result in a subjective response to the click rather than to the pure tone presented.

15. *If a hearing loss is present*, particularly at the frequencies of 1000 Hz or higher, *each threshold should be rechecked and recorded.*

16. All threshold readings should be recorded in *5 dB multiples.*

## MASKING

When an individual wishes to test vision in only one eye, he/she merely close the other eye or cover it with a patch to exclude it from the test. It is not as simple to test hearing in only one ear because sound waves, unlike light waves, travel in all directions and are not stopped easily by merely plugging the opposite ear. When a person hears normally in both ears, it is easy to test each ear separately because he hears the very weak threshold tones in one ear long before they become loud enough to be heard in the opposite ear. However, when there is a difference in threshold between the two ears, the test tone intended for one ear could be heard by the other ear instead. This phenomenon that prevents correct measurement of the ear being tested is called shadow hearing, shadow response, crossover, and cross hearing. The only way to keep the other ear from participating in the test is to keep it busy with a masking noise. The noise produces a temporary artificial loss in the non-test ear. We want to distract the non-test ear sufficiently so that tones presented to the test ear are heard by the test ear only. However, we do not want to use so much masking noise in the non-test ear that it also raises the threshold of the test ear—an error called overmasking. Ideally, proper masking isolates the two ears from one another—the test signal is heard in the test ear, and the masking noise is heard in the masked ear—and neither is heard in both.

## WHAT STARTING LEVEL OF MASKING SHOULD BE USED?

## AIR CONDUCTION TESTING

The starting masking level should be based on the air conduction thresholds for the frequency being tested in the masked ear plus ~30 dB HL. Interaural attenuation of sound is dependent on use of transducer. Supraaural headphone use will generally have an interaural attenuation of ~40 dB HL. Insert earphones have a larger interaural attenuation, around 60 dB HL. Therefore, the use of contralateral masking will be needed more commonly while testing with headphones versus insert earphones to overcome interaural attenuation.

## BONE CONDUCTION TESTING

Interaural attenuation for bone conducted sounds is generally considered to be 0 dB HL. Because of this, the likelihood for bone conduction masking is higher than air conduction due to sound crossover. Masking is used in bone conduction testing when an air–bone gap of 15 dB or larger exists. The starting masking level should be the air conduction threshold plus 15 dB plus occlusion effect compensation. Recommended occlusion effect compensation is greater in the low frequencies and smaller in the high frequencies and requires the addition of approximately 20 dB HL occlusion effect masking at 500 Hz, 15 dB HL at 1000 Hz, and minimal effects at 2000 Hz and 4000 Hz. In conductive losses, the occlusion effect has already compensated and should not be counted twice.

## WHAT TYPE OF MASKING DOES YOUR AUDIOMETER HAVE?

The type of masking noise produced by many audiometers are narrowband noise, speech spectrum noise, and white noise. The temporary hearing loss produced by masking noise is not the same for all frequencies at a particular dial setting of the masking control. It follows, then, that the numbers appearing on the masking control should be regarded as practically meaningless unless appropriate correction tables are compiled, and formulas are applied.

There is a way, however, of determining proper masking without going through the complicated process of establishing masking tables and formulas. The procedure is referred to variously as the plateau method, the threshold shift method, or the shadow method.

## WHAT IS THE PLATEAU METHOD OF MASKING?

The following procedure applies to both air and bone conduction threshold determinations:

1. Obtain air and bone conduction thresholds in both ears without masking.
2. If there is a possibility that shadow responses were obtained for the poor ear at some or all test frequencies, those frequencies will need to be retested with masking in the non-test, or better, ear.
3. Inform the subject that a steam-like noise will be heard in the ear to be masked. The subject also will be listening to the test tones heard previously and is to respond only to the test tones and not to the noise.
4. With the selector switch turned to "bone conduction," the masking noise automatically will be directed to one of the earphones. Determine which one is the masking earphone when doing bone conduction testing. When masking is used in air conduction testing, the noise automatically is directed to the earphone opposite the one in which the

earphone selected is placed. Earphone select in "right" means the test tone goes to the right ear and masking noise to the left ear.

5. When performing air conduction with masking, be sure to place the headset snugly against the ears to prevent leakage of the noise to the opposite side.
6. If performing bone conduction with masking, first place the vibrator on the prominent portion of the mastoid area behind the ear. Be certain that the vibrator does not touch the ear. Put the masking earphone on the opposite ear and the deadened earphone on the temple of the side of the head where the vibrator was placed. Do not permit the headbands of the vibrators and the earphones to touch. Recheck the bone vibrator for proper position. Be sure that the vibrator is flat against the mastoid.
7. Introduce masking into the non-test ear at a 30- to 40-dB effective level above the patient's threshold of the non-test ear. Obtain a threshold (do not record it yet). If this produces a threshold shift from the unmasked level, increase the masking by another 5 dB and obtain another threshold. If the threshold shifts 5 dB, you are still undermasking. Continue this procedure until the threshold stabilizes, even though masking is increased by three more 5-dB steps. At this point, you probably have found the true threshold of hearing (the plateau). At some point, further increases in masking will start to shift thresholds again. This is the point of overmasking.
8. Air conduction masking requires the tester to introduce masking into the non-test ear at a 15-dB effective level above the patient's threshold of the non-test ear. Obtain a threshold. Masking of the non-test ear should then be increased in 5-dB increments and increased over a 15- to 20-dB level to reach plateau. Each time a subject responds, increase the masking noise in 5-dB increments until noise is increased by 15–20 dB without a shift in threshold. Further masking at this level will begin to shift thresholds, causing overmasking.
9. Bone conduction masking requires compensation of occlusion effect at test frequencies

500–1000 Hz. An addition of ~20 dB of masking is suggested for 500–1000 Hz to account for occlusion. Little occlusion is noted at 2000 Hz and above. The tester may then identify the plateau for air conduction masking.

If the initial introduction of masking is not sufficient, and two or more successive increases in masking do not shift threshold correspondingly, you still may not have reached the plateau because the threshold in the masked ear has not been shifted successfully.

## WHEN IS MASKING USED?

## AIR CONDUCTION TESTING

Generally, masking should be used whenever there is a difference of ≥ 40 dB between the air conduction reading in the poorer ear and the *bone* conduction threshold in the better ear. For example, if the air conduction thresholds in the better ear are normal, it follows that the bone conduction thresholds are also normal. Then, when testing air conduction of the poorer ear, masking will be necessary if the difference between ears is ≥ 40 dB (each frequency is compared individually) (**Tables 6.1** and **6.2**).

When using insert earphones, masking should be used when there is a difference of > 60 dB between the air conduction reading in the poorer ear and the bone conduction threshold in the better ear.

If you have not performed bone conduction testing and there is a difference of ≥ 40 dB between the left and right ears, masking should be used in the better ear while testing the poorer.

Table 6.1  Masking needed in right ear when testing the left

| Frequency (k/Hz) | Right ear | | | | | | |
|---|---|---|---|---|---|---|---|
| | 0.5 | 1.0 | 2.0 | 3.0 | 4.0 | 6.0 | 8.0 |
| | 5 | 5/5 | 10 | 10 | 15 | 15 | 5 |
| | Left ear | | | | | | |
| | 0.5 | 1.0 | 2.0 | 3.0 | 4.0 | 6.0 | 8.0 |
| | 50 | 55 | 50 | 55 | 55 | 55 | 50 |

One can assume that the right ear has normal bone conduction.

Table 6.2  Masking needed in right ear at 2000–8000 Hz when testing the left

| Frequency (k/Hz) | Right ear | | | | | | |
|---|---|---|---|---|---|---|---|
| | 0.5 | 1.0 | 2.0 | 3.0 | 4.0 | 6.0 | 8.0 |
| | 40 | 35 | 45 | 40 | 40 | 45 | 40 |
| | Left ear | | | | | | |
| | 0.5 | 1.0 | 2.0 | 3.0 | 4.0 | 6.0 | 8.0 |
| | 40 | 40 | 90 | 85 | 90 | 85 | NR |

As yet, bone conduction of the right ear is unknown, but about a 40-dB difference exists at frequencies 2000–8000 Hz.

## BONE CONDUCTION TESTING

The purpose of the mastoid vibrator in bone conduction testing is to present the test tone directly to the inner ear using the cranial bones instead of the ossicles to transmit sound.

Bone conduction testing is performed to determine whether an elevated air conduction threshold of hearing is caused by problems in the outer or middle ear. Bone conduction testing should be performed whenever the air conduction hearing threshold in either ear exceeds 15 dB.

Unlike the 40-dB criteria in air conduction testing, there is little or no transmission loss between ears when tones are presented via the bone vibrator. In most cases, therefore, masking should be used routinely when doing bone conduction testing.

There are some occasions, however, when masking is not necessary during bone conduction testing. These include the following:

1. When bone conduction thresholds are equal to the air conduction threshold for that ear (no air–bone gap).
2. When bone conduction thresholds for the ear being tested are better than those of the opposite ear.
3. When there is no response at the upper bone conduction testing limits.

## WHAT FREQUENCIES SHOULD BE TESTED BY BONE CONDUCTION?

It is necessary to test only the frequencies 250–4000 Hz for bone conduction thresholds. It is not necessary to do bone conduction tests at frequencies where the air conduction thresholds are 15 dB or better. Many commercial audiometers are not calibrated for 250 Hz bone conduction testing.

## HOW IS RESIDUAL HEARING TESTED CLINICALLY?

Too frequently, a patient with unilateral deafness is tested with inadequate masking or no masking at all, and he/she is told he/she has residual hearing in an ear that is deaf. In some instances, the patient may even be misdiagnosed as having otosclerosis and be operated on with no chance of success. Such errors can be avoided through proper testing technique.

## SIMPLE METHODS OF MASKING

In clinical practice, several simple methods of masking are available to determine grossly whether an ear has some useful hearing or is profoundly deaf, as is commonly the case in unilateral hearing loss caused by mumps and in some ears postoperatively.

Frequently, patients are seen who have conductive hearing loss in both ears, often because of otosclerosis, but occasionally due to bilateral chronic otitis media. Some of these patients have had mastoid or stapes surgery in one ear only, and they seek the physician's help to determine whether it is possible to restore hearing in either ear. If the hearing level in both ears is ~50–60 dB, it is very difficult to mask either ear with commercially available masking devices. The important fact to be determined is whether the ear that had the surgery now is totally deaf or still has a good amount of residual hearing. The most effective way of ascertaining this in everyday practice is to strike a 500-Hz tuning fork, apply it to the operated ear by both air and bone conduction, and ask the patient whether he/she still hears it while a loud masking noise is placed in the other ear. If, while the fork

is still vibrating, the patient's hand comes down when the masking is turned on and then reappears when the masking is turned off again, the operated ear probably has little or no residual hearing, and further surgery is not warranted (**Figures 6.4** and **6.5**). Under such circumstances, it would be injudicious to operate on the opposite ear, for in the event of a surgical complication, the patient might lose the hearing in his/her only hearing ear and become totally deaf.

## HOW IS THE BONE CONDUCTION VIBRATOR CALIBRATED?

Major problems still exist in bone conduction testing. One involves calibration of the bone conduction vibrator; another concerns the relation of bone conduction threshold levels to the actual function of the sensorineural mechanism.

One method of calibrating the bone conduction vibrator is through the use of an artificial mastoid. The equipment necessary for this calibration procedure is fairly expensive and therefore usually is available only from the audiometer manufacturer or a well-equipped instrument laboratory. The authors prefer the biological method of checking vibrator responses.

Two biological techniques for calibration are used commonly. In the first, the manufacturer sets the bone conduction reference threshold level at 0 dB so that subjects with a 0 dB air threshold level get a 0 dB bone threshold level. In the second technique, the same reasoning is applied to patients who have sensorineural hearing loss so that the air and the bone conduction thresholds match. None of these techniques are really satisfactory, but they must be used until a more sophisticated and reliable method is developed.

The problems of bone conduction audiometry are numerous and complex. They include factors such as placement and pressure of the oscillator, thickness of the skin and underlying tissue, density of the petrous bone, the frequency being tested, noise conditions of the test room, condition of the ear not under testing, masking occlusion effect, and the vibrations of the skull and the bony otic capsule. Another important consideration is the air arising from the bone vibrator, especially

JOSEPH SATALOFF, M.D.
ROBERT THAYER SATALOFF, M.D.
1721 PINE STREET    PHILADELPHIA, PA 19103

**HEARING RECORD**

NAME _____    AGE ____

### AIR CONDUCTION

| | | | RIGHT | | | | | | | | LEFT | | | | | |
|---|---|---|---|---|---|---|---|---|---|---|---|---|---|---|---|---|
| DATE | Exam | LEFT MASK | 250 | 500 | 1000 | 2000 | 4000 | 8000 | RIGHT MASK | 250 | 500 | 1000 | 2000 | 4000 | 8000 | AUD |
| | | | -5 | -5 | -10 | -10 | -10 | -10 | - | 55 | 60 | 60 | 50 | 65 | 60 | |
| | | | | | | | | | 60 | 75 | NR | NR | NR | NR | NR | |
| | | | | | | | | | 80 | NR | NR | NR | NR | NR | NR | |
| | | | | | | | | | 100 | NR | NR | NR | NR | NR | NR | |

### BONE CONDUCTION

| | | | RIGHT | | | | | | LEFT | | | | | |
|---|---|---|---|---|---|---|---|---|---|---|---|---|---|---|
| DATE | Exam | LEFT MASK | 250 | 500 | 1000 | 2000 | 4000 | RIGHT MASK | 250 | 500 | 1000 | 2000 | 4000 | AUD |
| | | | | | | | | - | | 5 | 5 | 10 | 15 | 15 | |
| | | | | | | | | 60 | 25 | 35 | 50 | 60 | NR | |
| | | | | | | | | 100 | NR | NR | NR | NR | NR | |

### SPEECH RECEPTION

| DATE | RIGHT | LEFT MASK | LEFT | RIGHT MASK | FREE FIELD | MIC. |
|---|---|---|---|---|---|---|
| | | | | | | |

### DISCRIMINATION

| DATE | % SCORE | TEST LEVEL | LIST | LEFT MASK (RIGHT) | % SCORE | TEST LEVEL | LIST | RIGHT MASK (LEFT) | EXAM. |
|---|---|---|---|---|---|---|---|---|---|
| | | | | | | | | | |

### HIGH FREQUENCY THRESHOLDS

| | DATE | RIGHT | | | | | LEFT MASK | RIGHT MASK | LEFT | | | | |
|---|---|---|---|---|---|---|---|---|---|---|---|---|---|
| | | 4000 | 8000 | 10000 | 12000 | 14000 | | | 4000 | 8000 | 10000 | 12000 | 14000 |
| | | | | | | | | | | | | | |

| RIGHT | | WEBER | LEFT | | HEARING AID | | | |
|---|---|---|---|---|---|---|---|---|
| RINNE | SCHWABACH | | RINNE | SCHWABACH | DATE | MAKE | | MODEL |
| | | | | | RECEIVER | GAIN | | EXAM |
| | | | | | EAR | DISCRIM | | COUNC |

REMARKS

**Figure 6.4** Hearing record of patient with left total deafness caused by mumps. Right ear is normal. Without masking the right ear in testing the left, a threshold of ~60 dB seems to be present by air conduction, and bone conduction appears to be almost normal. These are shadow curves. With 60-dB white noise (WN) masking in the right ear, the shadow curve for air almost disappears, but it does not for bone conduction. With 80-dB WN in the right ear, the shadow curve for air is gone. With 100-dB WN in the right ear, there is no hearing for air or bone in the left ear. If, however, the 100-dB WN is put into the left ear during testing of the right normal ear, there is overmasking and the right ear will show a reduced threshold. WN in this case was measured above the zero average on the audiometer. *Abbreviation*: NR, no response.

when testing is done at the higher frequencies and intensities. A strong air signal emanating from the bone vibrator may be detected by air conduction before actual bone vibration takes place to elicit responses.

A strong air signal emanates from the bone vibrator. If a bone vibrator is calibrated on ears with pure sensorineural hearing loss and is used on ears with conductive hearing loss, it may not be of proper calibration at the higher frequencies and intensities. In these ears, the air signal may be suppressed, and this might produce poorer bone thresholds than the actual sensorineural losses of these patients would warrant.

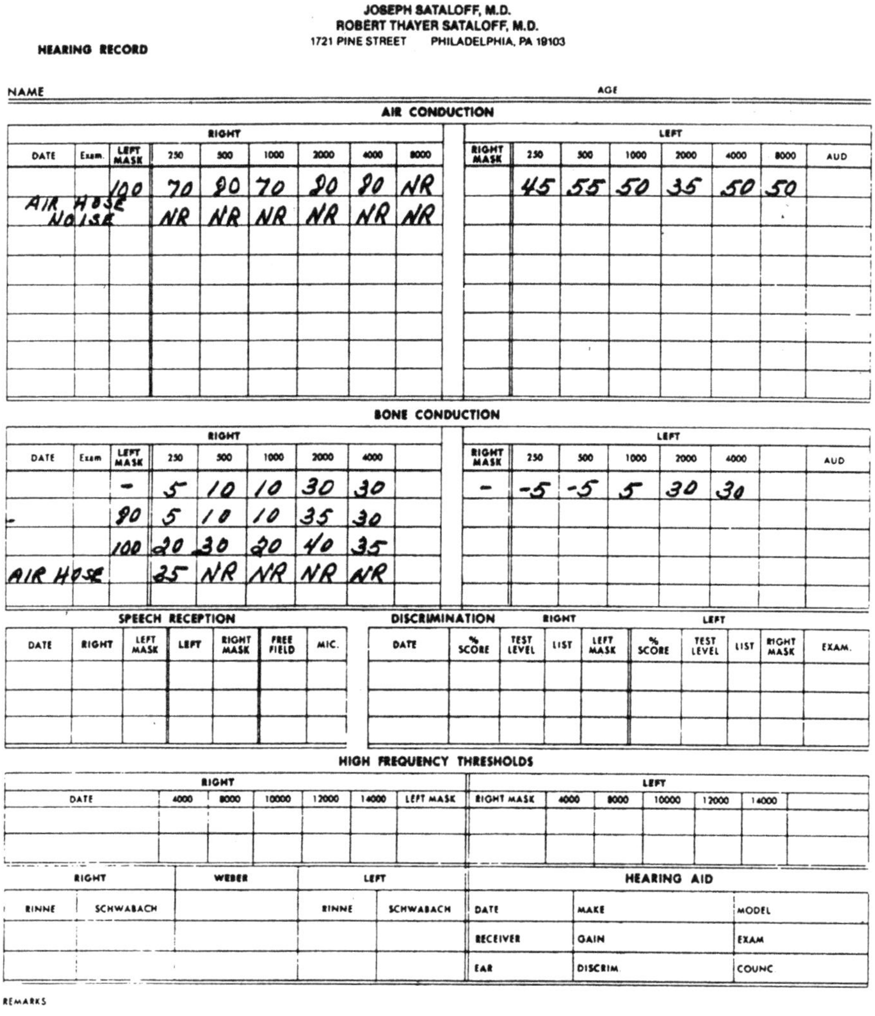

JOSEPH SATALOFF, M.D.
ROBERT THAYER SATALOFF, M.D.
1721 PINE STREET    PHILADELPHIA, PA 19103

HEARING RECORD

NAME _____    AGE _____

### AIR CONDUCTION

| | | | RIGHT | | | | | | | LEFT | | | | | | |
| DATE | Exam. | LEFT MASK | 250 | 500 | 1000 | 2000 | 4000 | 8000 | RIGHT MASK | 250 | 500 | 1000 | 2000 | 4000 | 8000 | AUD |
|---|---|---|---|---|---|---|---|---|---|---|---|---|---|---|---|---|
| AIR HOSE NOISE | | 100 | 70 | 90 | 70 | 20 | 80 | NR | | 45 | 55 | 50 | 35 | 50 | 50 | |
| | | | NR | NR | NR | NR | NR | NR | | | | | | | | |

### BONE CONDUCTION

| | | | RIGHT | | | | | | LEFT | | | | | |
| DATE | Exam | LEFT MASK | 250 | 500 | 1000 | 2000 | 4000 | RIGHT MASK | 250 | 500 | 1000 | 2000 | 4000 | AUD |
|---|---|---|---|---|---|---|---|---|---|---|---|---|---|---|
| | | – | 5 | 10 | 10 | 30 | 30 | – | -5 | -5 | 5 | 30 | 30 | |
| | | 90 | 5 | 10 | 10 | 35 | 30 | | | | | | | |
| | | 100 | 20 | 30 | 20 | 40 | 35 | | | | | | | |
| AIR HOSE | | | 25 | NR | NR | NR | NR | | | | | | | |

| SPEECH RECEPTION | | | | | | | DISCRIMINATION | | RIGHT | | | LEFT | | | |
| DATE | RIGHT | LEFT MASK | LEFT | RIGHT MASK | FREE FIELD | MIC. | DATE | % SCORE | TEST LEVEL | LIST | LEFT MASK | % SCORE | TEST LEVEL | LIST | RIGHT MASK | EXAM. |
|---|---|---|---|---|---|---|---|---|---|---|---|---|---|---|---|---|
| | | | | | | | | | | | | | | | | |

### HIGH FREQUENCY THRESHOLDS

| | RIGHT | | | | | | | LEFT | | | | |
| DATE | 4000 | 8000 | 10000 | 12000 | 14000 | LEFT MASK | RIGHT MASK | 4000 | 8000 | 10000 | 12000 | 14000 |
|---|---|---|---|---|---|---|---|---|---|---|---|---|
| | | | | | | | | | | | | |

| RIGHT | | WEBER | | LEFT | | | HEARING AID | | | |
| RINNE | SCHWABACH | | | RINNE | SCHWABACH | DATE | | MAKE | | MODEL |
|---|---|---|---|---|---|---|---|---|---|---|
| | | | | | | RECEIVER | | GAIN | | EXAM |
| | | | | | | EAR | | DISCRIM | | COUNC |

REMARKS

Figure 6.5 The right ear in this patient actually has no hearing, and it gives no caloric response; yet it gives a measurable threshold by air and bone conduction despite large amounts of masking. The reason is that the masking noise is not enough to overcome the conductive hearing loss in the left ear. Discrimination tests with masking are more helpful. The use of narrowband noise through an insert receiver effectively masks the left ear. With the present findings, a misdiagnosis of right conductive hearing loss with an air–bone gap could be made, and the patient could be operated on with no chance of success.

## WHAT IS THE RELATION OF THE BONE CONDUCTION THRESHOLD LEVELS TO THE FUNCTION OF THE SENSORINEURAL MECHANISM?

One may find that in a patient with a high-tone hearing loss, whose bone conduction even may be somewhat reduced, the cause is not in the sensorineural pathway but in the middle ear. Fluid in the middle ear is the most common cause, although often it produces a low-frequency hearing loss. Otosclerosis may also produce dip in bone conduction that is not due to sensorineural impairment (Carhart's notch).

When interpreting bone conduction audiograms, it is essential to bear in mind that the threshold obtained by bone conduction testing provides only a rough approximation of the function of the sensorineural mechanism. In certain cases of conductive hearing loss, especially in adhesive otitis and in the presence of fluid in the middle ears, the lower bone conduction values that frequently are obtained may not indicate true sensorineural loss but rather impaired mobility of the oval and the round windows.

Bone conduction audiometry on the mastoid bone often shows a reduction that is not borne out by testing on the upper incisor tooth with a 512-Hz tuning fork. In such instances, the better dental bone conduction is more likely to reflect the true sensorineural hearing than the poorer bone conduction via the mastoid bone. Of course, it is important to rule out tactile sensation in evaluating these conflicting findings. Another important factor in assessing bone conduction threshold is that the maximum intensity obtainable on commercial audiometers for bone vibrators is ~55 or 60 dB. Failure to obtain any bone conduction in routine testing does not necessarily indicate that the sensorineural mechanism is dead. It indicates only that the subject's hearing mechanism does not respond at the maximum intensity of the tone.

Problems in interpretation of bone conduction testing can result because stimulus in this type of testing is vibratory in nature. Many patients with very severe air conduction hearing losses give responses to bone conduction at 250 and 512 Hz as low as 20 or 25 dB. This gives the impression that an air–bone gap exists in these low frequencies, an impression that is not justified. Actually, in most patients with severe nerve deafness, the false thresholds at these low frequencies are probably a response to tactile sensation and not to auditory stimuli. On the basis of these low-frequency bone conduction findings alone, middle ear surgery is not warranted in these patients.

## HIGH-FREQUENCY AUDIOMETRY

High-frequency audiometry, also called ultrahigh-frequency audiometry and very high-frequency audiometry, refers to threshold testing of frequencies > 8000 Hz. Several commercially available audiometers include capabilities for testing at 10,000 and 12,000 Hz, and high-frequency audiometers are available to test hearing up to 20,000 Hz. High-frequency audiograms can help in early detection of hearing loss from ototoxicity and other conditions, revealing hearing damage before it is detectable at the frequencies measured routinely. In selected cases, high-frequency audiometry is also helpful in differentiating between hearing loss due to noise and that due to presbycusis. For example, in most cases of presbycusis, hearing levels continue to deteriorate progressively at higher frequencies. In noise-induced hearing loss, improvement in hearing levels may be seen at 10,000, 12,000, or 14,000 Hz, revealing an audiometric "dip" similar to that usually centered around 4000 or 6000 Hz.

## CONTINUOUS-FREQUENCY AUDIOMETRY

It is important to remember that routine audiometry samples hearing at only eight frequency regions out of thousands detected by the ear. Equipment is available to test the *in-between* frequencies, and such testing can be invaluable. For example, in a patient claiming to have tinnitus in one ear after exposure to a blast but who has normal hearing at 3, 4, 6, and 8 Hz, finding a 40-dB dip between 5240 and 5628 Hz provides useful confirmation that an organic problem is present.

# 7

# Special hearing tests

ROBERT THAYER SATALOFF, KERRIN E. RICHARD, AND PAMELA C. ROEHM

For the majority of patients who complain of hearing loss, the history, ear examination, tuning-fork tests, and air and bone conduction audiometry provide sufficient information to make at least a preliminary differential diagnosis. This information tells the physician how much hearing is lost and what frequencies are affected and even helps to determine whether the loss is conductive or sensorineural in nature.

These tests are adequate in most cases of conductive hearing loss. However, there are some cases of conductive hearing loss and many cases of sensorineural loss in which these tests do not disclose enough information to make an accurate diagnosis possible, and additional hearing studies become necessary.

Because air and bone conduction audiometry measures only thresholds for pure tones, it provides limited information. For instance, it does not help the physician to detect certain phenomena that aid in localizing the site of a lesion in sensorineural involvement or to assess a patient's capacity to use his/her residual hearing. Phenomena such as recruitment, tone decay, tone distortion, and the

patient's ability to discriminate speech, to localize sound, or to understand speech in a noisy environment give clues to the site of a lesion. To obtain this information, special hearing tests have been devised. These rarely are done by general practitioners or pediatricians, but many are carried out in an otologist's office, and most are performed in hospital or university hearing centers.

Although family doctors and occupational physicians may not perform all these tests, they should know when they are indicated, and they should be able to interpret the results.

## THE DIFFERENCE BETWEEN AUDIOMETRIC THRESHOLD LEVELS AND DISCRIMINATION

It is common practice to interpret a patient's ability to hear speech by averaging his/her pure-tone thresholds in the four speech frequencies in the audiogram. For example, if his/her hearing loss is

DOI: 10.1201/b23379-7

30 dB at 500 Hz, 40 dB at 1000 Hz, 50 dB at 2000 Hz, and 40 dB at 3000 Hz, his/her average hearing loss would come to 40 dB for the speech frequencies, and this would be called his/her hearing loss for pure tones and for speech. It is common practice to express this as an average and to tell the patient that he/she has a 40% hearing loss. This procedure has serious shortcomings and should be avoided in clinical practice. Percentages have some application in determining hearing impairment in compensation claims, but this is not the same as using them to describe a patient's hearing capacity, especially based directly on decibels measured, rather than calculated impairment percentages.

If a patient is told that he/she has a 40% hearing loss in the involved ear, he/she naturally infers that the ear has only 60% of its hearing left. This is not true, especially because maximum hearing does not stop at 100 dB (maximum output of some audiometers), but rather, the ear will respond to much higher intensities. Percentages are particularly deceiving in cases of sensory hearing loss with poor discrimination. When the physician tells a patient with Ménière's disease that he/she has a 40% hearing loss, the patient may reply that, as far as he/she is concerned, his/her hearing loss is nearly 100% because he/she cannot use that ear in telephone conversations and the patient gets little or no use of it in daily communication. The problem exists because the threshold determination shows a 40-dB hearing level for pure tones, whereas the patient is referring to his/her ability to distinguish or to discriminate what he/she hears. In some patients with Ménière's disease or with an acoustic neuroma, the ability to discriminate may be impaired so severely that the ear is useless even with only a 40-dB threshold level in the speech frequencies.

Still another shortcoming of expressing hearing loss on the basis of speech frequency averaging is demonstrated in **Figure 7.1**. Both patients, whose audiograms are shown in A and B, have an average hearing loss of 40 dB, but patient A can get along fairly well without the use of a hearing aid, whereas patient B needs a hearing aid to get along reasonably well.

The physician should explain to the patient the difference between audiometric threshold levels and discriminating ability. The patient also should be told the facts about his/her other difficulties, such as sound localization in unilateral hearing losses, recruitment, and hearing in the presence of noise.

## TESTING HEARING WITH SPEECH

## SPEECH RECEPTION TEST

In addition to pure tones for testing threshold and for calculating hearing acuity, the physician can use speech of electronically controlled intensity. What is measured by this test is called a speech reception threshold (SRT). This represents the faintest level at which speech is heard and repeated. The SRT is recorded in dB HL (decibels in hearing level). The results should be in good agreement with the average hearing levels obtained at 500, 1000, 2000, and 3000 Hz, the range that comprises the so-called speech frequencies, known as the pure-tone average. The pure-tone average and SRT normally vary from each other by no more than ~10 dB.

## Materials

Several types of speech material can be used to determine SRT. These include isolated words, individual sentences, and connected discourse. The most commonly used material is the standardized word list composed of spondaic words (spondees). These are two-syllable words equally stressed on both syllables, prepared in several lists (**Figure 7.2**).

## Administration

The test can be administered by recordings or by monitored live voice through a microphone attached to the speech audiometer. Earphones are placed on the patient's ears to test the hearing in each ear separately, or the patient may be tested through a loudspeaker, in which case binaural hearing is tested. The patient is instructed to repeat the spondaic words or sentences as they are presented. The patient should be told also that the

**HEARING RECORD**

JOSEPH SATALOFF, M.D.
ROBERT THAYER SATALOFF, M.D.
1721 PINE STREET     PHILADELPHIA, PA 19103

NAME _____   AGE _____

### AIR CONDUCTION

| | | | RIGHT | | | | | | | LEFT | | | | | |
|------|------|-------------|-----|-----|------|------|------|------|---------------|-----|-----|------|------|------|------|-----|
| DATE | Exam. | LEFT MASK | 250 | 500 | 1000 | 2000 | 4000 | 8000 | RIGHT MASK | 250 | 500 | 1000 | 2000 | 4000 | 8000 | AUD |
| (A) | | | 15 | 20 | 40 | 60 | 65 | NR | | | | | | | | |
| (B) | | | 50 | 50 | 40 | 30 | 30 | 35 | | | | | | | | |
| | | | | | | | | | | | | | | | | |
| | | | | | | | | | | | | | | | | |
| | | | | | | | | | | | | | | | | |
| | | | | | | | | | | | | | | | | |
| | | | | | | | | | | | | | | | | |
| | | | | | | | | | | | | | | | | |

### BONE CONDUCTION

| | | | RIGHT | | | | | | | LEFT | | | | | |
|------|------|-------------|-----|-----|------|------|------|---|------------|-----|-----|------|------|------|-----|
| DATE | Exam | LEFT MASK | 250 | 500 | 1000 | 2000 | 4000 | | RIGHT MASK | 250 | 500 | 1000 | 2000 | 4000 | AUD |
| | | | | | | | | | | | | | | | |
| | | | | | | | | | | | | | | | |
| | | | | | | | | | | | | | | | |
| | | | | | | | | | | | | | | | |
| | | | | | | | | | | | | | | | |

### SPEECH RECEPTION

| DATE | RIGHT | LEFT MASK | LEFT | RIGHT MASK | FREE FIELD | MIC. |
|------|-------|-----------|------|------------|------------|------|
| | | | | | | |
| | | | | | | |
| | | | | | | |

### DISCRIMINATION

| | | RIGHT | | | | LEFT | | | |
|------|---------|------------|------|-----------|---------|------------|------|------------|------|
| DATE | % SCORE | TEST LEVEL | LIST | LEFT MASK | % SCORE | TEST LEVEL | LIST | RIGHT MASK | EXAM. |
| | | | | | | | | | |
| | | | | | | | | | |
| | | | | | | | | | |

### HIGH FREQUENCY THRESHOLDS

| | RIGHT | | | | | | LEFT | | | | | |
|------|------|------|-------|-------|-------|-----------|-----------|------|------|-------|-------|-------|
| DATE | 6000 | 8000 | 10000 | 12000 | 14000 | LEFT MASK | RIGHT MASK | 4000 | 8000 | 10000 | 12000 | 14000 |
| | | | | | | | | | | | | |
| | | | | | | | | | | | | |
| | | | | | | | | | | | | |

| RIGHT | | WEBER | LEFT | | HEARING AID | | | |
|-------|-----------|-------|-------|-----------|----------|--------|-------|-------|
| RINNE | SCHWABACH | | RINNE | SCHWABACH | DATE | MAKE | | MODEL |
| | | | | | RECEIVER | GAIN | | EXAM |
| | | | | | EAR | DISCRIM | | COUNC |

REMARKS

Figure 7.1 Patients A and B have an average pure-tone loss of 40 dB, but patient A can get along well without the use of a hearing aid, whereas patient B will need amplification. *Abbreviation*: NR, no response.

words or the sentences will become fainter as the test proceeds but that he/she should repeat them until they are no longer audible.

## The significance of various SRTs

The point at which 50% of the items are heard correctly as the intensity is reduced is considered to be the SRT. In clinical practice, 5-dB steps of attenuation for every three words is a satisfactory rate. A person with normal hearing has an SRT of between 0 and 15 dB. An SRT up to ~25 dB usually presents no important handicapping hearing impairment. However, when the loss exceeds this level,

the patient may experience difficulties in everyday communication, and a hearing aid usually is recommended.

In general, thresholds for speech tests and thresholds obtained by averaging the pure tones in the speech frequency should differ by no more than 6 dB. Discrepancies may be found between the two in cases in which there is a sharp drop-off of pure-tone thresholds across the 500–3000 frequency range. Discrimination difficulty may result in a wide disparity between SRT and pure-tone average losses. There also may be a wide disparity in cases in which the loss is produced by emotional rather than organic causes.

| List A | List B | List C | List D | List E | List F |
|---|---|---|---|---|---|
| Greyhound | Playground | Birthday | Hothouse | Northwest | Padlock |
| Schoolboy | Grandson | Hothouse | Padlock | Doormat | Daybreak |
| Inkwell | Doormat | Toothbrush | Eardrum | Railroad | Sunset |
| Whitewash | Woodwork | Horseshoe | Sidewalk | Woodwork | Farewell |
| Pancake | Armchair | Airplane | Cowboy | Hardware | Northwest |
| Mousetrap | Stairway | Northwest | Mushroom | Stairway | Airplane |
| Eardrum | Cowboy | Whitewash | Farewell | Sidewalk | Playground |
| Headlight | Oatmeal | Hotdog | Horseshoe | Birthday | Iceberg |
| Birthday | Railroad | Hardware | Workshop | Farewell | Drawbridge |
| Duckpond | Baseball | Woodwork | Duckpond | Greyhound | Baseball |
| Sidewalk | Padlock | Stairway | Baseball | Cowboy | Woodwork |
| Hotdog | Hardware | Daybreak | Railroad | Daybreak | Inkwell |
| Padlock | Whitewash | Sidewalk | Hardware | Drawbridge | Pancake |
| Mushroom | Hotdog | Railroad | Toothbrush | Duckpond | Toothbrush |
| Hardware | Sunset | Oatmeal | Airplane | Horseshoe | Hardware |
| Workshop | Headlight | Headlight | Iceberg | Armchair | Railroad |
| Horseshoe | Drawbridge | Pancake | Armchair | Padlock | Oatmeal |
| Armchair | Toothbrush | Doormat | Grandson | Mousetrap | Grandson |
| Baseball | Mushroom | Farewell | Playground | Headlight | Mousetrap |
| Stairway | Farewell | Mousetrap | Oatmeal | Airplane | Workshop |
| Cowboy | Horseshoe | Armchair | Northwest | Inkwell | Eardrum |
| Iceberg | Pancake | Drawbridge | Woodwork | Grandson | Greyhound |
| Northwest | Inkwell | Mushroom | Stairway | Workshop | Doormat |
| Railroad | Mousetrap | Baseball | Hotdog | Hotdog | Horseshoe |
| Playground | Airplane | Grandson | Headlight | Oatmeal | Stairway |
| Airplane | Sidewalk | Padlock | Pancake | Sunset | Cowboy |
| Woodwork | Eardrum | Greyhound | Birthday | Pancake | Sidewalk |
| Oatmeal | Birthday | Sunset | Greyhound | Eardrum | Mushroom |
| Toothbrush | Hothouse | Cowboy | Mousetrap | Mushroom | Armchair |
| Farewell | Iceberg | Duckpond | Schoolboy | Whitewash | Whitewash |
| Grandson | Schoolboy | Playground | Whitewash | Hothouse | Hotdog |
| Drawbridge | Duckpond | Inkwell | Inkwell | Toothbrush | Schoolboy |
| Doormat | Workshop | Eardrum | Doormat | Playground | Headlight |
| Hothouse | Northwest | Workshop | Daybreak | Baseball | Duckpond |
| Daybreak | Greyhound | Schoolboy | Drawbridge | Iceberg | Birthday |
| Sunset | Daybreak | Iceberg | Sunset | Schoolboy | Hothouse |

Figure 7.2 Lists of spondees. (Auditory Test W-1, Spondee Word Lists, courtesy of Central Institute for the Deaf.)

# DISCRIMINATION TESTING

Determining the SRT is a rather imperfect measure of a person's ability to hear speech. Generally, it does not tell whether the patient is able to distinguish sounds that he/she hears, particularly difficult sounds. A special test to measure speech discrimination, devised to satisfy this need, differs from tests previously described in that it does not measure a minimal sound level but the *ability to understand speech* when it is amplified to a comfortable level.

Discrimination testing usually is done at 30 or 40 dB above the SRT. This level has been found to yield maximum discrimination scores. In some patients with a severe hearing loss, a level of 40 dB above the SRT is very difficult to obtain because most instruments cannot make sounds louder than 100 dB. For those patients, the discrimination score will be artificially decreased due to the limitations of the testing equipment. In other patients, sound levels 30–40 dB louder than the SRT may be painful or uncomfortable, or it might cause distortion in the instrument or the ear itself, resulting in invalid scores. In such cases, the level of presentation of the test material should be adjusted to a comfortable listening level for the particular subject with notation made of the testing limitation.

## Materials

The speech materials used to test discrimination ability are known as phonetically balanced (PB) word lists. These are lists of monosyllabic words balanced for their phonetic content so that they have about the same distribution of vowels and consonants as that found in everyday speech. The lists are made up of 50 words each, and because each list is balanced in a particular way, it is necessary to administer the full list of 50 words when the test is performed (**Figure 7.3**). Occasionally, the list is cut in half, but this leaves the resulting scores open to question.

## Administration

The test usually is administered through each earphone in order to test the discrimination ability of each ear individually. Testing can be done by means of a recording on which the PB word lists have been recorded or monitored live-voice testing through a microphone. Each word is preceded by an introductory phrase, such as, "Say the word \_\_\_\_\_," and the subject is asked to repeat the word that he/she thinks he/she hears.

## Rating

Only those words understood perfectly are counted as correct. Each word has a value of two points so that a perfect score would be 100 points. If 10 of the 50 words are repeated incorrectly, the patient has an 80% discrimination score. It is obvious, then, that an individual can suffer not only from a quantitative reduction in the ability to hear sounds but also from a reduction in discrimination ability so that even when the speech is well above his/her threshold, he/she still cannot understand what is being said.

| | List 4E | List 4F | List 3E | List 3F |
|---|---|---|---|---|
| 1. | Ought (aught) | Out (hour) | Add (ad) | West |
| 2. | Wood (would) | Art | We | Start |
| 3. | Through (thru) | Darn | Ears | Farm |
| 4. | Ear | Ought (aught) | Start | Out |
| 5. | Men | Stiff | Is | Book |
| 6. | Darn | Am | On | When |
| 7. | Can | Go | Jar | This |
| 8. | Shoe | Few | Oil | Oil |
| 9. | Tin | Arm | Smooth | Lie (lye) |
| 10. | So (sew) | Yet | End | Owes |
| 11. | My | Jump | Use (yews) | Glove |
| 12. | Am | Pale (pail) | Book | Cute |
| 13. | Few | Yes | Aim | Three |
| 14. | All (awl) | Bee (be) | Wool | Chair |
| 15. | Clothes | Eyes (ayes) | Do | Hand |
| 16. | Save | Than | This | Knit |
| 17. | Near | Save | Have | Pie |
| 18. | Yet | Toy | Pie | Ten |
| 19. | Toy | My | May | Wool |
| 20. | Eyes (ayes) | Chin | Lie (lye) | Camp |
| 21. | Bread (bred) | Shoe | Raw | End |
| 22. | Pale (pail) | His | Hand | King |
| 23. | Leaves | Ear | Through | On |
| 24. | Yes | Tea (tee) | Cute | Tan |
| 25. | They | At | Year | We |
| 26. | Be (bee) | Wood (would) | Three | Ears |
| 27. | Dolls | In (inn) | Bill | Ate (eight) |
| 28. | Jump | Men | Chair | Jar |
| 29. | Of | Cook | Say | If |
| 30. | Than | Tin | Glove | Use (yews) |
| 31. | Why | Where | Nest | Shove |
| 32. | Arm | All (awl) | Farm | Do |
| 33. | Hang | Hang | He | Are |
| 34. | Nuts | Near | Owes | May |
| 35. | Aid | Why | Done (dun) | He |
| 36. | Net | Bread (bred) | Ten | Through |
| 37. | Who | Dolls | Are | Say |
| 38. | Chin | They | When | Bill |
| 39. | Where | Leave | Tie | Year |
| 40. | Still | Of | Camp | Nest |
| 41. | Go | Aid | Shove | Raw |
| 42. | His | Nuts | Knit | Done (dun) |
| 43. | Cook | Clothes | No (know) | Have |
| 44. | Art | Who | King | Tie |
| 45. | Will | So (sew) | If | Aim |
| 46. | Tea (tee) | Net | Out | No (know) |
| 47. | In (inn) | Can | Dull | Smooth |
| 48. | Our (hour) | Will | Tan | Dull |
| 49. | Dust | Through (thru) | Ate (eight) | Is |
| 50. | At | Dust | West | Add (ad) |

Figure 7.3 Phonetically balanced word lists (PB lists).

## Arrangement of equipment

Ideally, pure-tone and speech tests should be conducted via a two-room arrangement, which provides a soundproof room with the necessary earphones, microphone, and loudspeakers, in which the patient is seated, and an adjacent control room housing the pure-tone audiometer, the speech audiometer, and the examiner's microphone. The examiner conducts the tests from this room. All electrical connections are accomplished through wall plugs, and the addition of an observation window between the two rooms permits the examiner to watch the patient's reaction during the testing period. The two-room arrangement is essential when monitored live-voice testing is done through a microphone; otherwise, the subject might very well hear the speech directly from the tester's voice rather than through the equipment that electronically controls the intensity of the speech. One other precaution is to have the subject seated so that he/she cannot observe the tester's lips during the procedure. Even a fair lipreader can render the speech tests inaccurate if the patient is allowed to complement the auditory signals with visual clues.

## Evaluation of discrimination score

It is essential to remember that the discrimination score cannot be translated directly into the percentage of difficulty that the patient will have in everyday life. A discrimination score provides only a rough idea of the patient's ability to distinguish certain sounds in a quiet environment. With experience, a broader interpretation can be made, but when this is done, other factors such as personal auditory needs and adaptability and the effects of environmental noise must be taken into consideration.

**Figure 7.4** compares the discrimination scores in a series of patients with about the same SRT but with different diagnoses. Discrimination scores between 90% and 100% are considered to be normal. Scores between 90% and 100% are seen for patients who have conductive hearing losses or those who have dips at high frequencies, such as a 40-dB dip at 3000 Hz; these scores are common also in cases in which the losses encompass only the higher frequencies of 4000, 6000, and 8000 Hz. Discrimination usually is not affected adversely when the loss is in this higher frequency range because most speech sounds are in the area < 4000 Hz. A slight reduction in the discrimination score may occur in patients with

sensorineural hearing loss involving ≥ 2000 Hz. Generally, patients with these high-frequency losses experience more difficulty in daily conversation than their discrimination score would suggest.

In the interpretation of a discrimination score, it should be recalled that the test was done in a quiet room and therefore does not measure the patient's ability to discriminate against a noisy background. In such an environment, discrimination probably would be worse because consonants are masked by the noise. At present, there is no completely reliable method of measuring an individual's ability to get along in everyday conversation under varied circumstances.

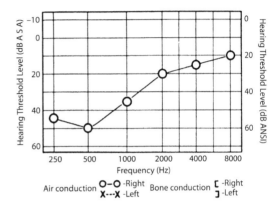

Figure 7.4 One patient had this audiogram as a result of otosclerosis. The discrimination score was 98%. Another patient had this same audiogram as a result of acoustic neuroma. The discrimination score was 42%. Still another patient had an identical audiogram as a result of Ménière's disease. The discrimination score was 62%. *Abbreviations*: ANSI, American National Standards Institute; ASA, American Standards Association.

## Causes of reduced discrimination

Discrimination scores are lower in patients with hearing loss due to presbycusis or most congenital causes. Severe reductions in discrimination are associated particularly with two principal causes, Ménière's syndrome and acoustic neuroma.

In Ménière's syndrome, the discrimination difficulty generally is attributed to the distortion produced in the cochlea, that is, distortion in loudness, pitch, and clarity of speech. The characteristic finding in severe Ménière's syndrome is that the discrimination score becomes even worse as speech is made louder (**Figure 7.5**).

Discrimination scores generally remain good in hearing loss caused by noise alone. They are rarely much <85%, although they may be slightly lower in far advanced cases.

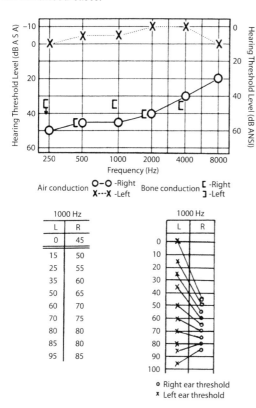

Figure 7.5 Audiogram of patient with Ménière's disease in right ear. Discrimination score: 62% at 70 dB, 42% at 80 dB, and 30% at 90 dB. ABLB testing (lower graphs) demonstrate hyper recruitment. Note that not only does the 1000-Hz tone sound equally loud in both ears at 80 dB but also an 85-dB tone in the bad right ear sounds as loud as a 95-dB tone in the normal left ear. Diplacusis is marked, with the higher-sounding and distorted tone in the right ear. *Abbreviations*: ABLB, alternate binaural loudness balance; ANSI, American National Standards Institute. ASA, American Standards Association.

When discrimination is significantly worse, other causes should be considered. Noise damages primarily outer hair cells, as discussed in Chapter 14.

In acoustic neuroma, the damage to the auditory nerve fibers may produce very little reduction in the hearing threshold level for pure tones but a disproportionately large reduction in the discrimination score. This disproportion is an important clue to the presence of acoustic neuroma, one that should be watched for in every case of sensorineural hearing loss, especially unilateral cases.

## The glycerol test

This test is used by some physicians to help establish a diagnosis of Ménière's syndrome and to help predict response to diuretic therapy or endolymphatic sac operation. Pure-tone and speech audiometry is performed immediately before and 3 hours after a single oral dose of glycerol, 2.3 mL/kg of body weight of 50% glycerol solution. Pure-tone threshold improvement of at least 10 dB in three adjacent octave bands and/or a speech discrimination improvement > 12% constitutes a positive test and suggests reversibility of the inner ear hydrops. Agents other than glycerol also may be used.

## Masking

Because masking often is overlooked in discrimination testing and speech reception testing, its importance must be reiterated. If the nontest ear is not masked properly, serious errors in diagnosis can be made (**Figure 7.6**).

## Etiology

From the examples in **Figures 7.4–7.6**, it is obvious that it is not always possible to predict the discrimination score from the pure-tone audiogram. The etiology is of the utmost importance in assessing the discrimination.

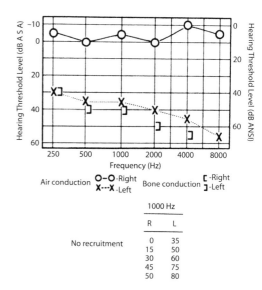

Figure 7.6 Audiogram of patient with an acoustic neuroma. There was abnormal tone decay in the left ear during the 60-second test (right ear masked). *Abbreviations*: ANSI, American National Standards Institute; ASA, American Standards Association.

## Clues to discrimination

These tests require equipment that may not be available in the offices of many practitioners. Nevertheless, even a careful history and examination will give a rough estimate of a patient's ability to hear and to distinguish speech. For example, the patient should be asked how well he/she does with each ear when using the telephone. The patient may volunteer that though voices sound loud enough, he/she cannot understand conversations on the telephone. This usually indicates a reduction in discrimination ability.

Another important clue to discrimination ability is whether the patient experiences more difficulty in noisy environments. If he/she does, it is probably because he/she has reduced discrimination, which is aggravated further by environmental noise that masks out the normally weak consonants. He/she also may have trouble with understanding higher-pitched female voices. The physician who has no hearing testing equipment in his/her office may obtain a fair idea of a patient's discrimination score by asking the patient to repeat words in the PB lists when the physician presents them without letting the patient see the examiner's face. The words should be spoken at a normal level of intensity and enunciated normally. If the loss is unilateral, the better ear must be masked with noise intense enough to prevent its participation in the test. The same precaution is necessary during testing with audiometric equipment. Scores obtained without masking the opposite ear can result in a wrong diagnosis.

## TESTS FOR RECRUITMENT

The phenomenon of recruitment has been defined elsewhere in this book as a disproportionate increase in the sensation of loudness of a sound when its intensity is raised. The principal value of detecting recruitment is that it helps to trace the site of the lesion in the auditory pathway to the hair cells of the cochlea. The patient often provides clues to the presence of cochlear damage when he/she is questioned about hearing difficulty. The patient may say that loud noises are very bothersome in his/her bad ear or that the sound seems to be tinny, harsh, and very unclear. He/she may volunteer that music sounds distorted or flat. These complaints should not be confused with the annoyance voiced by a neurotic patient who hears well but is bothered by such noises as the shouting of children. A well-defined sensorineural hearing loss is prerequisite to utilize recruitment as a basis for localizing an auditory deficit to the cochlea.

## TUNING FORK

Recruitment can be detected in some cases with the aid of a 512-Hz tuning fork if a hearing loss affects the speech frequencies, as often occurs in Ménière's disease. The test is done by comparing the growth of loudness in the good ear with that in the bad ear. The fork is struck once gently and held up to each of the patient's ears, and he/she is asked in which ear the tone sounds louder. Naturally, he/she will say the tone is louder in the ear that has better or normal hearing. Then, the intensity of the tone is increased by striking the fork once again quite hard (but not too hard, or the tone may be distorted). The patient then is asked again to indicate in which ear the tone now sounds louder, with the fork held first near the good ear and then quickly moved to about the same distance from the bad ear. If hyperrecruitment is present, the patient will now exclaim in surprise that the tone is as loud or louder in the bad ear. This means that there has been a larger growth in the sensation of loudness in the bad ear, in spite of a hearing loss.

## ALTERNATE BINAURAL LOUDNESS BALANCE TEST

Testing for recruitment with a tuning fork is a rather rough technique, but it may help in diagnosing recruitment. More precise tests have been devised to test for recruitment, but most of these are suitable for use only when one ear is impaired and the other is normal. The technique in common use is called the alternate binaural loudness balance (ABLB) test, which matches the loudness of a given tone in each ear.

This is done with an audiometer and involves presenting a tone of a certain intensity to the good ear and then alternately applying it to the bad ear at various intensities; the patient is asked to report when the tone is equally loud in both ears. Initially, a brief tone 15 dB above threshold is applied to the good ear. Then, the tone is presented briefly to the bad ear 15 dB above its threshold, and the patient is asked whether the tone was louder or softer than that heard in the good ear. According to the response, necessary adjustments are made to the intensity going to the bad ear until a loudness balance is obtained with the good ear. Then, the intensity to the good ear is increased by another 15 dB, and another balance is obtained with the bad ear. Loudness balancing is continued in 15-dB steps until sufficient information is obtained about the growth of loudness in the bad ear. This technique requires that the same frequency be balanced in the two ears and that the tone be presented alternately to the good ear, which serves as the reference. Also, the difference in threshold between the two ears should be at least 20 dB for this test to be valid.

If the difference in loudness level between the two ears is unchanged at higher intensities, recruitment is absent. If the loudness difference gradually decreased at higher intensities, recruitment is present. If the loudness difference completely disappears between the two ears at higher intensities, the condition is called complete recruitment and is indicative of damage to the inner ear. There may be hyper-recruitment, in which the tone in the bad ear sounds even louder than the tone in the good ear at some point above threshold. Recruitment may occur at varying speeds. If it continues regularly with each increase of intensity, it is called continuous recruitment, and this is indicative of inner ear damage. Recruitment that is found only at or near-threshold levels is not necessarily characteristic of inner ear damage but occurs often in patients with sensorineural hearing impairment. **Figures 7.5** and **7.7** show two cases that exhibit recruitment, with methods of recording the result.

## DETECTION OF SMALL CHANGES IN INTENSITY

Another method of demonstrating recruitment involves the patient's ability to detect small changes in intensity. A recruiting ear detects smaller changes in intensity than normal ears or those with conductive hearing loss. At levels near threshold, a normal ear is likely to require a change of ~2 dB to recognize a difference in loudness, but in an ear that recruits, only a 0.5-dB increase may be necessary to detect the loudness change. As the intensity of the tone then increases in normal ears, the change necessary for detecting the difference in loudness becomes smaller, whereas the recruiting ear requires about the same change as it did near-threshold level.

## SHORT-INCREMENT SENSITIVITY INDEX TEST

Another test for localizing the site of damage to the cochlea is the short-increment sensitivity index (SISI) test. It measures the patient's ability to hear small, shortchanges of sound intensity. The test is done monaurally by fixing the level of a steady tone at 20 dB above the patient's threshold at each frequency to be tested and superimposing on this steady tone 1-dB increments of ~200 milliseconds duration, interspersing the increments at 5-second intervals. The patient is to respond each time he hears any "jumps in loudness." If he/she hears five of the 1-dB increments, his/her sensitivity index is 25%. A score of between 60% and 100% at frequencies > 1000 Hz is positive for cochlear disorders, whereas a score <20% is considered to be negative. Scores between 20% and 60% are inconclusive.

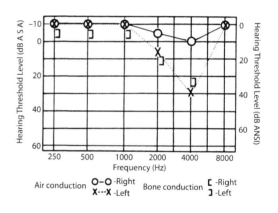

Air conduction: O—O -Right, X---X -Left  Bone conduction: [ -Right, ] -Left

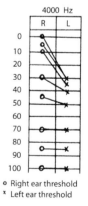

| 4000 | Hz |
| --- | --- |
| R | L |
| 0 | 30 |
| 5 | 30 |
| 10 | 35 |
| 30 | 40 |
| 45 | 50 |
| 70 | 70 |
| 85 | 85 |
| 100 | 100 |

o Right ear threshold
x Left ear threshold

**Figure 7.7** Audiogram of 21-year-old male with acoustic trauma of the left ear caused by explosion of a firecracker. Two methods of recording results of loudness balance tests (ABLB) are shown. *Abbreviations*: ANSI, American National Standards Institute; ASA, American Standards Association.

A revised form of the test called the high-intensity SISI uses a similar technique but with very loud tones rather than near-threshold tones. In high-intensity SISI testing, patients with cochlear hearing loss and those with normal hearing will exhibit a high percentage of responses to the short-increment increases. However, patients with retrocochlear disease, such as an acoustic neuroma, will continue to have low percentage scores. Thus, both the classical SISI and the high-intensity tests help to differentiate not only between cochlear and non-cochlear but also cochlear and retrocochlear pathology. However, the SISI test has many shortcomings and is of limited value.

## OTHER TESTS

There are more tests using speech discrimination and Békésy audiometry that also help to determine the presence of cochlear damage; these are supplementary to the basic tests described here. They are especially helpful when both ears have a hearing loss because a "control" ear is not essential to the test procedure. Stapedius reflex testing also is useful in these cases (see *Impedance Audiometry* section).

## TESTING FOR DIPLACUSIS— DISTORTION OF PITCH

Another simple and fairly reliable office test can be done with a tuning fork to help to localize the site of auditory damage in the cochlea. This test explores not distortion of loudness (recruitment) but distortion of pitch, which is called diplacusis. Distortion is the hallmark of hair cell damage.

A 512 Hz tuning fork is struck and held near the normal ear and then near the opposite ear. If the damage is localized in the cochlea, the patient may report that the same tuning fork has a different pitch when it is heard in the bad ear. Usually, he/she will say that the pitch is higher or lower and not as clear but rather fuzzy. It is important to clarify to the patient when this test is performed that he/she is being asked to evaluate pitch, not loudness; otherwise, inaccurate results may be obtained. This test may be performed with tuning forks of various frequencies. It is not rare for pitch distortion to be located primarily at frequencies that are affected by hearing loss.

## HEARING TESTS USING SPEECH TO DETECT CENTRAL HEARING LOSS

Special tests using modified speech are becoming very useful in deciding whether a hearing loss is caused by damage in the central nervous system. Lesions in the cortex do not result in reduction in pure-tone thresholds, but brainstem lesions may cause some high-frequency hearing loss. Routine speech audiometry is almost always normal in cortical lesions. Sometimes it is impaired in brainstem lesions but without a characteristic pattern. As neither pure tone nor routine speech tests help to localize damage in the central nervous system, more complex tests have been developed to help to provide this information.

A chief function of the cortex is to convert neural impulses into meaningful information. Words and sentences acquire their significance at the cortical level. Because quality, space, and time are factors governing the cortical identification of a verbal pattern, the tests are designed so that they explore the synthesizing ability of the cortex when one or more of these factors is purposely changed.

## BINAURAL TEST OF AUDITORY FUSION

One such test of central auditory dysfunction is the binaural test of auditory fusion. Speech signals are transmitted through two different narrowband filters. Each band by itself is too narrow to allow recognition of test words. Subjects who have normal hearing show excellent integration of test words when they receive the signals from one filter in one ear and the other filter in the other ear. Poorer scores are made by patients with brain lesions and are indications of a functional failure within the cortex.

## SOUND LOCALIZATION TESTS

Sound localization tests also are being used in the diagnosis of central lesions. Deviation of the localization band to one side points to a cerebral lesion on the contralateral side or to a brainstem lesion on the ipsilateral side.

## OTHER TESTS

*Distorted-voice, interrupted-voice,* and *accelerated-voice tests* likewise are used in detecting central lesions. In the distorted-voice test, PB words are administered ~50 dB above threshold through a low-pass filter that is able to reduce the discrimination to ~70% or 80% in normal subjects. Patients with temporal-lobe tumors present an average discrimination score that is poorer in the ear contralateral to the tumor.

The interrupted-voice test presents PB words at ~50 dB above thresholds, interrupting them periodically 10 times/second. Subjects with normal hearing obtain ~80% discrimination; those with temporal-lobe tumors have reduced discrimination in the ear contralateral to the tumor.

In the accelerated-voice test, when the number of words per minute is increased from ~150 to ~350 words, discrimination remains near 100% in subjects who have normal hearing, but threshold is raised by 10–15 dB. In patients with tumors of the temporal lobe, there is a normal threshold shift, but the discrimination never attains 100% in the contralateral ear. In cortical lesions, the impairment always seems to be in the ear contralateral to the neoplasms and moderate in extent. Brainstem lesions exhibit ipsilateral or bilateral impairments.

Ipsilateral and contralateral stapedius reflex tests also may be abnormal in the setting of central nervous system diseases affecting hearing.

## NEUROPSYCHOLOGICAL TESTING

When central auditory processing disorders are suspected, it is often helpful to refer the patient for formal neuropsychological testing. This approach helps map the site of brain dysfunction, confirms the auditory processing ability, and detects any other cognitive deficits. Neuropsychologists' treatment recommendations also may be extremely useful in the care of these patients.

## TESTING FOR FUNCTIONAL HEARING LOSS

Whenever a patient claims to have a hearing loss that does not seem to be based on organic damage to the auditory pathway, or whenever the test responses and the general behavior of the patient appear to be questionable, a variety of tests can be performed to help determine whether the loss is functional rather than organic.

## SUGGESTIVE CLUES

The most suggestive findings are inconsistencies in the hearing tests. For instance, one such typical patient has a hearing threshold level of 70 dB in one test and a 40-dB threshold when the test is repeated several minutes later. Another common scenario is when the patient replies to soft speech behind his/her back but has an audiogram of a patient show a 60-dB average hearing loss bilaterally, but the patient inadvertently replies to soft speech behind his/her back. Other common "tells" of functional hearing loss include mismatches of SRT and pure-tone averages and excellent speech discrimination ability in the setting of hearing loss with absent or poor responses on bone conduction tests. However, care must be exercised in these judgments. Certain organic conditions such as Ménière's disease, multiple sclerosis, and severe tinnitus also may cause inconsistent responses on audiometric testing.

In addition, the patient's behavior may not be consistent with the degree of loss claimed, especially in cases of bilateral functional hearing loss. Usually, a patient with severe bilateral deafness is very attentive to the speaker's face and mouth in order to benefit from lipreading. A functionally deaf person may not show this attentiveness. He/she also may have unusually good voice control, which is not consistent with the degree of loss. Occasionally, a functionally deaf person will assume an incompetent attitude or repeat part of a test word correctly and labor excessively over the last half of the word. These and other clues should alert the examiner to the possibility of the presence of a purely functional hearing loss or a functional overlay on an organic hearing loss.

## LOMBARD OR VOICE-REFLEX TEST

When a patient claims deafness in one ear, but it is suspected of being functional, several simple tests are available to determine the validity of the loss. The patient is given a newspaper or a magazine article to read aloud without stopping. While he/she is reading, the tester presents noise to the good ear. This may be done by rubbing a piece of thin paper over the patient's good ear. If the patient's voice does not get significantly louder, it is highly suggestive that he/she can hear in the supposedly "bad" ear. Because hearing also serves as a feedback mechanism that informs the speaker how loud he is speaking, a person with normal hearing will speak more loudly in a very noisy area in order to be heard above the noise. If the patient does not raise his/her voice when noise is applied to one ear, it means that he/she is hearing their speech in the other ear, and consequently that ear does not have the marked hearing loss indicated on the pure-tone or speech audiogram. A Bárány noise apparatus or the noise from an audiometer noise generator is extremely effective in this test because the level of the noise can be controlled. This type of test is called the Lombard or voice-reflex test, and although it does not help to establish thresholds, it does give the examiner some idea of whether or not the hearing loss is exaggerated.

## STENGER TEST

The Stenger test also is used for detecting unilateral functional hearing loss and evaluating the approximate amount of residual hearing. This test can be done with tuning forks or with an audiometer, the latter being the more reliable.

The Stenger test depends on a given pure tone presented to both ears simultaneously. The tone will be perceived in the ear where it is louder. If the sound in one ear is made louder, then the listener will hear it in that ear and will not realize that a weaker sound exists in the other ear.

A tone is presented to the good ear ~10 dB above threshold and, at the same time, 10 dB below the admitted threshold in the bad ear. If the patient responds, the test is a negative Stenger because he/she heard the tone in the good ear without realizing there was a weaker tone in the bad ear. If the patient does not respond, it is a positive Stenger because he/she heard the sound in the assumed bad ear without realizing there was a tone of weaker intensity presented to the good ear.

This test can be done with speech as well as pure tones. There must be a difference of at least 30 dB between thresholds of the good and allegedly bad ear for the test to be effective. Also, a two-channel audiometer is needed to administer the test.

The Stenger test also enables the examiner to obtain an approximation of the patient's true thresholds in the bad ear (1). This is done by presenting the pure tone 10 dB above threshold in the good ear and presenting a pure tone at 0 Hz in the bad ear. The tone in the bad ear is increased in 5-dB steps until the patients stops responding. The Stenger pure-tone threshold of the bad ear is ~15 dB above his or her true threshold.

## REPETITION OF AUDIOGRAM WITHOUT MASKING

Still another test to indicate whether a patient really has a severe or total unilateral hearing loss or may be malingering is to repeat the audiogram but this time without masking the good ear. As a pure tone presented to the test ear can be heard also in the nontest ear when the loudness of the tone is 50–55 dB above the threshold of the nontest ear, at least some shadow curve should be present in the absence of masking. If the patient does not respond when the intensity levels reach this point, then the chances are that he/she has a functional deafness in the test ear or is malingering. If the patient does report hearing the tone, he/she should be questioned carefully about its location. Again, total lack of response is an indication of the dilemma that the functional patient faces when he/she feels that his/her claim is threatened with exposure.

## DELAYED AUDITORY-FEEDBACK TEST

The monitoring effect of an ear also can be disrupted if a person listens to himself/herself speak through earphones while the return voice is delayed in time. A delay of 0.1–0.2 second causes symptoms similar to stuttering. If this occurs when the feedback level is lower than the admitted threshold, functional loss or malingering is present. In the delayed talk-back test (also called the delayed auditory-feedback test), which is done through a modified tape recorder, it is possible to detect hearing losses of sizable degree but not the minor exaggerations that occur occasionally in medicolegal situations. This is so because delayed feedback affects the rhythm and the rate of the patient's speech at levels averaging 20–40 dB above threshold.

## PSYCHOGALVANIC SKIN RESPONSE TEST

The psychogalvanic skin response (PGSR) test is close to being an objective test of hearing, though it still has many shortcomings. This technique is based to some extent on the traditional lie detector method. The patient is conditioned so that each time he/she hears a tone, it is followed about a second later by a definite electric shock through an electrode strapped to the leg. Through electrodes placed on the patient's fingers or palms, it is possible to measure the change in skin resistance elicited by the electric shock in the patient's leg. Each time that the patient receives a shock, the skin resistance is altered and can be read on a meter or recorded on a moving graph. After the patient is conditioned well, the electric shock is stopped, and only the sound is given. In a well-conditioned patient, about a second after the sound is applied, he/she will "expect" the shock again and show a typical change in the electrodermal responses. It can be concluded, then, that each time the patient gives a positive reading on the recording equipment after a sound is given, he/she has heard the sound. By lowering the intensity of the stimulus, a threshold level can be obtained. At certain intervals, it is necessary to reinforce the conditioned response mechanism by reapplying the electric shock.

Many complicating factors make PGSR testing far from a completely reliable method of measuring a hearing threshold level objectively and reliably. It may be helpful in establishing whether or not a hearing loss is organic or nonorganic if it is used in conjunction with a battery of other tests. PGSR is currently rarely used.

## BRAINSTEM EVOKED-RESPONSE AUDIOMETRY IN MALINGERING

Brainstem evoked-response audiometry (BERA) is discussed in greater detail later in this chapter. However, because BERA testing is objective, the technique may provide valuable information in malingerers and patients with functional hearing loss. Despite its limitations, BERA testing may be helpful in assessing auditory function in patients who are unable or unwilling to cooperate.

## USE OF EXCELLENT AUDIOMETRIC TECHNIQUE

One of the most effective methods of obviating intentional functional hearing loss, particularly in industry and in school hearing testing programs, is to use excellent audiometric technique. Malingering and inaccurate responses are discouraged by a tester who uses excellent technique. Malingering normal hearing also is possible. If a patient is given a sound and is asked repeatedly, "Do you hear it?" he/she will be tempted to say, "yes," even if he/she does not hear it, whenever some advantage or remuneration is at stake, such as obtaining employment.

### Responsibility of the tester

The question as to what a tester in industry or in a school should do when he/she suspects or detects a malingerer or someone with functional hearing loss is important. It is not the tester's responsibility to accuse or even to imply to the subject that he/she is suspected of giving inaccurate responses. Quite often, inaccurate responses are the result of disturbances in the auditory tract or nervous pathway, or the loss may be the result of conversion disorder or other psychiatric disability. The tester may not be qualified to express so sophisticated a judgment. The tester's only responsibility is to suspect that the audiogram does not represent the accurate threshold of hearing of the individual tested.

The subjects should be handled in a routine manner, and subsequently the findings should be brought to the attention of the physician in charge of the hearing testing program. If the physician is suitably trained to study the patient on a more comprehensive basis, he/she should proceed to do so. If not, the patient should be referred to an otologist or a hearing center that is equipped to study the problem.

## TESTING FOR AUDITORY TONE DECAY

Just as marked recruitment usually is indicative of damage in the inner ear, abnormal tone decay (abnormal auditory fatigue) usually is a sign of pressure on or damage to the auditory nerve fibers. This phenomenon may be of particular importance in that it can be an early sign of an acoustic neuroma or some other neoplasm invading the posterior fossa.

## ADMINISTRATION OF TEST

The test for abnormal tone decay is very simple to perform and should be considered in every case of unilateral sensorineural hearing loss, especially when no recruitment is found. The test is based on the fact that whereas a person with normal hearing can continue to hear a steady threshold tone for at least 1 minute, the patient who has a tumor pressing on his/her auditory nerve is unable to keep hearing a threshold tone for this length of time. The test is performed monaurally with an audiometer. A frequency that shows reduced threshold is selected, and the patient is instructed to raise a finger as long as he/she can hear the tone. The tone then is presented at threshold or 5 dB above threshold, and a stopwatch is started with the presentation of the tone. Each time the patient lowers his/her finger, the intensity is increased 5 dB, and the time is noted for that period of hearing. The tone interrupter switch never is released from the "on" position during any of the intensity changes. The test is 1 minute in duration.

## FINDINGS

A person with normal tone decay usually will continue to hold up his/her finger during the entire 60 seconds. Occasionally, he/she may require a 5-or 10-dB increase during the first part of the test, but he/she then maintains the tone for the remainder of the time. A patient who has abnormal tone decay may lower the finger after only ~10 seconds, and when the tone is raised 5 dB, he/she may lower his/her finger again after another 10 seconds and continue to indicate that the tone fades out repeatedly, until after 60 seconds there may be an increase of ≥25 dB above the original threshold. Some patients may even fail to hear the tone at the maximum intensity of the audiometer after 1 minute, whereas originally, they may have heard the threshold tone at 25 dB. Masking may be required. This finding of abnormal tone decay is highly suggestive of pressure on the auditory nerve fibers. **Figure 7.6** describes a typical case. A tuning fork can also be used to detect abnormal tone decay by testing for threshold, then fatiguing the ear and retesting for threshold. Modifications of this method can also be used.

## DIAGNOSTIC SELF-RECORDING AUDIOMETRY

## BÉKÉSY AUDIOMETRY

Another method of measuring abnormal tone decay is with a Békésy audiometer. This is a type of self-recording audiometer that is used for threshold and special testing. Similar but less well-controlled and potentially less accurate audiometric self-testing can be performed with computer and smartphone apps.

## PROCEDURE AND MECHANISM

This method of establishing pure-tone thresholds permits the patient to trace his/her own audiogram as the tone or tones are presented automatically. Each ear is tested separately. The patient holds a hand switch and has a set of earphones through which he/she hears the tone. As soon as he/she hears the tone, he/she presses the switch, which causes the sound to decrease in loudness, and holds it down until the tone is gone. This procedure continues until the full range of frequencies has been tested.

The switch controls the attenuator of the audiometer that decreases or increases the intensity of the tone. A pen geared to the attenuator makes a continuous record on an audiogram blank of the patient's intensity adjustments. The audiogram is placed on a table that moves in relation to the frequency being presented. Several methods of frequency selection are available. The audiometer can be set up to produce the frequency range continuously from 100 to 10,000 Hz, or it can be arranged to test hearing in a two-octave range or, if desired, to test threshold for a single frequency for several minutes.

The test signal can be continuous, that is, without interruption, or pulsed at a rate of ~2½ times/second. Operation of the patient's hand switch attenuates the signal at a rate of ~2.5–5 dB/second according to the speed selection made by the examiner. Thus, a test routinely performed with Békésy self-recording audiometry can determine thresholds with both pulsed- and continuous-tone presentations. It is important that the patient not see recording of the audiogram while it is being performed; awareness of the recordings may affect his/her responses and result in an invalid audiogram.

## VALUE

With proper instruction to the patient, Békésy audiometry not only provides an accurate picture of thresholds but also supplies other valuable information. By comparing the thresholds for the pulsed and the continuous tone, the physician can get a reasonably good indication of the site of the lesion within the auditory system.

## TYPES OF BÉKÉSY AUDIOGRAMS

In normal or conductively impaired ears, the pulsed and continuous tracings overlap for the entire frequency range tested. This is a type I audiogram. In the type II audiogram, the pulsed and continuous tones overlap in the low frequencies, but between 500 and 1000 Hz, the continuous-frequency tracing drops ~15 dB below the pulsed tracing and then remains parallel with the high frequencies. Type II audiograms occur in cases of cochlear involvement. Sometimes the difference between pulsed and continuous audiograms narrow to ~5 dB in the higher frequencies. Cases of cochlear involvement sometimes also show type I tracings.

In the type III audiogram, the continuous tracing drops suddenly away from the pulsed tracing and usually continues down to the intensity limits of the audiometer. Eighth-nerve disorders usually show type III audiograms. Another type of audiogram found in eighth-nerve disorders is the type IV tracing, in which the continuous-tone tracing stays well below the pulsed tracing at all frequencies.

## INTERPRETATION OF THE BÉKÉSY AUDIOGRAM

There is some feeling that the amplitude of the Békésy audiogram provides considerable information about the presence or the absence of recruitment. For example, tracings of very small amplitude might lead one to believe that the patient can detect changes in intensity much smaller than the average subject and that he/she therefore has recruitment. Unfortunately, this is not the case. It is more likely that tracings of small amplitude are suggestive of abnormal tone decay rather than of recruitment. A great deal of the interpretation depends on the on-and-off period of the tone presented. **Figures 7.8 and 7.9** show examples of Békésy audiograms.

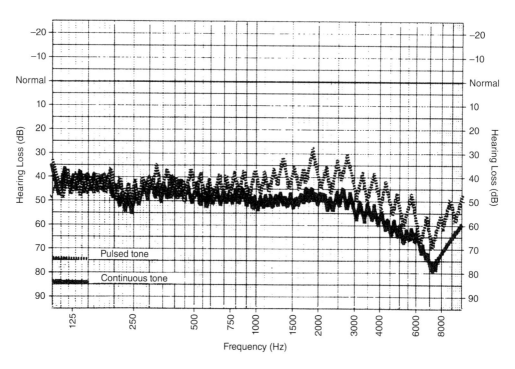

Figure 7.8 Békésy tracings of a patient with Ménière's disease. A slight separation of the pulsed- and the continuous-tone tracings appears only in the higher frequencies.

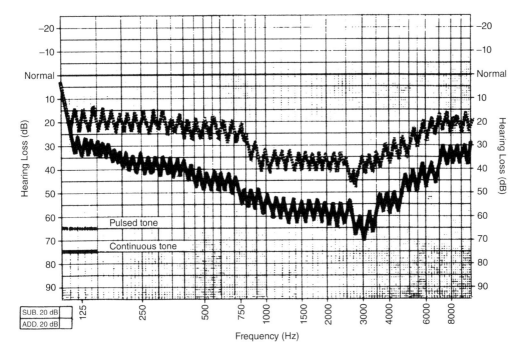

Figure 7.9 Békésy tracings in a case of acoustic neuroma. Tone decay is demonstrated by a large gap between the pulsed- and the continuous-tone tracings. In some cases, the continuous-tone tracing may break completely away at ~500 Hz, and the tone may not be heard even at the maximum output of the audiometer.

## NONDIAGNOSTIC SELF-RECORDING AUDIOMETRY

Whereas the Békésy audiometer is used in the battery of diagnostic tests, other self-recording audiometers are used for establishing pure-tone thresholds only. These self-recording audiometers present discrete individual frequencies that are changed automatically at 30-second intervals and can present both pulsed and continuous tones at the option of the operator. **Figure 7.10** shows an example of an audiogram obtained with a self-recording audiometer.

There is a feeling that hearing thresholds obtained with self-recording audiometers in the industrial setting may be more legally acceptable because the operator does not participate in the test. There are, however, specific procedures that must be adhered to if validity and reliability are to be assured. These include proper instructions to the subject and monitoring the test in the beginning and at intervals as the test proceeds (a common misconception is that the operator can "walk

away" from the area while the audiogram table and recording pen cannot be observed by the subject). When the test is completed, the tracings should be studied by the operator to ascertain that all are acceptable.

A trained, experienced technician generally can recognize an unreliable or invalid self-recorded audiogram or a reticent subject by using certain clues. (a) Barring a language problem, an employee may refuse to follow the directions of the operator or claim he/she does not understand the instructions about his/her role in performing the hearing test. Repeated attempts to instruct the subject do not result in improved operation. (b) On repeat tests, the employee may be unable to give reasonably similar responses, and this will result in a wide disparity between threshold tracings. (c) The subject may not respond at all to the tones, as though totally deaf, yet will be able to carry on a normal conversation with the examiner. (d) The audiogram may show extremely wide tracing sweeps, which makes it impossible to ascertain the actual threshold. There should be at least six crossings of threshold at each frequency, and a line drawn through the midpoints should be parallel to the time axis on the audiogram (horizontal). (e) Occasionally, an employee may show a moderate=-to-severe, mostly flat, loss, which ordinarily would cause little doubt as to its validity in the mind of the operator, except that such a pattern is uncommon and should raise the suspicion that perhaps the subject was pressing and releasing his/her hand switch in a perfectly timed sequence. (f) In some types of self-recording audiometers, it is possible to feign normal hearing by keeping the button depressed during the entire test sequence. If the operator has difficulty in communicating with the subject (again barring a language problem) and yet the audiogram indicates extremely keen hearing, there is reason to doubt the accuracy of the audiogram. Should any pattern appear suspicious, the questionable frequencies or the entire audiogram should be repeated. If responses remain unsatisfactory, the test should be repeated in the manual mode if the audiometer is so equipped, or it should be repeated on a backup manual audiometer.

Self-recording audiometers do allow some mobility of the technician (although this aspect tends to be abused) and permit one technician to test several people at the same time. As in all modes of hearing testing, proper audiometer calibration and satisfactory ambient-noise levels in the test area must be maintained. All technicians, no matter what test method is employed, should be properly trained and certified.

## IMPEDANCE AUDIOMETRY

Impedance audiometry is a comparatively new evaluation tool. It supplements otoscopic and audiometric findings and adds new capabilities to hearing evaluation.

Impedance audiometry is an objective method for evaluating the integrity and function of the auditory mechanism. It includes four separate types of measurement and has the potential for a much wider role as research in its use continues. The procedures most often used are as follows: (a) tympanometry, (b) static compliance, (c) physical volume (PV), (d) acoustic reflex thresholds, (e) acoustic reflex decay and other impedance test, (f) continuous-frequency audiometry, (g) tinnitus matching, and (h) high-frequency audiometry.

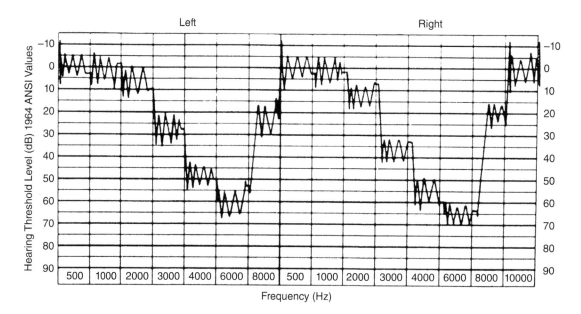

Figure 7.10 Self-recorded audiogram showing normal hearing in the low frequencies and at 8000 Hz and impairment at 3000, 4000, and 6000 Hz. *Abbreviation*: ANSI, American National Standards Institute.

# TYMPANOMETRY

The eardrum and ossicles comprise a mechanism that should transfer vibrating energy efficiently. Tympanometry measures the mobility of this system. It is analogous to pneumatic otoscopy. If the system becomes stiffer and more resistant because some condition impedes its free movement, we are able to measure the abnormal impedance (or its reciprocal "compliance"). The impedance of the middle ear system is measured by its response to variations in air pressure on the eardrum. The entrance of the ear canal is sealed with a probe tip containing three holes: one for supply of air pressure, one for a low-frequency probe tone (usually of 220 Hz), and the third opening connected to a pick-up microphone. As controlled degrees of positive and negative air pressure are introduced into the sealed ear canal, the resulting movement of the mechanism is plotted or automatically graphed on a chart called a tympanogram (**Figure 7.11**).

## STATIC COMPLIANCE

Static compliance is a measure of middle ear mobility. It is measured in terms of equivalent volume in $cm^3$, based on two volume measurements. (a) C1 is made with the tympanic membrane (TM) in a position of poor compliance with +200 mm $H_2O$ in the external canal. (b) C2 is made with TM at maximal compliance. C1 − C2 = static compliance, which cancels out the compliance due to the column of air in the external canal. The remainder is the compliance due to the middle ear mechanisms.

Static compliance is low when the value is < 0.28 $cm^3$ and high when > 2.5 $cm^3$. Its major contribution is to differentiate between a fixed middle ear and a middle ear discontinuity.

**Tympanogram Type A**

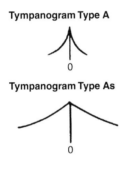

0

Normal middle ear function.
Normal compliance.
Normal middle ear pressure at the point of maximum compliance.

**Tympanogram Type As**

0

Normal middle ear pressure.
Limited compliance.
Seen in otosclerosis, thick or scarred tympanic membranes and occasionally in tympanosclerosis.
Indicative of "stiffness" or shallow curve.

**Tympanogram Type Ad**

0

Excessive compliance.
Seen in discontinuity of the ossicular chain or thinly healed tympanic membrane.
Indicative of "disarticulation" or deep curve.

**Tympanogram Type B**

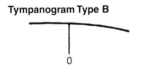

0

Little or no compliance.
Seen in serous and adhesive otitis media, congenital middle ear malformation, clogged ventilating but occluded ear canals and perforate tympanic membranes.

**Tympanogram Type C**

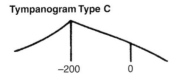

−200        0

Near normal compliance.
Negative air pressure.
Seen in poor eustachian tube function and otitis media.

Figure 7.11 Characteristic tympanograms.

## PHYSICAL VOLUME

The PV test uses a signal of fixed intensities in the ear canal. With an intact TM, the meter will balance at a $cm^3$ value of 1.0–1.5 in an adult and 0.7–1.0 in a child. If the eardrum is not intact, the PV measures will be large, often exceeding 5.0 $cm^3$. It is helpful in ruling out a non-observable perforation and can help to identify obstruction of a ventilating tube.

## ACOUSTIC REFLEX THRESHOLDS

This test determines the level in dB at which the stapedius muscle contracts. Normally, the reflex for pure tones is elicited at ~90 dB above the hearing threshold. For broadband noise, it occurs at ~70 dB above threshold. The contraction occurs bilaterally, even when only one ear is stimulated. In patients with cochlear damage and associated recruitment, the reflex may occur at sensation levels < 60 dB above the auditory pure-tone threshold (Metz recruitment). In bilateral conductive losses and in some unilateral losses, the acoustic reflex may be absent bilaterally. In a unilateral cochlear loss not > 80 dB, acoustic reflexes may appear unilaterally when the stimulation earphone is on the "dead ear" side. These factors then can be diagnostically important, especially when masking is impractical.

## ACOUSTIC REFLEX DECAY AND OTHER IMPEDANCE TESTS

In the normal ear, contraction of the middle ear muscles to a sound 10 dB above the acoustic reflex threshold can be maintained for at least 45 seconds without detectable decay or adaptation. In the presence of an acoustic neuroma or other retrocochlear lesion, however, the middle ear muscle contraction may show fatigue or decay in <10 seconds. In some cases, it may be entirely absent.

Other impedance tests include the *ipsilateral reflex test* for the differential diagnosis of brainstem lesions; *facial nerve test* for localizing the site of a lesion in facial paralysis; *eustachian-tube tests* for determining eustachian-tube function; *fistula test* in which positive air pressure will cause dizziness and deviation of the eyes if a fistula into the inner ear exists; and a test for presence of a *glomus tumor* in which meter variations in synchrony with the pulsebeat can be observed.

Impedance audiometry is especially useful in difficult-to-test patients such as very young children, the mentally impaired, the physically disabled, and the malingerer. Like all other tests, it is not 100% accurate and must be interpreted with expertise.

## CONTINUOUS-FREQUENCY AUDIOMETRY

It must be remembered that audiograms merely sample hearing at selected frequencies, leaving many frequencies between them untested. In some cases, it is helpful to test these frequencies. This can be done with a Békésy audiometer, or with several commercially available audiometers that permit either continuous-frequency testing or testing at ~60-Hz intervals. This kind of test may be useful, for example, a person who complains of ringing tinnitus and fullness in one ear but whose routine audiogram is normal. Continuous-frequency testing may reveal a dip at an in-between frequency, say 6450 Hz, which helps establish the cause of the symptom.

## TINNITUS MATCHING

Several devices are available to help quantify tinnitus, and some newer audiometers include tinnitus-matching capabilities. These tests allow reasonably good quantifications of tinnitus pitch and loudness. Interestingly, tinnitus that is reported by patients as "very loud" is rarely > 5–10 dB above threshold.

## HIGH-FREQUENCY AUDIOMETRY

It is often useful to test hearing thresholds > 8000 Hz, as discussed in Chapter 6. Testing to 12,000 or 14,000 Hz provides the desired information; in most cases, testing at frequencies >14,000 Hz presents special difficulties. High-frequency testing is especially valuable for differentiating presbycusis from occupational hearing loss and detecting early effects of ototoxic drugs. This technique can be useful in selected trauma cases (such as those with tinnitus and normal routine audiograms).

# ELECTROCOCHLEOGRAPHY

This method of assessing difficult-to-test patients involves placing an electrode in the ear and measuring directly the ear's electrical response to a sound stimulus. Most commonly, the electrode is placed through the eardrum into the promontory. In children, this may require a short general anesthetic. Newer electrodes permit high-quality testing with the electrode placed in the ear canal rather than through the TM. With electrodes placed in the ear canal, normal values may vary depending upon electrode type. An ear canal electrode that makes contact with the TM usually yield an abnormal summating potential to action potential (SP/AP) ratio of greater than 35%. For electrodes placed in the ear canal more laterally, an abnormal SP/AP ratio greater than 50% is typical.

Electrocochleography has proven clinically valuable particularly for confirming wave I in the brainstem response if the BERA results are equivocal, and for confirming endolymphatic hydrops in patients with Ménière's syndrome. The SP/AP ratio is used to help determine whether hydrops is present. If the electrode is placed through the eardrum in contact with a promontory, SP/AP ratio of greater than 30% is considered abnormal. This topic is covered in greater detail in Chapter 8.

# PROMONTORY STIMULATION

The promontory stimulation test is suitable for patients with profound deafness and is rarely appropriate in patients with occupational hearing loss. The test involves placement of an electrode through the TM. The electrode is placed against the promontory, and the cochlea is stimulated electrically. The test is used most commonly when assessing patients for possible cochlear implant candidacy.

# EVOKED-RESPONSE AUDIOMETRY

Accurate hearing testing in infants, mentally deficient patients, neurologically disabled patients, and others who cannot or will not volunteer accurate responses is a special problem. A few objective tests (those requiring no patient cooperation) are now available. Impedance audiometry is objective, but it is difficult to determine hearing thresholds from it in some cases. These tests can also be used to confirm hearing thresholds in patients with non-organic hearing loss.

Evoked-response audiometry is similar to electroencephalography or brainwave testing. A darkened, soundproof room is used for testing. Painless electrodes are attached to the patient. A computer is required to isolate the auditory response from the rest of the electrical activity from the brain. Pure-tone or broadband stimuli can be used. There are two types of evoked-response audiometry. More information on evoked responses appears in Chapter 8.

# CORTICAL EVOKED-RESPONSE AUDIOMETRY

This method focuses on electrical activity at the cerebral-cortex level. It allows measurement not only of auditory signals but also of other brainwave variations that are associated with the perception of sound. Therefore, it may prove a valuable tool in evaluating not only thresholds but also whether or not a sound actually reaches a level of perception in the brain. Cortical evoked responses occur at ~200 milliseconds after the stimulus. Unfortunately, they are of limited value for threshold testing because they can be affected volitionally. For example, responses are better if a patient concentrates on an auditory signal than if he/she attempts to ignore it. Cortical evoked responses may also be altered substantially by drugs and state of consciousness.

# MIDDLE LATENCY RESPONSES

Middle latency responses (MLRs) are electrical potentials whose origins are still uncertain. They are thought to be generated by sites central to the brainstem generators, such as the primary auditory cortex, association cortex, and thalamus. Although responses ~40 milliseconds are considered most common, MLRs may be observed between 8 and 50 milliseconds following stimulus onset. MLRs appear to be somewhat more amenable to use for special testing than brainstem responses, but they are also more subject to extraneous influence. Although MLR testing still appears to hold promise for special populations who are difficult to test by traditional means, shortcomings of this procedure have limited its clinical applicability.

## BRAINSTEM EVOKED-RESPONSE AUDIOMETRY

BERA or auditory brainstem responses (ABR) occur within the first 10 milliseconds of the sound-evoked EEG, and they are unaffected by behavior, attention, drugs, or level of consciousness. In fact, BERA can be measured under general anesthesia or during deep coma. They give information about the ear and central auditory pathways at the brainstem level, although not about cortical perception of hearing. BERA has become very popular because it is objective, consistent, and provides a great deal of valuable information. The test measures electrical peaks generated in the brainstem along the auditory pathways. The sites of origin of the waves are still controversial. Traditionally, the following scheme has been believed: Wave I is actually generated at the junction of the hair cell and VIII nerve, but the measured peak occurs in the distal auditory nerve where it leaves the bone and enters the cerebrospinal fluid (CSF) and the internal auditory canal; Wave II comes from the proximal portion of the acoustic nerve, although previously it was believed to originate at the cochlear nucleus; Wave III, at the superior olive; Wave IV, probably at the level of the lateral lemniscus in the pons; Wave V, at the inferior colliculus; Wave VI, probably at the thalamus; and Wave VII, possibly at the cortical level. Although there is good research to support these beliefs, other opinions remain possible. The most common alternate schema is as follows: Wave I, as above; Wave II, proximal portion of the auditory nerve; Wave III, cochlear nucleus; Wave IV, contralateral superior olivary complex; and Wave V, lateral lemniscus. At present, only Waves I–V are used clinically for audiological purposes. Absence or distortion of peaks, or delay between peaks, can help localize lesions in the auditory pathway. For example, difference in latency between a patient's two ears of > 0.2 milliseconds currently are one of the most sensitive audiological tests for detecting acoustic neuromas (2). Nevertheless, it must be stressed that BERA is not sensitive enough to be relied on or to rule out acoustic neuroma and may miss ~40% of tumors ≤1 cm. However, BERA can have other localizing value. The presence of Wave I with absence of later waves may occur following a brainstem vascular accident with normal peripheral hearing and damaged central pathways. Increasing interwave latencies with clear separation of Waves IV and V (which usually overlap) occurs in conditions that cause conduction delay, such as multiple sclerosis. In demyelinating disease, one also sees degradation of later waves aggravated by higher rates of stimulation. Testing can be done with pure tones, broadband noise, or clicks. Approximate threshold levels can be determined. The tests can be used on infants and children and has been used for routine screening in newborn nurseries.

## OTOACOUSTIC EMISSIONS

In 1977, Kemp discovered that the cochlea was capable of producing sound emissions (3). Specifically, Kemp proposed that a biomechanical amplifier within the organ of Corti underlies these properties. This amplifier is the origin of otoacoustic emissions (OAEs) that are generated as a byproduct of the traveling wave-initiated amplitude enhancement of basilar membrane vibration. There are four categories of OAEs: spontaneous, evoked, stimulus frequency, and distortion product. Two groups of OAEs appear to hold promise for future clinical use. Evoked OAEs may be conceptualized as an echo in response to a sound stimulus. They may produce consistent patterns in cochlear pathology with involvement of the outer hair cells such as noise-induced hearing loss, ototoxicity, and hereditary hearing loss. These emissions are also generally absent in hearing loss >30 dB and so are used as a hearing screening tool for infants and other patients who are unable to perform voluntary hearing tests.

Distortion product otoacoustic emissions (DPOAEs) are generated in response to paired pure tones and are felt to be more frequency specific (4). Some researchers feel that DPOAEs can accurately assess boundaries between normal and abnormal hearing with losses up to 50 dB. This category of OAEs may be clinically useful in monitoring changes in the cochlea due to hereditary hearing loss, progressive disease, and ototoxic agents. Research in the area of OAEs is still ongoing. However, they are utilized fairly often clinically. Chapter 8 provides more detail on this subject.

## REFERENCES

1. Rintelmann W, ed. Hearing Assessment. Baltimore, MD: University Park Press, 1979: 404–406.

2. Schmidt RJ, Sataloff RT, Newman J, Spiegel JR, Myers DL. The sensitivity of auditory brainstem response testing for the diagnosis of acoustic neuromas. Arch Otolaryngol Head Neck Surg 2001; 127:19–22.

3. Kemp OT. Stimulated acoustic emissions from within the human auditory system. J Acoust Soc Am 1978; 64:1386–1391.

4. Lonsbury-Martin BL, Harris FP, Stanger BB, Hawkins MD, Martin GK. Distortion product emissions in humans I. Basic properties in normally hearing subjects. Ann Otol Rhino! Laryngol 1990; 99:3–14.

# 8

# Auditory-evoked phenomena: Theory and clinical applications

MARK T. AGRAMA, ROBERT THAYER SATALOFF, AND THOMAS O. WILLCOX Jr.

The diagnosis and evaluation of hearing disorders is one of the foundations of modern otology. Much of our evaluation of hearing consists of a variety of audiometric tests (1). Audiometry helps to identify, characterize, and quantify hearing loss with great accuracy. Traditional audiometry, however, requires the patient to be an active participant in the process. These behavioral tests have only limited utility when the patient cannot or will not provide a subjective response. Examples of these patients include infants, the unconscious, and malingerers (2, 3).

As we have expanded our understanding of the cochlea and its neural pathways, we have developed various objective measures that reflect hearing function. These tests do not rely on the behavioral response of the patient. Instead, they record various electrical and sound phenomena produced by the ear in response to sound stimulus. Electrocochleography (ECOG) provides a measurement of the electrical potentials in the cochlea and the auditory nerve (4). Auditory brainstem response (ABR) measures the electrical potentials in the auditory nerve and higher brainstem structures (5). The testing of otoacoustic emissions (OAEs) consists of recording the sounds produced in the cochlea either spontaneously or in response to sound stimuli (6). Each of these physiologic tests

has specific limitations, yet they provide a powerful complement to traditional audiometry.

This chapter will begin with a brief overview of the history of auditory theory. Each of the three tests of auditory-evoked phenomena, ECOG, ABR, and OAEs, will be reviewed in detail. The description will include their basis in anatomy and physiology and the methods for their recording and analysis. Current and potential applications of auditory-evoked phenomena will then be discussed in the context of the clinical practice of otolaryngology.

## HISTORY OF AUDITORY THEORY

Helmholz described the resonance theory of cochlear function in 1862 (7). He studied acoustics using a series of sound resonators. He theorized that, similar to the strings on a harp, each location on the basilar membrane of the cochlea was tuned to a specific frequency.

In 1944, von Békésy presented his traveling wave theory (8). Using cadaveric cochleas, he showed that the basilar membrane vibrates maximally at different places along its length in response to pure-tone stimulation. The resulting pattern of vibration

DOI: 10.1201/b23379-8

appears as a wave traveling from the base to the apex. The stiffer and less massive basal end is more responsive to higher frequencies, whereas the more flexible and massive apex vibrates more in response to lower frequencies. The peak of the amplitude of the traveling wave corresponds with the point on the basilar membrane most tuned to that frequency.

Although von Békésy's traveling wave theory describes an overall frequency organization of the cochlea, it fails to account for its fine-tuning mechanism. Cadaveric cochleas produce waves that distribute energy passively over a broad section of the basilar membrane. Yet the amount of vibration at the peaks of the traveling waves seen in live animals is much greater than mechanically possible for a passively vibrating system.

In 1948, Gold (9) argued that the cochlea must use active mechanical processes to augment its sensitivity to slight differences in pitch and sound intensity. He theorized that the cochlea expends energy to actively vibrate a narrow segment of the basilar membrane in response to a specific frequency. Gold described a cochlear amplifier which enhances the sensitivity of the cochlea to specific frequencies at low intensity. In addition, he predicted that these vibrations would transmit in reverse to the middle ear, where they would resonate as sound. Gold never proved the existence of these vibrations, however, because of the limitations of his testing equipment.

It was not until 1978 that OAEs were recorded by Kemp (6). He delivered click stimuli to the ears of both normal hearing and cochlear deaf patients. He found "cochlear echoes" that are present only in normal hearing subjects. Using loop diuretics and noise trauma, he was able to suppress what he called "acoustic emissions." Kemp demonstrated what Gold had hypothesized: The cochlea not only transduces acoustic energy into nervous impulses but also produces its own detectable sounds.

In 1983, Brownell (10) showed that the outer hair cells will reversibly change their length in response to electrical stimulus. The outer hair cells have high actin content, numerous mitochondria, and extensive smooth endoplasmic reticulum. Resembling skeletal muscle cells, they function as cellular motors. The outer hair cells appear to be the anatomic basis of the cochlear amplifier. They enhance both the fine frequency selectivity of the cochlea as well as its sensitivity and ability to detect very faint sounds.

The cochlea receives both afferent and efferent innervation (11, 12). Most of the afferent neurons travel from the inner hair cells and carry sensory potentials to the brainstem. Efferent nerve innervation travels from the olivocochlear bundle and reaches the outer hair cells near the inferior vestibular nerve (13). Of the efferent fibers, 90% synapses directly onto outer hair cells, with the remaining 10% synapsing on the afferent fibers arising from the inner hair cells. Presumably, the efferent innervation regulates outer hair cell function and generates the active tuning mechanism of the cochlear amplifier (14).

## ELECTROCOCHLEOGRAPHY

ECOG is the measurement of electrical potentials arising in the cochlea and the auditory nerve (4, 15, 16). The cochlea is transiently stimulated either with a wide-band click or a specific frequency toneburst sound. The wide band click produces more robust potentials by stimulating the entire cochlea. Tone-burst stimulation produces potentials that are more accurate indicators of hearing levels at specific frequencies. Recordings are made by placing electrodes either through the tympanic membrane directly onto the promontory or noninvasively within the external auditory meatus (16, 17). The accuracy of these recordings improves as the electrodes are placed closer to the cochlea. The three potentials recorded are the cochlear microphonic, the summating potential (SP), and the eighth nerve compound action potential (AP) (4, 15). The fourth cochlear potential, the endolymphatic potential, represents the baseline direct current battery of the endolymph produced by the stria vascularis. It is not recorded during clinical ECOG.

The cochlear microphonic is an alternating current potential (16). It represents the changing potassium currents that flow through the outer hair cells. The alternating current shifts mimic the waveform of the auditory stimulus. As the basilar membrane vibrates, the outer hair cell resistance is altered, generating a current.

The SP is a direct current potential generated not only by the outer hair cells but also by the inner hair cells (16). The current is possibly reflective of basilar membrane distention. The SP can be observed as the baseline shift in the cochlear microphonic.

The compound AP represents the average response of the discharging neurons in the auditory nerve (16). Each auditory nerve fiber produces a very small amplitude biphasic pulse. Continuous stimuli tend to cause a random firing sequence of neurons. Because they are biphasic, they tend to cancel one another. Transient stimuli, however, produce a synchronized response of APs in neurons that tend to sum with one another. This effect creates the measurable compound AP.

One of the most important applications of ECOG is in the diagnosis of Ménière's disease (17–20). Ménière's is a fluctuating, progressive process that manifests with variable hearing loss, tinnitus, aural fullness, and vertigo. In addition to the distention of Reissner's membrane by endolymphatic hydrops, there is a significant loss of hair cells and cochlear neurons. Early in the disease course, stretching of Reissner's membrane is thought to increase the SP. Conversely, hydrops is thought to progressively kill sensory neurons, leading to an absolute decline in the compound AP. An SP/AP ratio of > 0.45–0.5 is considered to have a 95% specificity for Ménière's disease, but its sensitivity is reported to be only 56%–68%. Other clinical indicators include increases in the absolute summating potential and increases in the latency of the compound action potential.

Monitoring of ECOG potentials can also be performed intraoperatively (21, 22). Their presence or absence reflects the status of the cochlea. They have been used during operations on acoustic neuromas to monitor hearing. ECOG has exquisite sensitivity to disruption of cochlear blood supply. It is limited, however, to monitoring only the peripheral auditory function of the cochlea. It cannot detect changes to the intracranial portion of the auditory nerve.

## AUDITORY BRAINSTEM RESPONSE

Jewett et al. (5) first described ABR in 1970. The ABR is generated by transient acoustic stimuli, either clicks or tone bursts, similar to ECOG. Surface electrodes are placed on the forehead and near the ears, with the contralateral mastoid acting as a ground. These electrodes record the electrical activity of the auditory pathways which occurs in the first 10–15 milliseconds after a sound stimulus. The signal is filtered to eliminate ECG and EEG interference. Multiple stimuli are presented to the ear each second, and a computer is used to average the electrical responses. Reliable waveforms are produced from the average of hundreds of responses.

A series of five distinct waveforms is typically identified (23). Each succeeding waveform is thought to represent neural activity at progressively higher auditory structures. ECOLI is a mnemonic developed for the waveforms, roughly corresponding with the distal and proximal Eighth nerve, Cochlear nucleus, superior Olivary body, Lateral lemniscus, and Inferior colliculus.

In normal hearing ears, wave V is the largest and most consistent component of the ABR. Normative data also has been collected to describe the absolute latencies for Waves I, III, and V. The Wave I latency is 1.5 milliseconds, the interval between Wave I and Wave III is 2 milliseconds, and the interval between Wave III and Wave V is also 2 milliseconds.

The applications of ABR include threshold testing (24), neonatal screening (25), site of lesion diagnosis (26), and intraoperative monitoring (27).

Threshold testing with ABR relies upon the first appearance and latency of Wave V (24). As stimulus intensity decreases, Wave V latency increases, while the amplitude decreases until it disappears below threshold. The threshold corresponds with the lowest intensity level that produces a Wave V. ABR correlates well with the behavioral audiogram at frequencies between 1000 and 4000 Hz but is still deficient in accurately predicting hearing loss in the lower frequencies.

Objective threshold testing is valuable for testing infant hearing. Because of its reliability, ABR is considered by many to be the most objective method of evaluating neonates (24, 25). It remains, however, a relatively expensive and time-consuming method that requires an otolaryngologist or trained audiologist to interpret the results. A 1993 National Institutes of Health consensus panel recommended ABR screening of infants who fail an initial test, such as OAEs (28). Automated machines also have been developed that extract Wave V data and provide a "pass" or "refer" response based on comparison with normative data. This enables untrained professionals to screen large populations of infants with a reported sensitivity between

93% and 100% for potential hearing disorders. Patients who are referred after failed initial screening undergo a full ABR test.

Site of lesion testing with ABR relies upon Waves I, III, and V (26). Wave I serve as the benchmark for peripheral auditory function. A prolonged wave I latency with normal waveforms and interwave latencies correlates with conductive hearing loss. A prolonged wave I latency with abnormal waveforms with otherwise normal latencies suggests sensory hearing loss. A normal Wave I latency with delayed Wave I to Wave III interval suggests retrocochlear pathology. An isolated prolongation of the Wave III to Wave V interval suggests isolated axial brainstem pathology. While acoustic neuroma is the tumor best identified by ABR, other cerebellopontine angle tumors such as meningioma, cholesteatoma, and facial neuromas are detected with 75% sensitivity.

Several findings are particularly suggestive of acoustic neuroma. The most common is an interaural difference in the Wave V latency of 0.2 millisecond. The absence of all waves with the presence of only mild to moderate hearing loss (60 dB levels) in the high frequencies or the exclusive presence of Wave I suggests acoustic neuroma. Earlier estimates of the sensitivity of ABR for acoustic neuromas were ~95%. With the introduction of high-resolution MRI, however, ABR has a high false-negative rate for small tumors, with a reported sensitivity of only 85%–90% overall (29).

ABR also has found use during neuro-otologic procedures for acoustic neuromas and other lesions (27, 30–32). The presence of robust waves correlates with the physiologic integrity of both the cochlea and auditory nerve. A preoperative baseline is obtained from which to compare intraoperative recordings. Changes in the recordable potentials may correspond with injury caused by surgical manipulation. With sufficient warning, it is assumed that reversal of the specific surgical manipulation can reverse or at least halt the progression of the injury.

Most investigators have followed the recommendations of Grundy et al. (30), who advocate, for reasons of expediency, the measurement of only wave V. There is a practical trade-off between generating a more complete picture vs. faster real-time results. Wave V ABR has been shown to increase postoperative hearing preservation in surgery for acoustic neuromas ≤3 cc. Slavit et al. (32)

conducted a case–control study of intraoperative ABR monitoring. A total of 60 consecutive patients who underwent acoustic neuroma resection with ABR were compared with a matched group of 60 controls. Overall, 42% of those monitored vs. 25% of the controls had preserved hearing. Monitoring during operations for tumors <2 cm resulted in an even higher relative percentage of hearing preservation. Intraoperative monitoring has significantly improved the preservation of hearing during operations for tumors <3 cm.

## OTOACOUSTIC EMISSIONS

OAEs are sounds produced by the active vibration of the basilar membrane generated by the outer hair cells (6, 10, 33). Unlike the electrical potentials of ECOG and ABR, OAEs are mechanical auditory phenomena. In response to acoustic stimulus, the olivocochlear bundle activates the efferent nerves to the outer hair cells. Stimulation of the outer hair cells causes them to vibrate the basilar membrane. These vibrations are driven through the cochlea, through the ossicular chain, to produce sound at the tympanic membrane. In theory, the outer hair cells act as the cochlear amplifier as their vibrations enhance the tuning of the traveling wave. OAEs are thought to be a byproduct of this cochlear amplifier.

OAEs are either spontaneously produced or evoked by external stimuli (34, 35). Spontaneous OAEs can be recorded intermittently in the ears of subjects in the absence of external stimuli. A 50–60% of normal-hearing ears are reported to produce spontaneous OAEs. Their incidence in women is twice that of men. They are not associated with pathological conditions and are probably indicative of normal hearing function.

Evoked OAEs come in two forms (35). Transiently evoked OAEs were the first type recorded by Kemp (6). These emissions occur in response to brief acoustic stimuli such as a click or a tone burst. Because of the broad spectrum of the stimulus, most of the basilar membrane is involved. The responding emissions consist of a broad spectrum of frequencies at varying intensity. Conditions known to cause sensorineural hearing loss have been shown to reduce or eliminate transiently evoked OAEs at thresholds of 30 dB or worse.

In contrast, the presence of these emissions implies gross hearing thresholds of 30 dB or better.

Distortion product OAEs are single-frequency emissions produced in response to two simultaneous stimulus tones, F1 and F2 (36). The emission is called a distortion product because it originates from the cochlea at a frequency which is not present in either of the stimulus tones. Several distortion products are produced in response F1 and F2, but the largest is found at their cubic difference of 2F1–F2. As the primary frequencies are incremented from 500 to 8000 Hz, a distortion product audiogram can be generated similar to a pure-tone audiogram. Distortion product OAEs are suppressed at hearing thresholds of 50 dB or worse (37).

To generate robust emissions, multiple samples of transiently evoked and distortion product OAEs are obtained by repeatedly stimulating the external ear canal with sound (36). Transiently evoked involves one sound stimulus, whereas distortion product requires two sustained stimuli. The evoked responses are recorded serially by a probe microphone in the external canal. The recorded signals are then amplified, averaged, and processed by fast Fourier transform. A frequency spectrum of the OAEs is produced. The quality of the OAEs can be affected by poor stimulus delivery as well as internal and ambient noise. These factors can be minimized with proper equipment controls, noise floor thresholds, and patient cooperation.

OAE testing can also be affected by pathologic conditions involving the external and middle ear (35). Inflammation of the external ear canal can prevent comfortable placement of the stimulus and microphone probes. Middle ear effusion or ossicular discontinuity can prevent passage of the stimulus or production of the emission. OAEs are measurable in only a small percentage of children with middle ear effusion and flat tympanograms (38). After myringotomy, OAEs usually become measurable or show larger amplitudes than preoperatively.

Numerous clinical applications exist for OAEs in everyday otologic practice (35, 39, 40). These include the screening of newborns (2, 41, 42), assessment of sensorineural hearing loss (43, 44), ototoxicity monitoring (35, 39), pseudohypacusis testing (39), and site of lesion diagnosis (35, 39).

The screening of newborns has perhaps the highest volume of clinical application of OAEs (2, 41, 42). As discussed previously, ABR testing is considered the most objective current screening method. Rhodes et al. (2) conducted a study comparing the utility of transiently evoked, distortion product OAEs, ABR, tympanometry, and acoustic stapedial reflex for initial screening, followed by ABR testing for confirmation of those who failed. Distortion product OAE testing had an 89% initial pass rate and a 92% pass rate with ABR. Infants who failed the initial distortion product test also had the highest proportion of failures on subsequent ABR. Validation of these studies remains a difficult problem, however, because there is no acceptable gold standard.

OAEs are sensitive to sensorineural hearing loss and can augment traditional audiometric diagnosis (40, 43, 44). The presence of transient OAEs indicates a hearing threshold of 30 dB or better for the frequency range in their spectrum. Distortion product OAEs reveal amplitude decreases at hearing thresholds >15 dB and are generally absent at thresholds of ≥50 dB. Kimberley (40) used multivariate statistical analysis of distortion product OAEs amplitude to demonstrate up to 85–90% accuracy of predicting pure-tone thresholds as normal or abnormal, where normal is a 30 dB pure-tone threshold or better. The association between thresholds and distortion product OAEs, however, is not strong enough to extrapolate audiometric thresholds directly from a distortion product audiogram.

The presence or absence of OAEs can also help to distinguish pseudohypacusis from true hearing loss (35). Because behavioral audiometry relies upon accurate responses from patients, malingerers can provide false responses in an effort to receive compensation or attention. In addition to the Stenger test and ABR, OAE can provide objective results to confirm or reject the patient's claim of hearing loss.

Another role for OAEs is monitoring for dynamic changes in cochlear function and ototoxicity (35, 39). Noise trauma and ototoxic agents have been shown to affect outer hair cell function in animals. Distortion product OAEs have been shown to correlate well with the typical 4000-Hz notch pattern associated with noise-induced hearing loss. OAEs also have been shown to be an early and sensitive indicator of the ototoxic effects of cis-platinum and aminoglycosides. Serial monitoring of OAEs in workers in noisy environments or patients receiving ototoxic agents may provide a simple and objective measure of hearing loss.

OAEs may have some utility in site of lesion diagnosis of cochlear and retrocochlear pathology. Bonfils and Uziel (45) studied OAEs and conventional audiometry in 24 patients with acoustic neuromas. They discovered several emission patterns in which the OAE activity associated with the tumor was purely cochlear involvement (54%), solely retrocochlear (33%), or associated with mixed cochlear and retrocochlear symptoms (3%). For initial diagnosis, however, OAEs are not as sensitive as either ABR testing or MRI. Their role in the initial diagnosis of cerebellopontine tumors is adjunctive.

Distortion product OAEs may also have a role in the management of these tumors (39). Preoperative testing of smaller tumors (< 3 cm) may assist in predicting the success of hearing preservation surgery. Robust emissions would indicate a high likelihood of cochlear viability.

## CONCLUSIONS

Auditory-evoked phenomena provide a valuable adjunct to audiometric testing because they rely upon physiologic rather than behavioral measurements. One of their primary uses is evaluating hearing in patients who are unable or unwilling to provide behavioral responses. These phenomena also can be used in conjunction with traditional audiometric tests to provide objective confirmation.

In addition, auditory-evoked phenomena can provide information about subclinical hearing loss, occult tumors, and the real-time status of the cochlea and auditory pathways. Because ECOG, ABR, and OAEs provide a window to cochlear mechanics and auditory pathways, future research may lead to more precise understanding of sensorineural hearing loss.

## REFERENCES

1. Hall JW III, Mueller HG III. *Audiologists' Desk Reference Volume I*. San Diego: Singular Publishing Group, 1997.
2. Rhodes MC, Margolis RH, Hirsch JE et al. Hearing screening in the newborn intensive care nursery: comparison of methods. *Otolaryngology Head Neck Surgery* 1999; 120:799–808.
3. Sataloff RT, Spiegel JR. Neurotologic evaluation and treatment following minor head trauma. In Mandel S, Sataloff RT, Schapiro SR. *Minor Head Trauma*. New York, NY: Springer-Verlag; 1993:159–202.
4. Davis H. Principle of electric response audiometry. *Annals of Otology, Rhinology and Laryngology* 1976; 85(suppl 28):5–96.
5. Jewett DL, Romano MN, Williston JS. Human auditory evoked potentials: possible brain stem components detected on the scalp. *Science* 1970; 167:1517–1518.
6. Kemp DT. Stimulated acoustic emissions from within the human auditory system. *J Acoust Soc Am* 1978; 64:1386–1391.
7. Helmholtz HLF. Die Lehre von den Tonempfindungen als Physiologische Grundlage fur die Theories der Musik. In: Ellis AJ, ed. *On the Sensations of Tone*. 3rd ed. London, UK: Longmans, 1863.
8. von Békésy G. Experiments in Hearing. New York, NY: McGraw-Hill, 1960.
9. Gold T. Hearing II: the physical basis of the action of the cochlea. *Proceedings of the Royal Society B: Biological Sciences*. 1948; 135:492–498. [Database]
10. Brownell WE. Observations on a motile response in isolated outer hair cells. In: Webster WR, Aitken LM, eds. *Mechanisms of Hearing*. Melbourne: Monash University Press, 1983:5–10.
11. Kiang NY-S, Watanabe T, Thomas EC, Clark LF.. Discharge patterns of single fibers in the cat's auditory nerve. *MIT Res Monog* 1965; 35: 65.
12. Warr WB. Organization of olivocochlear efferent systems in mammals. In: Webster DB, Popper AN, Fay RR, eds. *Mammalian Auditory Pathway: Neuroanatomy*. New York, NY: Springer-Verlag, 1992.
13. Spoendlin H. Sensory neural organization of the cochlea. *Journal of Laryngology and Otology* 1979; 93:853–877.
14. Kemp DT. Otoacoustic emissions, traveling waves and cochlear mechanics. *Hear Res* 1986; 22:95–104.
15. Brackmann DE, Don M, Selters WA. Electric response audiometry. In: Paparella MM, Shumrick DA, eds. *Otolaryngology*. 3rd ed. Philadelphia, PA: WB Saunders, 1991.

16. Eggermont JJ. Electrocochleography. In: Keidel WD, Neff WD, eds. Handbook of Sensory Physiology. Vol. V. Part 3. Berlin, Germany: Springer-Verlag, 1976.

17. Margolis RH, Rieks D, Fournier EM et al. Tympanic electrocochleography for diagnosis of Ménière's disease. Arch Otolaryngol Head Neck Surg 1995; 121:44–55.

18. Coats AC, Jenkins HA, Monroe B. Auditory evoked potentials—the cochlear summating potential in detection of endolymphatic hydrops. Am J Otol 1984; 5:443–446.

19. Dauman R, Aran JM, Charlet de Sauvage R et al. Clinical significance of the summating potential in Ménière's disease. Am J Otol 1988; 9:31–38.

20. Ferraro J, Best LG, Arenberg IK. The use of electrocochleography in the diagnosis, assessment, and monitoring of endolymphatic hydrops. Otolaryngol Clin North Am 1983; 16:69–82.

21. Levine RA. Short-latency auditory evoked potentials: intraoperative applications. Int Anesthesiol Clin 1990; 28:147–153.

22. Sabin HL, Bentivoglio P, Symon L et al. Intraoperative electrocochleography to monitor cochlear potentials during acoustic neuroma excision. Acta Neurochir 1987; 85:110–116.

23. Moller AR, Jannetta PJ. Neural generators of the auditory brainstem response. In: Jacobson JT, ed. The Auditory Brainstem Response. Boston, MA: College-Hill Press, 1985.

24. Mahoney TM. Auditory brainstem response hearing aid applications. In: Jacobsen J, ed. The Auditory Brainstem Response. San Diego, CA: College-Hill Press, 1985.

25. Bluestone CD. Universal newborn screening for hearing loss: ideal vs. reality and the role of otolaryngologists. Otolaryngol Head Neck Surg 1996; 115:89–93.

26. Selters WA, Brackmann DE. Acoustic tumor detection with brain stem electric response audiometry. Arch Otolaryngol 1997; 103:181–187.

27. Moller AR. Intraoperative neurophysiologic monitoring. In: Brackman DE, Shelton C, Arriaga MA, eds. Otologic Surgery. Philadelphia, PA: WB Saunders, 2001.

28. National Institutes of Health. Early identification of hearing impairment in infants and young children. Int J Pediatr Otorhinolaryngol 1993; 27:215–217.

29. Wilson DF, Hodgson RS, Gustafson MF et al. The sensitivity of auditory brainstem response testing in small acoustic neuromas. Laryngoscope 1992; 102:961–964.

30. Grundy BL, Jannetta PJ, Procopio PT et al. Intraoperative monitoring of brainstem auditory evoked potentials. J Neurosurg 1982; 52:674–681.

31. Telischi FF, Mom T, Agrama M et al. Comparison of the auditory-evoked brainstem response wave I to distortion-product otoacoustic emissions resulting from changes to inner ear blood flow. Laryngoscope 1999; 109:186–191.

32. Slavit DH, Harner SG, Harper M et al. Auditory monitoring during acoustic neuroma removal. Arch Otolaryngol Head Neck Surg 1991; 117:1153–1157.

33. Brownell WE. Outer hair cell electromotility and otoacoustic emissions. Ear Hear 1990; 11:82–92.

34. Martin GK, Probst R, Lonsbury-Martin BL. Otoacoustic emissions in human ears: normative findings. Ear Hear 1990; 11:47–61.

35. Lonsbury-Martin BL, Martin GK, McCoy MJ et al. New approaches to the evaluation of the auditory system and a current analysis of otoacoustic emissions. Otolaryngol Head Neck Surg 1995; 112:50–63.

36. Lonsbury-Martin BL, Harris FP, Stagner BB et al. Distortion product emissions in humans I. Basic properties in normally hearing subjects. Ann Otol Rhinol Laryngol Suppl 1990; 99:3–14.

37. Martin GK, Ohlms LA, Franklin DJ et al. Distortion product emissions in humans III. Influence of sensorineural hearing loss. Ann Otol Rhinol Laryngol Suppl 1990; 99:30–42.

38. Lonsbury-Martin BL, Martin GK, McCoy MR et al. Otoacoustic emissions testing in young children: middle ear influences. Am J Otol 1994; 15(suppl 1):13–20.

39. Balkany T, Telischi FF, McCoy MJ et al. Otoacoustic emissions in otologic practice. Am J Otol 1994; 15(suppl 1):29–38.

40. Kimberley BP. Applications of distortion-product emissions to an otological practice. Laryngoscope 1999; 109:1908–1918.

41. Choi SS, Pafitis IA, Zalzal GH et al. Clinical applications of transiently evoked otoacoustic emissions in the pediatric population. *Ann Otol Rhinol Laryngol* 1999; 108:132–138.

42. Norton SJ. Emerging role of evoked otoacoustic emissions in neonatal hearing screening. *Am J Otol* 1994; 15(suppl 1):4–12.

43. Ohlms LA, Lonsbury-Martin BL, Martin GK. Acoustic-distortion products: separation of sensory from neural dysfunction in sensorineural hearing loss in human beings and rabbits. *Otolaryngol Head Neck Surg* 1991; 104:159–174.

44. Schweinfurth JM, Cacace AT, Parnes SM. Clinical applications of otoacoustic emissions in sudden hearing loss. *Laryngoscope* 1997; 107:1457–1463.

45. Bonfils P, Uziel A. Evoked otoacoustic emissions in patients with acoustic neuromas. *Am J Otol* 1988; 9:412–417.

# 9

# Conductive hearing loss

ROBERT THAYER SATALOFF AND PAMELA C. ROEHM

## DIAGNOSTIC CRITERIA

Certain findings are characteristic of conductive hearing loss. The most essential ones are that the patient hears better by bone than by air conduction and that the bone conduction is approximately normal. It would seem that these observations should suffice for classifying a case as conductive. Unfortunately, they are not always reliable because some patients have conductive hearing loss and yet also have reduced

DOI: 10.1201/b23379-9

bone conduction, as it now is measured. The difficulty is that bone conduction tests alone do not always provide an accurate assessment of the sensorineural mechanism. Other tests often are necessary. It is therefore essential to have a clear understanding of the symptoms and the features that characterize a conductive hearing loss. They should also be placed in context with the many other conditions that can affect the ear discussed throughout this book, some of which are summarized in Appendix II.

## CHARACTERISTIC FEATURES

These features are provided by the history, the otologic examination, and the hearing tests:

1. The history may reveal a discharging ear or a previous ear infection. A feeling of fullness, as if fluid were trapped in the ear, may accompany the hearing loss, or a sudden unilateral hearing loss may follow an effort to clean out wax with a fingertip. There may be a history of a ruptured or perforated eardrum or of head trauma. Often the hearing loss is of gradual onset and may have worsened during pregnancy. The hearing loss may have been present at birth or noted in early childhood.
2. Tinnitus may be present and may be continuous or pulsatile.
3. If the hearing loss is bilateral, the patient generally speaks with a soft voice, especially if the etiology is otosclerosis.
4. The patient hears better in noisy areas (paracusis of Willis).
5. Occasionally, the patient claims he/she does not hear well when eating foods that make loud noises when chewed, such as celery or carrots (because these noises are easily transmitted to the ears by bone conduction and produce a masking effect, with the result that he/she cannot hear airborne speech as well).
6. The hearing loss by air conduction may be greater in the lower frequencies.
7. The bone conduction threshold is normal or almost normal.
8. An air–bone gap is present.
9. Otologic examination may reveal abnormality in the external auditory canal, the eardrum, or the middle ear. Sometimes bubbles or a fluid level may be seen behind the eardrum. When only the ossicular chain is involved, the visible findings through an otoscope may be normal.
10. There is no difficulty in discriminating speech if it is loud enough.
11. Recruitment and abnormal tone decay are absent.
12. If the two ears have different hearing levels, the tuning fork lateralizes to the ear with the worse hearing.
13. The maximum hearing loss possible in pure conductive hearing impairment is ~70 dB.
14. The patient's hearing responses often are indecisive when they are tested at threshold during audiometry. This is in contrast to sharp end points in testing for sensorineural hearing losses.
15. Impedance audiometry may show abnormal findings.

It is helpful to understand the reasons for these characteristics so that they may be logically interpreted rather than merely memorized for classifying a clinical case.

When the patient's history reveals external or middle ear infections associated with hearing impairment, conductive hearing loss may be suspected. Complaints may include a draining ear, an infected external or middle ear, impacted wax, and a feeling of fluid in the ear accompanied by fullness. Often the fluid seems to move and hearing improves with a change in position of the head. These symptoms justify a suspicion of conductive hearing loss and suggest the need for confirmatory tests. Too hasty a classification may lead to an error. It is wise to recall that fluid in the middle ear, as in secretory otitis media, produces not only a reduced air conduction threshold but may affect bone conduction as well—especially at high frequencies—even though the sensorineural mechanism is intact. When the fluid is removed surgically, both air and bone conduction levels quickly return to normal.

The hard-of-hearing patient's answers to the physician's questions invariably provide essential clues to both classification and etiology, as discussed elsewhere in this book.

Among the distinguishing features of conductive hearing loss elicited by careful questioning are the following (in addition to those listed earlier):

1. The patient has no difficulty in understanding what he/she hears as long as people speak loudly enough (because in uncomplicated conductive hearing loss, only the threshold is affected, not the discrimination).
2. The patient often hears better in noisy areas such as on a bus or at a cocktail party. The reason for this is that people speak louder in noisy places, and the patient can hear the speaker's voice better above the background noises.
3. Another related finding in conductive hearing loss, but most prominent in otosclerosis, is the patient's remarkably soft voice. A soft voice in the presence of insidious hearing loss immediately should suggest otosclerosis, particularly if a low-pitched tinnitus is present. The voice is soft because the patient's excellent bone conduction gives the impression that his/her voice is louder than it actually is. Consequently, he/she lowers his/her voice to such a soft level that often it is difficult to hear the patient. Tinnitus rarely is present in conductive hearing loss, except in otosclerosis. When otosclerosis is present, there is frequently a family history of similar hearing loss. Otosclerotic hearing impairment may be worsened during or after pregnancy.

When inspection of the external ear canal or middle ear reveals any obstructive abnormality, a conductive hearing loss should be suspected. Prior to deciding on this classification, one should first rule out a possible sensorineural loss, which also may be present. Bone conduction studies can help resolve this question. If otologic findings are normal, and there is a significant air–bone gap (i.e., if the bone conduction is better than the air conduction), there is a conductive loss—probably caused by some defect in the ossicular chain. Occasionally, fluid causing a conductive hearing loss escapes otoscopic detection because of its position, and the hearing loss is attributed to a defect in the ossicular chain rather than to the fluid. Tympanometry may be helpful in such cases.

Whenever a hearing loss is substantially in excess of 70 dB (American National Standards Institute [ANSI]), some other type of damage is superimposed on the conductive hearing loss. The reason for this is that even total disruption of the sound transmission mechanism of the middle ear produces a loss of only ~70 dB (ANSI). For example, an ossicular discontinuity may occur after surgery or a fracture of the temporal bone, or in the presence of congenital aplasia.

## FINDINGS IN VARIOUS TESTS

In a pure conductive hearing loss, the bone conduction is normal or almost normal because there is no damage to the inner ear or the auditory nerve. We say "almost normal" for good reason. In some cases of pure conductive hearing loss, there is a mild reduction in bone conduction, especially in the higher frequencies, even though the sensorineural mechanism is normal. This observation emphasizes a significant blind spot in bone conduction tests; they really are not a completely valid measure of the function of the sensorineural mechanism or cochlear reserve, and reduced bone conduction sometimes may be due to purely mechanical reasons. In otosclerosis, a dip often occurs at ~2000 Hz in bone conduction ("Carhart's notch"). This is called a *stiffness curve.*

An air–bone gap is present in uncomplicated conductive hearing loss because the air conduction threshold is reduced, but the bone conduction threshold is essentially normal. A simple and excellent way to demonstrate this is to take a 512-Hz tuning fork and strike it gently. To a patient with a conductive hearing loss, the fork will sound weak when it is held close to his/her ear, but he/she will hear it better when the shaft is placed so that it presses on the mastoid bone or the teeth. This test is so useful that it should be used in every case of hearing loss, no matter how many other tests an audiologist or a technician may perform. In the hands of the experienced otologist, the tuning fork is an essential diagnostic instrument. This is the basis of the Rinne test.

If there is a conductive loss in only one ear or if the conductive loss is considerably greater in one ear than in the other, a vibrating tuning fork pressed against the skull will be heard in the ear with the greater hearing loss (Weber test). Tests depending on *lateralization*, as this phenomenon is called, are not as reliable as some other tuning-fork tests, such as those comparing the efficiency of air and bone conduction.

In every case, carefully done hearing tests are analyzed to confirm the classification of type of hearing loss. Air and bone conduction audiometry are fundamental but should be corroborated by tuning-fork tests. If there is still any doubt as to the classification, impedance audiometry, recruitment studies, discrimination, and special tests are performed. In this type of loss, there will be no evidence of recruitment or abnormal tone decay. The patient's ability to discriminate is always excellent in conductive hearing loss. Impedance changes, as described in Chapter 7, may be found. It is helpful to do all these tests routinely in every case, but this is not always possible in private practice. There are some audiologic centers in which an entire battery of hearing tests is carried out on all patients, even before they are examined and questioned. The experienced clinical physician performs only sufficient tests to make the classification or diagnosis reasonably certain. This selectivity saves the patient money and saves the patient and clinician considerable time.

## PROGNOSIS

In the vast majority of clinical cases of conductive hearing loss, the prognosis is excellent. With available medical and surgical treatment, most conductive hearing losses can be corrected.

## AUDIOMETRIC PATTERNS

There is a popular impression that the different classifications of hearing loss are characterized by distinctly shaped audiometric patterns. One cannot be sure whether the loss is conductive or sensorineural merely by inspecting an air conduction audiogram. However, it is true that many conductive hearing losses often have audiometric patterns of a distinctive appearance. One characteristic audiogram generally is described as an ascending curve, indicating that the hearing loss is greater in the lower than in the higher frequencies. This classic audiogram, illustrated in **Figure 9.1**, demonstrates almost all of

the findings characteristically present in conductive hearing loss resulting from otosclerosis or chronic serous otitis media.

Another audiometric pattern commonly found in conductive defects is shown in **Figure 9.2**, which illustrates the audiologic findings in chronic otitis media.

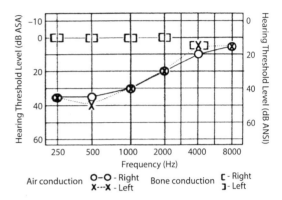

Figure 9.1 Ascending audiogram typical of conductive hearing loss. Bone conduction is better than air conduction and is normal. Discrimination is excellent. *History:* A 24-year-old woman complaining of insidious hearing loss and buzzing tinnitus over 10 years. One aunt uses a hearing aid. She has trouble hearing soft voices but understands clearly when voice is loud. She hears better at cocktail parties and in noisy places. Voice is soft and barely audible. *Otologic:* Normal. *Audiologic:* Vague responses during audiometry, and fluctuating hearing levels. Bilateral air–bone gap present. Opposite ear masked during bone conduction tests. *Speech reception threshold:* Right 30 dB and left 35 dB. *Discrimination score:* Right 100% and left 100%. Bone conduction prolonged and better than air conduction by tuning fork. Vague lateralization to right ear. *Classification:* Conductive. *Diagnosis:* Otosclerosis. Confirmed at surgery and hearing restored. *Aids to diagnosis:* The combination of the patient's ability to hear better in noisy places and soft voice indicates a conductive lesion, which was confirmed by audiometric testing (air–bone gap). Normal otologic findings suggest stapes fixation (otosclerosis). *Abbreviations:* ANSI, American National Standards Institute; ASA, American Standards Association.

Not every case of conductive hearing loss presents all distinctive characteristics. For example, **Figure 9.3** illustrates a case of secretory otitis media in which there is a high-frequency loss and reduced bone conduction, even though the sensorineural mechanism is normal.

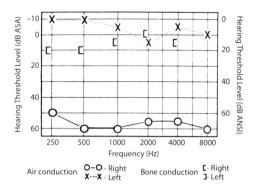

Figure 9.2 Flat audiogram found in conductive hearing loss caused by chronic otitis media. Bone conduction and discrimination are normal. *History:* An 8-year-old girl with discharge from right ear since age of 6 months. *Otologic:* Right tympanic membrane eroded with putrid discharge in middle ear. Ossicles absent at surgery. *Audiologic:* Reduced air and normal bone conduction responses in right ear with left ear masked. Tuning fork lateralizes to right ear. *Speech reception threshold:* Right 60 dB. *Discrimination score:* Right 98%. *Expected impedance findings:* Type B curve with bilateral, absent stapedius reflexes. *Classification:* Conductive. *Diagnosis:* Chronic otitis media. *Abbreviations:* ANSI, American National Standards Institute; ASA, American Standards Association.

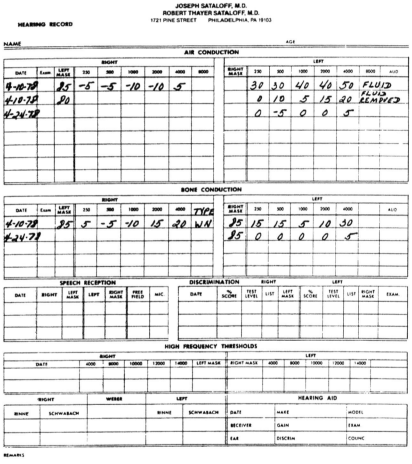

Figure 9.3 A typical audiogram in conductive hearing loss caused by thick fluid in the middle ear. The bone conduction is reduced but returns to normal after fluid is removed. *History:* Recurrent fullness in left ear with hearing loss for past 6 months. *Otologic:* Eardrum not freely mobile with air pressure. No fluid level seen. Thick, clear jelly in middle ear. Removed with myringotomy and suction. *Audiologic:* Reduced air and somewhat reduced bone conduction thresholds in left ear. Normal discrimination. Bone thresholds returned to normal after removal of fluid. Tuning fork lateralizes to left ear. *Expected impedance findings:* Type B tympanogram on the left. There is stapedius reflex with high-intensity stimulus in the left ear and none when stimulus tone is in right ear. *Classification:* Conductive. Initial testing indicated some sensorineural involvement because of the reduced bone thresholds. Removal of the fluid allowed bone responses to return to normal. *Diagnosis:* Secretory otitis. *Aids to diagnosis:* Immobile eardrum; fluctuating hearing loss with slightly reduced bone conduction; normal discrimination and lateralization to left ear suggest fluid in middle ear. Tympanogram will show abnormal findings.

## THE DANGER OF INCOMPLETE STUDIES

These cases illustrate the inadvisability of making a classification of conductive or any other type of hearing loss solely on the basis of the air conduction alone or even on the air and the bone conduction combined. Without a careful otologic history and examination, some of these patients may be classified inaccurately and thus may be treated incorrectly or deprived of effective therapy and relief from their hearing handicap.

## ESSENTIAL CRITERIA

To qualify as an uncomplicated conductive hearing loss, a case must have these features:

1. The bone conduction must be better than the air conduction.
2. The air–bone gap must be ~15 dB, especially in the lower frequencies.
3. The bone conduction must be normal or near normal.
4. The discrimination must be good.
5. The hearing threshold should not exceed ~70 dB (ANSI).
6. Although tests for recruitment and abnormal tone decay rarely are performed in the presence of the above features, both these phenomena should be absent.
7. Acoustic reflexes should be absent.
8. In many instances, impedance audiometry helps to confirm the site and the type of damage in the middle ear.

## VISIBLE OBSTRUCTION OF THE EXTERNAL AUDITORY CANAL

If a patient's audiologic findings show a conductive hearing loss and an obstruction is seen in the external canal, the cause of his/her hearing loss may be one of the following: congenital or acquired atresia of the external auditory canal, Treacher Collins syndrome, stenosis, exostosis, impacted cerumen, fluid in external canal, collapse of ear canal, external otitis, foreign body, carcinoma, granuloma, cysts, or other causes.

## CONGENITAL AURAL ATRESIA

When the external auditory canal is absent at birth, the condition is called congenital external auditory canal atresia or aplasia. It is the result of a defect in fetal development. When the physician is examining an atresia in an infant, or young child, he/she may wonder whether the neural mechanism also is defective. It is helpful to recall that the outer ear and the sensorineural apparatus are of different embryonic origins. The sound-conducting mechanism of the middle ear develops from the branchial system, whereas the sensorineural mechanism is derived from the ectodermal cyst. Therefore, it is rare to find embryonic defects in both the conductive and the sensorineural systems in the same ear. Malformations associated with syndromes are discussed in Chapter 13.

## EMBRYONIC DEVELOPMENT

Another interesting question concerns the ability to predict from the appearance of the outer ear the likely presence of ossicles in the middle ear. The auricle starts forming in 6 weeks of embryonic life and is almost complete after 12 weeks. In some patients, there is a small pit just in front and above the meatus of the canal. This shows the point at which the hillocks from the first and the second branchial arches fused to form the auricle. The embryonic structure occasionally may persist as a fistula or as a congenital preauricular cyst. The eardrum and the external auditory canal start forming about the end of 2 months of fetal life and are complete by ~7 months. First, the eardrum is formed, and a short time later, the meatus. It is possible, but uncommon, to find an aplasia of the meatus with a normal eardrum and ossicles. The ossicles begin to form from cartilage during 8 weeks of fetal life and are fully developed by 4 months, although not ossified until shortly before birth.

## CONGENITAL ABNORMALITIES

All the causes of congenital abnormalities are not yet known, and the variety is great. There may be only a membranous layer closing the canal, while everything else is normal, or there may be no canal, no eardrum, no ossicles, and even very little middle ear. Often the aplasia is unilateral, but even in such cases, evidence of a slight congenital defect may be found in the other ear.

It is not always possible to predict preoperatively whether a functioning eardrum and normal ossicles are present in congenital aural atresia. High-resolution CT of the temporal bones can yield a substantial amount of this information; however, due to the size of the structures involved, this study may not reveal all of the critical aspects of the anatomy. This can be obtained only through surgery. However, the shape of the auricle does provide some indication of the condition of the deeper structures in the ear. As the auricle is formed completely by the third month of fetal life, a deformed auricle suggests probable deformities of the eardrum and the ossicles. The chances of improving hearing are better when the auricle is well formed.

## THE QUESTION OF SURGERY

The question of what can be accomplished by surgery is of decisive importance in congenital aplasia and other malformations. Parents always are anxious to know how much hearing their children lose as a result of these conditions and whether hearing can be restored.

If the atresia is unilateral and the other ear is normal, surgery becomes an elective procedure. In bilateral aural atresia, early surgery is desirable to restore hearing in at least one ear so that the child can learn to speak at the normal stage in his/her development. If for any reason surgery is inadvisable or should be postponed for several years, a bone conduction hearing aid should be fitted on children as young as 3 months of age or even younger.

In the past, the results of surgical procedures were often disappointing, and, consequently, physicians may find cases of unilateral congenital aural atresia in adults. With new surgical approaches, the results are much more rewarding. The great variety of abnormal conditions that may be found at surgery and the distortion or the absence of landmarks make this surgery very difficult. It should be undertaken only by trained and experienced otologists.

## STUDYING THE EXTENT OF INVOLVEMENT

Although the diagnosis of aplasia may be made by simple inspection, the extent of involvement must be determined by careful study. CT scans or other imaging studies can be helpful in demonstrating the presence of an external auditory canal, ossicles,

and semicircular canals. CT can show the shape of the ossicles but not their function (**Figure 9.4**). The absence of semicircular canals makes the prognosis for restoring hearing very poor because this indicates a defect in the labyrinth. Hearing studies are essential, though these are difficult to perform in an infant. Nevertheless, a reasonable estimate of the child's hearing level can be obtained by a comprehensive study. For example, if a child consistently turns his/her head in the direction of a vibrating tuning fork that was not struck too forcefully, there is a reasonably good basis for optimism about restoring hearing. If there is no response to this simple test, it does not necessarily mean that hearing is absent. More elaborate tests are then indicated.

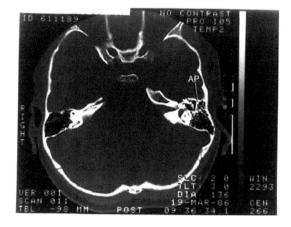

Figure 9.4 CT scan of the left ear showing partial bony atresia with an atresia plate (AP), and malleus and incus with a well-developed joint (white arrow).

## TREACHER COLLINS SYNDROME

One type of congenital aural atresia is so distinctive that it warrants separate consideration. In Treacher Collins syndrome, both auricles are deformed, and there is complete absence of both external auditory canals and eardrums; the malleus and the incus are also deformed. In addition, the patient's eyes are slanted downward at the lateral corners. Congenital defects, known as colobomas, are observed in ocular structures such as the iris, the retina, or the choroid. The mandible is small, and the lower jaw markedly recedes. The cheeks are pulled in, causing the lower eyelids and the face to droop.

Although intellectual disabilities do not accompany this syndrome, children afflicted with it present such a strange appearance that they generally are taken to be "backward." A contributory factor to this impression is the marked conductive hearing loss resulting from the aplasia. Because these children hear so poorly, they are slow in developing speech, and this in turn often is attributed unjustly to lack of mental acuity. These children usually have normal sensorineural mechanisms, and their hearing can be improved by successful surgery or by the early use of a bone conduction hearing aid. Preferably, this help should be provided in infancy to avoid retardation of speech development and thus to obviate any resulting psychological problems. The hearing level usually is ~70 dB for all frequencies. Preoperatively, it is very difficult to ascertain even by CT scan the condition of the ossicles or the presence or absence of an eardrum.

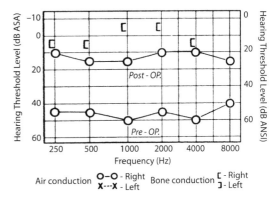

Air conduction **O—O** - Right **X---X** - Left  Bone conduction **[** - Right **]** - Left

Figure 9.5 *History:* A 6-year-old boy with right congenital aplasia. *Otologic examination:* Left ear normal. Mild microtia of right auricle. Meatus of right external auditory canal completely occluded by firm, thick skin. X-ray showed normal ossicles. At surgery, the aplasia was corrected, and the eardrum was found to be almost normal. *Abbreviations:* ANSI, American National Standards Institute; ASA, American Standards Association.

## STENOSIS OF THE EAR CANAL

Stenosis is diagnosed readily when otoscopic examination reveals complete obstruction of the external auditory canal leading to the eardrum. This obstruction may occur anywhere along the length of the canal. Occasionally, a skin layer is the only blockage present; this causes a hearing loss of ~40 dB (sometimes more) in the speech frequency range (**Figure 9.5**). More often, however, there is a bony wall behind the skin, and the hearing loss then may range from 50 to 60 dB in all frequencies.

Stenosis of the ear canal generally is detected on routine otologic examination in infancy. Sometimes, however, it is not picked up until a hearing loss is revealed in a school hearing test, after which physical examination shows closure of the ear canal.

Stenosis is not always congenital. It may be a sequela of infection, or it may result from complications from surgery on the ears or the result of trauma to the ear canal (including burns). In these instances, the obstruction usually is fibrous.

In some instances, stenosis is not complete, but it narrows the opening of the ear canal to such an extent that any small accumulation of wax or debris causes impaction and hearing loss. In such cases, the canal can be enlarged, and the hearing problem can be resolved. However, it is essential to enlarge the canal in such a manner that it does not close again.

Correction of a stenotic ear canal generally is advisable so that in the event of a subsequent middle ear infection necessitating myringotomy or ear treatment, the eardrum can be visualized adequately for diagnosis and treatment.

## EXOSTOSIS OF THE EAR CANAL

In exostosis of the ear canal, bony projections can be seen arising from the walls of the canal. They are not uncommon in adults, but they are rare in children. Although the cause of this condition is unknown, it seems to occur more frequently in individuals whose ears are exposed excessively to cold water, such as swimmers.

When it is recalled that the outer portion of the external ear is cartilaginous, it becomes logical that bony exostoses are found only in the bony or inner portion of the canal. Typically, these growths are small and do not of themselves occlude the lumen completely. However, they do narrow it to such a degree that any slight accumulations of water, wax, or dead skin or any infection may cause complete blockage and immediate hearing loss. These types of episodes may be so frequent in some patients that surgery is necessary to prevent recurrent hearing loss and infections.

The hearing loss is generally ~30–40 dB when the lumen of the canal becomes occluded. The loss is not as great as in complete atresia, possibly because some of the sound waves apparently traverse the flexible material that completes the closure of the ear canal. The loss is predominantly in the lower frequencies. Upon removal of the wax or the debris, hearing returns to normal. Utmost care is necessary in examining ear canals with exostoses because trauma to the very thin skin covering these growths can readily produce bleeding, swelling, infection, and further hearing loss.

In such cases, if water enters, it is very difficult for the patient to remove it by ordinary means. The water accumulates in the pockets between the exostoses and the eardrum. A diagnosis of hearing loss caused by exostoses must be based on the findings in the ear canal and the audiologic testing.

With local anesthesia in the ear canal skin, exostoses can be removed easily by elevating the skin off the bony projections, removing them with a surgical drill, and replacing the skin. If frequent or severe otitis externa has occurred in these ears leading to fusion of the skin, a split thickness skin graft may be required to keep the ear canal patent after removal of the exostoses.

## IMPACTED CERUMEN

## OCCURRENCE

As wax glands are situated only in the skin covering the cartilaginous or outer part of the ear canal, wax is formed exclusively in this outer area. If it is found impacted more deeply in the bony portion or against the eardrum, it probably was pushed in there, usually with a cotton swab or another object. Because of the structure of some ear canals and the consistency of the wax, the excess cerumen accumulates and plugs up the canal, causing hearing loss. This is common in infants because they have very narrow ear canals and because mothers are likely to use large, cotton-tipped applicators that push the wax into a baby's ear canal instead of removing it.

Obstruction caused by excessive cerumen occurs frequently among workers in industrial areas after being pushed in repeatedly due to use of ear plugs and also when dirt gets into their ear canals. Individuals with an abundance of hairs in the ear canal easily accumulate cerumen because it becomes enmeshed in the hairs and thus is prevented from falling out by itself.

Interestingly enough, the patient with impacted wax often gives a history of sudden rather than gradual hearing loss. The person may say that while chewing or poking a finger or a probe of some kind into the ear in an effort to clean it, he/she suddenly went "deaf" in that ear. The patient may have experienced some itching or fullness in the ear and, by probing into it with a large object, pushed the cerumen into the narrower portion of the ear canal until it caused an impaction. If the canal closes while the patient is chewing, it may be explained by the proximity of the temporomandibular joint to the cartilaginous portion of the ear canal. In such instances, pressure of the joint on the soft ear canal may displace wax from its normal position and block the narrow lumen of the canal.

## TINNITUS

If cerumen becomes lodged against the eardrum, the patient sometimes reports a rushing type of tinnitus or complains of hearing his/her own heartbeat. The tinnitus stops at once when the cerumen is removed. Hearing loss invariably is accompanied by a feeling of fullness, and the loss usually is greater in the lower frequencies. Rarely is the loss > 40 dB, and most often it is ~30 dB.

## RULING OUT AN ORGANIC DEFECT

Patients with hearing loss due to other causes commonly tell their physicians that wax in their ears probably is causing the loss. To help rule out another organic defect, it is essential to inquire whether the patient had impaired hearing and tinnitus before the present episode.

## TESTING

A common mistake is to look in an ear that has a large amount of cerumen and then to assure the patient that wax in the ear is his/her only trouble. Such a hasty diagnosis may necessitate an embarrassing retraction if the hearing loss persists after the wax is removed. Bear in mind that the severity of the loss cannot be estimated merely from the presence of a large amount of cerumen in the ear canal. Even if there is only a small pinpoint opening through the cerumen, the patient can hear almost normally, provided there is no other defect. It is only when the ear canal is blocked completely that the hearing loss occurs. Therefore, it is highly advisable to do at least air and bone conduction audiometry before venturing to establish the cause and the prognosis of any hearing impairment. It is also important to perform air conduction audiograms after removal of the wax to be certain that hearing has been restored fully.

## REMOVAL OF CERUMEN

If irrigation is used to remove impacted cerumen, the ear canal should be dried afterward; otherwise, some water may remain in the deeper area at the anterior–inferior portion of the ear canal, which might cause a feeling of fullness as well as a slight interference with hearing. **Figure 9.6** illustrates the type of hearing loss that frequently results from impacted cerumen. **Figure 9.7** illustrates an important reason for taking a careful history and doing audiologic testing before assuring a patient that his/her hearing loss can be cured merely by removing impacted cerumen. Note that in this case, some hearing loss still was present even though the ear canal was cleared entirely of cerumen.

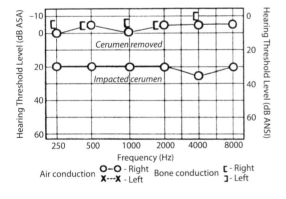

Figure 9.6 *History:* Fullness and hearing loss in right ear for several weeks after trying to clean ear with a cotton-tipped swab. *Otologic:* Right external auditory canal impacted with cerumen. Removal of cerumen revealed normal eardrum. *Audiologic:* Mild, flat hearing loss in right ear with normal bone conduction. Left ear masked. Removal of cerumen resulted in restoration of hearing to normal (upper curve). *Classification:* Conductive. *Diagnosis:* Impacted cerumen. *Abbreviations:* ANSI, American National Standards Institute; ASA, American Standards Association.

The removal of cerumen requires gentleness and patience and always should be performed with good illumination. The simplest method that suits the situation should be used. Firm plugs of wax can be removed best by gently teasing them out with fine forceps. The forceps or any other instrument should come in contact with the wax only and not with the skin of the canal, which is thin and tender. Soft wax can be wiped out with a curette or a very thin, cotton-tipped probe. Using cotton swabs to remove wax from a narrow canal only pushes it in further and impacts it. Sometimes, it may be necessary to irrigate wax from an ear canal, but this should be avoided if the canal is already inflamed. Irrigation should not be performed in the presence of a known perforation of the eardrum because this may result in otitis media. When irrigation is performed, the water used should be at body temperature to avoid stimulating the labyrinth and producing vertigo. The stream of water is most effective when it is directed forcefully toward one edge of the wax so that the water can get behind the plug and force it out. The ear canal should be dried carefully at the end of the procedure.

Harsh chemicals that are supposed to soften cerumen when introduced into the ear often irritate the tender skin of the canal and cause external otitis. They should be avoided or used with great caution.

## FLUID IN THE EXTERNAL AUDITORY CANAL

The external auditory canals in some people are angled such that when water gets in, it is very difficult to remove. This may be a problem after swimming, showering, or bathing, and it is common after people spray their hair with certain lotions and after they use shampoos. The reader may recall seeing a patient after a swim tilt his/her head, slap it on one side, then jump up and down—all this merely to get a little water out of an ear. People like this swimmer may have deformed ear canals or excess earwax that prevents water from coming out readily. Exostoses in the ear canal also may account for this difficulty. An example of hearing loss caused by fluid in

NAME _____

| DATE | RIGHT EAR AIR CONDUCTION | | | | | | | LEFT EAR AIR CONDUCTION | | | | | |
|---|---|---|---|---|---|---|---|---|---|---|---|---|---|
| | 250 | 500 | 1000 | 2000 | 4000 | 8000 | | 250 | 500 | 1000 | 2000 | 4000 | 8000 |
| | 45 | 50 | 40 | 50 | 65 | 60 | | 50 | 50 | 55 | 65 | 70 | 60 |
| AFTER REMOVAL OF WAX | 20 | 20 | 20 | 25 | 40 | 45 | | 20 | 25 | 35 | 35 | 45 | 50 |
| | | | | | | | | | | | | | |

| RIGHT EAR BONE CONDUCTION | | | | | | | LEFT EAR BONE CONDUCTION | | | | | |
|---|---|---|---|---|---|---|---|---|---|---|---|---|
| 10 | 10 | 10 | 10 | 40 | | | 5 | 10 | 10 | 20 | 50 | |

**SPEECH RECEPTION:** Right _____ Left _____     **DISCRIMINATION:** Right _____ Left _____

(Each ear is tested separately with pure tones for air conduction and bone conduction, if necessary. The tones increase in pitch in octave steps from 250 to 8,000 Hz. Normal hearing in each frequency lies between 0 and 25 decibels. The larger the number above 25 decibels in each frequency the greater the hearing loss. When the two ears differ greatly in threshold, one ear is masked with noise to test the other ear. Speech reception is the patient's threshold for everyday speech, rather than pure tones. A speech reception threshold of over 30 decibels is handicapping in many situations. The discrimination score indicates the ability to understand selected test words at a comfortable level above the speech reception threshold.)

Figure 9.7 *History:* Patient claims deafness started several months ago after attempt to remove wax from both ears. Occasional buzzing tinnitus. No vertigo. Denies family history of deafness. *Otologic:* Bilateral impacted cerumen. Removed. Eardrums normal. *Audiologic:* Bilateral reduced air conduction with near-normal bone conduction, except at 4000 Hz. Removal of cerumen closed the air–bone gap somewhat, but a residual conductive loss remained. *Classification:* Conductive. *Diagnosis:* Conductive hearing loss caused by impacted cerumen and an underlying condition of otosclerosis. *Aids to diagnosis:* Impacted cerumen does not typically cause such a severe conductive loss. Stapes fixation was found at surgery and bearing improved in left ear.

the external canal is seen in **Figure 9.8**. Note the high-frequency drop in air conduction that is so suggestive of sensorineural hearing loss, but also note that the bone conduction is normal. This example should be compared with a case showing fluid in the middle ear; in such a case, a drop in bone conduction usually accompanies the reduction in air conduction. When fluid in the external auditory canal is the only cause, removing it will restore normal hearing.

Occasionally, oily medicine dropped into a child's canal for treating an ear infection may be trapped there for a long time and cause hearing loss. It is well worth noting that if only air conduction testing is done, as is customary in most industrial and school hearing test programs, one might conclude erroneously that the two cases presented in **Figures 9.7** and **9.8** should be classified as sensorineural because the hearing loss was most pronounced in the higher frequencies.

## COLLAPSE OF THE EAR CANAL DURING AUDIOMETRY

In rare instances, auditory canals may be shaped in a way that when pressure is directed on the pinna, the canal wall completely collapses, and conductive hearing loss results. This condition may be produced when earphones are placed over the ears during a routine hearing test. Therefore, the examiner should adjust earphones to the ears carefully to avoid collapse of the canal and a spurious hearing level. Usually, the patient will complain that his/her ears feel full and he/she unable to hear well as soon as the earphones are placed over the ears. The patient also may make some effort to readjust the earphones. The examiner should be alert to this type of situation and correct it. In some cases, it is necessary to place small tubes in the ear canal to prevent collapse or use insert earbuds for hearing testing.

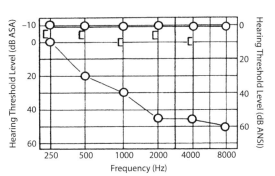

Figure 9.8 Conductive hearing loss induced in right ear by filling the external auditory canal with mineral oil. Note that the shape of the curve in this conductive loss is atypical because the greater loss is in the high frequencies. No recruitment is present with the ear filled with mineral oil. Hearing returned to normal after the mineral oil was removed. *Abbreviations*: ANSI, American National Standards Institute; ASA, American Standards Association.

**Figure 9.9** gives an example of such a circumstance in a patient who already had a sensorineural hearing loss. To demonstrate that there was a conductive overlay produced by the collapse of the ear canal, a plastic tube was inserted to keep the ear canal open, and the hearing level improved instantly.

If there is no collapse of the canal, and yet air conduction is reduced despite apparently normal speech reception (judged by the patient's response to conversation), functional hearing loss should be suspected.

## EXTERNAL OTITIS

## CAUSE

Occlusion of the auditory canal with debris or swelling due to inflammation of the surrounding skin is a common cause of hearing loss, particularly in summer and in tropical climates. The most common cause is prolonged exposure of the skin to water, especially during swimming, but inflammation may result also from excessive washing or irrigation of the ear. Trauma to the skin of the canal

during the removal of cerumen or foreign bodies may be another cause of external otitis, or it may result from dermatitis, infections, allergies, and systemic diseases.

## DIAGNOSIS

In diagnosing external otitis, the first consideration is to distinguish it from otitis media; this is difficult unless the eardrum is visible and appears to be normal. Occasionally, both external otitis and otitis media occur at the same time. When the eardrum is not visible, certain features aid in establishing the diagnosis. In external otitis, the skin of the auditory canal generally is edematous or excoriated. Tenderness around the entire ear is pronounced, and pain in the ear is aggravated by chewing or pressing on the ear. However, in most cases of otitis media, there is comparatively little swelling in the external canal unless mastoiditis is present or there is a profuse, irritating discharge from the middle ear. The pain in otitis media usually is very deep in the ear and is not aggravated by movements of the jaw during eating. However, sneezing and coughing often produce severe, sharp pain because of the increased pressure in the inflamed middle ear. If the discharge in an ear canal has a stringy mucoid appearance, as is found in the nose during rhinitis, it almost invariably indicates otitis media with a perforated eardrum.

Whenever a clear-cut diagnosis is not possible, therapy should be directed to both the external and middle ears. For external otitis, medication principally is applied locally to the outer ear; for otitis media, it is directed to the middle ear, the nasopharynx, and primarily systemically.

Overly forceful efforts to introduce an otoscope into a tender, inflamed ear canal should be avoided. In some instances, a preliminary diagnosis must be based on the history and the superficial examination, as well as the clinical experience, until the infection subsides, and visualization of the eardrum becomes possible.

## TREATMENT

Of the many successful methods of treating severe otitis externa, one of the best is to insert a large wick soaked in ear drops into the external auditory canal. The same wick should be kept in place and wetted

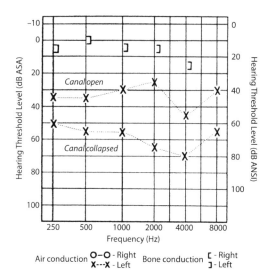

Air conduction O—O - Right / X---X - Left    Bone conduction [ - Right / ] - Left

Figure 9.9 *History:* A 37-year-old man with gradual progressive hearing loss. Occasional ringing tinnitus. Patient's maternal aunt is hard-of-hearing. *Otologic:* Ears normal. Stapes fixation confirmed at surgery. *Audiologic:* Right and left ears showed a moderately severe air conduction loss. The patient's responses to conversational voice did not seem to be in keeping with the pure-tone responses, and a functional hearing loss was suspected. After removal of the earphones, that patient reported that his/her hearing seemed to be blocked when the earphones were in place. A stock earmold used for hearing aid evaluations was placed in the left ear canal, the earphones were put on again, and the hearing was retested. Significant improvements in thresholds were obtained when the ear canal was held open with the earmold. Bone conduction thresholds were normal with the opposite ear masked. *Classification:* Conductive. *Diagnosis:* Otosclerosis. Inconsistencies in initial pure-tone thresholds and subjective responses to normal voice indicated a functional aspect to the problem presented. The patient's report pointed to the possibility of canal closure when earphones were worn. This was confirmed, and the original moderately severe loss actually was found to be mild in degree. *Comment:* In applying the earphones, care must be taken not to compress the ear canal. *Abbreviations:* ANSI, American National Standards Institute; ASA, American Standards Association.

with the same solution for at least 24–48 hours. The wick should not be allowed to dry. The drops may contain antibiotics with or without steroids or may contain acetic acid. This treatment (acetic acid) changes the pH in the ear canal and thus inhibits

the growth of certain pathogenic organisms while the ear is healing. More specific medication is indicated if this mild therapy does not resolve the infection. Too often, a resistant external otitis is misdiagnosed as a fungus infection; the fungus usually is a secondary invader, and more careful study will reveal a bacterial or an allergic problem. Steroid and antibiotic eardrops are helpful in treating severe external otitis.

The use of strong chemicals and overtreatment should be avoided, as should excessive manipulation in a swollen ear canal. Strong medications frequently will aggravate an external otitis, and prolonged use of medication will cause an infection to persist when it would have cleared up otherwise.

After the infection has subsided in the auditory canal and after the eardrum is visualized, it is advisable to perform a hearing test to be certain that there is no underlying hearing impairment from some other condition in the middle or the inner ear.

## FOREIGN BODY IN THE EAR CANAL

Hearing loss and fullness in the ear are often the only symptoms produced by a foreign body in the ear canal. It is surprising how long a patient can remain unaware of a piece of cotton or other foreign matter in the ear canal. Only when this foreign body becomes impacted with wax or swollen with moisture do fullness and hearing loss ensue, and then medical attention is sought. The hearing loss is caused by the occlusion of the canal; it is usually mild and greater in the lower frequencies.

The variety of foreign bodies removed from ear canals, especially in children, ranges from pencil erasers to peas. Most of these cause enough ear discomfort to attract attention before hearing loss becomes prominent, but not always. Caution always must be observed when attempting to remove a foreign body from the ear canal. Usually, special grasping instruments are essential, depending on the nature of the foreign body. General anesthesia may be advisable for a child unless the foreign body is obviously simple to grasp and to remove in a single painless maneuver. It is easy to underestimate the difficulty in removing a foreign body and to run into unexpected problems; excessive preparation is better than too little. Irrigation is contraindicated if the foreign body swells in water (which occurs with dried peas and water beads).

**Figure 9.10** illustrates the bearing loss and the findings in a man who was unaware that he had left a piece of cotton in his ear 3 months before. Only when shower water seemed to get trapped in his ear and cause fullness did he seek medical attention.

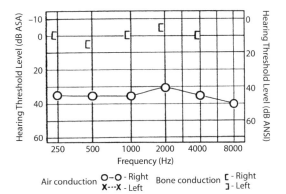

Air conduction  O–O - Right  Bone conduction  C - Right
            X···X - Left                    ] - Left

Figure 9.10  *History:* A 27-year-old man who complained of hearing loss in the right ear which had begun 3 months before. It started with itching and fullness in the canal. He did not seek medical attention until the ear had started to drain 2 days before. No tinnitus. *Otologic:* Left ear clear. Right ear had a putrid external otitis, and behind the discharge was a thick plug of absorbent cotton and debris. The patient recalled putting the cotton in the ear ~3 months previously. The foreign matter was removed. *Audiologic:* Right-ear air conduction thresholds revealed a flat, moderate loss. Bone conduction was normal with the left ear masked. Hearing returned to normal with removal of plug. *Classification:* Conductive. *Diagnosis:* Foreign matter in ear canal. *Note:* For an accurate diagnosis, the eardrums should be made visible by clearing out any debris that prevents inspection. *Abbreviations*: ANSI, American National Standards Institute; ASA, American Standards Association.

## CARCINOMA OF THE EXTERNAL CANAL

Whenever a granuloma or a similar mass is seen in the external canal, carcinoma should be suspected. Although carcinoma in this area is not common, the possibility is serious enough to warrant constant alertness. The most common complaints associated with carcinoma are fullness in the ear, hearing loss, pain, and bleeding from the canal. The mass does not have to be large to occlude the ear canal. Symptoms may have existed for only a short time so that it may be possible to diagnose the malignancy comparatively early, even though the prognosis in such cases is not always good. Hearing loss is an almost insignificant aspect of this important entity, but it is frequently the presenting symptom. Early attention to a complaint of hearing impairment may be essential to prompt diagnosis of carcinoma and early surgical intervention.

## GRANULOMA

Although granuloma in the external auditory canal is comparatively rare, it warrants special comment because hearing loss generally is the only presenting symptom. Occasionally, there may be some drainage from the ear caused by secondary infection, but more often, the patient complains of a gradual hearing loss for no apparent reason or possibly may attribute it to wax in the ear. A granuloma of the external auditory canal is seen readily by examination with an otoscope. This condition should not be mistaken for the fragile polypoid soft granulation tissue that arises in chronically diseased middle ears and sometimes extends into the canal. Granulomata are usually firm or hard masses that resemble neoplasms and may regenerate when they are removed. Occasionally, their cause and diagnosis are most difficult to determine; for example, in the case cited in **Figure 9.11**, the patient's chief complaint was an insidious hearing loss in the left ear, present for about a year, with no related symptoms or obvious cause. The right ear was normal, but the left showed an obvious complete atresia of the external canal a short distance from the opening.

The appearance was the picture of a stenosis with firm, thick, normal skin covering a bony undersurface. The major diagnostic feature was that the patient had had a normal audiogram and normal hearing in this same ear 2 years prior to his latest visit to the physician's office. This case illustrates the importance of considering the possibility of a granuloma as a cause of conductive hearing loss due to visible damage in the external canal.

The causes of granuloma include tuberculosis, eosinophilic granuloma, fungus infection, carcinoma, and others. Biopsies and special tests help to establish a definitive etiology.

## CYSTS IN THE EAR CANAL

A large variety of cysts can occur in the ear canal and may cause hearing loss by obstructing the lumen. The common types found in the canal are sebaceous and dermoid cysts, but others also are found.

Hematomas in the auricle may become large enough to extend into the external canal and completely occlude it, producing hearing loss. In a chronic type of hematoma that occurs in wrestlers' or boxers' ears, the opening of the canal can be so constricted by an old accumulation of blood and scar tissue that the canal is closed entirely, and hearing loss results.

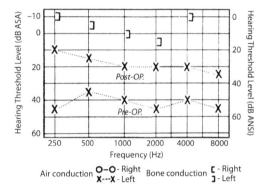

Figure 9.11 *History*: Prior otologic and audiologic examinations revealed normal findings. For the past year, the patient noted first intermittent, then gradual and constant fullness and hearing loss in left ear. No pain or tenderness in ear. *Otologic*: Complete atresia of left canal just inside opening. Under the thick skin was a firm bony layer that could not be penetrated with a needle. At surgery, a large, fibrous granuloma was removed from under the skin. The eardrum was thick and white but intact. A pathological diagnosis of foreign-body granuloma was established. The patient did not recall any event or symptom that might explain the diagnosis. X-ray films showed normal mastoid but bony occlusion in the left external canal. *Audiologic*: Reduced air and normal bone conduction thresholds in the left ear with masking in the right ear. Tuning fork lateralized to the left ear, and bone was better than air conduction. Postoperative air conduction responses were improved, but the air–bone gap was not closed completely. The eardrum was thick, opaque, immobile, and suggestive of a long-standing external otitis. *Classification*: Conductive. *Diagnosis*: Atresia with foreign-body granuloma. *Abbreviations*: ANSI, American National Standards Institute; ASA, American Standards Association.

## OTHER CAUSES

Other causes of conductive hearing loss with abnormal findings visible in the canal include furuncles, keloids, angiomas, papillomas, osteomas, acute infectious diseases, and malignancy. None of these is very common, but hearing impairment and fullness in the ear may be the chief or even the only symptoms to direct attention to the condition. The audiometric findings usually show hearing losses of <30 dB, with the lower frequencies involved to a greater extent.

## ABNORMALITIES VISIBLE IN THE EARDRUM

An abnormal appearance of the eardrum detected by otoscopic examination of patients with a conductive hearing loss may indicate a condition largely restricted to the drum itself. Conditions of this type are reviewed in this chapter. More often the abnormality visible in the eardrum is produced by injury or disease of the middle ear and communicating structures; such conditions are considered in this chapter. Careful inspection of the drum and the external ear also may reveal evidence of surgical procedures previously performed on the patient.

## MYRINGITIS

Occasionally, the eardrum is attacked by diseases without involvement of the rest of the external or the middle ear. This is called myringitis. In most cases, this condition is the result of a little-understood viral infection. The most common type is described as myringitis bullosa, in which blebs appear on the drum owing to pouching out of its outer layer with fluid. These blebs appear to be clear, and when punctured, they discharge a thin, clear, or slightly blood-tinged fluid. Sometimes the blebs may extend to the skin of the external canal. Myringitis starts rather abruptly and causes pain and fullness in the ear along with mild hearing loss. Usually, only one ear is involved. When the blister is punctured, the hearing promptly improves, and the feeling of fullness and pain diminishes.

The diagnosis occasionally is difficult because myringitis may be confused with a bulging drum caused by acute otitis media. The absence of an immobile eardrum or of any upper respiratory infection and the normal appearance of the portions of the drum not affected by blebs help to distinguish myringitis from a middle ear infection.

Furthermore, when a bleb is punctured carefully, no hole is made through the drum, and only the outer layer is incised, so that with air pressure in the canal or politzerization through the nose the intact eardrum moves. By contrast, after myringotomy because of the perforation, the drum does not move in response to a small difference in air pressure.

Bullous myringitis is commonly associated with mycoplasma infection. Herpes zoster, which can produce a picture somewhat similar to that of myringitis, is described in Chapter 10, as the sensorineural mechanism also is affected in many instances.

## RUPTURED EARDRUM

### DEFINITION

An eardrum is said to be ruptured when it is penetrated suddenly by a foreign body (like a hairpin) or when it tears from the force of a slap across the ear. Otherwise, a hole in an eardrum is called a perforation rather than a rupture. Usually, the edge of a rupture is more irregular, and it is not accompanied immediately by signs of inflammation.

### CAUSES

Most ruptures caused by penetrating objects are situated in the posterior portion of the drum because of the curve of the external canal and the slope of the drum. Ruptures caused by a sudden and intense pressure change, as by a blow to the side of the head or by an explosion, are more frequently in the anterior–inferior quadrant and occasionally in the pars flaccida. Another common cause of eardrum rupture is a slap or other impact on the ear while swimming under water. Because water gets into the middle ear, infections

are more likely to ensue. In all cases of ruptured eardrum, the history is most pertinent because marked pain, fullness, and ringing in the ear often are experienced.

### TREATMENT

Systemic antibiotics and eardrops may be useful in treating contaminated ruptures such as underwater injuries. Eardrops are not indicated for dry ruptures. Nose blowing should be avoided. In most cases, the small rupture heals spontaneously if infection is prevented. If healing does not take place, it may be necessary to encourage it by cauterization or by doing a myringoplasty at some future time. The hearing loss may be as large as 60 dB if the rupture was caused by a force severe enough to impair the ossicular chain, but usually the loss is > 30 dB and involves almost all frequencies. **Figure 9.12** shows an example of hearing loss caused by a ruptured eardrum.

### A TEAR IN THE EARDRUM

This may be considered a special type of rupture of the eardrum. It may result from a direct blow to the head that causes a longitudinal fracture of the temporal bone extending into the roof of the middle ear. Usually, the top of the eardrum is torn, blood gets into the middle and the outer ear, and occasionally the ossicular chain also is disrupted. Sometimes, there also may be a facial paralysis and cerebrospinal otorrhea. In longitudinal fractures, the CT may show a fracture line extending into the middle cranial fossa from the outer ear inward and parallel with the superior petrosal sinus. Because there is blood in the middle ear, bone conduction also is reduced but returns to normal after resolution occurs. If the fracture involves the sensorineural mechanism, bone conduction usually is affected more seriously and permanently.

## SPARK IN THE EARDRUM

In industry, a spark may hit the eardrum and have a severe effect on hearing. **Figure 9.13** points out what happens in such a case. Unfortunately, this is not a rare experience when workers are welding, grinding, chipping, or burning, and an occasional spark may find its way into the canal. It hits the drum with a devastating effect. Usually, the entire drum is destroyed cleanly, leaving only the handle of the malleus hanging down. Little or no infection accompanies this trauma. The pain is severe but of short duration. The hearing loss is usually ~50 or 60 dB and affects all frequencies. As in cases of ruptured eardrum, forceful nose blowing should be avoided after such an accident. Applying eardrops is not advisable. The spark cauterizes the area, and infection does not ensue if antibiotics are administered orally, and local probing is avoided. Myringoplasty usually is indicated, and the hearing usually can be improved or restored.

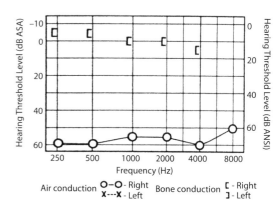

Figure 9.13 *History:* Patient works as a welder, and a spark flew into his right ear, causing severe burning pain and subsequent hearing loss. *Otologic:* Patient was seen 24 hours after accident. Right eardrum almost completely destroyed without evidence of inflammation. Handle of malleus visible as well as incudostapedial joint. External canal not affected visibly. *Audiologic:* Flat 60-dB loss with good bone conduction (left ear masked) and lateralization to right. *Classification:* Conductive. *Diagnosis:* Eardrum destroyed by hot spark *Abbreviations:* ANSI, American National Standards Institute; ASA, American Standards Association.

Wherever free sparks are produced in industry; steps should be taken to shield personnel from them. In places where this is not practical, as in some forges or foundries, it is essential to protect the ears with ear protection and the eyes with safety glasses.

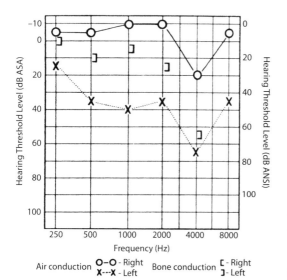

Figure 9.12 *History:* A 35-year-old man exposed to a firecracker explosion next to left ear. Intermittent ringing tinnitus. Had some previous exposure to gunfire in service. *Otologic:* Right, normal. Left ear had a large rupture of the eardrum without visible infection. *Audiologic:* The right ear had normal thresholds, except for a 20-dB dip at 4000 Hz (C-5 dip). The left ear had a moderate air conduction loss and a 65-dB C-5 dip. Masked bone conduction thresholds on the left ear showed a good degree of air–bone gap. *Classification:* Conductive. *Diagnosis:* Acoustic trauma with ruptured eardrum. The hearing returned to a level similar to that in the right ear after a myringoplasty. The ossicles were found to be functioning. *Abbreviations:* ANSI, American National Standards Institute; ASA, American Standards Association.

## PERFORATED EARDRUM

The role of the eardrum in hearing often is misunderstood, especially by lay people. Many believe that without an eardrum, it is not possible to hear at all. Some parents understandably become very concerned when a myringotomy is suggested for their child because they are fearful of having their hearing destroyed by a hole in the drum. There even are physicians who attribute marked hearing defects to such conditions as "hardening of the eardrum" and "too small an eardrum."

## EXTENT OF HEARING LOSS

Actually, it is possible to have very little loss in hearing though a large hole may be visible in the drum. In a nationwide study of school children, 60% of ears with dry perforations went undetected by hearing screening tests because the hearing loss of these children was < 20 dB. The hearing level in another 40% of the ears showing perforations was better than 5 dB on the audiometer. It really is not possible to predict the degree of hearing loss from the appearance of the tympanic membrane. In some cases, in which the membrane is perforated and even scarred, the hearing is nearly normal. There may be a severe hearing loss with only a pinpoint perforation. The cause of the pathology and its effect on the middle ear are more important criteria than the appearance of the eardrum.

However, the *location of the perforation* does have some *diagnostic meaning*. A persistent posterior perforation suggests associated mastoid infection, whereas an anterior perforation is not quite as serious. A superior perforation in Shrapnell's area also suggests that a fairly serious infection has been present.

A dry perforation in the tympanic membrane indicates that at some time infection probably was present in the middle ear. Only in rare instances does a perforation result from an infection in the external ear. Although the character and the location of the perforation are not reliable indications of the degree of hearing loss, they do play a certain role. For example, large perforations usually cause a greater loss. It appears that the principal effect of a perforation is a reduction of the surface on which sound pressure is exerted, the effect being proportional only to the area of the perforation. However, the relationship is not quite so simple.

Because the eardrum is effective only if it is in contact with the handle of the malleus, perforations affecting this area are especially damaging to the hearing. Perforations in the tense part of the eardrum, such as the anterior–inferior portion, affect the hearing more than those in the flaccid and superior portions because the tense part is largely responsible for the stiffness of the eardrum.

## TESTING FOR HEARING LOSS

An audiogram is the best way to determine the extent of the hearing loss when a perforation is found.

Caution should be exercised in correlating a perforation with the audiogram. It is natural for a physician to blame a hearing loss on a small perforation found in the eardrum, even if the loss is as severe as 60 dB; yet a perforation alone rarely produces such a marked degree of hearing loss. However, if the drum is entirely eroded and the ossicular chain has become ineffective, a hearing loss of 70 dB ANSI is to be expected. It is more than likely that there is some break in the ossicular chain when a severe degree of conductive hearing loss is found. This can be determined very simply by placing a small patch over the perforation, using Gelfoam or some other artificial material. If the hearing loss is a result of the perforation, then the hearing should be restored immediately.

This therapeutic test may be used when myringoplasty surgery is contemplated. If a hearing test shows that a temporary patch on the perforation in the drum fails to restore hearing, the otologist will know that further exploration of the middle ear is indicated to discover the major cause of the hearing loss because a simple myringoplasty would yield disappointing results.

## PERFORATIONS

### Demonstration

It is often difficult to be certain that a perforation actually is present in the tympanic membrane. Sometimes a large hole seems to be visible through the otoscope, but more careful scrutiny may reveal a very fine, thin, transparent film of epithelium covering the area. Such a film can be demonstrated best by gentle pressure on the ear canal with a pneumatic otoscope; by moving the eardrum, the light reflected from it will be visible on the covered perforation. Unless pressure is very gentle, the healed area may be broken readily. Spraying a fine, sterile powder into the ear also can outline a perforation or show an intact drum. It is also possible to fill an ear canal with water or ear drops and "pop" or politzerize the ear, looking for bubbles of an escaping through a tiny perforation.

### HEALING

Perforations in the eardrum heal in several ways. Most heal with a small scar that barely is visible. Others leave a somewhat thick, white scar which can be seen for many years. These scars in themselves produce no measurable hearing loss.

## RETRACTED DRUM WITH PERFORATION

In some ears, the drum is retracted so much that it envelops the promontory like a sheet of Saran Wrap, and yet it remains intact. In some cases, the retracted drum may have a perforation in it that is scarcely visible. The aperture can be visualized best by blowing camphor mist under pressure into one nostril while the other nostril is compressed, and the patient is asked to swallow. Through an otoscope, the mist can be seen coming out of the perforation. If the eardrum is intact, often it will push out a little bit, or it even may suddenly snap out quite sharply. In the latter case, the patient's hearing will improve suddenly.

## Methods of closing

Tympanic perforations cannot and generally should not be closed until the middle ear has been completely clear of infection and dry for at least several weeks; otherwise, the closure often breaks down. A small perforation that is not marginal (i.e., does not have an edge on the annulus) generally can be closed by repeated cauterization of its rim with trichloroacetic acid. This is done to destroy the edge of outer epithelium that has grown over the rim, thus preventing the middle (fibrous) layer from closing the hole spontaneously. The cauterization is repeated every few weeks until the closure is complete. Sometimes a long-standing perforation closes by itself after an acute attack of otitis media. In such cases, the edge of the perforation probably has been irritated and traumatized by the acute infection, and the trauma has stimulated growth of tissue around the edges of the perforation.

For large perforations and marginal ones, myringoplasty is necessary. This is often done under local anesthesia in adults. The epithelium around the edge of the perforation is removed, and a thin piece of skin, vein, fascia, fat, or other graft is applied. This technic produces excellent results. Sometimes in marginal perforations, a sliding skin graft from the external canal can be effective. In cases in which the preliminary closure of the perforation with Gelfoam or artificial membrane does not restore hearing, the middle ear and the ossicular chain should be explored during surgery, especially in cases in which the hearing loss exceeds 30 dB.

## RETRACTED EARDRUM

Physicians frequently attribute a marked conductive hearing loss, such as 50 dB, to a retracted eardrum, to adhesions in the middle ear, or to so-called catarrh. In most cases, these conclusions are unjustified. Rarely does any of these conditions alone cause a hearing loss > 40 dB. If the loss is substantially greater, there probably is some accompanying defect in the ossicular chain or the middle ear.

To understand why a retracted drum usually causes only a mild loss, it should be recalled that sound waves can be transmitted through the ossicles even if only part of the eardrum is present, particularly the portion around the malleus; therefore, even some badly retracted drums cause comparatively little hearing loss. In a few exceptional cases, a hearing loss > 40 dB is caused by retraction, and in these cases, hearing returns to normal with successful inflation of the middle ear. This is demonstrated in **Figure 9.14**.

Actually, a retracted eardrum is not pulled in; it is pushed in because the atmospheric pressure in the external canal is greater than that in the middle ear. Reduced middle ear pressure is produced most frequently by dysfunction in the eustachian tube. In children, hypertrophied adenoids and allergies are the chief causes. In adults, the principal causes are infections and allergies.

In any case, the eustachian tube becomes congested and blocks access to air needed to balance middle ear pressure with that in the external canal. The air already in the middle ear slowly is absorbed, and as a result, the eardrum gradually is pushed in toward the promontory. Sometimes the drum is so thin that when it is retracted, it envelops the promontory and is hardly discernible as a drum. By forced politzerization, it occasionally can be distended. If it does distend, it usually is flaccid and redundant, and later it retracts again unless the cause of the original retraction has been corrected.

In retracted drums, the reflected cone of light disappears, and the handle of the malleus appears to be prominent and shorter. Tinnitus rarely is caused by a retracted drum. If tinnitus is present, another cause should be suspected. Because a retracted eardrum often is associated with a perforation, it is important to use forced air pressure (pneumatic otoscopy) to be sure that the drum is intact.

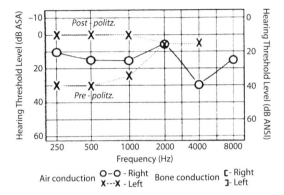

Figure 9.14 *History:* A 40-year-old woman with insidious hearing loss for past 3 years following an upper respiratory infection. Hears better intermittently. Has occasional pulsebeat tinnitus. *Otologic:* Scarred eardrums with healed perforations. Drums retracted. With politzerization the left eardrums ballooned out and hearing immediately returned to normal. *Audiologic:* Air conduction thresholds revealed a mild right hearing loss and a moderate left loss with greater loss in the low frequencies. After politzerization, the left ear thresholds returned to normal. *Impedance:* Type C tympanogram before politzerization. *Diagnosis:* Retracted and scarred eardrums caused by previous infections. *Abbreviations:* ANSI, American National Standards Institute; ASA, American Standards Association.

## FLACCID EARDRUM

A flaccid eardrum rarely causes hearing loss. The cause of the wrinkled and redundant eardrum is not always clear, but frequently it follows some long-standing malfunction of the eustachian tube, with alternate retraction and bulging of the eardrum resulting in the wrinkled appearance. Associated with a flaccid eardrum is a sensation of fullness, and occasionally the patient may report hearing his/her own breathing sounds. There is no general agreement on the best course of treatment, but politzerization and inflations generally should be avoided.

## THE SENILE EARDRUM

The appearance of a normal eardrum described in textbooks is always that of a young person. As human beings age, changes occur in the eardrum as they do in the eye and in the skin. The aged drum no longer reflects a cone of light, and it is no longer shiny. Its outer layer now appears to be thick and white or gray. It also loses its elasticity and becomes difficult to move with air pressure. White plaques and strands of fibrous tissue are evident in the middle fibrous layer of the drum.

It is difficult to ascertain how much hearing loss is caused by senile drum changes, but it probably is negligible. The high-frequency hearing loss associated with aging is caused by sensorineural changes. Usually, low-tone losses are negligible; if present, they too are likely to be sensorineural. Many aged patients whose eardrums show marked senile changes have normal hearing. However, it is important to expect senile changes in the drums of aged persons and not to attribute them to hearing losses which, in fact, have different etiologies.

## CAUSES IN MIDDLE EAR AND COMMUNICATING STRUCTURES

Although the causes of conductive hearing loss enumerated in this chapter originate in the middle ear, the eustachian tube, or the nasopharynx, they frequently can be detected by transilluminating the eardrum and looking not necessarily *at* the drum, but *through* it for telltale evidence of fluid, air bubbles, reflections, shadows, and the ossicles. The appearance of the drum itself also may be changed by the pathological conditions behind it. What the otoscope reveals must be interpreted using otologic experience.

## CATARRHAL DEAFNESS AND ADHESIONS

One may hear of a diagnosis of "catarrhal deafness." The pathology implied by this term is indefinite. Occasionally, it refers to a cloudy eardrum, which is blamed for a conductive hearing loss. Many times, the term is applied to any conductive hearing loss in which the drum appears to be slightly opaque or retracted. Typically, this is not catarrhal deafness but otosclerosis or tympanosclerosis with some incidental minor changes in the eardrum owing to malfunction of the eustachian tube. In all likelihood, the term catarrhal deafness was intended to apply to any one of the several conditions which today are identified separately as otitis media, secretory otitis media, and slight thickening and retraction of the eardrum suggesting middle ear adhesions. A better understanding of ear physiology and pathology now makes it possible to apply more specific and meaningful terms to these conditions.

There also is some doubt concerning the role of adhesions in the middle ear as a major cause of conductive hearing loss. Experience with stapes surgery has convinced otologists that occasional adhesions about the ossicles can produce negligible hearing loss. Even when many adhesions have to be cut during stapes surgery, very little of the hearing impairment seems to be attributable justly to this cause. Apparently, the ossicles transmit sound waves quite readily in spite of thin adhesions. However, in those instances in which the adhesions add weight and mass to the ossicular chain and drum, hearing is likely to be impaired measurably.

**Figure 9.15** illustrates the mild type of conductive hearing loss that probably is caused solely by adhesions in the middle ear. **Figure 9.16** shows a case that was diagnosed as catarrhal deafness by several otologists and proved on surgical exploration to be tympanosclerosis. Schuknecht reported a case of hearing loss caused by a bridge of bone binding the neck of the stapes and preventing mobility (**Figure 9.17**).

## AEROTITIS MEDIA (MIDDLE EAR BAROTRAUMA)

Hearing loss in aerotitis media usually is rather mild and temporary unless complications develop. The immediate cause of hearing impairment is retraction of the eardrum, but if the pressure disparity persists, fluid may accumulate in the middle ear and further aggravate the hearing loss.

The pressure disparity between the outer and middle ears almost invariably occurs during rapid descent in an airplane, when the atmospheric pressure increases rapidly as the plane comes down. If congestion prevents air from passing up the eustachian tube to equalize the increased pressure in the external canal, this pressure pushes in the eardrum toward the middle ear, causing sudden pain, fullness, and hearing loss. It occurs most frequently in people whose eustachian tubes are congested because of infection or allergy. To prevent aerotitis media, people with upper respiratory infections and acute allergies should be cautioned against flying. In adequately pressurized airplanes, aerotitis media is minimized.

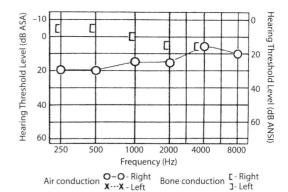

Air conduction O–O - Right / X---X - Left    Bone conduction [ - Right / ] - Left

Figure 9.15 *History:* A 42-year-old man with a history of recurrent otitis media in the right ear as a child. Nonprogressive. No tinnitus. No familial deafness. *Otologic:* Right eardrum was scarred and reflected previous infection, but it was intact and moved normally. No fluid visible. Hearing not improved after politzerization. Exploratory surgery on the right ear revealed multiple bands of scar tissue around incus and crura, binding ossicles to promontory. Stapes footplate was mobile. The ossicles were freed of the adhesions, and hearing in the right ear returned to normal. *Audiologic:* Mildly reduced low- and midfrequency thresholds with normal bone conduction thresholds in the right ear. Right ear bone thresholds were obtained with left ear masked. *Impedance:* Shallow type A tympanogram. *Classification:* Conductive. *Diagnosis:* Adhesive deafness. *Abbreviations:* ANSI, American National Standards Institute; ASA, American Standards Association.

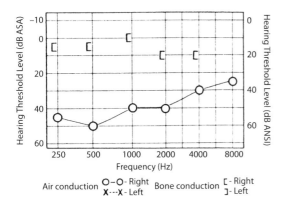

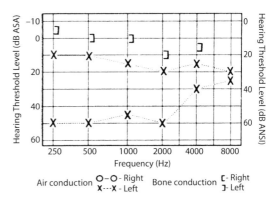

Figure 9.16 *History:* For a period of 6 years, patient had had chronic otitis media, which then had cleared up and remained so for the last 10 years. The original hearing loss has not progressed. Condition originally had been diagnosed as catarrhal deafness. *Otologic:* Right eardrum was intact but was thick, scarred, and had white calcific plaques. Exploratory surgery revealed no fluid in the middle ear but layers of tympanosclerotic bone around the footplate stapes. The plate was mobilized. *Audiologic:* Moderately reduced air conduction thresholds with normal bone conduction threshold in the right ear. Masking used in the left ear in testing for right-ear air and bone thresholds. Hearing improved with footplate mobilization. *Impedance:* Type A$_S$ tympanogram, stapedius reflex absent. *Classification:* Conductive hearing loss. *Diagnosis:* Deafness caused by tympanosclerosis rather than catarrhal deafness, as originally diagnosed. *Aids to diagnosis:* The severe, nonprogressive conductive hearing loss with white calcific deposits is suggestive of tympanosclerosis. *Abbreviations:* ANSI, American National Standards Institute; ASA, American Standards Association.

If a patient is seen soon after the onset of aerotitis media, the symptoms can be relieved by politzerization followed by steroids, or by decongestants and myringotomy, followed by administration of an oral decongestant and politzerization. When the air pressure in the middle ear is made equal to that in the outer ear, hearing is restored, and the feeling of fullness gradually disappears. **Figure 9.18** describes a classic example of aerotitis media with recovery. If a patient is seen several days after the onset of aerotitis media, it may be necessary to use antibiotics and steroids. In all cases, hearing should return to normal when the eardrum is restored to its normal position and the middle ear and the eustachian tube are clear.

Figure 9.17 *History:* Progressive hearing loss for 12 years. Patient had worn a hearing aid in the left ear for 5 years. *Otologic:* Normal eardrums. *Audiologic:* Air conduction thresholds revealed a moderately severe loss in the left ear and a moderate loss in the right ear. Tuning-fork tests indicated better hearing by bone conduction than by air conduction in the left ear. *Impedance:* Would have revealed type A$_S$ tympanogram with absent stapedius reflex. *Classification:* Conductive. *Diagnosis:* Bridge of bone that is binding the stapes visualized and corrected at surgery. *Abbreviations:* ANSI, American National Standards Institute; ASA, American Standards Association. (From Schuknecht [1].)

## HEMOTYMPANUM

Blood in the middle ear with an intact drum produces a dark-red or bluish hue. This is a common finding after head injury with fracture of the middle cranial fossa. Sometimes a fluid level is visible. If the sensorineural mechanism has not been injured, the conductive hearing loss generally is ~40 dB, usually involving all frequencies. Occasionally, the high frequencies are involved to a greater degree. Interestingly, the bone conduction shows a high-frequency drop (**Figure 9.19**) and prompts the erroneous belief that sensorineural damage has occurred. Both air conduction and bone conduction may return to normal as the blood is absorbed. Blood also may be seen in the middle ear for a short time following stapes surgery, and when this occurs, hearing improvement is delayed until absorption takes place.

The normal middle ear has a remarkable ability to remove fluid and debris by absorption, ciliary action, and phagocytosis. For this reason, it is usually unnecessary and often unwise to remove blood from the middle ear cavity by myringotomy and suction. This may introduce infection and cause complications. Whenever a red eardrum is seen and blood is suspected of being in the middle ear, a glomus jugulare tumor should be ruled out. Imaging studies and a good history are essential.

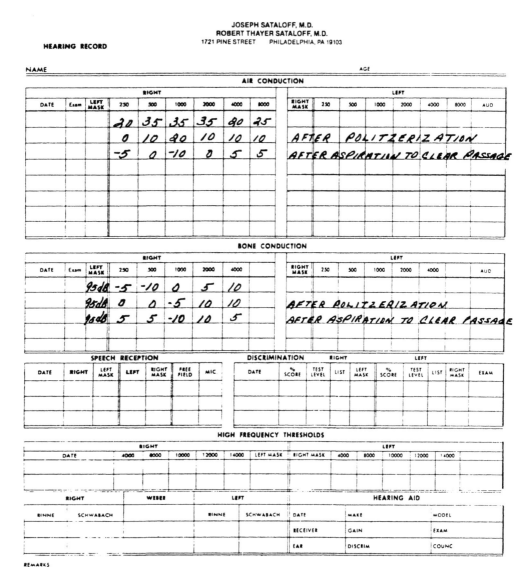

Figure 9.18 *History:* Patient developed fullness, pain, and hearing loss in right ear during descent in airplane. *Otologic:* Examination 2 days following the incident showed a slightly vascular handle of the malleus and bubbles in the right ear. The drum was retracted slightly and did not move freely. The patient had received an injection of penicillin 24 hours prior to the examination, and the eustachian tube seemed to be patent. The ear was politzerized, followed by a myringotomy and aspiration. *Audiologic:* Air conduction thresholds in the right ear revealed a mild loss and normal bone conduction. Hearing improved with politzerization and returned to normal after a myringotomy with aspiration. *Impedance:* Type B tympanogram before politzerization; Type C after politzerization. *Classification:* Conductive. *Diagnosis:* Aerotitis media. *Note:* Politzerization alone did not restore the hearing to normal because some fluid still remained in the middle ear.

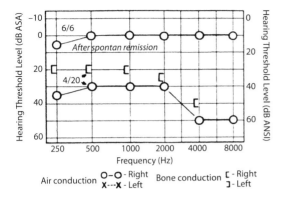

Air conduction O–O - Right  Bone conduction ⊏ - Right
                X--X - Left                    ⊐ - Left

Figure 9.19 *History:* A 24-year-old patient who sustained a head injury causing right middle ear to be filled with blood. *Otologic:* Tympanic membrane was intact but was deep red in color because of blood in the middle ear. The eardrum did not move well with air pressure. Resolution occurred spontaneously without myringotomy. *Audiologic:* Pure-tone thresholds in the right ear revealed a mild air conduction loss with reduced bone conduction (when left ear was masked). Note the greater loss in the high frequencies and the reduced bone thresholds because of the fluid in the middle ear. Hearing returned to normal at all frequencies after spontaneous resolution. *Classification:* Conductive; damage in middle ear. *Diagnosis:* Posttraumatic hemotympanum. *Aids to diagnosis:* A glomus tumor must be ruled out. Usually, the eardrum moves freely in a glomus tumor, and blanching may occur with positive pressure. Tympanogram may show pulsations. X-ray films are helpful if erosion is present. If a glomus tumor is suspected strongly, retrograde jugular venography may be performed. *Abbreviations:* ANSI, American National Standards Institute; ASA, American Standards Association.

## SECRETORY OTITIS MEDIA

In spite of considerable literature about secretory otitis media, neither the cause nor a specific cure is known. Secretory otitis media seems to have increased in incidence—a fact that has been related to the use of antibiotics.

## CHARACTERISTIC FEATURES

The major feature of the condition is accumulation of fluid in the middle ear, usually straw-colored and sometimes mucoid or gel-like in consistency. In many cases, the eustachian tube is patent, and the fluid can be removed readily by myringotomy and politzerization. However, the fluid continues to accumulate in spite of numerous myringotomies and various treatments, and hearing loss occurs concomitantly, usually greater in the higher frequencies (**Figure 9.20**). This can occur even with myringotomy tubes in place. Secretory otitis may be present in one or both ears, and it is found in babies as well as in adults.

Often the condition suddenly stops spontaneously, and the treatment used at that particular time is likely to get the credit. In some cases, the secretion continues to form and causes a perforation in the eardrum; the findings resemble those seen in chronic otitis media, but the discharge is free of infectious elements.

When the mucosa of the middle ear in secretory otitis media is examined by biopsy, it is found in most cases to be thickened. The thickened mucosa extends to the mouth of the eustachian tube in the middle ear, and perhaps this is a factor in the blockage. In many patients with secretory otitis, one can observe increased secretion in the nasal mucosa and in the nasopharynx as well; this suggests the possibility that secretory otitis may be more than a local middle ear phenomenon. Some ears fill with secretory fluid after removal of the soft palate for neoplasm. There seems little doubt that in such instances the condition is related to eustachian tube malfunction. Additionally, gastric reflux has been identified as a cause of middle ear fluid; and pepsin, a digestive enzyme from the stomach, has been recovered from the middle ear.

It often is difficult to distinguish secretory otitis from serous otitis. Caution in treatment is of the utmost importance, and unwarranted surgical procedures should be avoided. For example, it is injudicious to perform an adenoidectomy on an infant who has secretory otitis media without positive evidence that the adenoids are the principal cause of the difficulty, in which case it would be a serous otitis. Too frequently, secretory otitis will continue to recur after a T&A that was unjustified,

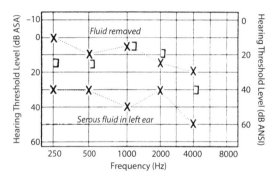

Figure 9.20 *History:* A 12-year-old boy with recurrent episodes of painless hearing loss in left ear. These occurred in the absence of upper respiratory infections. He had a tonsillectomy and adenoidectomy and an adenoid revision, allergy studies, desensitization, autogenous vaccines, and many courses of antibiotics and nose treatments. *Otologic:* The left eardrum was slightly scarred, but a fluid level was seen. The eustachian tube seemed to be patent. The eardrum did not move freely with air pressure. Exploration of the middle ear showed a thick, clear, gelatinous fluid, which was aspirated. The mucosa over the promontory was thick and hydropic. A myringotomy tube was placed in the eardrum and was removed after several months. The patient had had no recurrence since his surgery, but not all patients respond this well after the tube is removed. *Audiologic:* Pure-tone thresholds in the left ear revealed a mild air conduction loss with reduced bone conduction (right ear masked). After surgery, the air conduction thresholds returned to better levels than the original bone conduction thresholds at most frequencies. Reduced bone thresholds were caused by the thick fluid in the middle ear. *Impedance:* Type B tympanogram, absent stapedius reflex. *Classification:* Conductive. *Diagnosis:* Recurrent secretory otitis. *Aids to diagnosis:* Reduced bone conduction does not mean necessarily that a sensorineural bearing loss is present. An immobile drum, fluctuating hearing loss, and a feeling of fluid in an ear should suggest that reduced bone conduction may be due to middle-ear involvement rather than to sensorineural causes. *Abbreviations:* ANSI, American National Standards Institute; ASA, American Standards Association.

thereby placing the surgeon in an embarrassing situation. When adenoids are really the major cause of secretion in the middle ears (serous otitis), other symptoms usually are present, including recurrent otitis media and mouth breathing; furthermore, the hypertrophied adenoids can be felt and visualized in the lateral area of the nasopharynx. These findings often are not present if the cause is secretory otitis media.

## APPEARANCE AND TREATMENT

The appearance of the eardrum in secretory otitis often is characteristic, and yet sometimes it may be deceiving. Generally, it is easy to observe bubbles and a yellowish fluid behind the drum. Politzerization, which shows the eustachian tube to be patent, causes the fluid level to shift or even to disappear, and hearing suddenly improves (though it does not always return to normal).

Conductive hearing loss is usually present, and the bone conduction may be reduced somewhat in the higher frequencies. Myringotomy generally produces a gush of fluid, and the hearing improves markedly. The length of time that the hearing loss has been present is not a factor and may even be misleading because fluid can remain in the middle ear for many months or years. In many cases, it is advisable to insert a tube through an inferior myringotomy to maintain air in the middle ear.

## ANOTHER TYPE OF SECRETORY OTITIS AND ITS DIFFERENTIATION FROM OTOSCLEROSIS

Another type of secretory otitis media can lead to the erroneous diagnosis of otosclerosis because it is so difficult to observe abnormalities in the eardrum or in the middle ear. In this type, a gel-like mass of clear secretion or a very thick collection of mucoid secretion is located in the middle ear so that it causes hearing loss without any abnormality being visible through the drum. This leads to a diagnosis of otosclerosis. When the middle ear is exposed with the intention of doing stapes surgery, a thick secretion is found instead. Its removal causes the hearing to return to normal. Such a case is shown in **Figure 9.21**. A preliminary myringotomy and the introduction of a suction tip would have revealed the thick fluid.

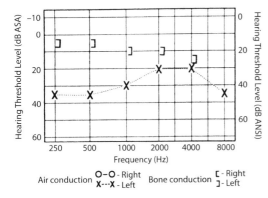

Air conduction **O–O** - Right  **X---X** - Left  Bone conduction **[** - Right  **]** - Left

Figure 9.21 *History:* A 27-year-old woman with gradual onset of hearing loss in the left ear for several years. Feeling of fullness and occasional heartbeat tinnitus in the left ear. Several members in the family have hearing loss. She denies any history of ear infections. The patient had been diagnosed as having unilateral otosclerosis. *Otologic:* Eardrums appeared to be normal (but did not move well with politzerization). When the eardrum was elevated, gelatinous fluid caused by secretory otitis was removed from the oval and the round windows. The stapes was found to be mobile. *Audiologic:* Air conduction thresholds in the left ear were reduced mildly in the lower frequencies. Bone conduction was almost normal with the right ear masked. The tuning fork lateralized to the left ear. Bone conduction was prolonged and better than air. Hearing returned to normal after removal of gelatinous mass. *Impedance:* Type B tympanogram, absent stapedius reflex. *Classification:* Conductive. *Diagnosis:* Secretory otitis. *Aids to diagnosis:* The original misdiagnosis of otosclerosis might have been avoided if the mobilization of the drum had been tested with politzerization and if a diagnostic myringotomy had been performed. Not all cases of fluid in the middle ear cause reduced bone conduction. *Abbreviations:* ANSI, American National Standards Institute; ASA, American Standards Association.

## SEROUS OTITIS MEDIA AND ADENOIDS

There is understandable confusion between serous otitis and secretory otitis media. In the first place, the etiology of secretory otitis is not known, and in the second place, the two conditions sometimes are hard to distinguish clinically. Even outstanding otologists have differences of opinion concerning the differential diagnosis and the distinguishing characteristics.

## DEFINITION

For present purposes, let us consider serous otitis media as a condition in which serous fluid accumulates in the middle ear because of obstruction or infection of the eustachian tube or the nasopharynx. If the middle ear becomes infected, the condition is called acute otitis media. The fluid is a secondary phenomenon and results from pathology external to the middle ear. This is in contrast to secretory otitis media, in which the pathology seems to originate in the middle ear.

## CAUSES

The chief cause of serous otitis in children is hypertrophied adenoids in the fossae behind the eustachian tube openings (Rosenmüller's fossae). The adenoids do not always grow over the mouth of the eustachian tube and instead often cause obstruction in its lumen by submucosal compression or congestion. For this reason, it is essential to resect this area of adenoid tissue carefully under direct visualization in doing an adenoidectomy for recurrent otitis media or hearing impairment. Merely removing the central adenoid in such cases leads to recurrent symptoms and the need for adenoid revisions.

Adhesions in the Rosenmüller's fossae may be caused by previous surgery or radiation to the nasopharynx and may lead to serous otitis by restricting the normal function of the mouth of the eustachian tube; the adhesions may result in hearing impairment. In cases caused by surgery, the adhesions must be removed meticulously under direct vision, and the tubal ends must be mobilized with care not to injure the submucosal layers or to cause further adhesions.

Nasopharyngeal neoplasms, nasopharyngeal radiation, and allergies also may produce serous otitis.

## DIFFICULT DETECTION

The diagnosis of serous otitis as a cause of hearing loss in children often is overlooked because the hearing loss rarely exceeds 40 dB, and usually is less than 25 dB, and children generally are addressed in a loud voice. Thus, hearing difficulty is not detected until a school hearing screen is performed or until the symptom has persisted a long time.

A fluid level and bubbles often are readily apparent through the drum. The serous fluid level may show no movement when the child's head is bent forward or backward. Sometimes the fluid is hidden or fills the ear so completely that it goes undetected even on otoscopic examination. In such a case, the eardrum is hypomobile and may not move even with air pressure. Fullness and dullness in the ear are common complaints. **Figure 9.22** shows a typical case of hearing loss caused by serous otitis that went undetected for many months until a routine school audiogram was performed.

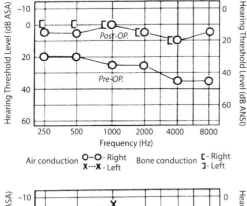

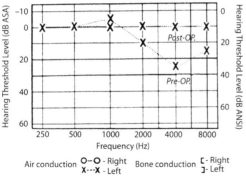

Figure 9.22 *History:* An 8-year-old child who failed to pass a school hearing test. No history of ear trouble. T&A performed at age 4. *Otologic:* Amber fluid in right middle ear. Slight amount of fluid in left middle ear also. Eustachian tube not clearly patent. Large mass of regrown adenoid tissue, especially in lateral pharynx. No response to a year of conservative therapy. The adenoidectomy was revised, and thin, clear fluid aspirated through myringotomy. *Audiologic:* Pure-tone thresholds in the right ear revealed a mild air conduction loss with normal bone conduction. The left ear had a mild loss in the higher frequencies. Hearing returned to normal after surgery. *Impedance:* Shallow type C tympanogram on the right; type A on the left. *Classification:* Conductive, *Diagnosis:* Hypertrophied adenoids with serous otitis media. *Abbreviations:* ANSI, American National Standards Institute; ASA, American Standards Association.

## AIM OF THERAPY

If only a myringotomy is performed in these cases, the hearing can improve temporarily because the cause still is present in the nasopharynx. Therefore, therapy should be directed to the causes as well as to provide immediate relief of symptoms in the ear.

## ACUTE OTITIS MEDIA

## EXTENT OF HEARING LOSS

In acute otitis media, hearing loss is temporary. Hearing improves when the inflammation subsides and the debris in the middle ear is absorbed. Depending on the stage of the infection, the hearing loss may be as great as 60 dB if the middle ear is filled with pus. Usually, all frequencies are involved if the fluid forms in the ear. If there is no fluid in the ear, sometimes only the lower frequencies are involved. An interesting paradox characterizes some cases of severe otitis media in which inflammation extends to the postauricular area. A tuning fork held to the mastoid region shows considerably reduced bone conduction. The same finding can be obtained by bone conduction audiometry on the mastoid region. It seems that sound waves are conducted poorly through the inflamed mastoid bone, but the sensorineural mechanism is not affected. When bone conduction is tested on the teeth or on a tongue blade clenched between the teeth, it is found to be normal.

The hearing loss in otitis media is caused by impeded sound transmission across the eardrum and the ossicular chain as a result of the additional mass in the middle ear. Tinnitus rarely is present; when it is reported, the patient reports hearing his/her own pulse. Although hearing loss during an attack of acute otitis media may be a cause for concern after the pain has subsided, the immediate and urgent problem is the relief of pain. However, what is most important in the long run is to treat otitis media adequately so that it resolves without leaving permanent hearing damage.

## THE QUESTION OF MYRINGOTOMY

The question arises whether myringotomy should be done in all cases of acute otitis media to prevent hearing impairment. There are avid supporters for myringotomy in all cases and equally enthusiastic supporters of the concept that myringotomy rarely should be done. Probably, the best approach lies somewhere in between. Whenever a middle ear contains pus and is causing the drum to bulge, myringotomy definitely is indicated to relieve pain and to prevent hearing loss. This is in keeping with the proven surgical principle that incision and drainage are advisable whenever pus is under pressure. In most bulging drums, there is an area of anesthesia in the eardrum created by the pressure in the middle ear, and if the myringotomy is done quickly in this area without pressing deeply into the drum, very little pain is experienced. Topical antibiotics also can be used to dull the discomfort of this procedure.

## ANTIBIOTICS

In spite of the excellent results that have been achieved in the prevention and treatment of acute otitis media by nonsurgical means, a large number of cases do progress to chronic otitis media. One of the causes for some of these failures is the use of inadequate doses or kinds of antibiotics. In many cases of otitis media, a much higher blood level of antibiotic is needed than is generally recognized because the infection has become walled off or is encased in bone and can be reached only by very high blood levels of the drug.

## DIFFERENCE BETWEEN ACUTE AND CHRONIC OTITIS MEDIA

Because acute otitis media frequently still leads to chronic otitis media and hearing loss, a more extensive discussion is in order. First, we should clarify the general difference between acute and chronic otitis media. Not infrequently, a patient is referred to an ear specialist with a diagnosis of "chronic otitis media," and the otologist finds the drum to be practically normal. The history may reveal that the patient has had repeated earaches and infections almost every 3 months. This is recurrent acute otitis media, not what is meant by chronic otitis media. Instead, otologists mean an ear that has been infected continuously for at least many months. An acute otitis media is an ear infection of comparatively short duration. If the acute otitis media does not respond

satisfactorily to therapy and the infection persists for many months, it then becomes a chronic otitis media.

If a patient has an acute otitis media that results in a persistent perforation in the eardrum and the infection clears up only to return again in a month or so, this should be considered to be a recurrent acute, not a chronic otitis media. As a matter of fact, this very situation is common in otologic practice. Many patients with perforations whose ears have been dry either get water in them or blow their noses improperly during an upper respiratory infection, and the ear becomes reinfected. In such cases, the otorrhea usually is stringy and mucoid and comes from the area of the eustachian tube. Hearing loss generally is minimal, and closure of the perforation often restores the hearing.

## COMMON CAUSES AND PREVENTION

The common causes of acute otitis media are upper respiratory infections and sinusitis, hypertrophied adenoids, allergies, and improper nose blowing and sneezing as well as eustachian tube blockage and possibly exposure to secondhand smoke in children. It is notable that all these causes are external to the ear itself so that in most instances acute otitis media is a secondary infection, and its prevention must be directed to its causes.

To prevent otitis media and hearing loss, patients should be cautioned to refrain from indiscreet nose blowing and sneezing. Forceful blowing or sneezing while pinching both nares causes a buildup of pressure in the nasopharynx; this pressure may force small amounts of infected mucus through the eustachian tube into the middle ear, with resulting otitis media. These facts should be impressed on patients with upper respiratory infections. In spite of the social stigma attached to the practice, sniffing is far safer than nose blowing. If the nose is blown, both nostrils should be left unpinched.

## POST-INFECTION HEARING EVALUATION

In all cases of acute otitis media, it is advisable to perform hearing tests after the infection has subsided to be certain that there is no residual hearing impairment that might be permanent or that might require further treatment.

## CHRONIC OTITIS MEDIA

When infection persists continuously in the middle ear for long periods of time, it is called chronic otitis media, and this is a very frequent cause of hearing impairment. The mechanism varies. There is invariably a perforation in the eardrum.

Occasionally, the entire drum is eroded, and much of the middle ear is visible through the otoscope. The more severe hearing losses are caused by erosion of some part of the ossicular chain. The most common ossicular defect is erosion of the long end of the incus so that it does not contact the head of the stapes. Occasionally, the handle of the malleus and even the stapedial crura are eroded. In some ears, the entire incus has been destroyed. Scarlet fever and measles are notorious causes of severe erosion of the ossicles and the eardrum.

Another cause of hearing loss in chronic otitis media is discharge in the middle ear. This naturally adds a mass which impedes transmission of sound waves. Strangely enough, a patient may say he/she hears much worse after the ear is cleared of discharge, and the audiogram often will substantiate this complaint. This result may be explained in several ways, but one of the more reasonable theories is that the discharge blocks sound waves bound for the round window niche and thereby permits some semblance of normal phase difference for sound waves hitting the inner ear. To make this clear, it may be pointed out that sound waves in normal ears selectively enter the oval window rather than the round window because of their direct transmission through the ossicular chain. When the eardrum is missing and the ossicular chain is not functioning properly, sound waves occasionally strike both the round and the oval windows almost simultaneously so that the waves may in part cancel each other before they can reach the inner ear. This causes hearing loss. A discharge in the middle ear sometimes may prevent this

effect by blocking sound waves that otherwise would reach the round window niche. Thus, the patient may hear better when his/her ear is moist. The same mechanism sometimes is used purposely to improve hearing in ears that are free of infection.

One type of prosthesis covers the round window opening so that sound waves cannot strike both the round and the oval windows simultaneously, thereby nullifying their effects in the inner ear and causing a hearing loss. Ointments can be used for the same purpose in some of these cases. Aquaphor ointment is an example. If the patient's eardrum is gone so that the round window niche is visible, a patient's hearing sometimes may be improved markedly by carefully applying a plug of Aquaphor ointment over the round window niche. In appropriate cases, this ointment maintains the hearing improvement for several weeks; occasionally, the patient can be taught to replace the ointment.

However, these considerations should not lead a physician to disregard discharge in the hope of achieving improved hearing because infection often can result in serious complications. There are more satisfactory methods to restore hearing after an infection has been controlled. When a perforation (especially a posterior superior perforation) is found in the eardrum with a putrid discharge, it generally means that mastoiditis is present. If the infection is allowed to continue, it may cause a number of complications, including erosion of the ossicles and severe hearing loss. A cholesteatoma may form that could erode the semicircular canals and the facial nerve and even produce a brain abscess. Sensorineural hearing loss often occurs in patients who have long-standing chronic ear infections.

It is important, therefore, to cure a chronic middle ear infection as rapidly as possible. Unfortunately, systemic antibiotics do not often succeed in clearing up cases of chronic otitis media because the chronically diseased mastoid cells in the middle ear have a poor blood supply. Consequently, it is necessary to treat the ear locally, and occasionally surgery must be performed when local therapy has been unsuccessful, and complications threaten.

**Figures 9.20–9.23** illustrate several audiometric patterns that may occur in chronic otitis media.

## TYMPANOSCLEROSIS

As a result of as yet undetermined causes, sclerotic changes occur in some chronically diseased middle ears. After infection has subsided, a shalelike layer of bony deposit remains over the promontory of the cochlea and around the oval window region.

Occasionally, the stapes and the incus are enveloped by stratified bone that can be peeled off in layers. This condition is called tympanosclerosis, and it produces hearing loss by fixing the stapes and the incus in a manner similar to that of otosclerosis. It differs markedly from otosclerosis in that its onset follows an infection, without a familial history of hearing loss. Furthermore, it is generally unilateral. In addition, pathological changes are visible in the eardrum in most cases of tympanosclerosis. The drums may show healed scars and are thick and yellowish-white with white areas that suggest sclerosis.

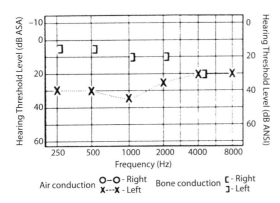

Figure 9.23 *History:* This patient had a discharging left ear for many years. X-ray study showed a cholesteatoma. *Otologic:* Large posterior marginal perforation. The ossicular chain was not disrupted; otherwise, the hearing loss would have exceeded 50 dB. Ossicular continuity was confirmed at surgery. *Audiologic:* Pure-tone thresholds in the left ear revealed a mild air conduction loss with a gradually decreasing air–bone gap at the higher frequencies. Right ear masked. *Impedance:* Type B tympanogram; pressure seal for probe maintained without difficulty at usual test pressures. *Classification:* Conductive. *Diagnosis:* Cholesteatoma with marginal perforation. *Abbreviations:* ANSI, American National Standards Institute; ASA, American Standards Association.

**Figure 9.16** describes a typical case of tympanosclerosis in which a stapes mobilization was performed. It is wise to point out that stapedectomies should be undertaken with great caution in cases of tympanosclerosis because for some unknown reason the incidence of "dead ears" and severe sensorineural loss may be substantial even when the surgery seems to be successful in the operating room. It has been suggested that an operation on an ear of this type should be done in two stages, in the first removing the tympanosclerosis and in the second mobilizing the stapes or doing a stapedectomy. The hearing loss may be mild or as severe as 65 dB when the fixation is complete. All frequencies usually are affected. In many long-standing cases, a sensorineural hearing loss develops.

## CARCINOMA

Carcinoma of the middle ear is rare, and frequently it is not recognized at its inception. Its onset resembles chronic otitis media as it causes at first a mild conductive hearing loss and later a loss of up to 60 dB as invasion or restriction of the ossicles ensues. Sometimes carcinoma occurs in an ear with chronic otitis that has been present for many years. This is even more difficult to detect because the change takes place below the typical surface of granulation and polypoid tissue and is not visible to the examiner. Even roentgenograms may be of little help. Biopsy of all granulation tissue is advisable but not always practical in office practice. However, it should be done in all cases of long-standing granulation with recurrent polypoid formation that resists conservative therapy or continues even after surgical intervention, especially when severe pain is present. If the tissue is harder than usual or bleeds readily, a biopsy is indicated. Usually, the eardrum perforates early, and chronic otitis media develops so that the appearance is not very distinctive. **Figure 9.24** shows an unusual case of carcinoma of the middle ear. Hearing is of secondary consideration in carcinoma of the middle ear, but it may be important as a presenting symptom to alert the physician to the presence of a serious condition. Malignancies of the ear are discussed in detail in Chapters 21 and 22.

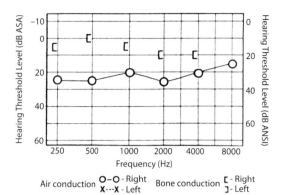

Figure 9.24 *History:* A 42-year-old woman complained of fullness and severe pain in right ear for several months. No vertigo or tinnitus. She had received antibiotics and myringotomies without satisfactory help. Imaging showed only a mild haziness in the right mastoid but not in the left. *Otologic:* The eardrum was slightly opaque but moved satisfactorily with air pressure. *Audiologic:* Mild conductive ascending hearing loss in right ear. Left normal. *Diagnosis:* After continued unsuccessful conservative therapy, the right ear was explored, and a carcinomatous invasion of the middle ear and the mastoid was found. The patient did not respond to cobalt irradiation, and, unfortunately, radical surgery was not done. *Abbreviations:* ANSI, American National Standards Institute; ASA, American Standards Association.

## NASOPHARYNGEAL TUMORS

Unilateral conductive hearing loss frequently is commonly the first presenting symptom of a tumor in the nasopharynx. The mechanical cause of the resulting hearing loss resembles that described in serous otitis media: gradual obstruction of the eustachian tube. The possibility that such a serious condition may exist adds emphasis to the importance of doing a nasopharyngoscopic examination in all cases of conductive hearing loss, especially when they are unilateral and associated with middle ear fluid. The hearing loss by air conduction is comparatively mild in the beginning and may progress to ~40 dB, and bone conduction usually is normal. The nasopharyngeal examination shows a fullness that is sometimes clear-cut but in other cases uncertain with poor delineation, depending on the nature of the tumor. A better perspective

of the tumor generally is obtained through a nasopharyngeal mirror below the soft palate or using fiber-optic endoscopes.

In the early stages, when the hearing loss is mild, the eardrum appears to be normal. Later, retraction of the drum or serous fluid becomes visible. When there has been recurrent fluid formation in one ear and multiple myringotomies are necessary, it is essential to rule out a nasopharyngeal mass.

## ALLERGY

Allergy plays a somewhat vague role in hearing loss of middle ear origin. Undoubtedly, allergic conditions can lead to congestion of the eustachian tube and the middle ear, with resultant serous otitis media. A few cases of hearing loss have been reported that appear to result primarily from allergy in the middle ear. When the allergy is treated, hearing improves. If judgment is based on experience and a review of the literature, this type of case is not very common unless fluid is present in the middle ear.

Certainly, allergic swelling of the eardrum or the mucosa of the middle ear does occur and may produce hearing loss, but this does not happen as frequently as one might expect from the known frequency of allergies of the upper respiratory tract. Medical treatment of the allergy is of major help in clearing up many cases of serous otitis media.

Hearing loss resulting from allergy of the middle ear is mild. If it exceeds ~20 dB, fluid probably is present in the middle ear, or some other causative factor is present.

## X-RAY TREATMENTS

Irradiation to the region of the nasopharynx frequently produces malfunction of the eustachian tube. Hearing loss along with serous otitis media often is present. The radiation may have been directed to the thyroid, the face, the skull, or the nasopharynx. The hearing loss produced is mild and rarely exceeds 30–35 dB. After months of conservative therapy, the malfunction may subside, and the hearing may return to normal (**Figure 9.25**).

An extraordinary incidence of conductive hearing loss caused by irradiation for a brain tumor was encountered by the author. Notable was an aseptic mastoid cell necrosis that occurred >20 years after the treatment. The severe conductive loss was caused by two factors: a large erosive defect in the posterior external canal wall and profuse serous discharge from the middle ear. The hearing was improved slightly by occluding the perforation in the canal wall.

## SYSTEMIC DISEASES

Certain systemic diseases are known to affect the middle ear and to cause conductive hearing loss. The most common of these are measles and scarlet fever. Both are notorious for the marked otitis media that they can cause, with erosion of the eardrum and the ossicles. This complication is not nearly as common now as it was years ago, but the hearing losses resulting from these conditions still are encountered in practice. **Figure 9.26** shows an example of conductive hearing loss following scarlet fever in childhood. The eardrum and the ossicles in such cases typically are eroded, and the hearing level is ~60 dB.

Letterer–Siwe disease, xanthomatosis, eosinophilic granulomatosis, and other granulomata are additional causes of conductive hearing loss. Although not very common, they can damage the middle ear and cause handicapping hearing loss, as discussed in Chapter 13.

## GLOMUS JUGULARE AND GLOMUS TYMPANICUM

Glomus jugulare tumors are rare, but when they are present, hearing loss and tinnitus frequently are the only symptoms. This neoplasm arises from cells around the jugulare bulb and expands to involve neighboring structures. In doing so, it most frequently extends to the floor of the middle ear, causing conductive hearing loss and pulsating tinnitus (**Figure 9.27**). As the disease progresses, it may appear as chronic otitis media and may even extend through the eardrum and appear to be granulation tissue in the ear canal. Unsuspecting biopsy of this apparent granulation tissue may result in profuse bleeding because of the striking vascularity of glomus tumors. As the disease extends, it may destroy portions of the temporal bone and jugular bulb and may spread intracranially.

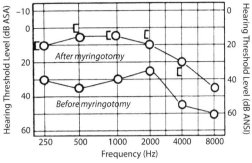

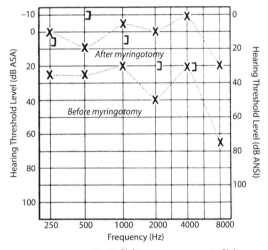

Figure 9.25 *History:* A 51-year-old woman with acromegaly who received X-ray radiation to the pituitary gland. Several weeks later, she noted insidious hearing loss, and her own heartbeat sounded loud in both ears. She was treated with tranquilizers with little relief. *Otologic:* Normal eardrums, but highly congested nasopharynx and eustachian tubes. Eardrums mobile but difficult to politzerize. Amber fluid evacuated from both ears through myringotomy, with restoration of hearing. Tinnitus disappeared. *Audiologic:* Right and left ears showed mild conductive losses with normal bone conduction in the low- and midfrequency range. After both middle ears were aspirated, air conduction thresholds returned to preoperative bone levels in the right ear and battered these levels in the left ear. Reduced bone conduction thresholds were caused by fluid in middle ears. *Impedance:* Type C tympanogram. *Classification:* Conductive. *Diagnosis:* Otitis media caused by X-ray treatment to pituitary for acromegaly. *Abbreviations:* ANSI, American National Standards Institute; ASA, American Standards Association.

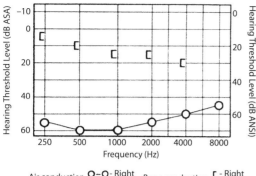

Air conduction O–O - Right / X---X - Left   Bone conduction Γ - Right / Ⅎ - Left

**Figure 9.26** *History:* A 20-year-old man who had scarlet fever as a child with right chronic otitis for 1 year. Since that time, the hearing has been reduced, but the ear drained only after swimming or a bad cold. *Otologic:* The entire eardrum was eroded, and the handle of the malleus was gone, except for a small remainder. The incus and the stapedial crura also were eroded. *Audiologic:* Air conduction thresholds in the right ear revealed a moderately severe loss and slightly reduced bone conduction thresholds. The mild reduced bone conduction does not mean necessarily a sensorineural involvement in such a case. *Classification:* Conductive. *Diagnosis:* Right chronic otitis media caused by scarlet fever. *Abbreviations:* ANSI, American National Standards Institute; ASA, American Standards Association.

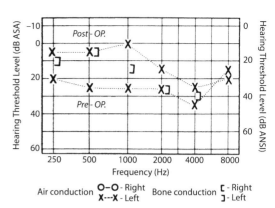

Air conduction O–O - Right / X---X - Left   Bone conduction Γ - Right / Ⅎ - Left

**Figure 9.27** *History:* A 57-year-old woman with sudden discomfort in the left ear 6 months before. Thumping tinnitus for past 6 months. No facial paralysis. Some hearing loss. No pain. *Otologic:* Right ear clear. Left middle ear was red and inflamed, but eardrum moved freely. Needle aspiration produced bleeding, which was controlled quickly. *Audiologic:* Left ear air conduction thresholds revealed a mild, flat hearing loss. Bone conduction thresholds showed an air–bone gap at 500, 1000, and 2000 Hz only. Left ear discrimination was 96%. *Classification:* Conductive with high-frequency sensorineural involvement. *Diagnosis:* Glomus jugulare tumor, removed surgically; tympanogram showing pulsations, radiologic evidence of bone erosion, and obstruction or retrograde jugular venogram generally confirm the diagnosis preoperatively. *Abbreviations:* ANSI, American National Standards Institute; ASA, American Standards Association.

Glomus tumors also may arise from cells along the promontory or medial wall of the middle ear. These are called glomus tympanicum tumors and are generally easier to manage surgically. It is essential to distinguish between glomus tympanicum and glomus jugulare before attempting surgical intervention.

As in any expanding neoplasm, early diagnosis of a glomus tumor facilitates surgical cure. As conductive hearing loss may be the only symptom for a long time, the physician is obligated to establish the cause for every case of unilateral conductive hearing loss.

Physical examination may disclose a pink mass in the middle ear. Positive pressure on the eardrum may reveal blanching of the mass. Pulsating tinnitus may be audible to the examiner by using a

Toynbee tube or a stethoscope placed over the ear. The finding of objective tinnitus may occur not only with glomus tumors but also with carotid artery aneurysms, intracranial arteriovenous malformations, carotid artery stenosis, and other conditions. Glomus tumors must be distinguished from other masses that may be present in the middle ear, such as carotid artery aneurysms, high jugular bulbs, meningiomas, and adenomas.

Radiological evaluation is now the mainstay of glomus tumor diagnosis. Biopsy rarely is indicated. CT and MRI of the temporal bone are used to assess bone erosion and soft tissue extent and arteriography and retrograde jugular venography are used to define the extent of the neoplasm.

Four-vessel arteriograms or CT angiogram are recommended by some otologists because of the high incidence of associated tumors. Up to 10% of patients with glomus tumors will have associated bilateral glomus tumors, glomus vagale, carotid body tumor, or thyroid carcinoma. The vast majority of glomus patients are female, and the tumor is extremely rare in children. If the diagnosis is entertained seriously in a child, biopsy then may be appropriate to rule out other lesions. Biopsy also is used in patients who are not surgical candidates prior to instituting palliative radiation therapy.

## CAUSES WITH APPARENTLY NORMAL EARDRUMS AND MIDDLE EARS

The following are some of the causes of conductive hearing loss in which the external auditory canals, the eardrums, and the middle ears appear to be normal on otoscopic examination:

1. Congenital ossicular defects
2. Acquired ossicular defects
3. Otosclerosis
4. Tympanosclerosis
5. Paget's disease
6. van der Hoeve's syndrome
7. "Invisible" fluid
8. Malfunction of the eustachian tube
9. Superior canal dehiscence syndrome

## CONGENITAL OSSICULAR DEFECTS

A variety of defects may arise in the ossicular chain during fetal development and produce a conductive hearing loss of 60–70 dB even though the eardrum and middle ear appear to be normal during physical examination. The impairment, if bilateral, usually is discovered by the time the child is 3 years old, but the discovery may be delayed if the defect affects only one ear.

A congenital ossicular defect should be suspected when a young patient with an apparently normal eardrum "has had a hearing loss all his/her life," when it is conductive and in the range of 50 dB or more, and particularly when it is unilateral and nonprogressive. Complaints of tinnitus are rare.

If the hearing loss is bilateral, careful questioning usually will disclose that speech development was delayed, and that the patient reacted to the impairment in one of two ways: poor schoolwork or a behavioral problem related to the child's inability to hear and to respond. Although the nonprogressive character of the hearing loss is of considerable diagnostic importance, the hearing may fluctuate during upper respiratory infections, allergies, and similar conditions, as is true also of hearing losses of other etiologies.

**Figure 9.28** shows an audiogram of a patient whose hearing loss is highly suggestive of congenital ossicular defect. Reference to this audiogram at this point serves to emphasize the importance of a careful and critical appraisal of the otologic findings in conjunction with audiology, especially a meticulous inspection through the drum.

In case in which an ossicular defect is suspected, the procedure of choice is to elevate the eardrum and to examine the ossicular chain. A defect can be found in almost any part of the chain. One of the most common is congenital fixation of the stapes. Another is congenital absence of the long process of the incus and no connection between the incus and the head of the stapes. General malformation of the stapedial crura also has been found to be responsible for hearing loss in some of these cases. There are other congenital defects that challenge the ingenuity of the surgeon who attempts to establish a functional continuity of the ossicular chain.

## ACQUIRED OSSICULAR DEFECTS

It is possible for the ossicular chain to be disrupted or damaged without causing visible changes in the tympanic membrane. **Figure 9.29** shows an interesting example of ossicular damage following head injury in an industrial accident. A similar defect can be produced during myringotomy in childhood if the myringotomy is too high and the knife penetrates too deeply and damages the incus. After the operation, the eardrum may heal without scarring, but the damage to the incus remains.

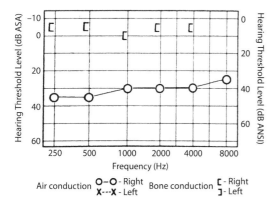

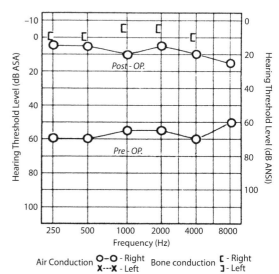

Figure 9.28 *History:* A 16-year-old boy with right ear hearing loss following an ear infection at age 7. Ear was lanced at that time. There have been no further infections, and the hearing loss has not progressed. No tinnitus. *Otologic:* Eardrums almost normal with only slight evidence of scarring. At surgery, the end of the incus was found to have been fractured and to have healed with fibrous union. This damage probably was caused by a myringotomy knife. A plastic tube was used to improve the incudostapedial connection. *Audiologic:* Right-ear air conduction thresholds revealed a mild, flat hearing loss, with normal bone thresholds. *Impedance:* Deep type A tympanogram; probably not type $A_D$ because of the fibrous union. *Classification:* Conductive. *Diagnosis:* Ossicular disruption. *Aids to diagnosis:* Normal bone conduction thresholds are an important criterion in the diagnosis of ossicular defect (e.g., not depressed as the result of fluid or stapes fixation). *Abbreviations:* ANSI, American National Standards Institute; ASA, American Standards Association.

Figure 9.29 *History:* A 50-year-old man who had normal hearing until an industrial head injury. He lost consciousness, but there was no fracture of the skull. No tinnitus or vertigo, but a marked right-ear hearing loss resulted from the injury. *Otologic:* Normal eardrums and middle ears. Exploration revealed a complete dislocation of the end of the incus from the head of the stapes. Continuity was restored and hearing improved. *Audiologic:* Air conduction thresholds in the right ear revealed a moderately severe hearing loss. Bone conduction thresholds were normal. The air–bone gap was maximal for a conduction lesion. Tuning fork lateralized to the right ear, and air was better than bone conduction. *Impedance:* Type $A_D$ tympanogram. *Classification:* Conductive. *Diagnosis:* Ossicular disruption caused by head trauma. *Abbreviations:* ANSI, American National Standards Institute; ASA, American Standards Association.

**Figure 9.30** shows another case in which a patient heard well following a stapedectomy but suffered a sudden hearing loss when she received a sharp blow to the operated side of her head.

Examination of the middle ear showed that the prosthesis had been dislodged from its proper position by the blow. In a contrary experience, another patient failed to gain better hearing from a stapedectomy and vein graft. A sudden and hard stop in a descending elevator several months later caused her hearing to return immediately. Apparently, the prosthesis was moved into a better position, and the hearing improved. In all these cases, the

change in hearing was sudden in comparison with the long history of deafness in congenital defects and otosclerosis.

Occasionally, there is fixation of the malleoincudal joint or of the malleus itself. This may occur after a mild infection without evidence in the eardrum and may be congenital, or there may be no obvious cause. Two ossicles may become so fixed that they do not transmit sound waves, and a substantial hearing loss may result.

In some instances, the incus or the stapedial crura may be broken by a blow to the head, and healing takes place by fibrous rather than bony union (**Figure 9.28**). In such cases, the hearing loss may be comparatively mild. The hearing loss resulting from an ossicular defect generally involves all frequencies, and tinnitus is absent. The precise diagnosis seldom is made until the ossicular chain is examined surgically. The vast majority of these defects can be repaired, and the hearing can be restored.

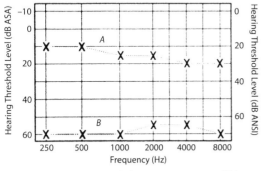

Figure 9.30 *History:* Patient had good stapedectomy result (A). Fifteen months postoperative she received a sharp blow to the left ear and the side of the face. Sudden deafness followed (B). No vertigo was experienced. *Otologic:* Exploration revealed the polyethylene type prosthesis was dislodged and lay free in the middle ear. This was removed and replaced with a steep piston and wire around the incus. *Audiologic:* Posttraumatic air conduction thresholds represented a 35- to 50-dB reduction in hearing from those obtained after a successful stapedectomy. Hearing was restored with a new prosthesis. *Classification:* Conductive. *Diagnosis:* Dislocated prosthesis. *Abbreviations:* ANSI, American National Standards Institute; ASA, American Standards Association.

One other type of ossicular defect with normal otoscopic findings is the damage that may be done either to the end of the incus or to the stapes during stapes surgery. In some cases in which stapes mobilization is attempted by pushing down on the end of the incus or in which a wire prosthesis is too tight, the end of the incus is weakened or split off. This impairs the efficiency of the incudostapedial joint and may cancel the benefits of successful mobilization or even make hearing worse.

Fracture of the head of the stapes or its crura is another cause of acquired ossicular defect. In some such instances, an initial hearing loss of 30 dB may be increased to 50 dB. The bones rarely heal sufficiently for the hearing to improve noticeably, and stapedectomy or replacement of the crura and the end of the incus with a stapes prosthesis then becomes necessary.

Stapedectomies also may be unsuccessful because, after removal of the stapes and replacement with an artificial stapes, the prosthesis may slip or make poor contact, or the oval window may close over, and the hearing loss may become worse than it was before surgery.

## OTOSCLEROSIS

When conductive hearing loss is present in an adult, and the eardrum and the middle ear appear to be normal through the otoscope, the most likely diagnosis is otosclerosis. The cause of otosclerosis is hereditary but otherwise unknown, but in some people, a gradual fixation of the stapedial footplate in the oval window occurs because of abnormal changes in the cochlear bone. Actually, the term "otosclerosis" is misleading, for it is not initially a sclerotic process; it is more like a vascularization in the bone with formation of spongy-appearing bone. This stage of the disease is called otospongiosis, and the mature, less active, later stage is otosclerosis. In common practice, the term otosclerosis is used to include both. Such changes have been reported only within the bony labyrinth and are not found in the rest of the body.

## CLINICAL OTOSCLEROSIS

There are many more people with otosclerosis than there are patients who seek medical advice for their hearing loss and receive the benefit of diagnosis. For instance, otosclerosis has been found at autopsy in the ears of many individuals who gave no evidence of hearing impairment while they were alive. It is present in up to 10% of Caucasian Americans but symptomatic in only ~1%. Conductive hearing loss is absent when otosclerotic changes affect areas of the body labyrinth other than the oval window. It is only when the oval window and the stapes are involved that conductive hearing loss develops, and then it is called clinical otosclerosis. For our purposes, we shall call it simply otosclerosis because the condition does not concern us clinically until hearing impairment develops. Fixation of the stapes may occur over a period of many months or even years. The hearing gradually diminishes as the footplate becomes more fixed. **Figure 9.31** shows a serial audiogram of a patient with otosclerosis whose hearing level has been followed repeatedly for years. Otosclerosis can be confused with Paget's disease and osteogenesis imperfecta. Distinguishing features are summarized in Appendix III.

## Extent of hearing loss

In some cases, the hearing loss stops progressing after reaching only a very mild level. We do not know why this occurs. More frequently, the hearing deteriorates until it stabilizes at ~70 dB. The hearing deficit classically starts in the lower frequencies and gradually progresses to the high ones. Eventually, all frequencies are involved. In numerous patients, the high frequencies continue to deteriorate even more than the low frequencies because of superimposed sensorineural hearing loss. Profound loss can occur in *far advanced otosclerosis.*

## Characteristic features

There are many intriguing and challenging features about otosclerosis. For example, it is far more common in females than in males, and it is generally noted first around the age of 18. Often the hearing loss is accompanied by a very annoying buzzing tinnitus; both symptoms usually are aggravated by pregnancy. The tinnitus commonly subsides over a period of many years.

**Psychological Aspects.** Of particular interest is the psychological complex present commonly in otosclerotic patients. Some of them become suspicious and feel that people are talking about them. Many become introspective and have marked personality changes. They retreat into their own shells. Some try to appear to be lighthearted and even humorous, but the attempt lacks conviction. Perhaps these symptoms are related to the gradual onset of otosclerosis; yet comparable reactions rarely are observed in patients with hearing loss from other causes, even though these also may

have a gradual onset. One of the vital reasons for trying to restore hearing early with surgery or amplification is to prevent adverse psychological changes.

**Familial Aspects.** Otosclerosis is familial to some extent. It often is found in several people in the same family. In contrast, many patients with otosclerosis deny any hearing loss in their families for as many generations as they may recall. It is not possible to predict on genetic principles who in a family will exhibit clinical otosclerosis, but on theoretical grounds, marriages between members of two families both of which have clear-cut cases of otosclerosis seem to be inadvisable. It is possible that none of their offspring will develop a hearing loss although generally it follows an autosomal dominant inheritance pattern with variable penetrance. Certainly, there is no justification for a therapeutic abortion in a pregnant woman with otosclerosis merely because her hearing loss might be aggravated during pregnancy. Some older textbooks took a contrary view, but it is unwarranted in the light of what we now know about otosclerosis.

**Effect of Excellent Bone Conduction.** As noted previously, patients with otosclerosis have excellent bone conduction. This explains why these patients speak in very soft and modulated voices, a prominent feature in otosclerosis. A patient may complain that his/her hearing is worse when chewing crunchy foods. The reason is that excellent bone conduction causes the crunching noises to interfere with the ability to hear conversation.

## Differentiation

During pure-tone audiometry, patients with otosclerosis often are uncertain whether or not they really hear the tone when they are being tested at threshold. In contrast, patients with sensorineural hearing loss generally are sure when they hear and when they do not.

In spite of the classic symptoms that otosclerotic patients present, many cases still are misdiagnosed as catarrhal deafness, allergic deafness, adhesive deafness, or deafness due to eustachian tube blockage. Because of these errors in diagnosis, the authors emphasized that these nonotosclerotic conditions produce only mild hearing loss and that they rarely are accompanied by

JOSEPH SATALOFF, M.D.
ROBERT THAYER SATALOFF, M.D.
1721 PINE STREET    PHILADELPHIA, PA 19103

**HEARING RECORD**

NAME _____    AGE _____

### AIR CONDUCTION

| | | | RIGHT | | | | | | | LEFT | | | | | | |
|---|---|---|---|---|---|---|---|---|---|---|---|---|---|---|---|---|
| DATE | Exam | LEFT MASK | 250 | 500 | 1000 | 2000 | 4000 | 8000 | RIGHT MASK | 250 | 500 | 1000 | 2000 | 4000 | 8000 | AUD |
| 1st YR. | | | 35 | 35 | 30 | 20 | 10 | 5 | | 35 | 40 | 30 | 20 | 5 | 5 | |
| 2nd YR. | | | 45 | 40 | 40 | 20 | 10 | 10 | | 40 | 40 | 30 | 20 | 10 | 10 | |
| 3rd YR. | | | 50 | 50 | 50 | 25 | 15 | 15 | | 40 | 45 | 35 | 20 | 15 | 15 | |
| 4th YR. | | | 55 | 55 | 50 | 40 | 20 | 25 | | 45 | 45 | 40 | 35 | 30 | 25 | |
| 7th YR. | | | 60 | 55 | 50 | 50 | 40 | 35 | | 50 | 55 | 50 | 45 | 45 | 40 | |
| 9th YR. | | | 60 | 55 | 55 | 60 | 65 | 50 | | 55 | 55 | 55 | 55 | 60 | 45 | |

### BONE CONDUCTION

| | | | RIGHT | | | | | | LEFT | | | | | |
|---|---|---|---|---|---|---|---|---|---|---|---|---|---|---|
| DATE | Exam | LEFT MASK | 250 | 500 | 1000 | 2000 | 4000 | RIGHT MASK | 250 | 500 | 1000 | 2000 | 4000 | AUD |
| 1st YR. | | | 0 | 0 | 0 | 5 | 5 | | 0 | 0 | 0 | 5 | 5 | |
| 4th YR. | | | 0 | 5 | 5 | 10 | 15 | | 0 | 5 | 10 | 10 | 15 | |
| 9th YR. | | | 0 | 10 | 20 | 25 | 30 | | 0 | 10 | 25 | 20 | 35 | |

### SPEECH RECEPTION

| DATE | RIGHT | LEFT MASK | LEFT | RIGHT MASK | FREE FIELD | MIC |
|---|---|---|---|---|---|---|
| 1st YR. | 30 | | 35 | | | |

### DISCRIMINATION

| | RIGHT | | | | LEFT | | | | |
|---|---|---|---|---|---|---|---|---|---|
| DATE | % SCORE | TEST LEVEL | LIST | LEFT MASK | % SCORE | TEST LEVEL | LIST | RIGHT MASK | EXAM |
| | 100 | 70 | | | 100 | 75 | | | |

### HIGH FREQUENCY THRESHOLDS

| | RIGHT | | | | | | LEFT | | | | |
|---|---|---|---|---|---|---|---|---|---|---|---|
| DATE | 4000 | 8000 | 10000 | 12000 | 14000 | LEFT MASK | RIGHT MASK | 4000 | 8000 | 10000 | 12000 | 14000 |
| | | | | | | | | | | | | |

| RIGHT | | WEBER | | LEFT | | HEARING AID | | |
|---|---|---|---|---|---|---|---|---|
| RINNE | SCHWABACH | | | RINNE | SCHWABACH | DATE | MAKE | MODEL |
| | | | | | | RECEIVER | GAIN | EXAM |
| | | | | | | EAR | DISCRIM | COUNC |

REMARKS

Figure 9.31 Progressive hearing loss in otosclerosis. Patient refuses surgical intervention and gets along well with a hearing aid. Note that bone conduction is becoming reduced, even though this patient was 38 years old at the time of the last audiogram.

tinnitus or a family history of deafness. Whenever a patient with normal otoscopic findings has conductive hearing loss exceeding 45 dB in the speech frequencies, the cause in all probability is otosclerosis or ossicular defect, even though there may be a marked allergic history and changes in the nose, or slight retraction of the eardrum or even a demonstrably blocked eustachian tube. It is important to remember that few, if any, causes other than otosclerosis produce progressive conductive hearing losses of >45 dB accompanied by tinnitus and a familial history.

## Variable progress in the hearing loss of each ear

Otosclerosis sometimes does occur unilaterally, with normal hearing in the other ear. The progress of the hearing loss in each ear, when otosclerosis is present in both ears, may differ widely so that most of the time a patient complains of hearing better with one ear than with the other. This difference may change, however, and the patient often says, "My left ear used to be the better ear, but it has gotten so bad that the right ear is now the better one." This subjective experience, corroborated by hearing tests, may determine which ear should be operated on when an attempt is made to restore hearing by stapes surgery.

## Other types

There are many other types of otosclerosis that the otologist can classify. One is the so-called malignant type, which is most disturbing. It may occur in young patients and is noted for a rapidly progressing hearing loss which, often in 1 or 2 years, reaches handicapping proportions and is accompanied by diminished bone conduction as a result of sensorineural involvement (**Figure 9.32**). Frequently, these cases are not seen until the sensorineural damage is already so pronounced that the otosclerotic origin is largely obscured, and surgery is of more limited value.

Although a connection has not yet been proven, the frequency with which sensorineural hearing loss accompanies otosclerosis suggests a relationship between them. Otosclerotic changes found in the sensory area of the cochlea, particularly mean the stria vascularis, are believed to be responsible for the sensorineural impairment.

Another type of otosclerosis is illustrated in **Figure 9.33**. This is hardly recognizable as otosclerosis, and yet the patient has all the classic history and symptoms, with the exception that the hearing loss is >60 dB, and sensorineural loss also is present. Many features of this type of otosclerosis are discussed in Chapter 10. This is definitely otosclerosis, and the hearing can be improved by surgery, as seen in the audiogram. The absence of responses to audiometric testing does not mean necessarily that the ear is "dead." It means merely that the threshold is beyond the limits of the audiometer. Another unusual but severe type of otosclerosis occurs when both the oval window and the round window are obstructed. Here again, the bone conduction is reduced.

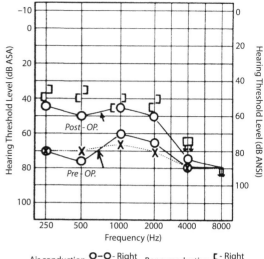

Air conduction  O–O - Right  X---X - Left     Bone conduction  Ը - Right  ]- Left

Figure 9.32 *History:* A 24-year-old woman with insidious hearing loss only 3 years from onset. Marked roaring tinnitus and some imbalance. No familial deafness. Voice normal. *Otologic:* Ears normal. Right stapedectomy improved the hearing after removing a thick, white otosclerotic fixed footplate. *Audiologic:* Pure-tone air conduction thresholds revealed a severe bilateral loss. Bone conduction also was reduced. Preoperative tuning-fork tests showed bone better than air conduction in both ears and no lateralization. Postoperatively, air equaled bone conduction in the right ear. Pre- and postoperative discrimination scores in the right ear were in the low 40% range. The air–bone gap in the right ear was closed with surgery. (A similar result was obtained later in the left ear.) *Impedance:* Type A tympanogram. *Classification:* Mixed hearing loss. *Diagnosis:* Otosclerosis with sensorineural involvement. The presence of mild imbalance is not uncommon in this type of otosclerosis with sensorineural involvement. *Abbreviations:* ANSI, American National Standards Institute; ASA, American Standards Association.

The above cases of otosclerosis that have a sensorineural component are not considered to be purely conductive but, rather, cases of mixed hearing loss. They are included in this chapter because the conductive element predominates.

Occasionally, there will be minimal visible abnormalities in the appearance of the eardrum, yet marked tympanosclerotic changes will be found in the middle ear. This condition, called tympanosclerosis, can cause ossicular damage or fixation and hearing loss.

The hearing loss in Paget's disease may be either conductive or sensorineural. Conductive hearing loss occurs as a result of stapes fixation when calcium deposits prevent normal movement of the stapes footplate. These deposits form in the annular ligament of the stapes at its attachment to the oval window and present a hearing loss pattern similar to that which occurs in otosclerosis (**Figure 9.34**).

Sensorineural hearing loss develops because of changes in the labyrinth or narrowing of the internal auditory meatus and pressure on the auditory nerve. Other established findings in patients with Paget's disease are discussed in Chapter 13 and Appendix III.

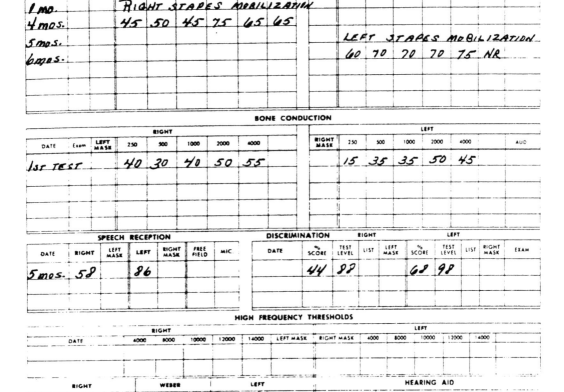

Figure 9.33 *History:* A 67-year-old woman with insidious hearing loss for >30 years. Refuses to wear hearing aid and communicates only in writing. No familial history of deafness. No tinnitus or vertigo. *Otologic:* Normal. *Audiologic:* There is severe sensorineural hearing loss, but the patient has an air–bone gap. Reduced discrimination. Hears tuning fork well by teeth. *Impedance:* Type A tympanogram. *Aid to diagnosis:* The excellent results obtained by stapes mobilization emphasize that these ears are not "dead" but have hearing beyond the audiometer's limits.

In van der Hoeve's syndrome, the patient exhibits a combination of a generalized bone disorder, osteogenesis imperfecta (Lobstein's disease), with blue sclera and hearing loss. In this condition, cartilages throughout the body are softened, and the teeth become transparent in a few of these patients. It is common to find several members of the same family having hearing loss and blue sclera. Although the audiologic findings closely resemble those of otosclerosis, the impression during stapes mobilization surgery suggests that the stapes fixation is of a different consistency than that found in otosclerosis (see Chapter 13 and Appendix III).

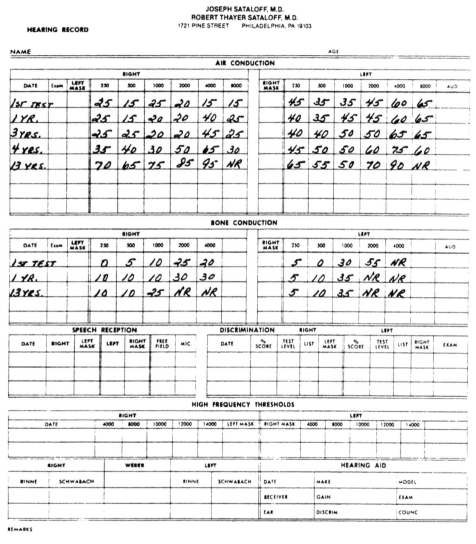

Figure 9.34 *History:* A 59-year-old man first noticed beginning impairment in hearing in the left ear at the age of 44. Hearing loss gradually progressed with increasing discrimination difficulty and occasional tinnitus. Diagnosed as having far-advanced Paget's disease at the age of 46. Tinnitus started in the right ear 6 months after diagnosis was made. Wearing hearing aid in left ear since age 52. Had periods of fleeting imbalance for the past few years. Speech normal. Skull roentgenograms revealed a narrowing of the internal auditory canal and no visualization of the right canal. Neither cochlea could be made out clearly. *Otologic:* Both eardrums were slightly opaque. *Audiologic:* Air and bone conduction thresholds measured over a period of 13 years show a slowly progressive hearing loss with greater loss in the higher frequencies. An air–bone gap was always present in the lower frequencies but not in the higher frequencies. No recruitment was found. *Classification:* Low-frequency conductive loss and subsequent sensorineural involvement in the middle and higher frequencies. *Diagnosis:* Paget's disease.

# EUSTACHIAN TUBE AND ITS RELATIONSHIP TO CONDUCTIVE HEARING LOSS

## Action of the eustachian tube

The eustachian tube generally is straight, but sometimes it has a slight curve and a little twist where the bony portion from the middle ear joins the cartilaginous portion in the nasopharynx. In addition, the opening of the tube is wide in the nasopharynx and in the middle ear, but the lumen narrows down considerably at the bony cartilaginous junction. Normally, the eustachian tube is not open except during swallowing, sneezing, yawning, or forceful nose blowing. Behind the opening of the eustachian tube in the nasopharynx is a deep depression called the fossa of Rosenmüller. Excessive growth of adenoid tissue in this area often compresses the tube and prevents normal aeration of the middle ear. Congestion and infection in the nasopharynx and the adenoid region also can cause closing of the tube by upward progression along the tubal mucosa and the submucosal areas.

**Functions.** The eustachian tube normally has two important functions: one is to allow drainage from the middle ear into the nasopharynx and the other is to maintain equal air pressure on both sides of the eardrum. The mucous membrane of the middle ear absorbs air, though slowly. As the eustachian tube normally is closed, it is essential that the eustachian tube be opened at intervals to maintain pressure equilibrium. This is done during swallowing not only when eating but also continually throughout the day and night as saliva and mucus collect in the pharynx and stimulate the swallowing reflex.

**Methods of Evaluating Function.** One simple way to demonstrate that the tube opens during swallowing is to hold a vibrating tuning fork in front of the nostrils. The sound perceived by the patient will be weak until swallowing, and then it will be much louder as the sound waves travel up the eustachian tube into the middle ear.

Another way of determining whether the tube is functioning and opening properly is to use Politzer's method. A large nasal tip on a pressure bottle containing camphor mist (or only air) is inserted snugly into one nostril while the other is occluded, and the patient is told to say "kick" or "cake." Pronouncing the "k" sound causes closure of the nasopharynx by lifting the soft palate, and the air or the mist then is forced up the eustachian tube, causing the eardrum to push out slightly. It is helpful to watch the eardrum through an otoscope during this procedure. The normal eardrum will move out very slightly and then return to its original position. Abnormal results may include a slow return of the eardrum to its initial position, persistent pouching out of large blebs, or failure of the drum to move at all. These irregularities suggest abnormal conditions in the tube and the middle ear. Caution must be exercised not to use too much air pressure, as this may rupture a weakened eardrum or cause dizziness. The whole procedure is contraindicated if infection is present in the nose or the nasopharynx.

Other methods of evaluating the function of the eustachian tube include direct examination through a nasopharyngoscope and catheterization. Politzerization also is especially helpful if a small perforation is suspected in the eardrum but cannot be visualized through the otoscope. The camphor mist can be seen coming out of the small perforation, thereby pinpointing its site. If air is used, water or ear drops can be placed in the ear and the perforation can be located by watching for bubbles.

Impedance audiometry can demonstrate eustachian tube function by recording changes in middle ear pressure while swallowing. When a perforation is present, tubal function can be measured directly.

# EXTENT OF HEARING LOSS WITH EUSTACHIAN TUBE INVOLVEMENT

No part of the auditory system has been incriminated more wrongly and mistreated more than the eustachian tube. This was understandable before there was clear understanding of the physiology of hearing, of the function of the eustachian tube, and of otosclerosis. At the present time, however, there should be no reasonable excuse for blaming or mistreating the eustachian tube when the cause of the hearing loss actually lies elsewhere.

Malfunction of the eustachian tube causes only conductive hearing loss. If sensory hearing loss is present, the eustachian tube generally should not be the target for treatment, even though politzerization or tubal inflation may give the patient a subjective sense of well-being and an apparent hearing improvement for a few moments. Such treatment can delay the patient's aural rehabilitation.

In general, simple blockage of the eustachian tube causes only a comparatively mild hearing loss not exceeding ~35 dB; most of the time it is much less than that. The loss is greater in the lower frequencies than in the higher. The most common causes are acute upper respiratory infections and allergies in which the eustachian tube becomes boggy and obstructed owing to congestion and inflammation. This condition makes the ears feel full, and the individual appears to be slightly hard-of-hearing. If the obstruction in the tube persists, the air in the middle ear is absorbed by the mucosal lining, and the eardrum becomes slightly retracted aggravating hearing loss, sometimes even up to measurable levels (~ 35 dB). If fluid forms in the middle ear, there may be an even greater hearing loss, including higher frequencies. This frequency change is caused by the addition of the fluid mass to the contents of the middle ear. When there is fluid in the middle ear, the bone conduction also may be slightly reduced, and this reduction may suggest a false diagnosis of sensorineural hearing loss. However, removal of the fluid restores both air and bone conduction to normal.

There are exceptions to these generalizations. When the tube has been closed for many months or years, the drum may become retracted so completely that it becomes "plastered" to the promontory, a condition that causes a hearing loss of ~50 dB, or if the fluid is thick and gelatinous, the loss may be slightly greater. In general, eustachian tube obstruction *per se* causes only a mild hearing loss. The loss increases only when complications arise in the middle ear, such as the presence of a fluid, retraction of the drum, or infection. Therefore, it is safe to conclude that if the hearing loss exceeds 35 dB and the eardrum and the middle ear appear to be practically normal, the fault does not typically lie in the eustachian tube. The cause is more likely to be found in the ossicular chain and especially in the stapes.

## INJURIES TO THE EUSTACHIAN TUBE

Trauma of the eustachian tube is not a frequent cause of hearing loss, but during armed conflicts, a number of patients were seen whose eustachian tubes were injured by gunshot or shrapnel wounds to the face. The damage generally is unilateral and can be visualized through the nasopharyngoscope.

Following trauma to the eustachian tube, the scar tissue that forms during healing narrows the tube and causes recurrent or persistent attacks of serous otitis media. Similar scarring and narrowing can occur after radiation therapy for nasopharyngeal cancers. In such instances, it is important to avoid harsh manipulation inside the eustachian tube, which eventually would aggravate the constriction. Repeated myringotomies, or a temporary tube in the eardrum, and the use of oral and local decongestants are the best alternatives in most cases. Patients usually complain of fullness in the affected ear and hearing loss, which clears up when the fluid is removed from the middle ear.

## PATULOUS EUSTACHIAN TUBE

In rare instances, a patient complains of a loud swishing sound in the ear whenever he/she inhales through the nose, and the ears also may feel full and the hearing muffled. The examination of the mouth of the eustachian tube through a nasopharyngoscope may reveal the opening to appear to be much larger and far more patent than normal. Such a condition is called a patent, or patulous, eustachian tube. The cause is not always clear, but it often appears to result from a depletion of fat around the eustachian tube. Anything that causes fat redistribution may produce this condition: weight loss, use of steroids, pregnancy, birth control pills, and other conditions.

Patients with a patulous eustachian tube are far more disturbed by their symptoms than are those with an obstructed eustachian tube. It can be very annoying to a patient to hear a swish in the ear with each breath. The condition is aggravated by exercise. The patient eventually may become obsessed with this symptom. The symptoms stop when breathing is done through the mouth. Another complaint is hearing one's own voice as if in a resonant chamber. This is called autophonia. Another unusual observation is to see the eardrum move in and out during respiration. This may be confirmed by tympanometry. Although the patient may believe that there is difficulty hearing in the involved ear, actually there is no hearing loss, and this condition is not a hearing defect. Although many treatments have been suggested for this abnormality, there is no one specific cure for these annoying symptoms. Weight gain, myringotomy and tube placement, and eustachian tube injection may be helpful.

## HYPERTROPHIED ADENOIDS

Serous otitis media is the most common cause of mild conductive hearing loss in children and can be caused by hypertrophied adenoids, allergy, and other conditions. School surveys in several states agree that ~3% of children have significant hearing losses in at least several frequencies. Well over 80% of these are conductive and may be associated with hypertrophied adenoids (**Figure 9.35**). Other possible causes of this condition are secretory otitis, cleft palate, allergies, nasopharyngitis, sinusitis, gastric reflux, and nasopharyngeal tumors, but even in some of these conditions, hypertrophied adenoids may be a contributing factor.

As audiograms are not always performed routinely in children, hearing loss is probably much more prevalent than commonly believed. Children usually are spoken to in a raised voice, and as a result, hearing losses seldom are noted until they approach 40 dB. These losses develop insidiously in many children and may be present for many months or even years before they are distinguished from childhood inattention. Hearing loss as mild as 15 dB can have a measurable effect on a child's behavior. Adenoidectomies often are performed because of mouth breathing or chronic ear infection without a preoperative audiogram; it seems reasonable to speculate that routine audiograms would reveal a substantial number of hearing losses in such children. Hence, universal screening has been advocated. In uncomplicated cases, hearing loss may subside under either conservative or surgical treatment without its existence ever having been noted by either the parent or the physician. Routine audiograms clearly are indicated in all children with recurrent attacks of otitis media, chronic inattention, history of mouth breathing, and earache especially in the presence of hypertrophied adenoids.

Opinions differ widely as to the indication for adenoidectomy in children. These differences range from the routine performance of adenoidectomies in almost all the children having upper respiratory infections to the opposite extreme of never removing the adenoids unless there is complete obstruction in the nasopharynx. Such marked differences of opinion concerning the effectiveness of adenoidectomy in dealing with this problem indicate the need for continuing reappraisal based on objective studies.

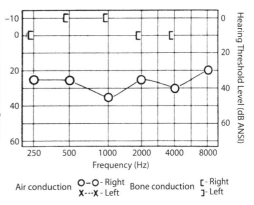

Figure 9.35 *History:* A 6-year-old child with recurrent earaches and hearing loss for the past year. The child is also a chronic mouth breather. The patient had had six myringotomies, allergic desensitization, and a T&A before being seen by the author. *Abbreviations:* ANSI, American National Standards Institute; ASA, American Standards Association.

Untreated childhood ear disease may result in hearing loss later in life. The sequelae of serous otitis are primarily conductive hearing losses. However, chronic, recurrent infectious otitis media appears to occur more often in people with serous otitis and may result in sensorineural hearing loss in selected cases. It is important to remember that the implications of serous otitis, especially unilateral serous otitis, are different in adults. Unilateral serous otitis with no apparent etiology should be considered carcinoma of the nasopharynx until proven otherwise. Serous otitis is often the presenting symptom of this disease because of unilateral malignant eustachian tube obstruction.

## EFFECTS OF EAR SURGERY

Procedures of middle ear surgery are beyond the scope of this book, but the physician who examines the ear of a patient with conductive hearing loss may discover evidence of previous ear surgery. He/she should be prepared to evaluate the relation of the patient's hearing deficit to past otologic surgical procedures. A brief review of these interventions and the visible traces they are likely to leave may be helpful.

## MICROSCOPES

Otologic microsurgery utilizes magnification, usually provided by an operating microscope. Many surgeons are not familiar with formulas that determine accurately the amount of magnification used, and it is often recorded incorrectly in operative reports. It is not unusual for surgeons to assume that the number on the indicator on the zoom control correlates with the number of times the image is magnified, but accurate determination is more complex than that. This author usually works with a Zeiss operating microscope (Oberkochen, Germany), and the information in this discussion refers specifically to Zeiss instruments. However, the principles are the same for microscopes by other companies. In order to determine the amount of magnification, the focal length of the binocular tube is divided by the focal length of the objective lens, and then multiplied by the magnification of the eye pieces (2). The result is then multiplied by the indicator on the magnification (zoom) knob of the microscope. Many current microscopes have internal zoom which is not specified. The focal length of the binocular tube is usually a number such as F125, F160, or F170. For example, the older Zeiss OPMI-6 microscope has a binocular tube with a focal length of F160, and the newer design with the wider angle of view has a focal length of F170. The focal length of the objective lens varies depending upon the surgeon's preference. For ear surgery, it is usually 250 or 300 mm. For laryngeal surgery, a 400-mm lens is commonly used. The usual eye piece magnification is either 10× or 12.5×. The indicator number ranges from 0.4 to 2.4. The OPMI-6-S, for example, provides a continuous magnification range of 1:4. Older Zeiss operating microscopes (such as the OPMI-1) have magnification changes that are step-like rather than continuous and have numbers that range from 6 to 40 next to the dial. These provide five magnification steps in a range of 1:6. These numbers should not be used in the formula noted earlier but can be converted as follows: 40 corresponds to 2.5, 25 corresponds to 1.6, 16 corresponds to 1.0, 10 corresponds to 0.6, and 6 corresponds to 0.4. So, for example, if a surgeon is using an OPMI-1 microscope with 10× eyepieces, a 400-mm objective lens, and the magnification set at 40 (maximum), image magnification is 7.8× (i.e., [125/400] 2.5 × 10 = 7.8×), not 40× as misstated commonly. Simply changing the eyepieces from 10× to 12.5× increases the magnification from 7.8× to 9.8×,

and using 20× eyepieces increases the magnification to 15.6×. Utilizing an objective lens with a shorter focal length also increases magnification but brings the microscope closer to the operating field. While this approach is used during ear surgery, it is not suitable for laryngeal surgery because the decreased space between the microscope and direct laryngoscope is not sufficient to permit unimpeded manipulation of long-handled laryngeal instruments. It is important for surgeons to be familiar with these principles in order to optimize surgical conditions for each surgery.

## MYRINGOTOMY

Incision and drainage through the eardrum is called myringotomy. This incision is made in the bulging part of the eardrum or in the posterior inferior or an anterior quadrant to avoid injuring any middle or inner ear structure in case the incision goes too deeply. This might occur if the patient moved inadvertently during the procedure.

Very rarely, the end of the incus and, even more uncommonly, the stapedial crura may be injured during myringotomy. **Figure 9.28** is a case report in which such an injury occurred in childhood and remained undiagnosed until surgery was performed many years later. These injuries may be avoided if the myringotomy is performed in the anterior–inferior quadrant.

In most instances, after myringotomy, the eardrum returns to normal, but sometimes permanent scar tissue is left. Hearing is not damaged by a myringotomy itself or by the scar tissue it occasionally leaves in the eardrum. A perforation may persist, especially when the myringotomy incision has been kept open with a synthetic tube. These perforations can be closed surgically.

## HEARING LOSS ASSOCIATED WITH EAR SURGERY

When many kinds of ear surgery are performed, prime consideration is given to preservation or restoration of hearing. Of course, in surgery for mastoiditis or chronic otitis media, the principal objective is to remove the infection, but the type of surgery done is determined to a great degree by efforts to preserve hearing. A number of surgical procedures that potentially are associated with hearing impairment produce visible changes in the eardrum, the mastoid, or the external ear. Some procedures, such as stapes surgery, leave little or no recognizable scarring, and even a skilled otologist may be unable to tell from looking that the ear has been operated on. Therefore, it is important to obtain a careful history of any previous surgery by questioning the patient.

## SIMPLE MASTOIDECTOMY

Extremely common several years ago, simple mastoidectomy for acute infection now is rare. Better management of otitis media by the general practitioner and the pediatrician has nearly eliminated the need for this procedure. It was done most commonly in children who had severe otitis media that extended to the mastoid bone and caused postauricular swelling, pain, and tenderness as well as hearing loss. Hearing loss was present because of the middle ear infection, not the mastoiditis.

A simple mastoidectomy consists of making a postauricular incision, removing the mastoid cell, and creating an opening into the tympanic antrum that leads to the middle ear. This opening allows aeration and drainage of pus. Essentially, this procedure is a complex type of incision and drainage for pus under pressure. As the middle ear is not disturbed deliberately, and the eardrum usually remains intact (after the infection subsides), hearing usually returns to normal. It is common to find patients with large postauricular scars who have retained normal hearing after having had several simple mastoidectomies.

Unfortunately, not all patients who have had simple mastoidectomies or myringotomies have normal hearing. Some have persistent hearing loss due to persistent perforation in the eardrum or other damage from the infection; still others have mild hearing losses caused by retraction of the eardrum, by middle ear adhesions, or other consequences of the infection.

The chief evidence of a previous simple mastoidectomy is the presence of a postauricular scar with a normal or almost normal eardrum and good hearing. Even if the eardrum is perforated, but the hearing level is better than ~30 dB, the surgery probably was a simple mastoidectomy that left an intact ossicular chain.

Simple mastoidectomy also is done for access to the endolymphatic sac, the facial nerve, or the nerves of the internal auditory canal and cerebellopontine angle, and a more extensive version is used widely for chronic otitis media and mastoiditis.

## MYRINGOPLASTY

When a perforation is found in the eardrum without any active infection, it is nearly always possible to close the perforation. If the hearing loss is due entirely to the perforation, the closure should restore the hearing. The improvement in hearing that can be expected by closing the perforation can be determined preoperatively by patching the hole with a small piece of cigarette paper, Gelfoam, or silastic film. Audiograms obtained prior to and after the patching show the amount of hearing improvement that can be expected from permanent closure with a graft. If no improvement occurs, it means the perforation is not the sole cause of the hearing loss. In either event, it is usually advisable to close the perforation, but the patient should be advised of the prognosis prior to the surgery. In cases in which the hearing loss is not caused by the perforation alone, a simple myringoplasty is inadequate as far as the hearing is concerned. Then, it is necessary to reflect the eardrum and explore the middle ear for ossicular problems or adhesions in addition to closing the perforation in the drum. **Figure 9.36** describes a case of simple myringoplasty.

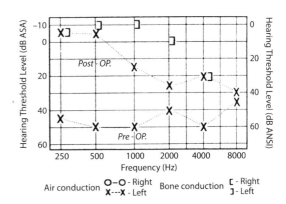

Air conduction  O–O - Right    Bone conduction  [ - Right
X---X - Left                  ] - Left

Figure 9.36 *History:* Intermittent discharge from left ear. *Otologic:* Large perforation in eardrum. Discharge was cleared up with conservative therapy, and later the large perforation was closed with a sliding flap from the external auditory canal. *Audiologic:* Left-ear air conduction thresholds revealed a moderate loss. Bone conduction thresholds were normal, except at 4000 Hz. After the myringoplasty, an air–bone gap remained at the two middle frequencies. *Classification:* Conductive. *Diagnosis:* Perforated drum corrected with myringoplasty. *Abbreviations:* ANSI, American National Standards Institute; ASA, American Standards Association.

The appearance of the eardrum following myringoplasty varies greatly. It is important to obtain a history of this type of surgical procedure from the patient; otherwise, a physician might be startled by the appearance of the eardrum and the hearing loss present and advise unjustified treatment. If a skin graft was used to close the perforation, the drum may appear to the thick and white, and redundant skin may be present so that the drum is flaccid and sometimes hardly delineated. If a vein graft was used, the drum may appear to be stranded and scarred and sometimes thickened and discolored. The appearance of the drum often depends on the graft used, its thickness, and the manner in which it "took." When a grafted eardrum appears flaccid and retracted, and the patient complains of a fluctuating hearing loss that becomes more noticeable every time there is a feeling of fullness in the ear, gentle politzerization often can restore hearing temporarily to an improved level. Sometimes a myringoplasty heals so well that it leaves the eardrum looking almost normal, and the examining physician is scarcely able to detect that any surgery has been done.

## OSSICULOPLASTY

The term "ossiculoplasty" denotes repair or restoration of the continuity of the ossicular chain. For example, in the case presented in **Figure 9.37**, closure of the perforation did not restore hearing. Therefore, at a later date, the then intact eardrum was elevated, and the ossicles were examined. Instead of a normal incus, the connection of the incus with the head of the stapes was fibrous, thin, and very weak, making poor contact. This condition probably resulted from the same infection that had caused the perforation. When the weak connection was replaced with an artificial joint, hearing improved markedly. The only reason that two surgical procedures were required in this case was that prior to the simple myringoplasty, no therapeutic test of closure with an artificial membrane had been done and the ossicular defects were not recognized initially.

The many types of deformities and defects sometimes found in the ossicular chain may test the ingenuity of the surgeon. The defects may be congenital or acquired and may involve any or all of the ossicles. The hearing loss can involve

practically all of the frequencies, and when there is complete disruption of the chain with an intact drum, the hearing loss is ~60–70 dB ANSI.

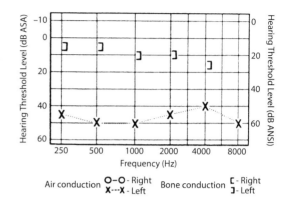

Air conduction O–O - Right  X---X - Left   Bone conduction Ⅽ - Right  ] - Left

Figure 9.37 *History:* A 44-year-old woman with a 2-year episode of left ear discharge when in her early 20s. No tinnitus. Had had a myringoplasty which did not restore hearing. *Otologic:* Large healed perforation. Further surgery revealed that the incus end was eroded and replaced with a thin band of fibrous tissue. The continuity of the chain was corrected with a plastic prosthesis. Hearing was restored with restoration of ossicular continuity. *Impedance:* Type A tympanogram; absent stapedius reflex. *Classification:* Conductive. *Diagnosis:* Ossicular disruption. *Abbreviations:* ANSI, American National Standards Institute; ASA, American Standards Association.

When the eardrum is normal and a nonotosclerotic ossicular defect is found, the etiology is often congenital. Exceptions do occur.

More commonly, however, there is a history of trauma or otitis media, and some abnormality is present in the drum. The diagnosis is not hard to make but is difficult to predict just which ossicle is involved prior to surgery.

Whenever a patient has a 60–70 dB hearing loss involving all of the frequencies and patching of the perforation does not improve the hearing, there is a good possibility that the ossicular chain is disrupted (if otosclerosis is excluded). If the hearing loss is only 40 dB and other circumstances are the same, it is more likely that the ossicular chain is intact but that some fracture or joint damage has healed with fibrous or weakened union or that one or more ossicles is partially fixed and not moving freely. The middle ear should be examined at least whenever there is any doubt that simple myringoplasty can restore hearing, and many surgeons recommend exploring the middle ear when repairing any perforation.

## STAPEDECTOMY

When the stapes is fixed by otosclerosis or congenital deformity, the resultant conductive hearing loss may be repaired by mobilizing the stapes or by removing it. When removed, it is replaced by a prosthesis (or "artificial bone") made out of titanium, Teflon, or a similar material. The prosthesis usually is connected to the incus, and it may be visible as a metallic reflection through the eardrum. This is not a problem and may be the only visible evidence of stapedectomy. Occasionally, if bone has been curetted for visibility, the posterior superior edge of the ear canal may be jagged, and the annulus may be displaced. However, most often there are no visible sequelae of stapes surgery.

## RADICAL MASTOIDECTOMY

Radical mastoidectomy is performed in selected cases of chronic otitis media and mastoiditis in which it is not advisable or possible to clear up the infection by more limited operations that preserve the ossicular chain and the eardrum, as well as hearing. Usually, in such cases, there is extensive cholesteatoma and erosion of the eardrum and the ossicles. Surgery can be done through an endaural or a postauricular incision. The mastoid air cells are removed, and the malleus and the incus are removed. The stapes (or at least its footplate) is carefully left in place. Because there is no ossicular chain or drum, the hearing level in ears after such surgery usually is between 35 and 70 dB at all frequencies. The appearance of the middle ear varies, but usually skin covers a large mastoid cavity, no eardrum is present, and one can see into the anterior part of the middle ear where the eustachian tube opening lies if it is not covered. Often, the eustachian tube orifice will be covered if possible, to prevent reflux of moisture from the nasopharynx into the middle ear These ears tend to collect debris and cerumen and require regular cleaning.

In many patients with radical mastoid cavities, it may be possible to improve hearing by tympanoplastic surgery that partly reconstructs the middle ear. The ear canal also can be rebuilt to eliminate the cavity.

## MODIFIED RADICAL MASTOIDECTOMY, TYMPANOPLASTY, AND INTACT CANAL WALL TYMPANOMASTOIDECTOMY

Hearing preserving surgeries may be performed to remove infection from the mastoid and middle ear. These surgeries include modified radical mastoidectomies, tympanomastoidectomies, and tympanoplasties. Among the most common procedures used to reconstruct hearing include ossiculoplasties, which those involve positioning of a prosthetic (or human) ear bone connecting the stapes or oval window with either a newly grafted eardrum or the malleus.

In modified radical mastoidectomies, the posterior ear canal wall is removed, but some portion of tympanic membrane, malleus, and/or incus is preserved. Some modified radical mastoidectomies and tympanoplasties are done through an endaural incision rather than postauricularly. Very little scar is left following endaural surgery, and this is seen as a fine line slightly above the tragus and directed upward toward the temple. The posterior position of the ear canal may have been removed, and thus an external ear canal larger than normal is created. The eardrum, usually present, generally is not normal because it has been scarred by infection and in most cases has been grafted to close a perforation.

Intact canal wall tympanomastoidectomy is the procedure of choice in many cases. This is similar to a simple mastoidectomy, but more extensive. A postauricular incision is used, and the mastoid cells are removed. Bone removal is carried anteriorly into the zygomatic root as far forward as the anterior ear canal wall. An extension from the mastoid into the middle ear may be created between the facial nerve and the bony external auditory canal. This is called a facial recess approach. The middle ear also is entered through a separate incision in the ear canal. When done properly, this somewhat more complicated technique permits eradication of disease, with preservation of the external auditory canal wall, eardrum (with or without graft), and any healthy ossicles. It permits the greatest chance for reconstruction of normal hearing. The disadvantage is that the ear is not exteriorized. So, when intact canal wall tympanomastoidectomy is performed for cholesteatoma, a "second-look procedure" is generally required 4–12 months later to remove any residual cholesteatoma while it is still small enough to be resected completely.

## FENESTRATION

Many ears were fenestrated in the past, but this complicated procedure has been superseded by stapes surgery. It is important to recognize a fenestrated ear, to be able to care for it, and to know the procedures available to improve hearing in an unsuccessful fenestration or in one in which the hearing has regressed.

Fenestrations were done in cases of otosclerosis with excellent bone conduction, and they usually were performed endaurally. The object was to circumvent the fixed stapes and to allow sound waves to impinge directly on a new window, bypassing the fixed oval window. The new window was made in the horizontal semicircular canal and was covered with a skin flap from the posterior canal wall continuous with the eardrum. Because of the depth and the difficulty of access to the operative site, the eardrum was relocated, and the incus and the head of the malleus were removed. On otoscopic examination, the external auditory canal is wider, and the eardrum is seen to be pushed back into the middle ear. Part of the mastoid bone also has been removed so that a cavity is visible. Because of the disruption of the ossicular chain and other factors, it was not common to obtain consistent hearing levels better than 15 or 20 dB in most fenestrated ears. **Figure 9.38** shows a typical successful result. Bone conduction had to be very good with a large air–bone gap to warrant fenestration. Occasionally, hearing regressed owing to closure to the fenestra.

In most of these cases, it is now possible to improve hearing by stapes surgery. In such cases, the stapes may be mobilized and connected to the

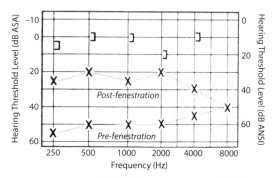

Air conduction O–O - Right, X⋯X - Left   Bone conduction Ⴀ - Right, Ⴈ - Left

**Figure 9.38** *History:* Gradual hearing loss and buzzing tinnitus > 10 years. Sister also hard-of-hearing. Soft voice and hears better in noisy room. *Otologic:* Normal. *Audiologic:* Left-ear air conduction thresholds revealed a moderate, flat loss. Bone thresholds were normal. Fenestration surgery reduced the air–bone gap, but because the ossicular continuity had been disrupted during this operation and the hearing pathway altered to go through a fenestration in the lateral semicircular canal, hearing rarely improved beyond the 15-dB level. *Classification:* Conductive. *Diagnosis:* Otosclerosis corrected with fenestration surgery. *Abbreviations:* ANSI, American National Standards Institute; ASA, American Standards Association.

eardrum or malleus remnant with a strut or wire. Another good procedure is to remove the stapes and place a prosthesis from the malleus to the oval window.

When cleaning debris from fenestrated ears, the physician should be careful while working deep in the ear. Vertigo is induced readily by pressing near the fenestrated area.

## REFERENCES

1. Schuknecht HF. Some interesting middle ear problems. Laryngoscope 1957; 67:395–409.
2. Hoerenz P. The operating microscope: optical principles, illumination systems, and support systems. J Microsurg 1980; 1:364–369.

# 10

# Sensorineural hearing loss: Diagnostic criteria

ROBERT THAYER SATALOFF, SKYLAR DREXEL, AND PAMELA C. ROEHM

Sensorineural hearing loss (SNHL) is a challenging problem confronting physicians. Millions of industrial workers and older citizens have this type of impairment. It generally is irreversible and often affects daily communication. The potential psychological implications place SNHL in the foreground of medical importance.

pinpoint the diagnosis specifically as being either a sensory or a neural type. If it can be established that the major damage to the auditory pathway is in the inner ear, the case is classified as a sensory hearing loss. If the chief damage is in the fibers of the eighth nerve rather than in the inner ear, it is classified as a neural hearing loss.

## CLASSIFICATION

The damage to the auditory pathway may take place both in the inner ear (sensory loss) and in the auditory nerve (neural loss). We emphasize that the damage may be in both areas (as the name sensorineural indicates), but it is possible in many cases to

## LIMITED INFORMATION

The precise cause or the detailed pathology of some cases is not known. It is difficult for investigators to explore the very small and intricate cochlea, deeply embedded in the temporal bone. Temporal bones from patients whose hearing characteristics have been studied are available only infrequently—hence the problem of correlating clinical findings with pathological observations. Animal experiments, although they are helpful, provide limited information and must be interpreted with caution.

## COROLLARIES TO CLASSIFICATION

Although it is not possible to specify the causes of all clinical cases of SNHL, merely classifying them as sensorineural provides important information. In the first place, such classification is a recognition that the site of the damage is not in the middle ear. This contraindicates surgical therapy in the middle ear in most cases. There is no logical ground for eustachian tube inflation, stapes surgery, or removal of adenoids and tonsils when the diagnosis is SNHL. Second, the prognosis is not nearly as optimistic as it is when there is a conductive type of loss. Many times the hearing deficit is irreversible, and it behooves the physician to tell the patient in a forthright manner that recovery of hearing is unlikely. The physician also is able to tell the patient whether the hearing loss is likely to be progressive or nonprogressive and what therapy is worthwhile. For example, the patient can be assured that the deafness will not progress if it can be established that it is of some congenital type or possibly a result of intense noise exposure. On the other hand, it is likely to grow progressively worse if it is due to presbycusis.

## RELATION OF PATHOLOGY TO NEURAL AND ANATOMIC MECHANISMS

Prominent investigators, such as Guild, Rasmussen, Fernandez, Lawrence, and Schuknecht, have broadened our understanding of the mechanisms underlying such phenomena of abnormal hearing as poor discrimination, recruitment, and pitch distortion (diplacusis). Because these symptoms are prominent in SNHL, it seems fitting to crystallize the available information for the purpose of visualizing the pathological conditions likely to be present when these findings are encountered in practice.

For many years, the endolymphatic sac has been considered important in maintaining various aspects of cochlear fluid, and it has been postulated as the site of pathology in patients with endolymphatic hydrops (Ménière's syndrome). Recently, the endolymphatic sac has been found to function as an endocrine gland. Its chief cells produce saccin, an inhibitor of sodium resorption in the kidneys. This discovery has led to a new theory of endolymphatic hydrops. This theory postulates that the endolymphatic duct becomes obstructed by debris. An increased volume of endolymph within the cochlea results from production of saccin. This, combined with the secretion of hydrophilic proteins within the sac, is believed to clear the obstruction, suddenly restoring longitudinal flow, and precipitating an attack of vertigo. This interesting speculation would explain clinical observations, but further research is required to determine whether it is accurate.

The organ of Corti in the inner ear contains ~25,000 cells resting on a basilar membrane. These hair cells are arranged in long rows conforming to the spiral shape of the organ of Corti. There are ~3500–5000 inner hair cells arranged in a single row and >20,000 outer hair cells which run in three to five parallel rows. There is a tunnel between the inner and outer hair cells (**Figure 10.1A** and **B**). There are also various types of supporting cells in the inner ear that relate to the nerve fibers as well as to the inner ear. About 95% of the auditory nerve fibers terminate on the inner hair cells, and only 5% go to the many outer hair cells (1). If there are adequate supporting cells in the inner ear, the nerve fibers do not seem to show much degeneration. However, if the hair cells and the supporting cells are damaged, the nerve fibers supplying them degenerate so that many cases of sensory hearing loss progress to the sensorineural type.

The hair cells change mechanical vibrations into electrochemical impulses that can be interpreted by the nervous system. As the hairs or cilia covering the tops of the inner and outer hair cells are deflected, an electrical current flow across the top of the cell, leading to a nerve impulse. Outer hair cells are in contact with the tectorial membrane, a gel-like structure that appears to assist in deflection and restoration of position. Contact between the cilia of the inner hair cells and the tectorial membrane is slight or possibly nonexistent (2). The hair cells are contained in the organ or Corti that rests on the basilar membrane in the cochlear partition. The partition itself also moves because of complex fluid phenomena. Acoustic vibrations result in a wave that travels through the cochlea (3). Motion of the cochlear partition is important to hearing, and impairment of motion may be responsible for some kinds of hearing loss, as discussed later in the section on presbycusis. At present, it is believed that the frequency selective properties of the auditory system are due to mechanical processes within the cochlea rather than to complex peripheral neural interactions. However, many of the mysteries of auditory physiology remain unsolved. For example, there is a suggestion that an active, energy-producing system exists in the cochlear partition and is responsible for the sharp mechanical tuning abilities of the ear (4). However, this structure has not really been identified or explained. In fact, even the roles of the inner and outer hair cells are not well understood. Several histological peculiarities of the outer hair cells remain unexplained. For example, there are many subsurface layers in the outer hair cells that appear to be specialized for calcium storage, and the cylindrical external surface is surrounded by the fluid of the organ of Corti (unlike inner hair cells which are closely juxtaposed to supporting cells). These outer hair cell findings are not commonly associated with sensory receptor cells, and they suggest that the outer hair cells may be serving functions yet undiscovered. The structures of the lateral wall of the outer hair cells are unusual. It is trilaminate, including a plasma membrane, cortical lattice, and subsurface cisternae. Outer hair cells can alter their length in response to voltage changes across the cell membrane. This phenomenon is called an electromotile response. It is believed to be due to conformational changes of Prestin, a membrane-bound protein molecule. When cell membrane potential is changed, axial stiffness and cell motility result, and intracellular anions act as extrinsic voltage sensors. Somatic motility involves both cochlear and vestibular hair cells. There is speculation that somatic motility plays a role in mechanical sound amplification. However, this remains to be proven or disproven. Nevertheless, when outer hair cells are damaged, hearing loss occurs, and the frequency of the hearing loss is directly related to the area of outer hair cell damage. Outer hair cell loss also damages or eliminates fine-tuning capabilities. In addition,

absence of the outer hair cells changes markedly the neural output from the cochlea, even though this outflow originates primarily from the inner hair cells.

Despite the small neural distributions of the outer hair cells, these cells are extremely important to hearing. They are also very fragile. Damage to the auditory system usually is first seen as outer hair cell injury, with noise and direct head trauma destroying the outer row of outer hair cells first. Interestingly, many ototoxic drugs tend to injure the inner row of outer hair cells. The maximum hearing loss (threshold shift) that occurs when the outer hair cells are lost is ~50 dB. The hearing loss exceeds 60 dB only when the inner hair cells also become damaged. When all the hair cells are lost, no stimuli are available to excite the nerve endings, and consequently there is no sensation of hearing, although the nerve itself may be entirely intact. Considerably more research is necessary to clarify the functions of even the hair cells, let alone the entire auditory system. The reader is encouraged to consult an excellent summary by Dallos for a review of other concepts in cochlear physiology (6).

In addition to the afferent bundles from the ear to the brain, there is also an efferent bundle of Rasmussen that carries impulses to the ear from the brain. This efferent tract appears to play a role in the inhibition of impulses, and its fibers appear to stimulate the outer hair cells causing a change in the mechanical properties of the organ of corti and cochlear partition.

The relation of the hair cells to the nerve is the basis for explaining the phenomenon of recruitment which is most evident in noise-induced hearing loss and Ménière's syndrome. It is found also in patients whose hearing has been damaged by certain drugs. The precise explanation for recruitment of loudness in its varying forms still is not clear. The essential element for recruitment is damage to the hair cells that is disproportionately large compared with the nerve fiber supply. The mechanism seems to be that sufficient hair cells are damaged to reduce the threshold, but enough remain so that when a certain individual-specific sound threshold is reached, a normal number of nerve fibers are excited as if all the hair cells were present. Although this explains most types of recruitment, it does not provide a satisfactory explanation for the phenomenon of hyperrecruitment, in which

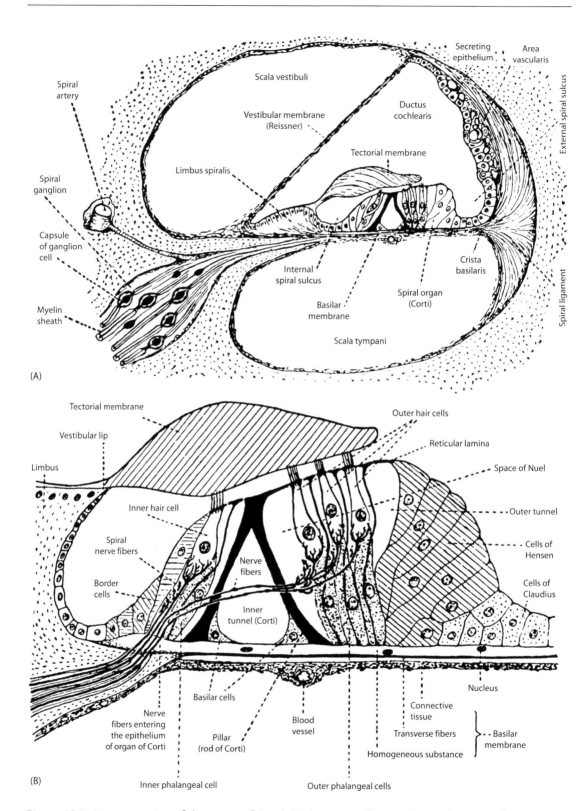

Figure 10.1 A cross-section of the organ of Corti. (A) Low magnification. (B) Higher magnification. (After Rasmussen [5].)

the sound in the damaged ear is not only as loud as that in the normal ear but is perceived by the patient as even louder. This suggests that the number of nerve impulses ascending the auditory nerve is even greater per unit of time than in the normal ear. Patients with hyperrecruitment complain habitually that almost all noises are very bothersome and exceptionally loud.

Some patients with damage to the inner ear and marked recruitment can detect very small changes in sound intensity, smaller than those which even the normal ear can detect. The ear seems to become ultrasensitive to loudness. This phenomenon technically is called reduced intensity difference-limen or, briefly, reduced difference-limen. Its occurrence has a logical explanation similar to that of recruitment.

Certain facts should be clarified about the ability of present-day hearing tests to detect damage to the sensorineural pathway. Although an audiogram may show a 0-dB hearing level, which is considered to be normal, it does not necessarily indicate that the sensorineural mechanism is undamaged. Crowe, Schuknecht, and others have shown that many nerve fibers can be destroyed without affecting threshold hearing for pure tones. As a matter of fact, as many as 75% of the auditory nerve fibers supplying a certain cochlear area can be sectioned without creating a substantial change in the hearing threshold level. This must be considered in the interpretation of hearing tests and in visualizing auditory pathway damage. It also should be borne in mind that when octave bands are measured, acuity in the many frequencies between the octave points measured (especially in the large area between 4000 and 8000 Hz) is unknown.

## CHARACTERISTIC FEATURES

## REDUCED BONE CONDUCTION: NEED FOR COMPLETE EXAMINATION

Because the damage is sustained by the areas that analyze sound waves and transmit nerve impulses, certain features result that are characteristic of SNHL. Another characteristic feature of SNHL is difficulty in hearing a vibrating tuning fork by bone conduction. It would seem reasonable to assume that this reduced bone conduction alone would sufficiently warrant classifying hearing loss as sensorineural, but in practice, this assumption is not consistently reliable. There are equivocal cases of conductive hearing loss in which bone conduction is reduced; these make it essential to do a complete otologic and audiologic examination in all cases of hearing loss to be certain of their classification.

## IMPAIRED DISCRIMINATION

In comparing the histories of patients with conductive hearing losses and those with SNHLs, one clinical difference immediately becomes evident. In addition to inadequate hearing ability for soft sounds, patients with SNHL can have the problem of impaired discrimination. Though they may hear people speak, they may be unable to distinguish words with similar vowel sounds but different consonants. This is predominant when the speech frequency range is involved, but it may be observed also when only the higher frequencies are affected. In a conductive hearing loss, the patient has no difficulty understanding someone if the speech is loud enough. By contrast, the patient with SNHL may mistake one word for another, although it is said in a loud voice. One of the most prominent complaints in these cases is the inability to understand speech, especially on the telephone: voices do not seem to be clear, and people sound as if they are always talking with loose dentures or cigarettes in their mouths. Foreign and unfamiliar accents are a special problem to these patients. Music and voices that compete with conversation make understanding especially difficult. The severity of hearing loss and degree of discrimination impairment are not always directly proportional. **Figure 10.2** shows the audiogram of a patient with a severe unilateral hearing loss, but his ability to discriminate is well preserved so long as sounds are loud enough. **Figure 10.58** shows the audiogram of a patient with much better hearing threshold who has poor discrimination caused by an acoustic neuroma.

Many different etiologies produce SNHL, and the characteristics vary accordingly. The most common etiology is presbycusis, which produces the prominent features associated with sensorineural loss.

JOSEPH SATALOFF, M.D.
ROBERT THAYER SATALOFF, M.D.
1721 PINE STREET      PHILADELPHIA, PA 19103

| DATE | RIGHT EAR AIR CONDUCTION | | | | | | | LEFT EAR AIR CONDUCTION | | | | | |
|------|-----|-----|------|------|------|------|--|-----|-----|------|------|------|------|
|      | 250 | 500 | 1000 | 2000 | 4000 | 8000 |  | 250 | 500 | 1000 | 2000 | 4000 | 8000 |
| 3/91 | 5 | 10 | 10 | 10 | 15 | 20 |  | 90 | 90 | 85 | 85 | 100 | 100 |
|      |   |   |   |   |   |   |  |   |   |   |   |   |   |
|      |   |   |   |   |   |   |  |   |   |   |   |   |   |

| | RIGHT EAR BONE CONDUCTION | | | | | | | LEFT EAR BONE CONDUCTION | | | | | |
|--|--|--|--|--|--|--|--|-----|-----|-----|-----|-----|-----|
|  |  |  |  |  |  |  |  | NR | NR | NR | NR | NR | NR |
|  |  |  |  |  |  |  |  |   |   |   |   |   |   |

SPEECH RECEPTION: Right _____ Left _____          DISCRIMINATION: Right _100%_ Left _96%_

Figure 10.2 This 39-year-old man was involved in a motor vehicle accident in which he suffered a head injury with unconsciousness for I–2 hours. He had a left oval window fistula which caused hearing loss and intractable dizziness. The dizziness improved following middle ear exploration and fistula repair, but the hearing loss persisted. Notice that despite severe left sensorineural hearing loss, discrimination was normal.

## GENERAL CHARACTERISTICS

General characteristics of SNHL are the following:

1. If the hearing loss is marked, bilateral, and of long duration, the patient's voice generally is louder and more strained than normal. This is particularly notable when the voice is compared with the soft voices of patients with otosclerosis.
2. If tinnitus is present, it usually will be described as high-pitched hissing or ringing.
3. The air conduction threshold is reduced.
4. The bone conduction threshold is reduced to about the same level as the air conduction so that there is no substantial air–bone gap. Often the tuning fork held to the skull is not heard at all even when it is struck hard.
5. The discrimination score is reduced decidedly when the speech frequencies are involved and to a lesser degree when only the high frequencies are involved.
6. The patient finds it more difficult to understand speech in a noisy environment than in a quiet one.
7. When the discrimination score is reduced, the patient will discriminate as well or slightly better when the intensity of the speech is increased (in contrast to some cases of sensory hearing loss caused by Ménière's disease).
8. In most cases, there is little, if any, evidence of abnormal tone decay (adaptation).
9. Recruitment generally is absent; if present, it is not marked and is found only in the region just above threshold (noncontinuous and incomplete).
10. The vibrating tuning fork lateralizes to the ear that has better hearing in patients who have a substantial difference in hearing level between the two ears.
11. Responses to audiometry are usually sharp and clear-cut.
12. Otologic findings are normal.

13. Little or no separation is found between the interrupted and the continuous Békésy audiograms.
14. If the hearing loss originally was sensory but has progressed to a sensorineural loss, some characteristics of sensory hearing loss may persist, such as mild recruitment and diplacusis.
15. The prognosis for recovery with treatment is poor, with rare exceptions.

## ASPECTS OF CRITERIA

## LOUDNESS OF VOICE

Many of these criteria have interesting backgrounds. For instance, the loudness of voices depends on many factors such as personality, the distance from a listener, the eagerness to be heard, the amount of background noise, and what the individual has been taught to regard as socially acceptable.

Individuals control the loudness of their voices mainly by hearing themselves speak. They do this by both air and bone conduction to varying degrees. It is a feedback system whereby the individual hears his/her own voice, and if it seems too loud, he/she lowers it, or if too soft, he/she raises it. In otosclerosis, the patient hears his/her own speech chiefly by bone conduction because it is far better than the air conduction, and so, he/she tends to keep the voice soft; otherwise, the patient thinks he/she is shouting. Furthermore, in otosclerosis, the patient does not have the urge to raise his/her voice above the background level because the background noise is hardly heard.

In marked SNHL of long duration involving both ears, the patient cannot hear his/her own voice by either air or bone conduction. When continued efforts fail to hear one's own voice and thus to obtain the feedback control to which one has become accustomed, the voice often becomes louder and more strained.

However, not all patients with severe, long-standing sensorineural hearing impairment develop loud and strained voices. We have seen patients who, despite becoming progressively deaf as adults until no residual hearing remains, have been able for many years to maintain almost normal speech levels. Speech and voice therapy, their own conscious efforts, and tactile feedback have enabled these patients to fix a certain loudness reference level for their own voices similar to what they used when they had normal hearing. However, it becomes strikingly evident that such patients do not lower or raise their voices in different noise environments as most people with normal hearing do. Some of them will inadvertently speak loudly in a quiet room and softly in a noisy one.

## SPEECH DISCRIMINATION

Another intriguing aspect of SNHL concerns understanding speech. In otologic practice, the physician frequently sees patients whose findings are similar to those described in **Figure 10.3**. This important industrialist's only complaint was that he could not discern what was said at meetings or in groups in which several people spoke at the same time. Many people who have losses chiefly > 2000 Hz complain of "hearing trouble" when they actually mean discrimination trouble. In a routine audiologic evaluation, tests usually do not duplicate the circumstances under which the patient noted this handicap, such as in noisy areas and in multiple conversations or on the telephone. Some of these difficulties can be attributed to psychological causes as well as hearing losses. Such cases are merely mild examples of the common type of SNHL involving a bilateral high-frequency loss and measurable reduction in discrimination. One reason for reduced discrimination is a patient's inability to distinguish certain consonants that fall within the frequency range of the hearing loss. As consonants help give meaning to words, and the patient has trouble distinguishing certain consonants, the patient misunderstands certain key words and thus at times misinterprets the speaker. If the speaker talks fast and fails to enunciate well, or if noise masks already quiet consonants, the patient with high-frequency loss could have even greater difficulty understanding conversation. This type of discrimination difficulty is different from that encountered in the sensory hearing loss produced by Ménière's syndrome, in which there is marked distortion and fuzziness of speech sounds that worsen when the speech becomes louder.

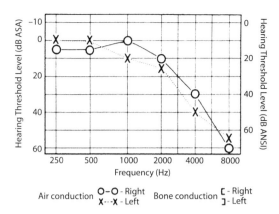

Air conduction O–O - Right, X··X - Left   Bone conduction [ - Right, ] - Left

Figure 10.3 *History:* A 64-year-old industrialist complaining of difficulty in understanding people who speak, especially at important meetings. He found it necessary to resign as board chairman of a large corporation because of his hearing handicap and personal stress. *Otologic:* Normal. *Audiologic:* Patient has typical high-frequency hearing loss of presbycusis. Discrimination score is 86%, but he has more trouble in a noisy background. *Classification:* Sensorineural hearing loss. *Diagnosis:* Presbycusis. *Aid to diagnosis:* Two years later, the pure-tone threshold dropped only slightly, but the discrimination score fell to 65%, indicating more neural damage. *Abbreviations:* ANSI, American National Standards Institute; ASA, American Standards Association.

## TESTS AND THEIR SHORTCOMINGS

In SNHL, another shortcoming of hearing tests occurs in interpreting discrimination testing. In some cases of mild high-frequency loss, discrimination testing shows an excellent score of 90% despite the patient's complaint of difficulty understanding speech. It must not be concluded that the patient's complaint is always unwarranted. Rather, it should be realized that the discrimination test was done under very quiet conditions in a sound-treated room and with a tester who enunciated very clearly and spoke slowly through an expensive amplification system. Under such conditions, the patient did well. However, in everyday experiences such favorable conditions are rare. Usually, there is some loud distracting noise to mask what the speaker says. Furthermore, few people speak slowly and enunciate clearly. If the speech is coming through an amplification system (e.g., at a train station), it often is distorted and even muffled. It is

no wonder that the patient has complaints under such circumstances.

When a physician talks to a patient, it is common to underestimate the patient's discrimination difficulty because he/she communicates so well in an office setting. A tendency to underrate the patient's difficulty should be avoided, for most patients visit a physician only after such symptoms have persisted and become disturbing. To brush aside the patient's complaint on the strength of a brief face-to-face conversation is to show a lack of understanding of hearing and psychological problems which gives the patient ample motive for discouragement.

Testing bone conduction with a tuning fork in a case of SNHL sometimes may confuse the physician. Occasionally, the physician sees a patient with about a 70-dB hearing loss who absolutely denies hearing a tuning fork by bone conduction regardless of how hard it is struck. Does this mean the nerve is dead? It cannot be completely dead, or there would be no hearing by air conduction. It must be borne in mind that bone conduction is not always a valid test for sensorineural function and also that the ear is ~60–70 dB more sensitive to air conduction than to bone conduction so that the fork would have to produce a very loud tone to be heard by the deafened patient. Some tuning forks are unable to reach this intensity even when they are struck very hard.

In patients with unilateral SNHL, the tuning fork placed on the skull or the teeth sounds louder in the good ear. This is a result of a reduced bone conduction in the ear with SNHL. The physician also will observe that he/she can hear the fork on his/her own skull (if the doctor's hearing is normal) much better than the patient with SNHL can hear it. When testing for this, it is necessary to mask the patient's good ear with noise so that the patient will not report erroneously that hearing was present in the bad ear when the vibrations were conducted through the skull to the good ear.

## RECRUITMENT AND PERCEPTION OF INTENSITY

Recruitment is the outstanding feature of sensory rather than neural hearing loss. However, there may be some degree of recruitment in neural hearing loss, particularly if the loss originally started as sensory and progressed to involve the nerve endings. In such cases, the recruitment is mild, and the abnormal increase in loudness occurs near the threshold. It rarely continues into the high intensities to equal the loudness in the ear that has normal hearing; when it does, this is referred to as "complete recruitment." When the loudness in the recruiting ear exceeds that of the normal ear for the same tone, the condition is called "hyperrecruitment."

It has been pointed out previously that during audiometry the patient with conductive hearing loss waivers in his/her responses as if he/she is uncertain whether sounds are heard near threshold, whereas in sensorineural cases, the responses are sharper and more decisive. The reason is that the patient with sensorineural loss often has a keener ability to detect small differences in intensity than either a patient who has normal hearing or one with conductive hearing loss.

## HYPERACUSIS

Hyperacusis may be related to recruitment, but the phenomenon is not well understood. The term describes painful hypersensitivity to sounds. It may occur in patients with little measurable hearing loss and no measurable recruitment. Patients with hyperacusis are excessively disturbed by common sounds of intensities routinely encountered in daily life. The term hyperacusis does not imply "super hearing," or the ability to detect sounds softer than normal thresholds, although it is occasionally defined this way in some sources. It is not clear whether hyperacusis is caused by peripheral, central, or psychological factors or a combination, and problems involving inhibitory pathways have been proposed as causal, as well.

## ALMOST SYMPTOMLESS TYPES

Some types of sensorineural hearing impairment are almost symptomless and are detected only by audiometric examinations. The early noise-induced dips and the early high-frequency hearing losses are typical.

## MEDICAL TREATMENT

An often-repeated maxim is that SNHL is irreversible, and damage to the auditory nerve fibers cannot be cured. Although the generalization may be true in many cases, the catch lies in the term "damage." In some cases of sensorineural hearing impairment,

the patient gets better spontaneously, but medication may be of help. What the maxim really means is that there is no cure for permanent damage to the auditory nerve. It is not true that all sensorineural damage is permanent. The simplest example of the reversibility of sensorineural damage is auditory fatigue following exposure to gunfire. There can be a marked SNHL that gradually reverts to normal. There are many other cases of SNHL which have all the characteristics of being permanent, and yet they improve dramatically, often with medication or even without. SNHL can be very severe and yet return to an excellent level, as demonstrated in **Figure 10.4**. The chief lesson to be learned from such examples is that it is possible for some cases of SNHL to improve, but at present, there is not sufficient knowledge to forecast consistently when this will happen, nor is there any specific therapy known to promote the return of hearing consistently in many cases. One generalization needs to be considered of value. The cases more likely to be reversible are those of sudden onset rather than those that develop slowly over a period of months. As we have gained experience with conditions such as luetic labyrinthitis and autoimmune SNHL, we have realized that this generalization is not a good one. The onset of hearing loss of the sensorineural type is often helpful in establishing its possible cause. Included in this chapter is a chart showing the known and likely causes of SNHL of sudden and insidious onset. Examples of each cause in the list are found in the following chapters.

The classic example of SNHL is presbycusis because it invariably occurs bilaterally and almost symmetrically. Occupational hearing loss is another common example. The unilateral losses are always interesting and challenging, and it is occasionally difficult to be certain of their cause.

Sensorineural hearing impairment frequently is attributed to factors such as viruses, vascular spasm, vascular embolus, and thrombosis, although sometimes it is difficult to definitively identify a cause for an individual patient.

A SNHL may occur unilaterally or more commonly bilaterally, either simultaneously or at different rates in each ear. A sudden onset of hearing loss almost always motivates the patient to seek a physician's advice as quickly as possible. The patient with hearing loss of gradual onset infrequently seeks help until he/she has experienced many difficulties in communication or has developed disturbing tinnitus or vertigo.

JOSEPH SATALOFF, M.D.
ROBERT THAYER SATALOFF, M.D.
1721 PINE STREET    PHILADELPHIA, PA 19103

**HEARING RECORD**

NAME _____                                      AGE _____

## AIR CONDUCTION

| | | | RIGHT | | | | | | | LEFT | | | | | | |
|------|------|------|------|-----|------|------|------|------|------|------|------|------|------|------|------|------|
| DATE | Exam | LEFT MASK | 250 | 500 | 1000 | 2000 | 4000 | 8000 | RIGHT MASK | 250 | 500 | 1000 | 2000 | 4000 | 8000 | AUD |
| 7th day post-op. | | | 60 | 55 | 45 | 50 | 50 | 70 | | 60 | 55 | 40 | 50 | 45 | NR | |
| 9th day post-op. | | | 15 | 10 | 20 | 25 | 20 | 30 | | 25 | 15 | 15 | 25 | 10 | 20 | |
| 16th day post-op. | | | 10 | 5 | 5 | 0 | 5 | 25 | | 5 | 0 | 5 | 5 | 5 | 10 | |
| | | | | | | | | | | | | | | | | |
| | | | | | | | | | | | | | | | | |
| | | | | | | | | | | | | | | | | |
| | | | | | | | | | | | | | | | | |

## BONE CONDUCTION

| | | | RIGHT | | | | | | LEFT | | | | | |
|------|------|------|------|-----|------|------|------|------|------|-----|------|------|------|------|
| DATE | Exam | LEFT MASK | 250 | 500 | 1000 | 2000 | 4000 | RIGHT MASK | 250 | 500 | 1000 | 2000 | 4000 | AUD |
| 7th day post-op. | | | 35 | 45 | 40 | 40 | 50 | | 35 | 40 | 35 | 45 | 55 | |
| 9th day post-op. | | | 10 | 10 | 15 | 15 | 20 | | 10 | 15 | 15 | 10 | 15 | |
| 16th day post-op. | | | 0 | 0 | 0 | 0 | 5 | | 5 | 0 | 5 | 0 | 0 | |

## SPEECH RECEPTION

| DATE | RIGHT | LEFT MASK | LEFT | RIGHT MASK | FREE FIELD | MIC. |
|------|-------|-----------|------|------------|------------|------|
| | | | | | | |

## DISCRIMINATION

| DATE | % SCORE | TEST LEVEL | LIST | LEFT MASK | % SCORE | TEST LEVEL | LIST | RIGHT MASK | EXAM |
|------|---------|------------|------|-----------|---------|------------|------|------------|------|
| | | | | | | | | | |

## HIGH FREQUENCY THRESHOLDS

| | | RIGHT | | | | | | | LEFT | | | | |
|------|------|------|-------|-------|-------|-----------|------------|------|------|-------|-------|-------|
| DATE | 4000 | 8000 | 10000 | 12000 | 14000 | LEFT MASK | RIGHT MASK | 4000 | 8000 | 10000 | 12000 | 14000 |
| | | | | | | | | | | | | |

| RIGHT | | WEBER | | LEFT | | HEARING AID | | | |
|-------|-----------|-------|-------|-----------|-----------|-------------|---------|-------|------|
| RINNE | SCHWABACH | | | RINNE | SCHWABACH | DATE | MAKE | | MODEL |
| | | | | | | RECEIVER | GAIN | | EXAM |
| | | | | | | EAR | DISCRIM. | | COUNC |

REMARKS

Figure 10.4 A 28-year-old woman had undergone a tonsillectomy. During the first 6 days following surgery, she took 200 tablets of aspirin for what she called "terrific pains." On the seventh postoperative day, she complained of hearing loss, recurrent tinnitus, and a recurrent sensation of unsteadiness. Examination showed normal eardrums. Audiometric studies indicated bilateral, symmetrical, severe hearing loss by both air conduction and bone conduction and evidence of recruitment. The aspirin was stopped, and the hearing showed considerable improvement 2 days later. The patient was aware of the improved hearing, and the tinnitus ceased altogether. Vestibular tests performed the same day showed no evidence of vestibular disturbance. Audiometric studies revealed normal hearing 9 days after the first hearing test. (From Walters [7].)

## CHARACTERISTIC AUDIOMETRIC PATTERNS

The audiogram considered to be the classic example of SNHL is the high-frequency loss shown in **Figure 10.3**. An audiogram of this shape has come to be called a "nerve-type audiogram" because it is found so often in presbycusis.

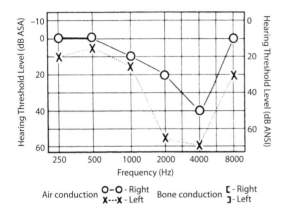

Air conduction  O-O - Right  Bone conduction  [ - Right
X---X - Left  ] - Left

Figure 10.5 Exposure to small arms gunfire. Complete recruitment present at 2000 Hz.

| R | L |
|---|---|
| 60 | 70 |
| 80 | 80 |

*Classification:* Sensorineural. *Diagnosis:* Repeated acoustic trauma. *Abbreviations:* ANSI, American National Standards Institute; ASA, American Standards Association.

Another audiometric pattern characteristic of sensorineural hearing impairment is the high-frequency dip shown in **Figure 10.5**. This is caused frequently by exposure to intense noise, particularly rifle fire. Initially, this type of loss is sensory rather than sensorineural. Then, as the damage grows more extensive, and the supporting cells and nerve fibers become affected by various factors, the classification becomes sensorineural, but the classic subjective symptoms of SNHL are not so well defined. The same explanation applies to still other audiometric patterns found in sensorineural loss. For instance, **Figure 10.6** shows an audiogram of SNHL associated with otosclerosis.

Although these patterns, especially the first, are highly suggestive of damage in the sensorineural mechanism, it must be remembered that other possibilities exist. For instance, an audiometric pattern similar to that shown in **Figure 10.3** can be obtained after merely dropping oil into an ear canal, and this scarcely affects the sensorineural mechanism. The ascending curve and the flat audiogram certainly are more common in conductive hearing loss. This phenomenon demonstrates that a diagnosis cannot be made reliably solely on the basis of the air conduction audiogram.

The paramount audiometric characteristic of SNHL is that the bone conduction curve is not normal and usually assumes the same shape and level as the air conduction curve. The Békésy audiograms show no singular features. Continuous and interrupted Békésy tracings usually reveal little or no separation. Neither marked recruitment nor abnormal tone decay is present.

## DIFFERENTIATING SENSORY HEARING LOSS FROM NEURAL HEARING LOSS

Until recently, when bone conduction was found to be reduced, a case could be classified only as sensorineural or, as it was more commonly called, perceptive or nerve deafness. With the development of improved tests based on a clearer understanding of auditory pathology, it is now possible in some cases to determine whether the damage is primarily in the sensory or in the neural mechanism. The designations "sensory" and "neural" have become more meaningful as knowledge of ear pathology has improved. The distinction is not possible in every case because many patients actually have damage both in the inner ear and in the nerve and thus have a sensorineural loss. In some patients, the hearing loss has its origin in the inner ear and satisfies all the criteria for sensory hearing loss, but later the damage extends to the nerve, and the classification then becomes sensorineural. Certain criteria, when available, are helpful in differentiating between sensory and neural types. These include recruitment, abnormal tone decay, and discrimination. If a patient demonstrates marked recruitment and diplacusis, the site of his auditory damage is most likely in the inner ear, and the hearing loss is classified as sensory. Patients with nerve deafness rarely have this marked degree of recruitment. If a patient demonstrates clear-cut evidence of abnormal tone decay, the damage is in the fibers of the auditory nerve, and the classification then is neural hearing loss. Cases of sensory hearing loss usually do not show abnormal tone decay. This does not necessarily mean that every case of sensory hearing loss must show marked recruitment, but when these phenomena are present, they are highly suggestive. Except for Ménière's syndrome, labyrinthitis, and a few other conditions, low discrimination scores are more indicative of damage to the nerve rather than the inner ear, especially the outer hair cells.

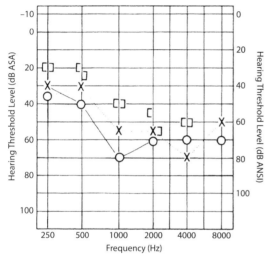

Figure 10.6 *History*: A 37-year-old man with insidious hearing loss for 10 years. No tinnitus or vertigo. A brother and a sister had successful stapes surgery. The patient uses hearing aid successfully. *Otologic*: Normal. *Audiologic*: Bilateral mixed hearing loss. Hears tuning fork only by teeth. *Classification*: Sensorineural hearing loss. *Diagnosis*: Otosclerosis with sensorineural involvement. *Abbreviations*: ANSI, American National Standards Institute; ASA, American Standards Association.

The availability of these criteria is limited. Recruitment tends to disappear when neural factors complicate sensory hearing loss. Abnormal tone decay can be elicited only when damage to the nerve fibers is only partial, whereas it cannot be elicited in those cases in which nerve fibers have presumably lost all function, as in congenital nerve deafness and most cases of advanced presbycusis.

The tests used to establish the presence of recruitment and abnormal tone decay are described in Chapter 7. One testing procedure of increasing importance is continuous- and fixed-frequency audiometry, which was done traditionally with a Békésy-type audiometer. This instrument is rather expensive and at present is used very little even in large hearing centers. However, other instruments are available now to provide similar information. For this reason, the emphasis in this book is on the results of the tests and their interpretation rather than the details of technique.

## SENSORY HEARING LOSS

The classification of sensory hearing loss includes all cases in which, according to the best information available, the damage to the auditory pathway is in the inner ear. The damage usually is in the hair cells and sometimes in labyrinthine fluid systems.

## CHARACTERISTIC FEATURES OF SENSORY HEARING LOSS

1. Some patients give a history of recurrent attacks of labyrinthine vertigo associated with fullness in the ear, ocean-roaring tinnitus, and intermittent hearing loss. This history is highly suggestive of the syndrome variously called Ménière's syndrome or disease, cochlear hypertension, labyrinthosis, or labyrinthine hydrops.
2. In Ménière's syndrome, the hearing loss is more likely to be unilateral.
3. In Ménière's syndrome, if tinnitus is present, usually it is described as roaring; it may be likened to the sound of a seashell held against the ear. In cases of hearing loss caused by exposure to loud noises, the tinnitus is said to sound like a high-pitched ring. Occasionally, the history will reveal exposure to intense noise accompanied by ringing tinnitus.
4. In Ménière's syndrome, there may be a reduction in the threshold of hearing during an attack and a return of hearing when the attack has subsided. The hearing loss eventually becomes permanent.
5. The patient's voice usually is of normal loudness.
6. The otologic examination is normal.
7. There is a hearing loss by air conduction.
8. There is a hearing loss by bone conduction.
9. There is no air–bone gap.
10. If the hearing loss is moderate or marked in the speech frequencies, speech discrimination is reduced.

11. Frequently, discrimination gets worse when the patient is addressed in a loud voice.
12. Marked recruitment is present; it may be continuous and complete, and occasionally there even may be hyperrecruitment.
13. Diplacusis is present.
14. The threshold of discomfort for loud sounds is lowered.
15. There is no abnormal tone decay or stapedius reflex decay.
16. With some exceptions, the tuning fork lateralizes to the ear that has better hearing when struck softly. When struck forcefully, the tuning fork may lateralize to the bad ear because of recruitment.
17. There is a type II Békésy tracing.

The reasons for some of these distinguishing features will be described briefly because almost all are discussed in the chapter on hearing testing (see Chapters 5, 6, 7, and 8).

The history is helpful because it is distinctive in two notable causes of sensory hearing loss: noise-induced hearing loss and Ménière's disease. The patient with noise-induced hearing loss generally will volunteer the information that the hearing loss and ringing tinnitus started after exposure to gunfire, exploding firecrackers, or industrial noise. In Ménière's disease, the hearing impairment usually will be unilateral and accompanied by ocean-roaring, or seashell, tinnitus and a feeling of fullness in the ear. Vertigo may or may not be a feature, and this as well as the hearing loss will be intermittent at first, though later it may become persistent. Many patients with Ménière's disease, even when it is unilateral, will not say that they do not hear, but they will complain that they are unable to distinguish the exact words they hear. *Bath* sounds like *path* and *bomb* like *palm*. This indicates a reduction in discrimination. Along with this, they will say that speech and sounds are distorted and irritating, especially if loud. A baby's cry may sound unbearably loud. (This indicates a lowered threshold of discomfort due to recruitment, although hyperacusis may produce a similar complaint.)

According to most authorities on Ménière's disease, this disorder is characterized by a pathological change in the endolymph, which then affects the hair cells. This causes damage which at first is temporary and reversible but later results in permanent damage inside the cochlea, and, ultimately,

degeneration of the auditory nerve fibers takes place, making the result a SNHL.

If both ears have been involved markedly for many years, the patient's voice then becomes loud because bone conduction is affected. However, it usually is not as loud as in some cases of long-standing neural deafness because many sensory hearing losses are unilateral.

There is no air–bone gap because the bone conduction hearing level usually is about the same as the air conduction hearing level. In Ménière's disease, the patient's ability to distinguish or to discriminate between words that sound somewhat alike often gets worse instead of better when the voice is raised. Much of this is caused by recruitment and increased distortion with higher intensities. The otologic findings are normal because the damage is restricted to the inner ear.

The comment regarding lateralization with a tuning fork is of special interest. If the tuning fork is struck gently and held to the forehead or the teeth in a case of unilateral sensory hearing loss, it will sound louder in the normal ear. However, if marked recruitment is present in the bad ear, and the tuning fork is struck hard, there is a good chance the tone will sound even louder in the bad ear than in the normal ear. For this reason, testing for lateralization in cases of unilateral hearing loss should be performed with deliberate control of the sound intensity of the tuning fork while caution is observed in technique and interpretation of results.

Distortion is an outstanding feature of sensory hearing loss. Pure tones, such as those produced by a tuning fork or a piano, sound raspy and of different pitch in the bad ear than in the unaffected ear—hence the phenomenon of diplacusis. This sensory distortion affects not only pure sounds but also voices and noises generally, and it represents a source of much irritation, frustration, and emotional strain to the patient, a problem insufficiently understood by many physicians.

Patients with bilateral sensory hearing loss are less able to use hearing aids in a satisfactory manner. The amplification provided by the aid may add to speech distortion and thus makes voices even less intelligible, especially in noisy areas.

The prognosis for sensory hearing impairment is better than it is for the neural type but not nearly as favorable as for conductive hearing loss.

In the early stages, many cases of sensory hearing loss seem to be reversible. For example, there are recurrent intermittent attacks of hearing loss with Ménière's disease alternating with periods of better hearing. There is, however, a great need for more facts and information concerning this point.

## AUDIOMETRIC PATTERNS IN SENSORY HEARING LOSS

As in conductive hearing loss, the shape of the air conduction audiogram in sensory impairment depends to a great extent on the cause and the pathology. However, two audiometric patterns are typically associated with the two common causes of sensory hearing loss.

**Figure 10.7** shows the audiometric pattern found in a classic early case of Ménière's disease. This is described as an ascending air conduction hearing level with a reduced bone conduction hearing level. During the loudness balance test, the patient reported that the tone in the left ear was not as clear as the tone in the good ear and there was pitch distortion and was confirmed with a tuning fork This is diplacusis and is an important symptom in inner ear pathology. The patient also had a lowered threshold of discomfort. There was no abnormal tone decay. This patient presented almost all the symptoms classically associated with sensory hearing loss secondary to Ménière's disease.

| 1000 Hz | |
|---|---|
| R | L |
| 0 | 40 |
| 10 | 45 |
| 20 | 50 |
| 30 | 35 |
| 40 | 55 |
| 50 | 60 |
| 60 | 65 |
| 70 | 70 |

During the loudness balance test, the patient reported that the tone in the left ear was not as clear as the tone in the good ear. This is diplacusis and is an important symptom in inner ear pathology. The patient also has a lowered threshold of discomfort. There was no abnormal tone decay. *Impedance Audiometry*: Normal tympanogram. Stapedius reflex would show Metz recruitment. *Diagnosis*: Ménière's disease. *Abbreviations*: ANSI, American National Standards Institute; ASA, American Standards Association.

| 1000 Hz | |
|---|---|
| L | R |
| −5 | 45 |
| 10 | 40 |
| 25 | 45 |
| 40 | 50 |
| 55 | 65 |
| 70 | 80 |
| 85 | 90 |
| 4000 Hz | |
| L | R |
| 10 | 45 |
| 25 | 45 |
| 40 | 55 |
| 55 | 60 |
| 70 | 65 |

Another example of alternate loudness balance testing for recruitment. *Interpretation*: The columns of figures indicate that, on pure-tone threshold testing, the left ear at 1000 Hz had a threshold of −5 dB, and the right ear had a threshold of 45 dB. When subsequently the intensity of the tone presented to the left ear was raised, and the patient was asked to match the loudness of the tone in the right ear with that in the left, it was noticed that the threshold difference tended to disappear. At 85 dB for the tone in the left ear, the intensity required to produce equal loudness in the right ear was 90 dB. Thus, the threshold difference, which was 50 dB, compares with a difference of only 5 dB when the tone intensity was increased to 85 dB (left) and 90 dB (right), respectively. This is a measure of recruitment. If the tone loudness in the two ears matched exactly at the same intensity, this condition would be called *complete recruitment*. If the tone sounded even louder in the bad ear than in the good ear at the same intensity, it would be called *hyperrecruitment*.

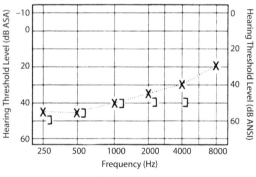

Air conduction O–O - Right  X···X - Left      Bone conduction Ⅽ - Right  ⅃ - Left

Figure 10.7 *History:* A 37-year-old man with recurrent sudden attacks of rotary vertigo accompanied by nausea, vomiting, and an ocean-roar tinnitus in the left ear. Between attacks the patient reports fullness and hearing loss, aggravated during attacks. The patient is annoyed by loud noise in the left ear, and voices sound fuzzy and unclear. *Otologic:* Normal. *Audiologic:* Moderate hearing loss with no air–bone gap. *Left ear discrimination:* 60%. Binaural loudness balance studies show complete recruitment in the left ear.

Another characteristic type of audiogram found in sensory hearing loss is shown in **Figure 10.8**. This is sometimes described as a C-5 dip, and in this instance, the cause was exposure to intense noise. It is the serial audiogram of a man who was exposed to extensive small-arms gunfire, with the result that he suffered a permanent high-frequency loss. It is appropriate to point out that the term "C-5 dip" is not very satisfactory. It is commonly designated this way because of the way audiograms are done. If the tests were to be made at several hundred Hertz on either side of 4000 Hz, the so-called C-5, the chances are that the dip would be found there as well. When testing is done with continuous-frequency audiometry, the dips can occur at 3000 Hz, at 5000 or 6000 Hz, or anywhere in between, without involving 4000 Hz. Consequently, the term "C-5 dip" should be replaced by the term "high-frequency dip," which really means that the hearing is relatively normal on either side of a sharp depression in the hearing level.

Although the range of frequencies involved in this high-frequency dip is comparatively small, recruitment studies often show complete and continuous recruitment. However, no significant reduction in speech discrimination is detectable with presently available tests. This is so because speech frequencies have not become involved. A high-frequency dip is not the only type of threshold shift that can be produced in the early stages of noise exposure, nor is noise the only etiology of dips in the hearing level, as discussed in Chapter 17.

Obviously, in sensory as in conductive hearing loss and, as will be noted, in neural hearing loss as well, certain characteristic patterns apparently are associated with each; this does not mean that other patterns do not occur or that one may not find a so-called characteristic pattern associated with nonclassical types of hearing loss.

## The basic audiologic features

In making a classification of sensory hearing loss, it is necessary to look for: (a) reduced threshold of hearing by air conduction and bone conduction, (b) the absence of any air–bone gap, (c) recruitment, (d) reduced discrimination if the speech frequencies are involved and still further reduction as the intensity of speech is increased, (e) lateralization of the sound of the tuning fork to the ear that hears better (with some exceptions), and (f) an absence of pathological adaptation. When these features are present along with a corroborating history and otologic examination, a case can be classified accurately as sensory hearing loss.

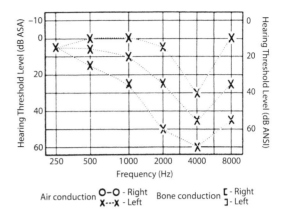

Air conduction O–O - Right  X---X - Left   Bone conduction [ - Right  ] - Left

Figure 10.8 Classic audiometric curves showing progressive hearing loss caused by extensive repeated exposure to gunfire. The hearing loss can continue beyond that shown in the upper threshold curve if the exposure continues and if the noise is very intense, as indicated in the two lower threshold curves. *Abbreviations*: ANSI, American National Standards Institute; ASA, American Standards Association.

## NEURAL HEARING LOSS

When hearing impairment results from damage to the fibers of the auditory nerve *per se*, the hearing loss is classified as a nerve or neural type of hearing loss.

## CHARACTERISTIC FEATURES OF NEURAL HEARING LOSS

Certain features are characteristic of neural hearing loss.

1. The history is variable. The deafness may be sudden in onset and practically complete in one ear, as may occur in fracture of the skull involving the internal auditory meatus, or it may be gradual and bilateral, as in progressive hereditary nerve deafness. It may follow many other patterns as well. A history of familial deafness often is helpful, but it should be borne in mind that a family history of hearing loss also is to be expected in otosclerosis. The patient's age is of little help because nerve deafness may occur in any age group. Vertigo is an important symptom.

If it is present, especially in the presence of a unilateral sensory hearing loss, its cause must be established: At least the presence of an acoustic nerve tumor (acoustic neuroma) must be ruled out. Tinnitus does not aid the differential diagnosis of nerve deafness *per se*, but if present, it is likely to be high-pitched.

2. Both air conduction and bone conduction are reduced.
3. There is no air–bone gap.
4. If the hearing loss is unilateral or more severe in one ear than in the other, the vibrating tuning fork is lateralized to the better-hearing ear.
5. Recruitment usually is absent, but if it is present, it is minimal and not complete.
6. There generally is a striking disparity between the hearing threshold level and the patient's ability to discriminate speech.
7. Abnormal tone decay is present except in cases of congenital nerve deafness and presbycusis. If this feature can be elicited, it localizes the damage to the auditory nerve fibers, and this is of great diagnostic value.

8. Stapedius reflex may be absent, or decay may be present.
9. Békésy audiometry in the presence of abnormal tone decay generally shows a separation between the continuous-tone and interrupted-tone tracings, and the continuous-tone tracings are of small amplitude (type III or IV).

The basic causes underlying some of these criteria have been traced by a study of proven cases of auditory nerve tumors. Of paramount importance is the finding of abnormal tone decay as has been recognized for many years (8). This phenomenon strongly suggests acoustic neuroma. Any injury that causes what one might call "partial damage" to the auditory nerve is likely to produce abnormal tone decay. A classic example is shown in **Figure 10.9**. Here, after the nerve was damaged by direct injection, all features of nerve damage were evident. It is notable also that temporary damage to the auditory nerve can occur; recovery from nerve damage is in fact not uncommon.

**HEARING RECORD**

NAME                                                                                      AGE

**AIR CONDUCTION**

| DATE | Exam. | LEFT MASK | RIGHT 250 | 500 | 1000 | 2000 | 4000 | 8000 | RIGHT MASK | LEFT 250 | 500 | 1000 | 2000 | 4000 | 8000 | AUD |
|------|-------|-----------|-----------|-----|------|------|------|------|------------|----------|-----|------|------|------|------|-----|
| 1st test | | | 15 | 10 | 0 | 0 | 20 | 15 | | | | | | | | |
| 17 days | | 85 | 90 | 95 | NR | NR | NR | NR | After injury to 8th nerve | | | | | | | |
| 1 yr. | | 95 | 65 | 50 | 40 | 30 | 30 | NR | | | | | | | | |
| | | | | | | | | | | | | | | | | |
| | | | | | | | | | | | | | | | | |
| | | | | | | | | | | | | | | | | |
| | | | | | | | | | | | | | | | | |
| | | | | | | | | | | | | | | | | |

**BONE CONDUCTION**

| DATE | Exam. | LEFT MASK | RIGHT 250 | 500 | 1000 | 2000 | 4000 | | RIGHT MASK | LEFT 250 | 500 | 1000 | 2000 | 4000 | | AUD |
|------|-------|-----------|-----------|-----|------|------|------|--|------------|----------|-----|------|------|------|--|-----|
| 1st test | | | 20 | 15 | 0 | 15 | 15 | | | | | | | | | |
| 17 days | | 85 | NR | NR | NR | NR | NR | | After injury to 8th nerve | | | | | | | |

Figure 10.9 *History:* A 43-year-old woman with recurrent attacks of severe pain in the right side of the face for years. No other complaints. Hearing was normal. *Otologic:* Normal. *Audiologic:* Normal hearing. After accidental surgical injection of the eighth nerve with boiling water for relief of the facial pain, there was near-total deafness, facial palsy, and absence of caloric response due to direct injury to the eighth nerve. *Classification:* Nerve deafness. *Diagnosis:* Injury to auditory nerve. Severe hearing loss persisted for several months, and then hearing gradually returned and showed no recruitment but marked tone decay in all frequencies. Return of hearing after such a severe injury and hearing loss is remarkable. (Modified from Harbert and Young [8].)

Another example of the reversibility of nerve damage is auditory fatigue or temporary threshold shift (TTS). It is generally assumed that TTS, like permanent threshold shift (PTS), results from damage to the hair cells of the inner ear. Although there is extensive proof that this is true for PTS, there is no conclusive evidence that it is true for TTS. Animal experiments have demonstrated that hair cells do not fatigue readily, and experiments with humans seem to indicate that TTS may be a reversible neural type of hearing loss.

## Comment on criteria

The onset of neural hearing loss is very variable. It may occur slowly, as in a typical case of acoustic neuroma, or suddenly, as is seen after herpes virus reactivation.

From what little is known about tinnitus, one would expect it to be an important feature accompanying neural hearing loss, but this is not borne out in practice. Many patients with acoustic neuromas complain little, or not at all, of noise in their ears. Even elderly patients who give evidence of a marked neural type of hearing loss do not complain of tinnitus very often. This is in contrast to patients having SNHL, who sometimes complain bitterly of hissing or ringing tinnitus.

The reduced bone conduction in nerve deafness is particularly marked. The vibrating tuning fork might not be heard even when struck very hard. This is especially true in older patients. The fork would be expected to lateralize to the ear that has better hearing.

One of the earliest findings in auditory nerve damage caused by pressure from a neoplasm is disturbance of the vestibular pathways. Although there may be no subjective vertigo, vestibular studies often show abnormal findings; such studies should be considered routinely in all cases of unilateral SNHL, especially when marked recruitment is absent.

Another singular feature in nerve deafness is the great discrepancy often found between a hearing threshold level and the patient's ability to discriminate. **Figure 10.10** illustrates an excellent example of a patient with a comparatively good hearing level but a disproportionately poor discrimination score. At surgery, an acoustic neuroma was removed. The reason for the good hearing threshold level despite so much auditory nerve damage must be borne in mind: almost three-quarters of the auditory nerve can be severed before the threshold for pure tones is affected markedly. The discrimination score and the patient's ability to understand what is heard, however, are affected by auditory nerve damage even when the hearing thresholds are not. It seems that the neural patterns carrying information to the auditory cortex are disturbed by the nerve damage so that the patient has great difficulty in understanding what is said. This problem is aggravated further by anything that interferes with understanding, such as ambient noise, distortion, and distraction.

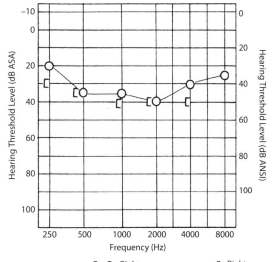

Figure 10.10 *History:* A 40-year-old woman with occasional imbalance and feeling of fatigue. She did not have tinnitus or rotary vertigo. She had noted progressive hearing loss in right ear for 2 years. *Otologic:* Normal. Vestibular studies showed no response in the right ear and perverted response of the vertical canals on the left side. *Audiologic:* Békésy audiometry-wide separation between pulsed- and continuous-tone tracings and small amplitude of continuous-tone tracings. No recruitment but marked tone decay. Moderate pure-tone loss with no air–bone gap. Right-ear discrimination was 42%. Left ear masked during all testing of right ear. *Classification:* Neural. Damage in auditory nerve fibers. *Etiology:* Right acoustic neuroma, removed at surgery. *Abbreviations:* ANSI, American National Standards Institute; ASA, American Standards Association.

As a rule, recruitment is not present in nerve damage, but it may be found occasionally, probably when there is also some cochlear damage not recognizable by available testing methods.

## AUDIOMETRIC PATTERNS IN NERVE DEAFNESS

It is difficult to describe definite characteristic patterns associated with pure nerve deafness, except for a cause such as acoustic neuroma. When actual nerve deafness develops in presbycusis, this often is preceded by degeneration in the inner ear, causing the typical high-frequency loss. This makes it difficult to determine precisely what the nerve deafness alone would cause. For our purposes, we can assume that the typical picture of nerve deafness is that of high-frequency hearing loss.

However, it is important to keep in mind that other types of audiometric patterns besides these two are possible in nerve deafness. For example, **Figure 10.11** shows an ascending type of nerve deafness in a very elderly patient. The cause was never established with certainty, but the findings were highly suggestive of nerve deafness.

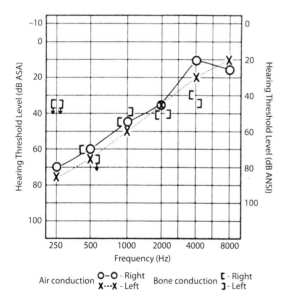

Figure 10.11 *History:* A 74-year-old woman with insidious hearing loss for 30 years. No tinnitus or vertigo. Soft speaking voice. *Otologic:* None. *Audiologic:* Moderate-to-severe loss in the low frequencies. No air–bone gap. *Discrimination score:* Right, 82%; left, 78%. *Classification:* Neural hearing loss. *Diagnosis:* Unknown. *Abbreviations:* ANSI, American National Standards Institute; ASA, American Standards Association.

## CAUSES OF SENSORINEURAL HEARING LOSS

The clinical pictures and causes of SNHL are numerous and varied. Different causes often produce the same clinical profile, and a single cause may produce a variety of clinical pictures. In some cases of SNHL, the cause is speculative or completely unknown. To complicate the problem further, physicians now are beginning to realize that in some patients with histories and audiologic findings highly suggestive of peripheral sensorineural impairment, the temporal bone findings at autopsy do not account for the hearing loss on the basis of any visible pathology.

To provide the reader with a comprehensive perspective of SNHL, we have included as many as possible of the characteristics of the conditions commonly encountered in practice. The cases are classified by causes and on the basis of whether the hearing loss is insidious, sudden, unilateral, bilateral, or congenital. However, patients are not always certain or able to give valid information about the onset of their deafness.

## CLASSIFICATION

### CAUSES OF SENSORINEURAL HEARING LOSS OF GRADUAL ONSET

1. Presbycusis
2. Occupational hearing loss
3. Sensorineural aspects of otosclerosis and chronic otitis media
4. Sensorineural aspects of Paget's and van der Hoeve's diseases
5. Effects of hearing aid amplification
6. Auditory nerve damage from chronic systemic diseases (diabetes, etc.)
7. Unknown causes

### CAUSES OF SUDDEN BILATERAL SENSORINEURAL HEARING LOSS

1. Meningitis
2. Infections
3. Functional hearing loss

4. Ototoxic drugs
5. Multiple sclerosis
6. Syphilis
7. Autoimmune diseases
8. Unknown causes

## CAUSES OF SUDDEN UNILATERAL SENSORINEURAL HEARING LOSS

1. Mumps
2. Head trauma and acoustic trauma
3. Ménière's disease
4. Viral infections
5. Rupture of round-window membrane or inner ear membrane
6. Vascular disorders
7. Following ear surgery
8. Fistula of oval window
9. Following general surgery and anesthesia
10. Syphilis
11. Some acoustic neuromas
12. Unknown causes

## CAUSES OF SENSORINEURAL CONGENITAL HEARING LOSS

1. Heredity
2. Rh incompatibility with kernicterus
3. Anoxia
4. Viruses
5. Unknown causes

## CAUSES OF SENSORINEURAL HEARING LOSS OF GRADUAL ONSET

## PRESBYCUSIS

The most common cause of SNHL is presbycusis, the gradual reduction in hearing with advancing age. The hearing loss takes place in a well-defined manner. It occurs gradually over a period of years, usually with the very highest frequencies affected first and the lower ones gradually following. Both ears are affected at about the same rate, but sometimes the loss in one ear may progress faster than the other. Whenever an older patient

is encountered who has a hearing loss much greater in one ear than in the other, a diagnosis of presbycusis should not be made without reservation, for it is likely that some other cause is also present.

## Development

The process of presbycusis starts quite early in life. Children can hear up to ~20,000 Hz. But many adults can hear only up to 14,000, 12,000, or 10,000 Hz. With advancing years, the ability to hear the higher frequencies becomes less acute, and by the age of 70, most people do not hear frequencies > 6000 Hz.

Because human beings make very little use of frequencies normally > 8000 Hz, they do not become aware of any loss in hearing until the frequencies < 8000 Hz are affected. These frequencies start to become affected typically around the age of 50. The rate at which presbycusis advances and the degree to which the individual becomes affected vary widely. To some extent, heredity plays a role, for early or premature presbycusis often is found in several members of the same family.

There is a form of early presbycusis in which the inner ear structures may be affected in such a manner that only the frequencies between 2000 and 6000 Hz become involved before there are any changes in the higher ranges. When this occurs, hearing loss does not progress to a marked degree before the higher frequencies also become involved. This audiometric picture closely resembles that of the hearing loss caused by intense noise exposure.

**A Typical Case and Average Values.** **Figure 10.12** shows the typical way presbycusis develops in one individual. This is a longitudinal study, as the same man has been examined for ~20 years. In most presbycusis cases in which 6000 and 8000 Hz are impaired, there is a greater loss in the higher frequencies, such as at 10,000 and 12,000 Hz. It is possible to find middle-aged people with marked presbycusis, whereas quite elderly people may be found who have very little hearing loss for pure-tone thresholds. Presbycusis should not be confused with hereditary progressive SNHL, which typically starts at a younger age and is more rapidly progressive.

JOSEPH SATALOFF, M.D.
ROBERT THAYER SATALOFF, M.D.
1721 PINE STREET     PHILADELPHIA, PA 19103

**HEARING RECORD**

NAME _____ AGE _____

## AIR CONDUCTION

| | | | RIGHT | | | | | | | | LEFT | | | | | |
|---|---|---|---|---|---|---|---|---|---|---|---|---|---|---|---|---|
| AGE | Exam | LEFT MASK | 250 | 500 | 1000 | 2000 | 4000 | 8000 | RIGHT MASK | 250 | 500 | 1000 | 2000 | 4000 | 8000 | AUD |
| 53 | | | 0 | 0 | 5 | 15 | 25 | 40 | | 0 | 0 | 0 | 10 | 20 | 35 | |
| 58 | | | 0 | 0 | 10 | 15 | 30 | 45 | | 0 | 0 | 5 | 10 | 25 | 40 | |
| 63 | | | 5 | 0 | 10 | 15 | 55 | 60 | | 0 | 0 | 10 | 15 | 40 | 55 | |
| 67 | | | 5 | 0 | 10 | 20 | 60 | 75 | | 5 | 0 | 10 | 20 | 55 | 65 | |
| 74 | | | 10 | 10 | 25 | 35 | 65 | 75 | | 10 | 5 | 15 | 30 | 65 | 70 | |

## BONE CONDUCTION

| | | | RIGHT | | | | | | | | LEFT | | | | |
|---|---|---|---|---|---|---|---|---|---|---|---|---|---|---|---|
| DATE | Exam | LEFT MASK | 250 | 500 | 1000 | 2000 | 4000 | | RIGHT MASK | 250 | 500 | 1000 | 2000 | 4000 | AUD |
| | | | | | | | | | | | | | | | |
| | | | | | | | | | | | | | | | |
| | | | | | | | | | | | | | | | |
| | | | | | | | | | | | | | | | |

## SPEECH RECEPTION

| DATE | RIGHT | LEFT MASK | LEFT | RIGHT MASK | FREE FIELD | MIC |
|---|---|---|---|---|---|---|
| | | | | | | |
| | | | | | | |
| | | | | | | |

## DISCRIMINATION

| | | RIGHT | | | | LEFT | | | |
|---|---|---|---|---|---|---|---|---|---|
| DATE | % SCORE | TEST LEVEL | LIST | LEFT MASK | % SCORE | TEST LEVEL | LIST | RIGHT MASK | EXAM |
| | | | | | | | | | |
| | | | | | | | | | |
| | | | | | | | | | |

## HIGH FREQUENCY THRESHOLDS

| | RIGHT | | | | | | | LEFT | | | | |
|---|---|---|---|---|---|---|---|---|---|---|---|---|
| DATE | 4000 | 8000 | 10000 | 12000 | 14000 | LEFT MASK | RIGHT MASK | 4000 | 8000 | 10000 | 12000 | 14000 |
| | | | | | | | | | | | | |
| | | | | | | | | | | | | |

| RIGHT | | WEBER | LEFT | | HEARING AID | | |
|---|---|---|---|---|---|---|---|
| RINNE | SCHWABACH | | RINNE | SCHWABACH | DATE | MAKE | MODEL |
| | | | | | RECEIVER | GAIN | EXAM |
| | | | | | EAR | DISCRIM | COUNC |

REMARKS

Figure 10.12 *History:* Routine audiograms were done on this patient while he was being treated for allergic nasal discomfort. At age 63, he started to complain of discrimination difficulty. No tinnitus or vertigo. *Otologic:* Ears clear. *Audiologic:* This is a longitudinal study of gradual progressive deafness due to aging. Important here are the comparatively small change in pure-tone thresholds at 500, 1000, and 2000 Hz between the ages of 63 and 74 and the dramatic change in discrimination ability during that same period.

| Discrimination score | | |
|---|---|---|
| Age 63 | Right 92% | Left 90% |
| Age 74 | Right 60% | Left 56% |

Bone conduction thresholds were at the same level as the air thresholds at all frequencies. *Classification:* Sensorineural hearing loss. *Diagnosis:* Presbycusis.

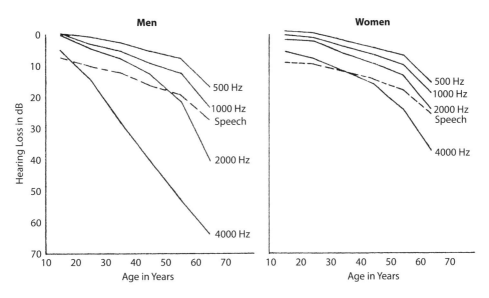

Figure 10.13  Average hearing loss by decades for men and women from age 10 to 70. Median loss in right ear and median loss in left ear were averaged. (Adapted from data collected by Research Center, Subcommittee on Noise in Industry, American Academy of Ophthalmology and Otolaryngology. Wisconsin State Fair Survey, 1954.)

**Figure 10.13** shows the average hearing loss in each frequency that can be expected with aging in the general population. These are average values to be used for statistical purposes; they do not necessarily hold for specific individuals.

## A COMPLEX PHENOMENON

Despite its simple definition and predictable development, presbycusis is a complex phenomenon. Even its classification is complicated. In the early stages of some cases of presbycusis, only the epithelial elements in the cochlea may be affected (sensory hearing loss); later, the nerve elements also are involved (sensorineural), and eventually, in the last decade of life, the cortex and the central pathways become involved, taking on the aspects of central hearing loss or central dysacusis. In still other cases of presbycusis, the nerve fibers seem to be damaged, making it chiefly neural hearing loss. In this way, a single etiology, presbycusis, can produce hearing loss that may fall into one of four different classifications. Schuknecht and Gacek's classification of presbycusis has shed light on this complex subject (9). **Sensory presbycusis** characteristically produces bilateral, symmetrical high-frequency hearing loss with an abruptly

sloping pattern. Discrimination depends upon the frequencies involved. The damage is primarily in the basal end of the cochlea, and sensory presbycusis appears to be genetically modulated. **Neural presbycusis** involves loss of neurons in all turns of the cochlea. It may begin early in life but does not usually become symptomatic until later in life. Normally, an ear contains ~37,000 neurons during the first decade of life, and only ~19,000 neurons in the ninth decade of life, losing ~2000 per year per decade. Discrimination correlates with the extent of neuron loss in the 15- to 22-mm region of the cochlea where the speech frequencies are represented. In neural presbycusis, loss of discrimination ability tends to be severe. Nerve loss is usually diffuse throughout the cochlear turns, and the audiometric pattern shows a gradually sloping loss involving all frequencies. **Strial presbycusis** is associated with atrophy of the stria vascularis causing a flat, pure-tone hearing loss, with good discrimination. The degree of strial atrophy correlates with the degree of hearing loss (10). **Cochlear conductive presbycusis** is associated with gradual, sloping high-frequency hearing loss that generally is noticed first during middle age. Discrimination depends upon the steepness of the audiometric pattern. The histologic correlate of cochlear conductive presbycusis has not been established with certainty, but Schuknecht and Gacek believed it is associated with thickening of the basilar membrane and stiffening of the cochlear partition that "are related to the physical-anatomic gradients that determine the resonance characteristics of the cochlear duct" (9).

The cause of presbycusis is also complex and not well understood. The simplest hypothesis is based on arteriosclerosis. However, this theory is not borne out by studies, most of which show no pertinent vascular changes in the ear to explain the clinical findings of sensorineural impairment. Still under debate are the factors that predispose to presbycusis or that produce the damage to the hearing mechanism. A study in Africa showed that elderly natives who had spent their lives in an atmosphere free of the everyday noises to which most human beings are exposed in modern society show little clinical evidence of presbycusis. This led a few investigators to propose that presbycusis may be the damage produced by exposure to the everyday noises of modern civilization, but there are many other incidental circumstances to be considered. Based on comparable physiological studies of the eyes, the skin, the brain, and so on, one would expect a natural wearing down of the hearing mechanism function with age. An interesting epidemiological study using the Framingham Heart Study Cohort looked at hearing loss in an elderly population trying to determine which variables had a significant impact upon hearing loss (11). Age was the most critical risk factor by far, although sex, illness, family history of hearing loss, Ménière's syndrome, and noise exposure were also significant population risk factors. Further study of this complex issue is needed.

## THE CLINICAL PICTURE

The sensorineural type of presbycusis is rather characteristic. The patient generally is >50 and usually >60 years of age. The major complaint is not difficulty in hearing but, rather, a gradual difficulty in understanding what has been said. At first, this happens only in noisy gatherings such as cocktail parties or when several people are speaking at the same time, particularly if the high-pitched voices of women are prominent.

As the loss continues to progress, the symptoms become more apparent. Now the patient may miss what is being said on the radio and television or at church or meetings. If the patient is a businessperson, there will be many difficult moments in cross-conversation, and generally he/she will have to ask with embarrassing frequency, "What did you say?" This difficulty may be even worse when the speaker talks softly, quickly, or has dentures that do not fit well. It is even more marked when the speaker has a foreign accent and poor enunciation. The audiogram by this same time shows that all the high frequencies have become affected, and the loss has extended into the speech range at 2000 Hz. The hearing threshold level at 2000 Hz usually has reached ~30 dB, and the higher frequencies are worse.

The patient's difficulty in understanding speech is like that in advanced cases of occupational hearing loss. The vowels are heard, but certain consonants that fall into the high-frequency range cannot be differentiated. For example, there is a problem in determining whether the speaker said, "yes," "yet," "jet," "get," or "guess." This inability to understand what is being said generally is mistaken for inattention or, in the case of an aging parent or a boss who is ready to retire, for "brain deterioration" or "signs of old age."

**Ways of Helping**. As a result of hearing difficulty, the senior citizen faces major psychological problems that demand better understanding from physicians and all people. Though physicians have no cure for presbycusis, this does not mean that we cannot help the patient who has discrimination difficulty. It reassures the elderly patient with presbycusis when we explain that the chief difficulty is not in the brain but merely in the hearing mechanism of the ears. The microphones are not working properly, and this is the reason that conversations at the dining-room table or in the living room are not clear.

If members of the patient's family can be made to understand this problem, they will obviate countless strained situations that breed insecurity, depression, and introversion in the senior citizen. Families deliberately should speak not-too-loudly, slowly, and clearly to parents or grandparents with handicapping degrees of presbycusis. Every effort should be made for the speaker and the listener to be in the same room so that the older person can see the face of the speaker. In this way, consonants that cannot be heard are seen on the lips, and conversation can be carried on much more readily and easily. It is difficult to adjust to the loneliness of old age after a successful career, and each family and physician must strive to help the senior citizen to communicate better.

If the loss in the speech frequencies is greater than ~35 dB, a hearing aid sometimes can be of considerable benefit to the elderly patient. Although the hearing aid does not improve the patient's discrimination, it helps the patient to hear with greater ease and less strain. Unfortunately, some elderly patients cannot adjust readily to using an aid and must be helped by repeated educational talks and reminders, in order to understand that their compliance is essential for improved communication.

**Tinnitus**. About 25% of healthy people > 65 have tinnitus. Occasionally, a patient will complain of ringing or hissing head noises, and sometimes these may even become a severe complaint. In the absence of specific therapy, symptomatic treatment may be necessary to reduce excessive reaction to head noises.

**Bone Conduction**. A common audiologic finding in presbycusis is inordinately poor bone conduction. The bone conduction threshold usually is much worse than the air conduction, and often the bone conduction cannot even be determined with a tuning fork or an audiometer. This does not necessarily mean that the patient's sensorineural mechanism is incapable of responding. It may mean that there is something in the skin or in the bone of the head that prevents the vibrating tuning fork or the audiometric oscillator from being heard. Frequently, if the tuning fork is placed on the patient's teeth or dentures, it will be heard more easily than when it is pressed against the skull. Bone conduction testing in older patients is a particularly poor indication of their sensorineural potential.

**The Eardrum**. In elderly patients, a change in the appearance of the eardrum is also seen often. The cause of SNHL must not be attributed to a thick, scarred, or white eardrum. This does not solve the difficulty and may lead the patient only to seek treatment of the eardrum while the real problem is disregarded.

**A Striking Feature**. A complaint of difficult hearing without a sufficient corresponding reduction in audiometric threshold is prominent in cases of presbycusis. Even the discrimination score sometimes is not reduced as much as the patient's complaints would lead one to expect. This is characteristic of elderly patients with presbycusis. In the central type of presbycusis and pure nerve damage, the results of tests are even more inconsistent with the patient's complaints. These patients may have a concurrent auditory processing problem as well.

## OCCUPATIONAL DEAFNESS

Exposure to hazardous noise in industry can result in hearing loss. For details, see Chapter 14.

## OTOSCLEROSIS (SENSORINEURAL SEQUELAE)

Otosclerosis is basically a disease of cochlear bone. When it reaches the oval window and the stapedial footplate, it can cause the classic clinical picture of conductive hearing loss known as clinical otosclerosis.

## BONE CONDUCTION

Unfortunately, the clinical findings are not always quite as classic or so simple. Many cases of otosclerosis, even in their incipient stage, do not have normal bone conduction. One feature of the reduced bone conduction associated with clinical otosclerosis is called the "Carhart notch." This is a 20- or 15-dB reduction in bone conduction at 2000 Hz. Its cause has been attributed to some defect in the transmission of sound conducted through bone at this frequency through the patient's skull because of the fixed footplate. When hearing is restored by surgery, the reduced bone conduction often improves to ~5 dB.

In most cases of otosclerosis in the authors' experience, bone conduction is rarely normal for all frequencies. Usually, there is some reduction in bone conduction at 2000 and 4000 Hz and even at some other frequencies. The frequent association of otosclerosis with reduced bone conduction has created a suspicion that there must be some relationship between the two. As yet, no experimental or valid clinical relationship has been established. Histopathological studies support this impression.

## SENSORINEURAL DAMAGE

There is little doubt that otosclerosis often leads to sensorineural damage. Cases of otosclerosis in which bone conduction and the sensorineural mechanism remain normal for years are in the minority. High-frequency hearing loss, associated with reduced bone conduction, and recruitment in the early stages are definite manifestations of this sensorineural damage. In many cases, the early perceptive effects seem to be only in the cochlea. However, in others the picture is one of SNHL associated with otosclerosis. In unilateral cases with sensorineural damage, it often is possible to demonstrate complete recruitment (**Figure 10.14**). Even the so-called Carhart notch may in some instances represent a sensorineural loss rather than a mechanical defect. This is especially true in cases in which the hearing and the bone conduction do not improve markedly after surgery or in which the improvement is only to 5 or 10 dB. The normal level for such an individual probably was −10 dB, and actually he/she has a 15-dB sensorineural hearing impairment in that frequency. Although there is impressive evidence that otosclerosis can cause SNHL, there still is no proof that surgical correction of otosclerosis prevents the development of sensorineural hearing impairment. A toxic effect on the sensory mechanism has been speculated but not proven, and sensorineural impairment seems to be associated with otosclerotic involvement of bone adjacent to the stria vascularis.

**Diagnostic Clues.** The onset of SNHL associated with otosclerosis generally is insidious. It may appear long after the conductive hearing loss has been recognized. Occasionally, otosclerosis and sensorineural impairment are diagnosed simultaneously (**Figure 10.15**). In a few such cases, the diagnosis of otosclerosis may seem to be far-fetched, but it is established at surgery, and hearing sometimes can be improved. The important clues in such cases are that bone conduction is present and better than air conduction (especially with the tuning fork in contact with the teeth), and there is reasonably good discrimination. The typical history of a soft voice is also helpful, particularly if the patient gets better results with a hearing aid than would be expected in a case of sensorineural loss. The fact that many cases of this type have been diagnosed successfully and operated on should in no way be misconstrued as encouragement for patients with sensorineural hearing impairment to demand middle ear surgery for possible otosclerosis. A diagnosis of otosclerosis must be made positively by hearing tests and history, not by surgical exploration, in nearly all cases.

**Surgical Complications.** So many patients with otosclerosis have had stapedectomies, and so many of these have had some postoperative high-frequency hearing loss and reduced bone conduction that it is

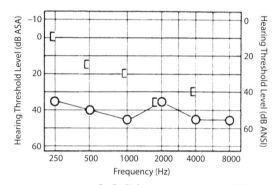

Air conduction O–O - Right / X---X - Left    Bone conduction [ - Right / ] - Left

Figure 10.14 *History:* A 22-year-old woman with right-ear hearing loss for 2 years. Occasional ringing tinnitus. No vertigo. *Otologic:* Normal. *Audiologic:* Left ear normal. Right-ear air conduction thresholds revealed a moderate and essentially flat loss. Bone thresholds were reduced, but an air–bone gap existed at all frequencies except 2000 Hz. The right ear had complete recruitment with diplacusis. There was no abnormal adaptation. Right-ear discrimination was 86%. Masking used in the left ear for all right-ear tests. *Classification:* Mixed hearing loss. *Diagnosis:* Unilateral otosclerosis with secondary sensorineural involvement. *Aids to diagnosis:* The presence of an air–bone gap, good discrimination, and negative otoscopic findings indicates middle ear damage, specifically, stapes fixation. The presence of recruitment, diplacusis, and reduced bone conduction indicates sensorineural involvement. Otosclerotic stapes fixation was confirmed at surgery and hearing improved postoperatively. *Abbreviations*: ANSI, American National Standards Institute; ASA, American Standards Association.

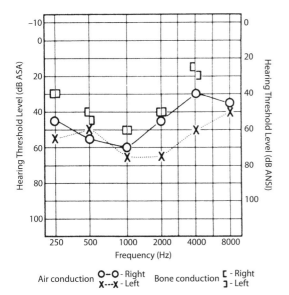

Air conduction O–O - Right / X---X - Left    Bone conduction Γ - Right / ] - Left

Figure 10.15 *History:* A 50-year-old woman who had a soft speaking voice and used a hearing aid in the left ear for insidious hearing loss occurring for several years. Initially, she had buzzing tinnitus, which gradually disappeared. Two sisters had hearing loss. No vertigo or ear infections. Patient says she is getting satisfactory results with her hearing aid. *Otologic:* Normal. *Audiologic:* Very little air–bone gap is present, but the patient hears better with the tuning fork on the teeth than by air conduction. Dental bone conduction is also better on the teeth than on the mastoid, where there is little or no response. *Discrimination score:* Right, 88%; left, 84%. *Classification:* Mixed hearing loss. *Diagnosis:* Otosclerosis associated with sensorineural hearing loss. *Aids to diagnosis:* Soft voice, satisfactory hearing aid usage, familial history of hearing loss, fairly good discrimination, and bone conduction better than air conduction by tuning fork all point to the possibility of initial conductive involvement. An exploration was done on the left middle ear, and the footplate was found to be markedly fixed, with otosclerosis in the oval window. Mobilization was achieved, and the patient said that she heard better. There was a 10-dB improvement at most frequencies postoperative. *Abbreviations:* ANSI, American National Standards Institute; ASA, American Standards Association.

now common to see cases like that in **Figure 10.16**. This patient probably had good bone conduction preoperatively and reduced bone conduction postoperatively. Seeing this patient for the first time

postoperatively, a physician may wonder why surgery was done in the first place, as there is little or no air–bone gap, and the diagnosis now is SNHL. The new examiner should always bear in mind that the bone conduction may not be the same now as it was preoperatively and may have been decreased by some complication. One such complication is a perilymph fistula or a leak of fluid between the inner ear and middle ear. This is particularly important because it may be repaired surgically. It is essential to recognize treatable and reversible causes of SNHL.

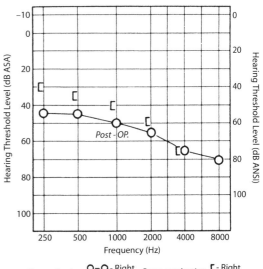

Air conduction O–O - Right / X---X - Left    Bone conduction Γ - Right / ] - Left

Figure 10.16 *History:* Patient had a right stapedectomy followed by vertigo, fullness, and tinnitus. The hearing worsened after surgery. There is a family history of otosclerosis. *Otologic:* Normal. *Audiologic:* Left ear normal. Right-ear air conduction thresholds are reduced moderately, as are the bone thresholds. Right-ear discrimination is 66%. There is complete recruitment with diplacusis. *Classification:* Mixed hearing loss. *Diagnosis:* Otosclerosis with postoperative labyrinthosis. *Aids to diagnosis:* Although this picture is highly suggestive of Ménière's disease, the history points to postoperative labyrinthosis as the etiology. *Abbreviations:* ANSI, American National Standards Institute; ASA, American Standards Association.

## CHRONIC OTITIS MEDIA

Ear infection may produce SNHL. The causal relationship is obvious when the hearing loss follows an acute infection that extends to the inner ear and/or auditory nerve. However, the relationship may be less apparent when associated with chronic ear disease. SNHL is a well-recognized concomitant of chronic otitis media, particularly in cases with recurrent otorrhea or cholesteatoma. Hearing loss is also not uncommon in the presence of tympanosclerosis involving the middle ear, another condition generally associated with chronic otitis media.

## PAGET'S AND VAN DER HOEVE'S DISEASES

Both Paget's and van der Hoeve's diseases can affect the auditory nerve pathway. In the early stages, usually only conductive hearing loss is produced, but as the disease progresses, the sensorineural mechanism becomes affected, often quite severely. The specific reason for this involvement is not completely clear, but generally there are degenerative processes in the inner ear and the nerve fibers. Sometimes the auditory nerve may be constricted by narrowing of the internal auditory meatus caused by Paget's disease. A toxic effect on the inner ear, such as that which probably exists in some cases of otosclerosis, also warrants consideration in Paget's and van der Hoeve's diseases. In some cases, the conductive and the sensorineural losses seem to start simultaneously and to progress in parallel. An interesting case is described in **Figure 10.17**. Note the characteristics of van der Hoeve's disease as a cause of hereditary deafness—blue sclera and fragile bones that sustain repeated fractures (see Chapter 13 and Appendix III).

## OTHER GENETIC AND SYSTEMIC CAUSES

Many other hereditary and nonhereditary conditions are associated with SNHL. Many of these are discussed in Chapter 13.

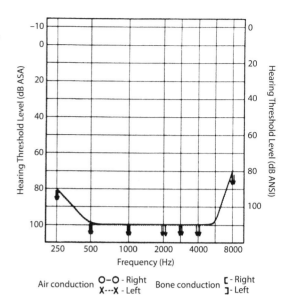

Air conduction O–O - Right, X---X - Left    Bone conduction ⊏ - Right, ⊐ - Left

Figure 10.17 *History:* A 70-year-old woman with hearing loss for >30 years. Wears a hearing aid in the right ear and seems to get along with some residual hearing. Other members of her family have long-term deafness. Both this patient and other members of the family have a history of having blue sclera and repeated fractures of the long bones. *Otologic:* Ears normal. *Audiologic:* No response to air conduction audiometry and only tactile response to bone conduction at the lower frequencies. *Classification:* Mixed hearing loss. *Diagnosis:* van der Hoeve's disease. *Aids to diagnosis:* Deafness, blue sclerae, fragile bones, and the hereditary features established the diagnosis. *Abbreviations:* ANSI, American National Standards Institute; ASA, American Standards Association.

## HEARING AID AMPLIFICATION

In a few cases, a person who has used a hearing aid has noted marked aggravation of hearing loss only in the aided ear. There seems to be no doubt about this causal relationship, but because only a few ultrasensitive ears are affected, advice against the use of hearing aids is unjustified. The hearing loss, usually associated with the use of a powerful hearing aid, is of a peculiar type. Ordinarily, in a typical picture there would be a temporary or even a permanent threshold changes as the result of amplification by the aid. This is not what we

JOSEPH SATALOFF, M.D.
ROBERT THAYER SATALOFF, M.D.
1721 PINE STREET     PHILADELPHIA, PA 19103

HEARING RECORD

NAME                                                                AGE

### AIR CONDUCTION

| DATE | Exam | LEFT MASK | RIGHT 250 | 500 | 1000 | 2000 | 4000 | 8000 | RIGHT MASK | LEFT 250 | 500 | 1000 | 2000 | 4000 | 8000 | AUD |
|---|---|---|---|---|---|---|---|---|---|---|---|---|---|---|---|---|
| 5/10/52 | | | 25 | 55 | 60 | 70 | 90 | AID | ON | 15 | 40 | 50 | 50 | 45 | | |
| 6/7/54 | | | | | | | | | | 70 | NR | NR | NR | NR | | |
| 6/21/54 | | | | | | | | AID | OFF | 50 | 70 | 85 | 85 | 75 | | RING. TIN. |
| 9/5/54 | | | | | | | | | | 30 | 55 | 60 | 55 | 50 | | |
| 10/2/54 | | | | | | | | AID | ON | 25 | 50 | 60 | 55 | 50 | | |
| 11/20/54 | | | | | | | | | | 60 | 85 | 95 | 85 | 70 | | |
| 12/4/54 | | | | | | | | AID | OFF | 30 | 50 | 60 | 60 | 50 | | |
| 4/2/55 | | | | | | | | AID | ON | 25 | 60 | 85 | 80 | 80 | | SUDDEN RING. |
| 4/8/55 | | | | | | | | AID | OFF | 15 | 50 | 60 | 60 | 50 | | PERSIST. |
| 9/4/56 | AID ON | | 25 | 50 | 65 | 70 | 85 | AID | ON | 55 | NR | NR | NR | NR | | RING. |
| 9/4/56 | ON | | | 50 | 65 | 70 | 85 | | | 60 | 90 | NR | NR | NR | | |
| 10/13/56 | | | 15 | 45 | 60 | 65 | 85 | AID | OFF | 20 | 50 | 60 | 70 | 60 | | |
| 1/20/57 | | | 20 | 45 | 65 | 70 | 90 | | | 25 | 45 | 65 | 70 | 70 | | |
| 4/6/57 | | | 15 | 40 | 60 | 75 | NR | AID | ON | 55 | NR | NR | NR | NR | | |
| 9/9/57 | | | 20 | 45 | 70 | 70 | NR | AID | OFF | NR | 45 | 40 | 75 | NR | | |

Figure 10.18 *History:* This boy was first seen at age 5 for a hearing loss that parents had noted since he was 3 years old. The child had a mild speech defect and had developed speech slowly. The diagnosis was congenital deafness of unknown origin. A hearing aid was placed on his left ear, and he did very well until he noted worse hearing in the left ear several years later. After numerous studies were done to rule out other causes, the hearing aid was removed, and his hearing improved. Each time the aid was used, the hearing got worse but then improved when the aid was removed. Finally, it was recommended that the aid be worn on the right ear, and the patient noted no adverse effect. *Diagnosis:* Sensorineural hearing loss caused by noise. *Note:* Even the low frequencies were affected in this case.

generally find, as is shown in the interesting case described in **Figure 10.18**. Although the hearing returned to its previous level after the hearing aid was removed, it took much longer to return than it would have taken in a TTS, and it did not have other classic characteristics of TTS.

Whenever a patient who uses a hearing aid complains that hearing is getting much worse in the aided ear, amplification should be suspected as a possible cause if the loss is sensorineural. In such instances, the hearing aid should be removed, and the hearing should be watched to see whether it returns to its original level. It may be necessary for the patient to use the aid in the other ear, and if this ear shows the same

sensitivity to amplification, a less powerful type of hearing aid might be indicated.

As in all cases of unilateral SNHL, the possibility of an acoustic neuroma always should be considered, and all necessary studies should be done.

## NEURITIS OF THE AUDITORY NERVE

Auditory neuritis is an inflammatory condition of the auditory division of the eighth cranial nerve. It causes hearing loss without dizziness, although tinnitus may be present. It is distinguished from vestibular neuritis which causes dizziness, without hearing loss. When hearing loss and balance disorders are involved in the presence of an inflammatory process, the diagnosis is usually either eighth nerve neuritis or labyrinthitis.

Auditory neuritis may follow systemic infections such as scarlet fever, influenza, typhoid fever, syphilis, and many other infectious diseases that produce high fevers. It is seen more frequently following less severe viral illnesses such as upper respiratory infections or herpetic infections such as those associated with cold sores or "fever blisters." The hearing loss may be noted immediately in conjunction with the infection, but the onset is often progressive over a period of days or weeks. It may be unilateral, or bilateral, but unilaterality or asymmetry is common. The condition often is associated with a feeling of fullness in the ear. In the early stages, hearing may improve following therapy with corticosteroids. Severity of the hearing loss varies from mild to profound. **Figure 10.19** shows the findings in a patient with a presumptive diagnosis of neuritis of the auditory nerve. **Figure 10.20** describes a case in which the diagnosis is more certain.

## VASCULAR INSUFFICIENCY

The labyrinthine artery which supplies the inner ear is a non-anastomotic end artery. That is, its branches do not intermingle with collateral vascular supply from other sources. Consequently, the inner ear appears to be more sensitive to vascular degeneration than most other organs. This problem is associated with generalized atherosclerosis, diabetes, and other conditions that alter blood flow to the ear. It may also occur without obvious systemic concomitants. More research is needed to clarify the process of hearing deterioration related to vascular degeneration.

## UNKNOWN CAUSES OF BILATERAL AND UNILATERAL SENSORINEURAL HEARING LOSS OF GRADUAL ONSET

There are cases of SNHL for which it is not possible to establish a specific cause. The accompanying series of examples, each of which emphasizes a different factor associated with the deafness,

JOSEPH SATALOFF, M.D.
ROBERT THAYER SATALOFF, M.D.
1721 PINE STREET     PHILADELPHIA, PA 19103

NAME J.F.

| DATE | RIGHT EAR AIR CONDUCTION | | | | | | | LEFT EAR AIR CONDUCTION | | | | | |
|---|---|---|---|---|---|---|---|---|---|---|---|---|---|
| | 250 | 500 | 1000 | 2000 | 4000 | 8000 | | 250 | 500 | 1000 | 2000 | 4000 | 8000 |
| | 45 | 80 | 80 | 85 | 90 | 70 | | 25 | 55 | 55 | 60 | 60 | 55 |
| | | | | | | | | | | | | | |
| | | | | | | | | | | | | | |

| RIGHT EAR BONE CONDUCTION | | | | | | | LEFT EAR BONE CONDUCTION | | | | | |
|---|---|---|---|---|---|---|---|---|---|---|---|---|
| 250 | 500 | 1000 | 2000 | 3000 | 4000 | | 250 | 500 | 1000 | 2000 | 3000 | 4000 |
| 35 | 60 | 75 | NR | NR | NR | | 25 | 40 | 35 | 55 | 55 | 55 |

SPEECH RECEPTION: Right 70 Left 35        DISCRIMINATION: Right 52% Left 80%

Figure 10.19 The findings in a patient with a presumptive diagnosis of neuritis of the auditory nerve.

**JOSEPH SATALOFF, M.D.**
**ROBERT THAYER SATALOFF, M.D.**
1721 PINE STREET   PHILADELPHIA, PA 19103

**HEARING RECORD**

NAME _____ AGE _____

**AIR CONDUCTION**

| | | | RIGHT | | | | | | | | LEFT | | | | | |
|---|---|---|---|---|---|---|---|---|---|---|---|---|---|---|---|---|
| DATE | Exam | LEFT MASK | 250 | 500 | 1000 | 2000 | 4000 | 8000 | RIGHT MASK | 250 | 500 | 1000 | 2000 | 4000 | 8000 | AUD |
| | | 95 | 30 | 35 | 40 | 40 | 55 | 60 | 95 | 40 | 50 | 55 | 60 | 65 | NR | |

**BONE CONDUCTION**

| | | | RIGHT | | | | | | LEFT | | | | | |
|---|---|---|---|---|---|---|---|---|---|---|---|---|---|---|
| DATE | Exam | LEFT MASK | 250 | 500 | 1000 | 2000 | 4000 | RIGHT MASK | 250 | 500 | 1000 | 2000 | 4000 | AUD |
| | | 95 | 25 | 30 | 40 | 40 | 50 | 85 | 35 | 45 | 50 | 50 | NR | |

**SPEECH RECEPTION**

| DATE | RIGHT | LEFT MASK | LEFT | RIGHT MASK | FREE FIELD | MIC |
|---|---|---|---|---|---|---|
| | 40 | 85 | 55 | 95 | 45 | |

**DISCRIMINATION**

| DATE | RIGHT %SCORE | TEST LEVEL | LIST | LEFT MASK | LEFT %SCORE | TEST LEVEL | LIST | RIGHT MASK | EXAM |
|---|---|---|---|---|---|---|---|---|---|
| | 65 | 70 | 4L | 85 | 52 | 85 | 4F | 95 | |

**HIGH FREQUENCY THRESHOLDS**

| | RIGHT | | | | | | | LEFT | | | | |
|---|---|---|---|---|---|---|---|---|---|---|---|---|
| DATE | 4000 | 8000 | 10000 | 12000 | 14000 | LEFT MASK | RIGHT MASK | 4000 | 8000 | 10000 | 12000 | 14000 |
| | 55 | 60 | NR | NR | NR | 85 | 95 | 65 | NR | NR | NR | NR |

| RIGHT | | WEBER | LEFT | | HEARING AID | | |
|---|---|---|---|---|---|---|---|
| RINNE | SCHWABACH | | RINNE | SCHWABACH | DATE | MAKE | MODEL |
| A>B | Poor | TO RIGHT | A>B | Poor | RECEIVER | GAIN | EXAM |
| | | | | | EAR | DISCRIM | COUNC |

REMARKS

Figure 10.20 *History:* A 55-year-old man with bilateral hearing loss following attack of flu during an epidemic. Loss has not progressed. No tinnitus or vertigo. *Otologic:* Normal. Caloric examination was normal. *Audiologic:* Bilateral hearing loss with no air–bone gap, reduced discrimination, and poor tuning fork responses. No recruitment or abnormal tone decay. *Classification:* Sensorineural hearing loss. *Diagnosis:* Neuritis of auditory nerve.

illustrates cases of this type (**Figures 10.21–10.23**). Vascular problems such as hypotension and hypertension are most prominent. In addition, Chapter 13 contains other examples of sensory and neural hearing loss. As has been pointed out, causes such as Ménière's disease, noise exposure, and occupational deafness may start as a sensory hearing impairment and later progress to sensorineural loss, especially in the presence of other superimposed conditions.

JOSEPH SATALOFF, M.D., D.Sc
ROBERT T. SATALOFF, M.D., D.M.A.
1721 PINE STREET • PHILADELPHIA, PA. 19103

**HEARING RECORD**

NAME _____ AGE _____

### AIR CONDUCTION

| DATE | Exam. | LEFT MASK | RIGHT 250 | 500 | 1000 | 2000 | 3000 | 4000 | 6000 | 8000 | RIGHT MASK | LEFT 250 | 500 | 1000 | 2000 | 3000 | 4000 | 6000 | 8000 | AUD |
|---|---|---|---|---|---|---|---|---|---|---|---|---|---|---|---|---|---|---|---|---|
| 1st test | | | 10 | 20 | 30 | 85 | | 90 | | NR | | 20 | 30 | 60 | 90 | | NR | | NR | |
| 4 years | | | 80 | 80 | 100 | NR | | NR | | NR | | 80 | 95 | 100 | NR | | NR | | NR | |
| 9 years | | | 75 | 85 | NR | NR | | NR | | NR | | NR | NR | NR | NR | | NR | | NR | |
| 10 years | | | 75 | NR | NR | NR | | NR | | NR | | NR | NR | NR | NR | | NR | | NR | |
| | | | | | | | | | | | | | | | | | | | | |
| | | | | | | | | | | | | | | | | | | | | |
| | | | | | | | | | | | | | | | | | | | | |
| | | | | | | | | | | | | | | | | | | | | |

### BONE CONDUCTION

| DATE | Exam | LEFT MASK | RIGHT 250 | 500 | 1000 | 2000 | 3000 | 4000 | RIGHT MASK | LEFT 250 | 500 | 1000 | 2000 | 3000 | 4000 | AUD |
|---|---|---|---|---|---|---|---|---|---|---|---|---|---|---|---|---|
| 1st test | | | 10 | 20 | 35 | NR | | NR | | 20 | 40 | NR | NR | | NR | |
| 9 years | | | NR | NR | NR | NR | | NR | | NR | NR | NR | NR | | NR | |
| | | | | | | | | | | | | | | | | |
| | | | | | | | | | | | | | | | | |
| | | | | | | | | | | | | | | | | |

### SPEECH RECEPTION THRESHOLD

| DATE | RIGHT | LEFT MASK | LEFT | RIGHT MASK | FREE FIELD | DATE | RIGHT | LEFT MASK | LEFT | RIGHT MASK | FREE FIELD |
|---|---|---|---|---|---|---|---|---|---|---|---|
| | | | | | | | | | | | |

### SPEECH DISCRIMINATION

| DATE | RIGHT % SCORE | TEST LEVEL | LIST | LEFT MASK | LEFT % SCORE | TEST LEVEL | LIST | RIGHT MASK | FREE FIELD | AIDED | EXAM |
|---|---|---|---|---|---|---|---|---|---|---|---|
| | | | | | | | | | | | |
| | | | | | | | | | | | |
| | | | | | | | | | | | |
| | | | | | | | | | | | |
| | | | | | | | | | | | |
| | | | | | | | | | | | |
| | | | | | | | | | | | |

COMMENTS:

Figure 10.21 *History:* Since the age of 18, this healthy 36-year-old man had known that he had a very mild high-frequency hearing loss. It was not progressing, and he participated in active military service. After the age of ~26 he became aware that his hearing was becoming worse, and despite extensive studies and a great variety of treatments, he continued to lose his hearing. No tinnitus or vertigo. There is no history of familial deafness. *Otologic:* Normal. Normal caloric responses. *Audiologic:* Rapid progressive bilateral hearing loss. *Classification:* Sensorineural hearing loss. *Diagnosis:* Unknown.

## CAUSES OF SUDDEN BILATERAL SENSORINEURAL HEARING LOSS

SNHL of sudden onset is of special interest to the otologist for at least two reasons. First, the cause is hard to establish, and second, it is not uncommon for the hearing to return. Certain causes more often affect both ears, whereas other causes affect only one ear. The severity of the hearing loss varies, but quite often it can be very profound. The common causes of sudden bilateral SNHL are as follows: (a) meningitis, (b) infections, (c) emotionally induced illness, (d) drugs, (e) multiple sclerosis, (f) autoimmune disease, (g) syphilis, and (h) unknown causes.

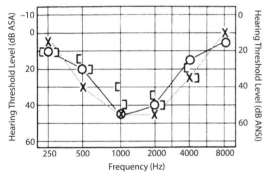

Air conduction O–O - Right X---X - Left   Bone conduction [ - Right ] - Left

Figure 10.22 *History:* A 50-year-old woman first noticed gradual hearing loss about a year ago and reports that it is progressing. She had not had ear infections or infectious diseases. No tinnitus or vertigo. No history of familial deafness. *Otologic:* Normal. *Audiologic:* Bilateral basin-shaped loss with no significant air–bone gap. Monaural two-frequency loudness balance tests indicate some recruitment in both ears. There was no abnormal tone decay. *Speech reception threshold:* Right, 38 dB; left, 42 dB. *Discrimination score:* Right, 100%; left, 94%. *Classification:* Sensorineural hearing loss. *Diagnosis:* Unknown. *Abbreviations:* ANSI, American National Standards Institute; ASA, American Standards Association.

## MENINGITIS

The sudden, profound irreversible bilateral deafness caused by meningitis makes this disease of great and singular concern to all physicians.

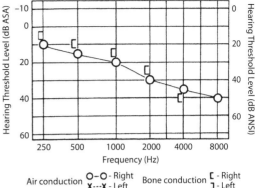

Air conduction O–O - Right X---X - Left   Bone conduction [ - Right ] - Left

Figure 10.23 *History:* A 45-year-old woman noted gradual onset of hearing loss in the left ear with slight ringing tinnitus. No vertigo. Blood pressure normal. *Otologic:* Normal. *Audiologic:* Left ear normal. Right ear had normal sloping to moderate hearing loss. No air–bone gap. No recruitment or abnormal tone decay. *Classification:* Unilateral sensorineural hearing loss, progressive. *Diagnosis:* No clear-cut cause for this progressive unilateral hearing loss. *Abbreviations:* ANSI, American National Standards Institute; ASA, American Standards Association.

**Figure 10.24** shows the typical, practically total loss of hearing that results when meningitis affects the sensorineural areas. Because the damage is irreversible, every effort must be exerted to prevent meningitis or to treat it vigorously and early to obviate such complications. Occasionally, a small amount of hearing remains, and a powerful hearing aid then is of some value. In these cases, the hearing aid will only assist in hearing sounds louder, not clearer or improving speech recognition. Tinnitus rarely is present, and rotary vertigo usually is of short duration.

Imbalance, particularly in a dark room, is common because of labyrinthine damage. Caloric studies, except in rare cases, reveal absent or poor vestibular function. In selected cases, cochlear implants (CIs) may be particularly helpful.

## ACUTE INFECTIONS

Systemic infections such as scarlet fever, typhoid fever, measles, and tuberculosis occasionally may cause bilateral SNHL. In the past, syphilis has been blamed for many cases of deafness that actually were because of other causes. At present, deafness is caused by syphilis more commonly than one might suspect, and in some cases, it can cause sudden bilateral hearing loss. Inner ear syphilis is a particularly important entity because it is treatable (see Chapter 11). Although a patient may have positive serological findings for syphilis along with sensorineural impairment, there may not be a causal relationship. The incidence of SNHL is so high that undoubtedly some of the people have syphilis without any relation between the two. Scarlet fever still causes a moderate degree of SNHL, usually accompanied by bilateral acute and later chronic otitis media. **Figure 10.25** shows a type that was much more prevalent prior to the use of antibiotics. Usually, the eardrum and the ossicles also were eroded.

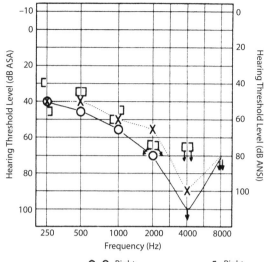

Air conduction O–O - Right X···X - Left  Bone conduction [ - Right ] - Left

Figure 10.25 *History:* A 48-year-old man with bilateral otitis media and draining ears since age 6 following scarlet fever. He had some ringing tinnitus but no vertigo. He used a hearing aid but has trouble because of ear discharge. *Otologic:* Both eardrums eroded and no evidence of ossicles. A putrid discharge is present in both middle ears. X-ray films show sclerotic mastoids but no cholesteatoma. *Audiologic:* Bilateral sloping audiogram shows moderate-to-severe hearing loss with no air–bone gap. Poor response to tuning fork even on the teeth. *Classification:* Sensorineural hearing loss. *Diagnosis:* Chronic otitis media and labyrinthitis involving the cochlea following scarlet fever. *Comment:* A bone conduction hearing aid usually is not recommended in losses of this type. However, the chronic otitis precludes the use of an air conduction aid, which requires an earmold in the ear. Use of a bone conduction aid when the ear is discharging might eliminate long periods of lack of amplification. *Abbreviations:* ANSI, American National Standards Institute; ASA, American Standards Association.

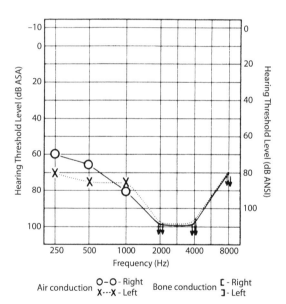

Air conduction O–O - Right X···X - Left  Bone conduction [ - Right ] - Left

Figure 10.24 *History:* A 16-year-old boy who had meningococcal meningitis at age 6. Speech shows marked evidence of deterioration. He went to school for the deaf but does not use a hearing aid. *Otologic:* Normal, but caloric responses are absent. *Audiologic:* Patient had some residual hearing in low tones. *Classification:* Sensorineural hearing loss. *Diagnosis:* Effect of meningitis on the cochlea. *Comment:* This boy could benefit from a powerful hearing aid and was urged to use one in his right ear. *Abbreviations:* ANSI, American National Standards Institute; ASA, American Standards Association.

## FUNCTIONAL HEARING LOSS

Some cases of bilateral sudden hearing loss are caused by emotional disturbances, and although there is no real damage to the sensorineural mechanism, the clinical findings strongly resemble this diagnostic entity. Hysteria is the outstanding feature of such cases, which are common during periods of marked emotional stress, as in wartime. Episodes of severe stress and tension can result in sudden hearing loss, with audiologic findings very similar to those found in sensorineural impairment attributable to other causes. The main distinguishing features are the history and the inconsistent audiologic findings. Because such cases sometimes do occur in civilian life, it is important to rule out functional hearing loss by obtaining consistent audiologic findings and an adequate history. Special audiometric tests are helpful in this diagnosis (see Chapter 7). **Figures 10.26** and **10.27** illustrate examples of functional hearing loss encountered in otologic practice.

JOSEPH SATALOFF, M.D.
ROBERT THAYER SATALOFF, M.D.
1721 PINE STREET     PHILADELPHIA, PA 19103

**HEARING RECORD**

NAME _____     AGE _____

**AIR CONDUCTION**

| | | | RIGHT | | | | | | | | LEFT | | | | | |
|---|---|---|---|---|---|---|---|---|---|---|---|---|---|---|---|---|
| DATE | Exam | LEFT MASK | 250 | 500 | 1000 | 2000 | 4000 | 8000 | RIGHT MASK | 250 | 500 | 1000 | 2000 | 4000 | 8000 | AUD |
| 1st Test | | | 40 | 45 | 50 | 50 | 50 | 55 | | 45 | 50 | 55 | 50 | 45 | 50 | |
| | | | 40 | 45 | 50 | 45 | 45 | 45 | | 40 | 45 | 50 | 45 | 50 | 50 | |
| 1 mo. | | | 45 | 50 | 40 | 50 | 40 | 55 | | 45 | 50 | 50 | 55 | 40 | 55 | |
| 4 mos. | | | 0 | -5 | 0 | 0 | -5 | 0 | | 0 | -5 | -5 | -5 | -5 | 0 | |

**BONE CONDUCTION**

| | | | RIGHT | | | | | | LEFT | | | | | |
|---|---|---|---|---|---|---|---|---|---|---|---|---|---|---|
| DATE | Exam | LEFT MASK | 250 | 500 | 1000 | 2000 | 4000 | RIGHT MASK | 250 | 500 | 1000 | 2000 | 4000 | AUD |
| 1st Test | | | 30 | 35 | 40 | 40 | 40 | | 35 | 35 | 40 | 40 | 40 | |
| 1 mo. | | | 35 | 30 | 40 | 45 | 40 | | 30 | 35 | 40 | 45 | 45 | |

**SPEECH RECEPTION**

| DATE | RIGHT | LEFT MASK | LEFT | RIGHT MASK | FREE FIELD | MIC. |
|---|---|---|---|---|---|---|
| 1st Test | 10 | | 10 | | | |
| 1 mo. | 10 | | 10 | | | |

**DISCRIMINATION** RIGHT                LEFT

| DATE | % SCORE | TEST LEVEL | LIST | LEFT MASK | % SCORE | TEST LEVEL | LIST | RIGHT MASK | EXAM |
|---|---|---|---|---|---|---|---|---|---|
| | 98 | 40 | | | 100 | 40 | | | |
| | 96 | 40 | | | 100 | 40 | | | |

**HIGH FREQUENCY THRESHOLDS**

| | RIGHT | | | | | | LEFT | | | | | |
|---|---|---|---|---|---|---|---|---|---|---|---|---|
| DATE | 4000 | 8000 | 10000 | 12000 | 14000 | LEFT MASK | RIGHT MASK | 4000 | 8000 | 10000 | 12000 | 14000 |
| | | | | | | | | | | | | |

| RIGHT | | WEBER | | LEFT | | HEARING AID | | | |
|---|---|---|---|---|---|---|---|---|---|
| RINNE | SCHWABACH | | | RINNE | SCHWABACH | DATE | MAKE | | MODEL |
| | | | | | | RECEIVER | GAIN | | EXAM |
| | | | | | | EAR | DISCRIM | | COUNC |

REMARKS

Figure 10.26 *History:* A 14-year-old girl whose hearing loss was suspected by teacher and confirmed by school nurse after audiometry. Her schoolwork deteriorated in the preceding year. No ear infections or related symptoms. *Otologic:* Normal. *Audiologic:* Note consistent hearing loss in air and bone conduction tests taken days apart, though the speech reception thresholds are normal (10 dB). The girl's normal hearing was confirmed by later testing. She had an emotional problem at school which was rectified by psychotherapy. *Classification:* Functional. *Etiology:* Emotional conflict.

## OTOTOXIC DRUGS

These are discussed elsewhere in this book. The severity and rapidity of onset of ototoxic hearing loss depend upon the patient's medical condition (renal, etc.), ototoxic potency of the drug, and method of administration. For example, certain diuretics such as furosemide administered in high doses through rapid intravenous push can cause sudden severe bilateral hearing loss associated with a high peak blood level of the drug. The same drug given over a longer period of time is less likely to result in similar otologic problems. Selected chemotherapeutic agents and other drugs also may cause bilateral hearing loss, in some cases sudden and severe.

## MULTIPLE SCLEROSIS

Multiple sclerosis is a rare cause of deafness, but it has been reported as a cause of sudden bilateral hearing loss and other patterns of sensorineural impairment. Usually, the deafness fluctuates, and hearing may return to normal even after a very severe depression. Susac's syndrome is commonly misdiagnosed as multiple sclerosis. Susac's syndrome includes the triad of microangiopathy of the brain and retina with SNHL in young women. Numerous cases have been recognized since the first report in 1979 (12).

## AUTOIMMUNE HEARING LOSS

Autoimmune hearing loss is discussed briefly in Chapter 11 and in greater detail here. **Figure 10.28** illustrates a case of autoimmune SNHL that developed following surgical manipulation of one ear.

Autoimmune SNHL was first described by McCabe (13) in 1979. In addition to hearing loss, he noted aural fullness and tinnitus and, rarely, destruction of external or middle ear structures. He defined this new entity on the basis of characteristic laboratory findings as well as its responsiveness to treatment with medications used classically for treatment of autoimmune disorders. McCabe's discussion stressed the importance of accurate diagnosis because of the availability of treatment options for this cause of SNHL.

The characteristics McCabe (13) described continue to be relevant even today, including asymmetric SNHL, occasionally involvement of balance organs, worsening over time, and responsiveness to steroids and other immunosuppressants such as cyclophosphamide. There is a spectrum of disease encompassed by the current terms autoimmune inner ear disease (AIED) and immune-mediated cochleovestibular disorders. The presentations include rapidly progressive SNHL, sudden deafness, and Ménière's syndrome (14). One of the authors (R.T.S.) has treated cases with virtually all audiometric patterns, including

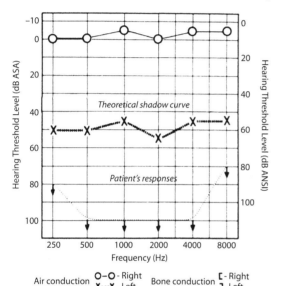

Figure 10.27 *History:* A 36-year-old man received a sharp blow behind the ear, lacerating the scalp but causing no unconsciousness. He claims sudden deafness in left ear following the industrial injury. No tinnitus or vertigo. *Otologic:* Normal. *Audiologic:* Patient denied hearing anything in his left ear when the right ear was unmasked. This led to a suspicion of nonorganic hearing loss. All malingering tests showed good hearing in left ear and did not substantiate a sudden hearing loss following head injury, as the man claimed. *Classification:* Functional hearing loss. *Diagnosis:* Malingering. *Aids to diagnosis:* When one ear is normal and the other is severely impaired, a shadow curve from the good ear (if unmasked) should appear when testing the impaired ear. This did not happen, and after much testing and discussion, the patient admitted he was fabricating his deafness, and eventually he gave a normal hearing audiogram in the left ear. *Abbreviations:* ANSI, American National Standards Institute; ASA, American Standards Association.

| NAME | CASE 2 | | | | | | | | | | AGE | | | | | | | | | |
|---|---|---|---|---|---|---|---|---|---|---|---|---|---|---|---|---|---|---|---|---|
| | | | | | | | | AIR CONDUCTION | | | | | | | | | | | | |
| | | | RIGHT | | | | | | | | | | | LEFT | | | | | | |
| DATE | Exam | LEFT MASK | 250 | 500 | 1000 | 2000 | 3000 | 4000 | 6000 | 8000 | RIGHT MASK | 250 | 500 | 1000 | 2000 | 3000 | 4000 | 6000 | 8000 | AUD |
| Pre-Op. | | | 40 | 35 | 45 | 25 | | 35 | | 50 | | 45 | 40 | 45 | 45 | | 65 | | NR | |
| Post-Op. | | | NR | NR | NR | NR | | NR | | NR | | NR | NR | NR | NR | | NR | | NR | |

Figure 10.28 *History:* This is a 26-year-old female who was born with choanal atresia, bilateral malformed ears, and poor vision. Right middle ear surgery was performed under local anesthesia. Her middle ear was shallow, and her facial nerve was dehiscent in the horizontal portion. The malleus and incus were slightly malformed, but the stapes and oval window were absent. A small fenestra was drilled through the promontory, and a stapes prosthesis was placed through the fenestra and crimped around the incus without difficulty. The patient's hearing improved substantially in the operating room, and there was no dizziness during the procedure. On the second postoperative day, she developed sudden deafness in her right ear. Four days later, she developed sudden deafness in her left ear. There was no evidence of infection. Comprehensive testing revealed no abnormalities. Immunophoresis was normal. Other immune system evaluation discussed below had not yet been described for autoimmune hearing loss. She did not respond to high-dose prednisone. Five years following surgery, she has no useful hearing in either ear. CI surgery was offered, but the patient declined. This is a rare case of sympathetic cochleitis, an autoimmune phenomenon.

total deafness and normal hearing with vestibular symptoms only.

To evaluate suspected autoimmune disease, it is most favorable to use organ biopsy as a diagnostic aid. Clearly, in the case of inner ear disease, the impossibility of biopsy results in a diagnostic dilemma (15). The initial laboratory tests discussed by McCabe (13) was the lymphocyte migration inhibition test, which was subsequently shown to have inconsistent results. The lymphocyte transformation test was introduced later by Hughes et al. (16) and showed high rates of specificity (93%) and sensitivity (between 50% and 80%). In addition, the indirect immunofluorescence test has been used to screen patients for inner ear-specific and inner ear-nonspecific autoantibodies. Veldman (17) demonstrated immunohistochemical proof of the immune-mediated reaction between spiral ganglia and patients' antibodies. The most definitive diagnostic test appears to be the Western blot assay for autoantibodies against cochlear antigens, but the sensitivity and specificity vary depending upon the method used.

Although the treatment proposed by McCabe (13) in his initial research consisted of the classic immunosuppressants corticosteroids and cyclophosphamide (Cytoxan), later research has confirmed the value of methotrexate (Rheumatrex) (18). Some of the most marked benefits of methotrexate

therapy include the improved side-effect profile compared with that of steroids and cyclophosphamide and its utility in patients who require long-term treatment.

When McCabe (13) described autoimmune hearing loss, initially, he defined it based on laboratory findings and clinical characteristics, such as its responsiveness to steroid therapy. The "typical" picture that has emerged since is that of a middle-aged female patient with bilateral progressive, asymmetric SNHL, with or without vertigo, and occasional systemic immune disease (16). However, in our experience, this description is far too limited.

Since the initial description of this entity, autoimmune SNHL has been found to occur in association with numerous immunologic and systemic autoimmune disorders, such as ulcerative colitis (19). Other diseases of a systemic nature that have been associated with otologic manifestations include connective tissue diseases (rheumatoid arthritis, polyarteritis, polymyositis, scleroderma, Sjögren's syndrome, amyloidosis), endocrine and associated organ diseases (Hashimoto's thyroiditis, Graves' disease, and pernicious anemia), and nonendocrine organ diseases (myasthenia gravis, glomerulonephritis, and Wegener's granulomatosis) (20). As a matter of fact, it has been demonstrated that otologic symptoms may be the harbinger of a systemic autoimmune disease that has yet to develop (21). However, the inner ear manifestations of these various diseases are identical. Although the exact mechanism of autoimmunity within the ear has not been elucidated fully, histologic studies have demonstrated the occurrence of an inflammatory reaction throughout the membranous labyrinth (19).

Previously, the presence of the blood–labyrinth barrier led to the notion of the inner ear as an immunoprivileged site. However, it has since been understood that under certain circumstances, immune cells may be present in the inner ear, particularly in the scala tympani (22). Occasionally, their presence is protective as against a viral infection; however, immune cells also may be destructive via a theoretical sensitization mechanism. The immune response likely occurs in the cochlea by the same mechanism as elsewhere throughout the body, with increased vascular permeability allowing the extravasation of leukocytes. The mechanism of this process was detailed by Ryan et al. (23). The endolymphatic sac appears to be important in the development of this reaction, although its precise role is undefined. It may represent as area for initial antigen presentation and processing, resulting in the production of the cytokines that trigger the increased vascular permeability and lymphocyte tracking that marks the remainder of the immune response (23). One of the authors (R.T.S.) has begun investigating cytokine system intervention (change from Th2 to Th1 control) as a possible treatment strategy for AIED.

The absence of HLA-DR4 is suggestive of AIED, as 80.6% of AIED patients lack this antigen (24). The other HLA findings that, when present, may indicate a propensity to develop AIED include B35, Cw4, and Cw7.

As described earlier, the lymphocyte transformation test had been used initially in the diagnosis of autoimmune SNHL. However, this test was determined to be insensitive, particularly after empiric corticosteroid treatment in patients in whom AIED was suspected (25). This test has since become an adjunct to the Western blot, which tests serum for antibodies against an inner-ear antigen. The sensitivity of the commercially available test (Immco Laboratories, Buffalo, NY) is only 42%; however, its specificity is 90% and its positive predictive value is 91% (25). Attempts to delineate the specific components responsible for the autoimmune reaction have consistently identified several proteins of similar weight. Most of these proteins are of the IgG type, with the rare IgA finding. They have been partially identified as antibodies to myelin protein PO (found in the spiral ganglion in the organ of Corti) and β-actin (in supporting cells and mechanosensory hair cells) (14).

Several antibodies still await identification, such as a 68-kDa protein that had previously been identified as heat shock protein 70 (hsp70) but recently has come into question (14). To attain a more accurate diagnosis, investigators have attempted to isolate the inner ear antigen that would be most closely linked to AIED (26). Although it has been identified repeatedly as the antigenic source, hsp70 has been questioned because of its ubiquity in human tissues. An autoimmune response related to this protein would likely have effects beyond simply the inner ear. The study produced the KHRI-3 antibody, which reacts strongly with supporting cells in the guinea pig organ of Corti. This protein migrates with a relative molecular mass of 65–68 kDa. Additionally, this protein, while abundant in inner ear extracts, is notably absent from extracts of other tissues. Testing of mice inoculated with KHRI-3 hybridoma revealed that mice carrying this hybridoma developed high antibody titers and exhibited a threshold shift on auditory brainstem response testing. High-frequency SNHL was also documented in most of these KHRI-3-bearing mice, and they had the highest degree of hearing loss and the highest circulating immunoglobulin levels. Further, *in vivo* testing of the guinea pig with an intracochlear mini-osmotic pump showed binding of antibody to organ of Corti supporting cells (including inner and outer pillar cells, phalangeal processes of out pillar cells, inner phalangeal cells, and phalangeal process of Deiters' cells). Outer hair cells were lost, as well as, in a few cases, inner hair cells. When the sera of patients suspected to have AIED were tested, the results were strikingly similar to those obtained with the KHRI-3 monoclonal antibody. There was also an observed relationship between the presence of antibodies to supporting cells and improvement in hearing after steroid therapy. However, the fact that this same relationship was not determined for antibody to the 68–70 kD a protein on Western blot led to the suggestion that Western blot assay may be less sensitive than immunofluorescence and that it may produce some false positives, but 89% of those patients who improved had antibody to supporting cells (positive immunofluorescence). Only 56% of Western blot-positive patients improved (26).

A positive Western blot also has a therapeutic implication, in that it has predictive value for the degree of corticosteroid responsiveness (25). Because of the low sensitivity of the Western blot, however, empiric corticosteroid treatment may be used in cases in which a high clinical suspicion exists. One must exercise caution, however, in overinterpreting responsiveness to steroid treatment, as several nonautoimmune processes similarly respond. For example, infectious processes such as syphilitic labyrinthitis and other inflammatory processes show improvement with steroid therapy (27). Another caution regarding steroid treatment is the plethora of side effects that accompany long-term use of high-dose corticosteroids. In addition, the response is rarely sustained. Moreover, failure to respond to steroids does not mean that the patient will not respond to cytotoxic drugs, and they should not be withheld on this criterion (24).

One other option that has been explored, cyclophosphamide, has proved to be moderately successful but again carries a high price in adverse effects, including susceptibility to infection, malignancy, and death (28). These risks prompted the search for an alternative therapy. Methotrexate had been used in the management of other autoimmune conditions, such as rheumatoid arthritis, with good efficacy and low toxicity (29). In a 1-year prospective study by Matteson et al. (30), methotrexate was started at 7.5 mg/week and increased to 17.5 mg/week over 4–8 weeks. Folic acid was given at 1 mg/day to minimize toxic effects. Of the 11 patients, 82% experienced a response to treatment (defined as improvement in pure tone average of > 10 dB or increased speech discrimination at > 15% in at least one ear) at 1-year of follow-up (30). A similar study performed by Salley et al. (31) described the response of 53 patients in methotrexate over an 8-year course. A response rate of 70% was found, according to response criteria similar to those of Matteson et al. (30) with the inclusion of a subjective reduction in vertigo or disequilibrium. Similar results have been observed in other studies (18, 32). A study conducted by Lasak et al. (24) involved cytotoxic therapy of Western-blot-positive patients with unresponsiveness to steroids or deterioration after steroid taper. These patients received 7.5–15 mg per week of oral methotrexate for at least 6 months or oral cyclophosphamide at 100 mg twice a day. Nonresponders were offered the other medication or azathioprine (Immuran) as an alternative. In total, 63% of patients who receive cytotoxic treatment responded, with modest improvement in mean pure tone average (4.5 dB) and marked improvement in mean speech discrimination (26.2%). Conversely, those patients treated solely with steroids experienced a marked improvement in mean pure-tone average (4.5 dB) but only a small improvement in mean speech discrimination (6.9%). On average, those who responded to steroids had less hearing loss before therapy than those who responded to cytotoxic therapy (24). Currently, various regimens are used in our center. Cytoxan is usually given as intravenous pulsed therapy, but Enbrel, CellCept, glutathione precursors, and, rarely, plasmapheresis are also used in the treatment of AIED.

Many of the mechanisms and signs of AIED remain unknown. For a brief period of time, it appeared that autoimmune SNHL might be associated with cochlear enhancement on the MRI. Zavod et al. (33) investigated this possibility and found that there was no correlation between the presence of antibodies to inner ear antigens in patients with hearing loss and cochlear enhancement on MRI scans.

Gupta and Sataloff (34) described a particularly interesting case of noise-induced autoimmune SNHL. This was the first reported case associating autoimmune SNHL with an environmental occurrence such as noise exposure. The patient was a 46-year-old woman who developed left-sided hearing loss after exposure to loud music at a party. Over the following decade, she had repeated episodes of temporary hearing loss, usually on the left side, precipitated by noise. Comprehensive neurotological evaluation was negative except for absence of HLA-DR4. Initially, Western blot for cochlear antibodies was negative, but a repeat Western blot was positive. Her hearing loss was steroid responsive, and her TTSs have been prevented for more than a decade by use of low-dose Imuran (50 mg daily). When she stopped the Imuran and was exposed to noise, she developed hearing loss. While she was taking the Imuran, noise exposure had no apparent effect on her hearing. This raises the question as to whether other cases of noise-induced hearing loss may involve an autoimmune mechanism. This question appears to warrant further research.

## CONGENITAL SYPHILIS

Congenital syphilis can cause sudden bilateral hearing loss (see Chapter 11). More often, it causes unilateral sudden hearing loss or bilateral, asymmetric progressive loss. However, if the patient is unaware that he/she is already deaf in one ear (as is often the case with deafness due to mumps in childhood), syphilitic sudden hearing loss in the other ear will make it appear as if the patient has experienced bilateral sudden hearing loss.

## UNKNOWN CAUSES

Bilateral sudden hearing loss occurs much less frequently than unilateral sudden hearing loss. Many cases of bilateral sudden hearing loss remain unexplained. Their causes have been attributed to viruses, vascular rupture or spam, or toxins, but as yet there is no certain knowledge of the precise mechanism. Cases like those illustrated in **Figures 10.29** and **10.30** occasionally are seen in clinical practice.

## CAUSES OF SUDDEN UNILATERAL SENSORINEURAL HEARING LOSS

Far more common than bilateral is unilateral sudden hearing loss. There is no satisfactory evidence to establish the specific cause for a large number of such cases. The degree of hearing impairment may range from a slight drop at 4000–8000 Hz

to total unilateral deafness. The hearing loss in some instances may disappear completely just as spontaneously as it appeared (and the medication used at the time generally gets the credit). Usually, if the hearing loss is going to improve, it does so within 2 or 3 weeks. About 65% of people with sudden unilateral hearing loss improve regardless of treatment. The outlook is not as good if the hearing loss is associated with vertigo. The cause of most of these cases is unknown, but viral and vascular etiologies are believed to be important. Syphilis always must be ruled out not only because it is one of the most readily treatable causes but also because, if left untreated, it may produce deafness in the other ear. Unilateral sudden hearing loss is, indeed, a most perplexing clinical picture.

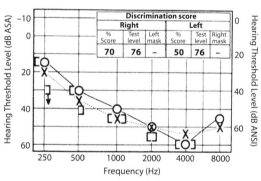

Air conduction O–O - Right, X---X - Left    Bone conduction [ - Right, ] - Left

Figure 10.29 *History:* This 40-year-old man noticed sudden deafness after getting chilled and sneezing repeatedly in an air-conditioned restaurant. He had rushing tinnitus but no vertigo. Sounds became fuzzy and distorted. The hearing loss did not clear up with time, nor did it get worse. *Otologic:* Normal. *Audiologic:* Air conduction and bone conduction were reduced. No abnormal tone decay. Recruitment could not be measured accurately. *Classification:* Unknown. *Cause:* Unknown. *Comment:* Sudden hearing loss of this kind with chills and vasospasm is not uncommon but rarely occurs bilaterally and permanently. The patient did not respond to vasodilators or histamine desensitization. A viral cause is unlikely. *Abbreviations:* ANSI, American National Standards Institute; ASA, American Standards Association.

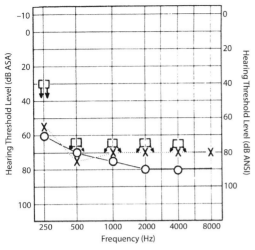

Air conduction O–O - Right / X---X - Left    Bone conduction Ⅽ - Right / コ - Left

Figure 10.30 *History:* This 8-year-old boy developed speech normally until the age of 5, when he awoke one morning and was severely deaf 1 week after a severe virus infection with high fever that might have been encephalitis. He had no other adverse effects. *Otologic:* Normal. No caloric responses. *Audiologic:* Severe air and bone conduction loss. *Classification:* Profound sensorineural hearing loss. *Diagnosis:* Unknown. *Comment:* Delayed deafness caused by virus infection occasionally occurs and may have been the cause here following encephalitis. No treatment is available, but speech therapy is essential to preserve good speech. A hearing aid is of some use. *Abbreviations:* ANSI, American National Standards Institute; ASA, American Standards Association.

## MUMPS

Sudden hearing loss may occur with mumps (see Chapter 11).

## DIRECT HEAD TRAUMA AND ACOUSTIC TRAUMA

They are discussed elsewhere in this chapter.

## MÉNIÈRE's SYNDROME

Ménière's syndrome may cause sudden hearing loss.

## VIRAL INFECTIONS

Comparatively little proof is available to show that viral infections produce partial sensory or sensorineural hearing impairment. It is known that mumps and herpes zoster can produce severe sudden hearing loss by attacking the cochlea and the auditory nerve. However, the mechanism is not known with certainty, nor the reason for the loss being almost invariably in one ear. As far as partial sensory or SNHL is concerned, there is a strong feeling among clinicians that patients may sustain this type of damage after such typical viral infections as head colds, mouth ulcers, and influenza. For this reason, many clinicians tell patients that their deafness probably was caused by some viral infection.

The authors have seen cases that seem to provide reasonable clinical proof that viruses can cause certain types of sensory hearing deficiency. For example, we were able to follow very closely an instance of sensory hearing loss associated with a viral upper respiratory infection in an audiologist. The case history is described in **Figure 10.31**. This is an interesting example of a cause of hearing loss that is undoubtedly more common than generally is realized. The symptoms of ringing tinnitus, fullness in the ear, and the measurable hearing loss associated with recruitment and diplacusis seem to be related to the typical upper respiratory viral infection that occurred in the patient. It appears that viruses can affect the inner ear and produce temporary partial deafness. The associated ringing tinnitus was found to match the frequency of the hearing loss and confirmed a common clinical impression that tinnitus can be produced by viral infections. The mechanism of these phenomena undoubtedly will be investigated much more extensively in the future. There seems to be justification, however, for considering a viral infection as the possible etiological factor in certain cases of partial sensory hearing impairment.

The clinical impression that viruses may cause sudden deafness in selected cases seems to be convincing (**Figure 10.31**). Although no viral studies were performed on this patient, the clinical picture was that of aphthous ulcers with stomatitis, a syndrome often associated with viral infection. The patient has had several recurrences of stomatitis because of the serious complication.

Herpes zoster is also known to cause sudden unilateral deafness of a severe degree. The authors have seen one instance of total loss of hearing that returned to normal in a few days. The patient had a typical case of shingles on his face.

JOSEPH SATALOFF, M.D.
ROBERT THAYER SATALOFF, M.D.
1721 PINE STREET    PHILADELPHIA, PA 19103

**HEARING RECORD**

NAME _____    AGE _____

## AIR CONDUCTION

| | | | RIGHT | | | | | | | | LEFT | | | | | |
|---|---|---|---|---|---|---|---|---|---|---|---|---|---|---|---|---|
| DATE | Exam | LEFT MASK | 250 | 500 | 1000 | 2000 | 4000 | 8000 | RIGHT MASK | 250 | 500 | 1000 | 2000 | 4000 | 8000 | AUD |
| 1ST TEST | | | 55 | 60 | 80 | 70 | 80 | 65 | ← | RIGHT STAPES MOBILIZATION. | | | | | | |
| 2 MOS. | | | 45 | 40 | 55 | 60 | NR | NR | ← | AFTER ATTACK OF APHTHOUS | | | | | | |
| 6 MOS. | | | 80 | 95 | 100 | 95 | NR | NR | ← | ULCERS OR HERPES. | | | | | | |

## BONE CONDUCTION

| | | | RIGHT | | | | | | | LEFT | | | | | |
|---|---|---|---|---|---|---|---|---|---|---|---|---|---|---|---|
| DATE | Exam | LEFT MASK | 250 | 500 | 1000 | 2000 | 4000 | RIGHT MASK | 250 | 500 | 1000 | 2000 | 4000 | AUD |
| 1ST TEST | | 90WM | 5 | 10 | 20 | 25 | 35 | | | | | | | |
| 6 MOS. | | 90WM | NR | 55 | NR | NR | NR | | | | | | | |

## SPEECH RECEPTION

| DATE | RIGHT | LEFT MASK | LEFT | RIGHT MASK | FREE FIELD | MIC |
|---|---|---|---|---|---|---|
| | | | | | | |

## DISCRIMINATION

| | | RIGHT | | | LEFT | | | |
|---|---|---|---|---|---|---|---|---|
| DATE | % SCORE | TEST LEVEL | LIST | LEFT MASK | % SCORE | TEST LEVEL | LIST | RIGHT MASK | EXAM |
| | | | | | | | | |

## HIGH FREQUENCY THRESHOLDS

| | RIGHT | | | | | | LEFT | | | | |
|---|---|---|---|---|---|---|---|---|---|---|---|
| DATE | 4000 | 8000 | 10000 | 12000 | 14000 | LEFT MASK | RIGHT MASK | 4000 | 8000 | 10000 | 12000 | 14000 |
| | | | | | | | | | | | |

| RIGHT | | WEBER | LEFT | | HEARING AID | | |
|---|---|---|---|---|---|---|---|
| RINNE | SCHWABACH | | RINNE | SCHWABACH | DATE | MAKE | MODEL |
| | | | | | RECEIVER | GAIN | EXAM |
| | | | | | EAR | DISCRIM | COUNC |

REMARKS

Figure 10.31 *History*: Patient with bilateral otosclerosis had a right stapes mobilization followed by mild vertigo for a few days postoperatively. The patient had a fair hearing improvement, but apparently mobilization was not adequate. About 4 months later, he developed either aphthous ulcers or herpes inside his buccal mucosa and on his tongue. During this period, he experienced sudden vertigo and roaring tinnitus in his right ear and deafness that has not improved. *Otologic*: Normal, and normal caloric response. *Audiologic*: There was marked depression of air conduction thresholds with no measurable bone conduction responses ("threshold" of 55 dB at 500 Hz is a tactile response). *Classification*: Sensorineural hearing loss. *Diagnosis*: Viral cochleitis and labyrinthitis.

Many cases of sudden unilateral hearing loss that now are attributed to blood vessel spasm or rupture may prove to be caused by viral infections. The peculiar reversibility of some cases of unilateral sudden hearing loss, even when they are very severe, is intriguing. Although now it is customary to consider SNHL to be permanent and incurable, many cases shed doubt on this maxim. Examples are shown in **Figures 10.4** and **10.32**. It is hard to believe that such a long-standing hearing loss as that in the subject of **Figure 10.32** can reverse itself. One is always suspicious in such examples and inclined to attribute the cause to psychological factors. In these and many other cases reported in the literature, this attitude merely diverts attention from finding the real cause and explanation for this phenomenon.

JOSEPH SATALOFF, M.D.
ROBERT THAYER SATALOFF, M.D.
1721 PINE STREET   PHILADELPHIA, PA 19103

**HEARING RECORD**

NAME                                                                  AGE

### AIR CONDUCTION

| | | | RIGHT | | | | | | | | LEFT | | | | | |
| DATE | Exam | LEFT MASK | 250 | 500 | 1000 | 2000 | 4000 | 8000 | RIGHT MASK | 250 | 500 | 1000 | 2000 | 4000 | 8000 | AUD |
|---|---|---|---|---|---|---|---|---|---|---|---|---|---|---|---|---|
| 1st TEST | | | 5 | 0 | 0 | 0 | 20 | 30 | | 0 | 0 | 0 | 0 | 10 | 25 | |
| 46 mos. | | 90-W | 45 | 40 | 40 | 15 | 25 | 45 | | 5 | -10 | -5 | -5 | 15 | 20 | |
| 48 mos. | | 90-W | 60 | 50 | 45 | 15 | 30 | 40 | | | | | | | | |
| 48 mos. | | 90-W | 30 | 15 | 10 | 10 | 10 | 35 | | | | | | | | |
| 55 mos. | | | 20 | 5 | 15 | 15 | 5 | 15 | | | | | | | | |
| | | | | | | | | | | | | | | | | |
| | | | | | | | | | | | | | | | | |
| | | | | | | | | | | | | | | | | |

### BONE CONDUCTION

| | | | RIGHT | | | | | | | LEFT | | | | | |
| DATE | Exam | LEFT MASK | 250 | 500 | 1000 | 2000 | 4000 | TYPE | RIGHT MASK | 250 | 500 | 1000 | 2000 | 4000 | AUD |
|---|---|---|---|---|---|---|---|---|---|---|---|---|---|---|---|
| 46 mos. | | 80 | 45 | 45 | 35 | 15 | 20 | WN | | | | | | | |
| 48 mos. | | 80 | 45 | 50 | 35 | 20 | 45 | WN | | | | | | | |
| | | | | | | | | | | | | | | | |
| | | | | | | | | | | | | | | | |
| | | | | | | | | | | | | | | | |
| | | | | | | | | | | | | | | | |

### SPEECH RECEPTION

| DATE | RIGHT | LEFT MASK | LEFT | RIGHT MASK | FREE FIELD | MIC |
|---|---|---|---|---|---|---|
| 46 mos. | 35 | 80 | | | | |
| 48 mos. | 40 | 80 | | | | |

### DISCRIMINATION

| | | RIGHT | | | | | LEFT | | | |
| DATE | % SCORE | TEST LEVEL | LIST | LEFT MASK | % SCORE | TEST LEVEL | LIST | RIGHT MASK | EXAM |
|---|---|---|---|---|---|---|---|---|---|
| 46 mos. | 65 | 65 | | 80 | | | | | |
| 48 mos. | 60 | 70 | | 80 | | | | | |

### HIGH FREQUENCY THRESHOLDS

| | | RIGHT | | | | | | LEFT | | | |
| DATE | 4000 | 8000 | 10000 | 12000 | 14000 | LEFT MASK | RIGHT MASK | 4000 | 8000 | 10000 | 12000 | 14000 |
|---|---|---|---|---|---|---|---|---|---|---|---|---|
| | | | | | | | | | | | | |
| | | | | | | | | | | | | |
| | | | | | | | | | | | | |

| | RIGHT | WEBER | LEFT | | HEARING AID | | |
| RINNE | SCHWABACH | | RINNE | SCHWABACH | DATE | MAKE | MODEL |
|---|---|---|---|---|---|---|---|
| T.F. 512 Hz   A>B | | → | | A>B | RECEIVER | GAIN | EXAM |
| B.C. Comparison to Normal - Poor | | | | | EAR | DISCRIM | COUNC |

REMARKS

Figure 10.32 *History*: A 50-year-old woman with recurrent attacks of hearing loss, rotary vertigo, and tinnitus in right ear for 2 years. Occasional vomiting with attacks. Marked diplacusis and distortion in right ear during attacks. *Otologic*: Normal. Normal caloric responses. *Audiologic*: Fluctuating hearing loss. Continuous and complete recruitment at 1000 and 2000 Hz during attacks. Normal discrimination when hearing returns to normal. *Classification*: Sensory hearing loss. *Diagnosis*: Ménière's disease. *Comment*: This sensory hearing loss persisted for over 2 months, and then hearing returned.

The influenza virus has been blamed for many cases of deafness, especially during major epidemics. Here, again, it is hard to find laboratory proof, but the clinical evidence is impressive. In all likelihood, many cases described as auditory neuritis could have been caused by viruses with a predilection for sensorineural tissue, as is true of mumps.

There also is evidence that viral infections during the first trimester of pregnancy can seriously affect the sensorineural mechanism of the fetus and result in congenital hearing loss.

## RUPTURE OF ROUND-WINDOW MEMBRANE, OVAL WINDOW MEMBRANE, OR INNER EAR MEMBRANE

The membranes of the inner ear or round oval window may rupture, causing hearing loss accompanied

at times by vertigo and tinnitus. This occurs most commonly in cases of barotrauma associated with activities such as flying, diving, or severe straining. An interesting case of sudden sensorineural unilateral hearing loss occurred in a patient who blamed it on an attack of severe sneezing (see **Figure 10.33**).

## VASCULAR DISORDERS

The role of blood vessel spasm, thrombosis, embolism, and rupture as causes of hearing loss still is not clear (see Chapter 11). It is common and logical to attribute a progressive SNHL in an older person to arteriosclerosis or thrombosis. Yet such an explanation rarely is confirmed by histopathological studies. Although physicians continue to blame terminal blood vessel occlusion in the ear for many causes of hearing loss, we do not have proof that this is so. Other causes also should be considered.

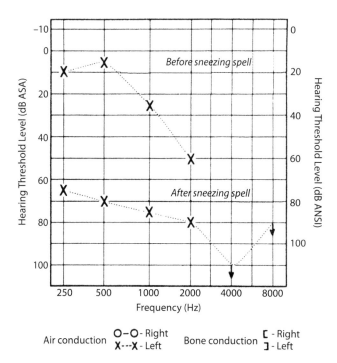

Air conduction  O–O - Right  X--X - Left    Bone conduction  C - Right  ] - Left

Figure 10.33 *History*: During a severe sneezing spell, this 56-year-old man noted ringing tinnitus in his left ear, and 2 hours later, his hearing became bad. The hearing continued to get worse for many months until the ear was practically deaf. He experienced no vertigo. *Otologic*: Normal, and normal caloric responses. *Audiologic*: No abnormal tone decay. Slight separation of Békésy fixed-frequency tracings. Left ear discrimination, 40%. Bone conduction poor; no air–bone gap. *Classification*: Sensorineural. *Diagnosis*: Ruptured round-window membrane observed at surgery. *Abbreviations*: ANSI, American National Standards Institute; ASA, American Standards Association.

Sudden unilateral hearing loss may be explained most reasonably on the basis of blood vessel spasm and rupture. In clinical practice, one sees quite a few patients with unexplained attacks of sudden unilateral deafness of short duration—or even of longer duration, an attack that may last for several weeks followed by a spontaneous return of hearing to normal or improved levels.

Often the hearing losses are accompanied by rotary vertigo, imbalance, and high-pitched tinnitus. In other cases, hearing loss is the only symptom other than a sensation of fullness in the ear. In still other patients, both deafness and tinnitus are permanent, but the imbalance disappears.

Cases of permanent sudden hearing loss in one ear often are blamed on vascular rupture of vascular occlusion, whereas those that recover are attributed to reversible vessel spasm. There are, however, some pitfalls in this explanation. For want of a better understanding at this time, most otologists continue to attribute such cases of deafness to circulatory difficulties, viral diseases, or membrane ruptures.

The role of hypertension and hypotension in deafness is also unknown. However, hypertension associated with hyperlipoproteinemia may be associated with hearing loss, as discussed in Chapter 13. Hypotension seems in some cases to be vaguely associated with progressive high-frequency SNHL. Usually, recurrent attacks of imbalance are also experienced by such patients. Hypotension may predispose to sudden losses in hearing, but here again, convincing proof is lacking. Patients with certain vascular disorders, such as endarteritis, Buerger's disease, diabetes, and others, should have a high incidence of sensorineural hearing impairment, but this has not been borne out by investigations.

The degree of hearing impairment present in patients with sudden unilateral hearing loss varies and may be only 15 or 20 dB and last only a few moments, as most individuals probably have experienced at one time or another when they have felt a sudden fullness and ringing in one ear, or the hearing loss may be up to 70 dB or even total, as described previously. Criteria have been defined to help predict the reversibility of sudden hearing loss. New medical therapies are being developed, and it is necessary for anyone treating this condition to be familiar with the latest literature.

## FOLLOWING EAR SURGERY

The increase in stapes surgery has brought with it a marked increase in the incidence of unilateral sudden hearing loss. Physicians are familiar with the sudden severe deafness that may result as a complication of mastoid and fenestration surgery. The loss is sudden and occurs either at the time of the operation owing to disturbance of the inner ear or shortly after surgery owing to infection. With the advent of stapedectomies, otologists have encountered sudden hearing loss in patients weeks, months, or even years after surgery. **Figure 10.34** is an example of a patient who became deaf in his operated ear 4 months after a stapedectomy. Surgical exploration showed invasion of the vestibule with white scar tissue from the middle ear. The hearing in another patient suddenly became poor several months after stapedectomy during a bad infection described as a virus. No unusual findings were encountered in the middle ear or the oval window during exploration, and the perilymphatic fluid in the inner ear appeared to be normal. It is important, therefore, in all cases to inquire about previous ear surgery, but one should not assume that the previous surgery is casually related to the hearing loss. Surgery for tympanosclerosis in which the oval window is opened is a common cause of sudden hearing loss, usually noted within 1 or 2 days postoperatively.

The sensorineural deafness that can follow ear surgery need not be severe or total. Most often it consists of a high-frequency hearing loss that did not exist preoperatively (**Figure 10.35**). We generally attribute this to injury to the inner ear during surgery or infection postoperatively. The patient's chief complaint in such situations is reduced ability to understand speech. This is a justified complaint, one that can be demonstrated with discrimination tests. Sometimes a patient with a very successful return of threshold hearing following stapes surgery will appear to be most unhappy about the hearing result and bewilder the surgeon. **Figure 10.36** shows such as case, and the discrimination scores show that despite the improved threshold level, this patient is far worse postoperatively than she was preoperatively.

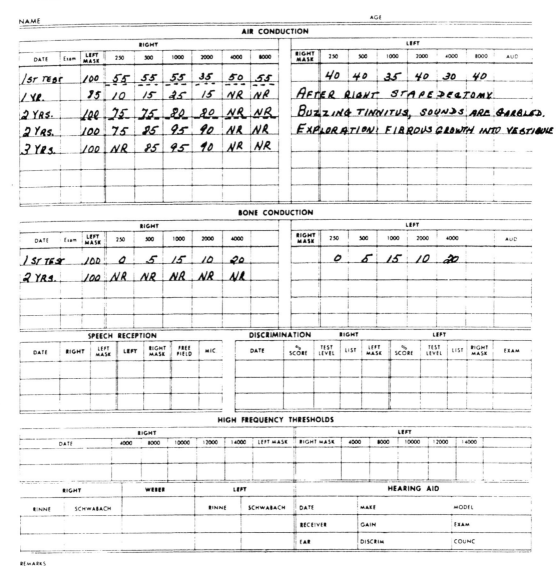

JOSEPH SATALOFF, M.D.
ROBERT THAYER SATALOFF, M.D.
1721 PINE STREET    PHILADELPHIA, PA 19103

Figure 10.34 *History*: Four months after a successful right stapedectomy, using a Teflon piston over Gelfoam, this 23-year-old man suddenly noticed a pop in his right ear, and his hearing improved. Several hours later, he noted a buzzing tinnitus and distortion. The next day, his hearing gradually diminished, became garbled, and was completely gone that evening. He had constant hissing tinnitus but no vertigo. Exploratory surgery showed that the prosthesis was in good position, but a fibrous tissue mass had invaded the labyrinthine vestibule. Removal of much of the mass failed to improve the hearing.

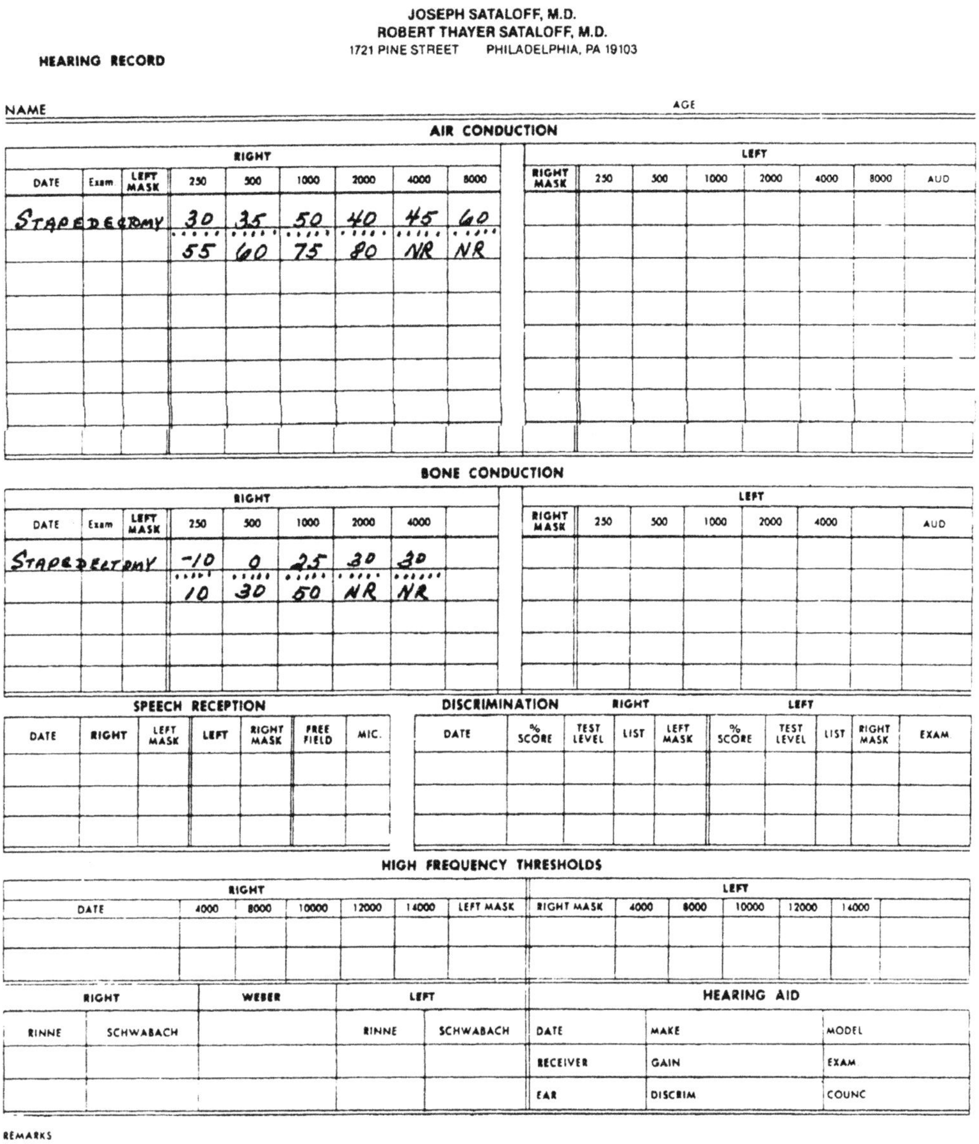

JOSEPH SATALOFF, M.D.
ROBERT THAYER SATALOFF, M.D.
1721 PINE STREET     PHILADELPHIA, PA 19103

**HEARING RECORD**

NAME _____     AGE _____

## AIR CONDUCTION

| | | | RIGHT | | | | | | | | LEFT | | | | | |
|---|---|---|---|---|---|---|---|---|---|---|---|---|---|---|---|---|
| DATE | Exam | LEFT MASK | 250 | 500 | 1000 | 2000 | 4000 | 8000 | RIGHT MASK | 250 | 500 | 1000 | 2000 | 4000 | 8000 | AUD |
| STAPEDECTOMY | | | 30 | 35 | 50 | 40 | 45 | 60 | | | | | | | | |
| | | | 55 | 60 | 75 | 80 | NR | NR | | | | | | | | |

## BONE CONDUCTION

| | | | RIGHT | | | | | | | LEFT | | | | | |
|---|---|---|---|---|---|---|---|---|---|---|---|---|---|---|---|
| DATE | Exam | LEFT MASK | 250 | 500 | 1000 | 2000 | 4000 | RIGHT MASK | 250 | 500 | 1000 | 2000 | 4000 | AUD |
| STAPEDECTOMY | | | -10 | 0 | 25 | 30 | 30 | | | | | | | |
| | | | 10 | 30 | 50 | NR | NR | | | | | | | |

## SPEECH RECEPTION

| DATE | RIGHT | LEFT MASK | LEFT | RIGHT MASK | FREE FIELD | MIC. |
|---|---|---|---|---|---|---|
| | | | | | | |
| | | | | | | |
| | | | | | | |

## DISCRIMINATION

| | | | | RIGHT | | | LEFT | | | |
|---|---|---|---|---|---|---|---|---|---|---|
| DATE | % SCORE | TEST LEVEL | LIST | LEFT MASK | % SCORE | TEST LEVEL | LIST | RIGHT MASK | EXAM |
| | | | | | | | | | |
| | | | | | | | | | |
| | | | | | | | | | |

## HIGH FREQUENCY THRESHOLDS

| | | RIGHT | | | | | | | | LEFT | | | | |
|---|---|---|---|---|---|---|---|---|---|---|---|---|---|---|
| DATE | 4000 | 8000 | 10000 | 12000 | 14000 | LEFT MASK | RIGHT MASK | 4000 | 8000 | 10000 | 12000 | 14000 | |
| | | | | | | | | | | | | | |
| | | | | | | | | | | | | | |
| | | | | | | | | | | | | | |

| RIGHT | | | WEBER | LEFT | | HEARING AID | | |
|---|---|---|---|---|---|---|---|---|
| RINNE | SCHWABACH | | | RINNE | SCHWABACH | DATE | MAKE | MODEL |
| | | | | | | RECEIVER | GAIN | EXAM |
| | | | | | | EAR | DISCRIM | COUNC |

REMARKS

Figure 10.35 *History*: A 62-year-old women who had a stapedectomy in right ear and heard well for 2 days. She then developed vertigo and roaring tinnitus and hearing deteriorated. She complained of distortion and being bothered by loud noise. *Otologic*: Normal. *Audiologic*: Reduced bone conduction postoperatively with recruitment, diplacusis, lowered threshold of discomfort, and reduced discrimination. *Classification*: Sensory hearing loss. *Diagnosis*: Postoperative labyrinthitis.

# FISTULA OF OVAL WINDOW

A postoperative fistula in the oval window can cause fluctuating hearing loss, recurrent vertigo, fullness, and tinnitus in the ear. This may occur even many years following the surgery. Spontaneous oval or round-window fistulas also can occur even in people who have never had ear surgery.

# FOLLOWING ANESTHESIA AND GENERAL SURGERY

Hearing impairment following anesthesia and general surgery has been encountered by some otologists, but evidence is unavailable as to which, if either, of these interventions is the immediate cause. It is not uncommon in otology to find patients who claim that they

JOSEPH SATALOFF, M.D.
ROBERT THAYER SATALOFF, M.D.
1721 PINE STREET     PHILADELPHIA, PA 19103

HEARING RECORD

NAME _____    AGE _____

**AIR CONDUCTION**

| | | | RIGHT | | | | | | | LEFT | | | | | |
|---|---|---|---|---|---|---|---|---|---|---|---|---|---|---|---|
| DATE | Exam | LEFT MASK | 250 | 500 | 1000 | 2000 | 4000 | 8000 | RIGHT MASK | 250 | 500 | 1000 | 2000 | 4000 | 8000 | AUD |
| 1ST TEST | | | 45 | 45 | 45 | 50 | NR | NR | | 65 | 70 | 65 | 65 | 85 | 75 | |
| 4 DAYS | | | | | | | | | | 10 | 25 | 60 | 65 | NR | 75 | |
| 6 DAYS | | | | | | | | | | 55 | 50 | 50 | 60 | 90 | 75 | |
| 10 DAYS | | | | | | | | | | 15 | 15 | 30 | 45 | 90 | 75 | |
| 20 DAYS | | | | | | | | | | 15 | 15 | 5 | 30 | 85 | 75 | |

**BONE CONDUCTION**

| | | | RIGHT | | | | | | LEFT | | | | | |
|---|---|---|---|---|---|---|---|---|---|---|---|---|---|---|
| DATE | Exam | LEFT MASK | 250 | 500 | 1000 | 2000 | 4000 | RIGHT MASK | 250 | 500 | 1000 | 2000 | 4000 | AUD |
| 1ST TEST | | | -10 | -10 | -10 | 25 | 50 | | 10 | 0 | -5 | 15 | 55 | |

| **SPEECH RECEPTION** | | | | | | | | **DISCRIMINATION** RIGHT | | | | LEFT | | | | |

| DATE | RIGHT | LEFT MASK | LEFT | RIGHT MASK | FREE FIELD | MIC | | DATE | % SCORE | TEST LEVEL | LIST | LEFT MASK | % SCORE | TEST LEVEL | LIST | RIGHT MASK | EXAM |
|---|---|---|---|---|---|---|---|---|---|---|---|---|---|---|---|---|---|
| 1ST TEST | | | 64 | | | | | 4 DAYS | 94 | 90 | | | | | | | |
| 10 DAYS | | | 34 | | | | | | 42 | 64 | | | | | | | |
| 20 DAYS | | | 12 | | | | | | 60 | 42 | | | | | | | |

**HIGH FREQUENCY THRESHOLDS**

| | RIGHT | | | | | | LEFT | | | | | |
|---|---|---|---|---|---|---|---|---|---|---|---|---|
| DATE | 4000 | 8000 | 10000 | 12000 | 14000 | LEFT MASK | RIGHT MASK | 4000 | 8000 | 10000 | 12000 | 14000 |
| | | | | | | | | | | | | |

| RIGHT | | WEBER | | LEFT | | HEARING AID | | |
|---|---|---|---|---|---|---|---|---|
| RINNE | SCHWABACH | | | RINNE | SCHWABACH | DATE | MAKE | MODEL |
| | | | | | | RECEIVER | GAIN | EXAM |
| | | | | | | EAR | DISCRIM | COUNC |

REMARKS

Figure 10.36 *History*: This patient had an excellent improvement in pure-tone threshold after a left stapedectomy, but she was very unhappy with the result because she could not use the left ear satisfactorily. Speech testing postoperatively showed a real drop in discrimination, which probably was caused by postoperative labyrinthosis. No satisfactory treatment for this is known to the author at present. Note that before surgery, she heard 94% of the test words, but after surgery, only 60%. When the test material was presented at a higher level, the discrimination score dropped to 42% owing to distortion.

suffered hearing loss or that their hearing loss was aggravated after some surgical procedure. A causal relationship may be possible, or it may be coincidental.

## ACOUSTIC NEUROMAS

Approximately 10% of acoustic neuromas present as sudden deafness. It is therefore essential that a complete evaluation be carried out on every patient

with sudden deafness searching for the cause that predisposed the deafened ear to injury.

## UNKNOWN CAUSES OF SUDDEN UNILATERAL SENSORINEURAL HEARING LOSS

Because unilateral sudden SNHL is so common in clinical practice, several additional examples are

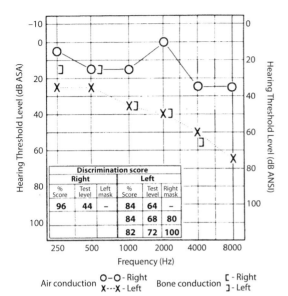

Because inner ear damage frequently progresses into the nerve elements, many cases originally starting as sensory progress to the sensorineural type.

The following causes are known to produce sensory hearing impairment. All are characterized, at least in their early stages, by some degree of recruitment and hearing distortion.

1. Ménière's disease
2. Prolonged exposure to intense noise (occupational deafness)
3. Acoustic trauma
4. Direct head trauma
5. Ototoxic drugs
6. Virus infections
7. Labyrinthosis following ear surgery
8. Congenital cochlear disease

Figure 10.37 *History*: A 50-year-old patient who developed sudden hearing loss in left ear 3 months before, accompanied by distortion and buzzing but no vertigo of any sort. All symptoms except deafness gradually subsided. *Otologic*: Normal. Only minimal response from both ears after caloric stimulation. No spontaneous nystagmus. *Audiologic*: Left ear hearing loss greater in higher frequencies with reduced bone conduction. Complete recruitment in all frequencies and diplacusis. No abnormal tone decay. *Classification*: Sensory hearing loss. *Etiology*: Unknown. *Comment*: Findings of complete recruitment and diplacusis and no abnormal tone decay localize the lesion to the inner ear. The patient's good discrimination score, which did not worsen with increased sound intensity, and the cessation of tinnitus and distortion are not indicative of Ménière's disease. Possible causes include vasospasm and viral cochleitis. *Abbreviations*: ANSI, American National Standards Institute; ASA, American Standards Association.

presented to help the physician make a better classification and diagnosis (**Figures 10.37–10.39**).

## CAUSES OF SENSORY HEARING LOSS

Certain causes of hearing impairment are known to affect the inner ear primarily and to produce findings characteristic of sensory hearing loss.

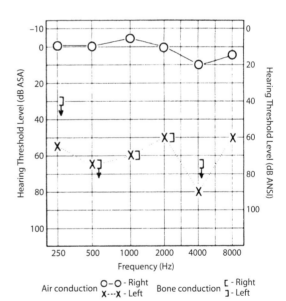

Figure 10.38 *History*: A 45-year-old man with sudden hearing loss in left ear on awakening one morning. Some ringing tinnitus but no vertigo. *Otologic*: Normal. *Audiologic*: Very little recruitment present and no abnormal tone decay. Discrimination was about 68% and no diplacusis. *Classification*: Sensorineural hearing loss. *Diagnosis*: Unknown. This damage possibly could be of vascular origin. *Abbreviations*: ANSI, American National Standards Institute; ASA, American Standards Association.

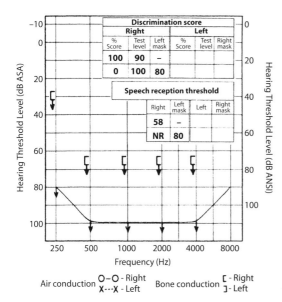

| Discrimination score | | | | | | |
|---|---|---|---|---|---|---|
| | Right | | | Left | | |
| | % Score | Test level | Left mask | % Score | Test level | Right mask |
| | 100 | 90 | – | | | |
| | 0 | 100 | 80 | | | |

| Speech reception threshold | | | | |
|---|---|---|---|---|
| | Right | Left mask | Left | Right mask |
| | 58 | – | | |
| | NR | 80 | | |

Air conduction  O–O - Right  X--X - Left    Bone conduction  [ - Right  ] - Left

Figure 10.39 *History*: A 45-year-old woman who for several years had experienced a pounding sensation in the right ear whenever she became nervous. Two weeks prior to her presentation, she developed complete deafness, accompanied by momentary severe dizziness and positional vertigo lasting 1 day. Since that time, she had buzzing tinnitus in the right ear. *Otologic*: Normal. Normal caloric response in right ear. *Audiologic*: No response to pure tones or speech testing with the left ear masked. *Classification*: Sensorineural hearing loss. *Diagnosis*: Unknown, but probably a vascular accident. *Abbreviations*: ANSI, American National Standards Institute; ASA, American Standards Association.

## MÉNIÈRE'S DISEASE

Ménière's disease presents all the classic symptoms and findings associated with a sensory hearing loss. There still is confusion concerning the criteria for diagnosing Ménière's disease. Part of the confusion centers around the original findings of the 19th-century otologist Prosper Ménière, who reported the autopsy findings on a patient who had suffered from dizziness and deafness. Apparently, what he described and what is now considered to be Ménière's disease are not the same. However, the confusion lies mostly in terminology and the tendency of some physicians to call all cases of vertigo of undetermined origin as Ménière's disease.

## Terms and definition

Research studies on patients with vertigo, tinnitus, and deafness have revealed histopathological findings suggesting hydrops of the labyrinth caused by distention with endolymphatic fluid. The cause of the presence of excessive fluid is unknown, but it has now come to be associated with subjective symptoms of Ménière's disease. Because of this hydrops, new names have been applied to the condition. It is variously called labyrinthosis (in contrast with labyrinthitis, which implies an inflammatory involvement) and even labyrinthine hypertension. Common clinical usage now restricts the condition named Ménière's disease to patients who have recurrent attacks of vertigo, hearing loss, and tinnitus. Most often the hearing loss fluctuates, especially in the lower frequencies and early in the course of the disease. Usually, the hearing loss is not total, and seashell-like tinnitus is often present.

Atypical Ménière's disease occurs most commonly in four forms. Cochlear Ménière's disease lacks the vertiginous episodes but is typical otherwise. Vestibular Ménière's occurs without the hearing loss. Sometimes these forms are present early but ultimately progress to typical Ménière's disease later. Lermoyez's syndrome is Ménière's disease in which vertigo and hearing loss fluctuate in reverse relationship to each other (one condition improves when the other becomes bad) rather than in the usual parallel fashion. Tumarkin's variant, or otolithic catastrophe, in which the patient has abrupt falling attacks of short duration, also is considered a form of Ménière's disease by some clinicians.

Ménière's disease is idiopathic. The diagnosis cannot be made until comprehensive evaluation has ruled out the many specific and often treatable causes of hydrops that produce the same symptoms (Ménière's syndrome).

## Symptoms and their effect on the patient

The characteristic findings in Ménière's disease are generally clear-cut, and all are present in most cases. The typical history is marked by a sudden onset of ear fullness, hearing loss, and a seashell-like tinnitus in one ear. This may last for a period of minutes or several days and then disappear. The same symptoms then may recur at varying time intervals. After several attacks, the hearing loss and the tinnitus may persist. The loss may not be severe, but voices begin to sound tinny and muffled on the telephone, and it becomes difficult for the patient to follow a conversation because of the inability to distinguish between different words that have related sounds. In addition, there is distortion of sound, and the threshold of discomfort for loud noises is reduced. Fullness in the ear is common.

## VERTIGO AND TINNITUS

Generally, the patient complains of recurrent attacks of vertigo, during which either the room seems to spin, or the patient feels as if he/she is spinning. Everything goes around, and the tinnitus is aggravated severely during the attack. Sometimes nausea and vomiting may occur.

The vertigo in Ménière's disease is of a specific type that involves some sort of motion. It is "subjective" when the patient has a sensation of moving or "objective" when things seem to move about the patient. Usually, the motion is described as rotary, especially during the acute attack. Occasionally, between acute attacks patients have a mild feeling of motion whereby they seem to fall to one side and have trouble keeping their balance. Less often, there is a strange up-and-down or to-and-fro motion. Other types of sensation, such as a feeling of faintness or weakness, or seeing spots before the eyes, or just vague "dizziness," should not be attributed to Ménière's disease. The possible causes for these subjective symptoms are numerous, but Ménière's disease is not one of them. There must be some evidence of hearing loss being, or having been, present for the diagnosis to be typical Ménière's disease. It is true that in the very early phases, hearing may be lost only during the acute attack and that it may be normal between attacks. But even in such cases, the patient will recall having experienced fullness and roaring in one ear. If these subjective symptoms are absent and no hearing loss is present, a diagnosis of Ménière's disease should be made only with the utmost caution, and further studies should explore the possibility of some other cause of the dizziness.

Patients are concerned more frequently about the vertigo and tinnitus than about their hearing loss. For an individual who works on scaffolding or drives a car or a truck, a sudden unexpected attack of vertigo beyond his/her control is indeed a serious problem. These patients are invariably apprehensive and gravely concerned. Anxiety is a prominent symptom in patients with Ménière's disease. Many of them seem to be much improved and less subject to attacks when they are relaxed and free of tense situations.

The ocean-roaring or seashell-like tinnitus also is a matter of great concern. When patients are in quiet surroundings or when they are under tension, the tinnitus may become so alarming to them that they often are willing to undergo any type of surgery, even if it means the loss of all their hearing in affected ear, provided that the noise can be made to disappear. Under such circumstances, the otologist should not let the patient influence him/her to perform irrational and sometimes unsuccessful surgery for the tinnitus. Other than cochlear implantation for patients with severe-profound hearing loss and tinnitus, physicians have no specific, reliable procedure to control tinnitus.

### Hearing loss

Generally, the hearing impairment is not as disturbing to the patient as the other two symptoms, but when it happens to a businessperson who uses the telephone to conduct business, it becomes an especially important issue.

### Audiologic findings

An audiogram of a typical case of Ménière's disease is shown in **Figure 10.7**. Note the low-frequency hearing impairment with reduced bone conduction. If the bone conduction were not reduced, this audiometric pattern would be typical of conductive instead of sensory hearing loss. There is no air–bone gap because both air conduction and bone conduction are reduced to the same degree. The patient's ability to discriminate in the bad ear is reduced so much that he/she can distinguish only 60% of the speech heard at ordinary levels of loudness. Furthermore, if speech is made louder (from 50 to 70 dB), the patient distinguishes even less (contrary to expectations). This brings out one of the most important features of Ménière's disease: distortion. Distortion explains many of the symptoms, not only the reduced discrimination but also the tinny character that speech assumes in the patient's ears, the inability to discriminate words on the telephone, and diplacusis.

## Recruitment

Another interesting phenomenon in patients with Ménière's disease is called a lower threshold of discomfort, and it is manifested by the patient's complaint that loud noises bother him/her. This difficulty is related partially to distortion but principally to the phenomenon of recruitment. Recruitment is a telltale audiologic finding in the diagnosis of inner ear hearing loss and particularly Ménière's syndrome. It stems from an abnormally rapid increase in the sensation of loudness, and when it is present to a marked degree, it permits the physician to classify a case with reduced bone conduction as being sensory and to localize the damage to the inner ear. In the absence of recruitment, the localization is uncertain, and the condition must be classified as sensorineural.

Continuous and complete recruitment and sometimes hyperrecruitment occur in Ménière's disease. These phenomena are hypothesized to have their origin in disturbances in the hair cells. A simple test for recruitment by means of a tuning fork should be done routinely in cases of reduced bone conduction. Note in **Figure 10.7** that this patient evidence all the phenomena associated with Ménière's disease, including marked recruitment. Abnormal tone decay is absent. The Békésy audiogram (see Chapter 7) also is often characteristic, without a gap between the continuous and the interrupted tone (type II).

## CLINICAL STUDIES

The case in **Figure 10.7** is typical Ménière's disease, but there are many cases in which the diagnosis is not quite so certain. For example, **Figure 10.40** shows a patient whose history is suggestive of Ménière's disease. In this patient, however, only the high frequencies were impaired. The audiologic findings were equivocal, except for complete recruitment, and for this reason, such a case may be classified as Ménière's disease. The diagnosis was established definitely as the disease progressed. **Figure 10.41** shows a difficult and frustrating type of case in which there is bilateral Ménière's disease. Note the comparatively mild

reduction in auditory threshold coupled with severe decreased discrimination. A hearing aid is of no value to this patient because it generally aggravates the distortion. The patient sometimes hears more poorly with the hearing aid and very rarely better. The psychological effects of not being able to understand what his customers were saying and the severe tinnitus drove this pharmacist to seek psychiatric attention.

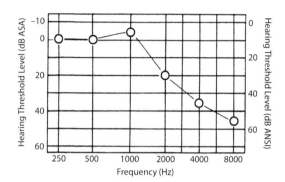

Figure 10.40 *History*: A 42-year-old man with sudden hearing loss and rushing tinnitus in the right ear. Symptoms present for 6 months when first seen for examination. Has slight difficulty distinguishing certain sounds. Feels occasional fullness in the right ear. No vertigo. *Otologic*: Normal with normal caloric responses. *Audiologic*: Left ear normal. Right has a high-frequency loss with complete recruitment at 2000 Hz. No abnormal tone decays. Diplacusis with 2000-Hz tone. *Discrimination score*: Right, 4%. *Classification*: Sensory hearing loss. *Diagnosis*: Ménière's disease. *Aids to diagnosis*: This man worked in a noisy environment, and his unilateral hearing loss originally was misdiagnosed as occupationally related deafness. The presence of complete recruitment, diplacusis, and discrimination difficulty point to sensory hearing loss and probably Ménière's disease without vertigo. In this case, the diagnosis was confirmed months later when the patient developed attacks of rotary vertigo. His hearing then changed to levels similar to those in **Figure 10.6**. Both the unilateral impairment with depression at 8000 Hz and the relatively low noise level (90 dB overall) in the allegedly "noisy plant" mitigated against a diagnosis of noise-induced hearing loss. *Abbreviations*: ANSI, American National Standards Institute; ASA, American Standards Association.

## Laboratory tests

Recent work has shown that a number of treatable diseases may be associated with symptoms like those found in Ménière's disease. Inner ear syphilis, hyperlipoproteinemia, diabetes mellitus, autoimmune SNHL, Lyme disease, and hypothyroidism are among the most prominent. These should be investigated, at least by history. Many physicians recommend an FTA-absorption test (not RPR or VDRL), thyroid profile, and screening tests for diabetes and hyperlipoproteinemia in this clinical picture. Collagen vascular disease work-up may also be appropriate.

## Labyrinthine tests

Rotary vertigo may occur in both sensory and neural deafness, and when it is essential to differentiate between unilateral inner ear hearing loss and unilateral nerve hearing loss (possibly due to a tumor), labyrinthine tests are necessary. Not infrequently a patient will experience the vertigo during examination in a physician's office. The patient will complain that the room, or he/she, is starting to turn and that there is a severe noise in his/her ear. At that time, examination of the eyes showed marked nystagmus with a slow and fast component. The nystagmus may be in almost any plane; it may even be oblique, and the direction also may vary. Such a strange type of nystagmus often suggests the presence of an intracranial tumor. However, careful watching usually reveals that the nystagmus soon subsides, and the vertigo stops (in contrast with most him/her cases of intracranial involvement). Caloric studies, which should not be performed during the attack, show either diminished or exaggerated labyrinthine responses with nausea and vomiting in Ménière's disease, but the direction and the type of nystagmus are normal with respect to amplitude and direction, unlike the findings in some posterior intracranial fossa neoplasms. Electronystagmograms may be helpful in diagnosing and documenting the vestibular disturbance.

## TREATMENT

It is beyond the intent of this book to describe treatment of Ménière's disease. However, no specific therapy is available. Many remedies have been suggested as curative, but the spontaneous remissions typical of this disease make it difficult to evaluate the

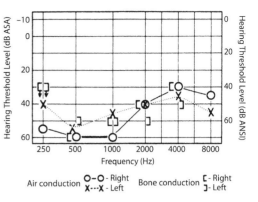

Air conduction O—O - Right X---X - Left   Bone conduction C - Right J - Left

**Figure 10.41** *History*: A 31-year-old man with insidious hearing loss for many years with ocean-roar tinnitus and rare mild vertigo. He complained of severe speech discrimination problems. He had great difficulty with telephone conversation and did not note improvement in hearing from a hearing aid in either ear because of distortion. *Otologic*: Normal. *Audiologic*: Bilateral loss with no air–bone gap. No abnormal tone decay. *Discrimination score*: Right, 32%; left, 36%. Discrimination was reduced when the intensity of the test material was >80 dB. *Classification*: Bilateral sensory hearing loss. *Diagnosis*: Bilateral Ménière's disease. *Abbreviations*: ANSI, American National Standards Institute; ASA, American Standards Association.

effectiveness of suggested cures. The authors believe that destructive surgery of an ear with Ménière's disease should be performed only as a last resort and, at that, very rarely. Even though discrimination is poor with the residual hearing in the diseased ear, there is always the chance that the other ear may become involved, and thus destructive surgery in the ear first affected could produce a serious handicap. Also, the chance that a specific cure might be found at some future time should be borne in mind and should deter indiscriminate destructive surgery. Vestibular nerve section and endolymphatic sac surgery may be a better option when surgery is warranted, unless the ear is profoundly deaf.

## PROLONGED EXPOSURES TO INTENSE NOISE (OCCUPATIONAL DEAFNESS)

Intense noise can produce hearing loss. If the exposure is brief, such as the effect on the ear of a single pistol shot, explosion, or firecracker, the sudden hearing loss produced is called acoustic trauma. If the exposure is prolonged, over many months and years, and the hearing loss develops gradually, the condition is called occupational industrial hearing loss. Acoustic trauma and occupational hearing loss are specific types of noise-induced hearing loss.

## Two components

Both acoustic trauma and occupational hearing loss have two components: one is the temporary hearing loss (auditory fatigue or TTS) that is of brief duration and clears up, and the other is the permanent hearing loss (or PTS) that remains. When we speak of occupational hearing loss, we really refer to the permanent loss of hearing from prolonged exposure, not the temporary loss.

## Clinical history and findings

The broad aspects of occupational deafness are discussed in detail in Chapter 14 because of the growing importance of the subject and because the physician will be called upon more and more to express an opinion in cases of this type. In this section, the clinical history and findings that the physician encounters in practice are presented.

The pattern of occupational hearing loss is such that physicians generally do not see patients with this complaint until the impairment has become somewhat disturbing in daily communication. This means that the high-frequency hearing loss is advanced and irreversible. These two points indicate the importance of preventing occupational deafness.

Occupational hearing loss generally develops in a well-defined manner. In the very early stage, only the frequencies around 3000, 4000, and 6000 Hz are affected. This is the C-5dip (so called because 4000 Hz corresponds to C-5, or the fifth C, in the normal audiometric testing range seen in the audiogram) (**Figure 10.8**). Note that the 8000 Hz frequency is normal. The fact that hearing at the higher frequencies remains normal is an important distinction from presbycusis, which classically progresses from the higher frequencies to the lower ones. This does not necessarily mean that all cases of dips are due to intense noise exposure; they are not (**Figures 10.42 and 10.43**). Nor does it mean that the hearing loss is not due to noise exposure if the highest frequencies are damaged because as exposure to intense noise continues, the frequencies on either side of 3000, 4000, and 6000 Hz also become affected. The classic course of progressive SNHL caused by noise exposure is illustrated in

**Figure 10.8**. This takes place generally over a period of many years. Susceptible subjects in rare instances may develop some hearing loss after a few months of exposure if the noise is exceptionally intense. There is no valid evidence that noises < 90 dB are responsible for clinically significant hearing losses, even after many years of exposure.

The C-5 dip pattern is the most common, but not the only early finding in noise-induced hearing loss. Exposure to certain types of noise produces the most damage principally in the speech frequencies (**Figure 10.44**). Communication handicaps manifest themselves much earlier in such a case.

The degree and the type of hearing loss depend on numerous factors such as the intensity and the spectral characteristics of the noise and the time relation of the noise (its suddenness), its intermittent or continuous character, the duration of exposure, and the individual's susceptibility to intense noise.

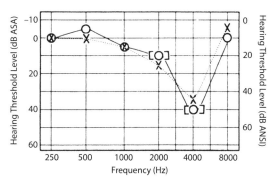

Figure 10.42 *History*: A 40-year-old woman with ringing tinnitus for the past year. No trauma. No noise exposure. The patient denied having had any serious illness or infection. Hearing loss was nonprogressive. *Otologic*: Normal. *Audiologic*: Normal thresholds, except for bilateral C-5 dip. *Classification*: Sensory hearing loss. *Diagnosis*: Unknown but probably viral cochleitis. *Abbreviations*: ANSI, American National Standards Institute; ASA, American Standards Association.

Extensive studies show conclusively that the early damage caused by intense noise takes place in the outer hair cells of the basal turn of the cochlea. The site of damage makes it a sensory hearing loss, and this diagnosis in a given patient is often confirmed by showing the presence of recruitment and diplacusis. As the damage progresses, and the loss exceeds ~50–60 dB, the inner hair cells also become involved, and then the supporting cells become damaged. In some cases, there also appears to be a decrease in the number of nerve fibers supplying the region of hair cell injury. However, clarification of the reason for and clinical significance of this observation requires additional research.

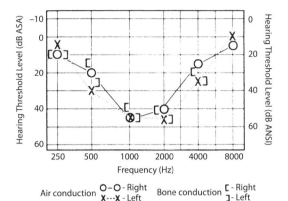

Figure 10.43 *History*: A 50-year-old woman noted gradual hearing loss I year ago. No exposure to intense noise. No vertigo or tinnitus. Hearing loss is progressive. *Otologic*: Normal. *Audiologic*: Hearing loss is chiefly in the speech frequencies, and discrimination also is reduced. *Classification*: Sensorineural hearing loss. *Diagnosis*: Unknown. *Abbreviations*: ANSI, American National Standards Institute; ASA, American Standards Association.

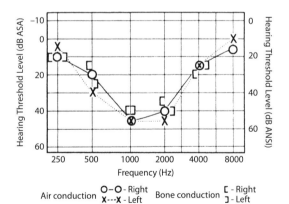

Figure 10.44 *History*: A 48-year-old man employed in a large mill with high noise levels. The noise spectrum is such that the speech frequencies are affected more than the higher frequencies. Fellow employees have similar hearing losses. *Otologic*: Normal. *Audiologic*: Bilateral middle frequency dip with no air–bone gap. There is some evidence of recruitment but no abnormal tone decay. *Classification*: Bilateral sensory hearing loss. *Diagnosis*: Noise-induced hearing loss. *Abbreviations*: ANSI, American National Standards Institute; ASA, American Standards Association.

In advanced cases of occupational hearing loss, it may be difficult to distinguish the portion of the loss caused by noise from the portion that is caused by presbycusis. If, in a specific case, a reasonably good hearing level can be recorded in the frequencies > 8000 Hz, the diagnosis could be noise-induced hearing loss. However, if the threshold level at 8000 Hz is about the same or worse than it is at 4000 Hz, then causes other than noise exposure should be considered, unless the employee was exposed for many years to high-frequency, high-intensity noise such as that from chipping and high-pressure air. Frequencies > 8000 Hz also should be tested.

Because auditory fatigue can be a factor, it is advisable to evaluate the amount of occupational hearing loss present after the employee has been free of exposure to intense noise for at least 14 hours.

Ringing tinnitus is found commonly in acoustic trauma but not very frequently in occupational hearing loss. Slight tinnitus may be present each night but disappears when the auditory fatigue subsides. Vertigo is never caused by long-term occupational noise exposure. If vertigo is present, its true cause should be sought.

Sudden hearing loss is not caused by continuous exposure to occupational noise. If deafness is sudden, and especially if it affects only one ear, another cause should be sought. Military as well as civilian personnel on gun firing duty, where the noise is intense, may experience much TTS after a day's exposure and perhaps some mild PTS, but more serious PTS involving the speech-frequency range occurs only after repeated exposure. When a person is taken out of a noisy environment, his/her hearing improves at least partially. If, after removal from noise, hearing continues to get worse over a period of months or years, other causes should be investigated.

The term "occupational hearing loss" is somewhat misleading. It implies the presence of obvious difficulties in the ability to hear speech. The difficulty more often lies in *understanding* speech rather than in *hearing* it. This results from loss of the hearing in the high frequencies, which is the characteristic finding in occupational hearing loss. As many of the consonants that give meaning to words occur in the higher frequencies, it is natural that people who do not hear these frequencies or hear them feebly should be handicapped in understanding certain speech sounds, especially when they are poorly enunciated or masked by a noisy environment. Some of these speech sounds are s, f, t, z, ch, and k. Therefore, unless one specifically looks for this lack of consonant discrimination, the presence of hearing loss is likely to be overlooked because intense efforts generally are made by the employee to compensate for his/her handicap of reduced discrimination.

## TEMPORARY HEARING LOSS

Although temporary hearing loss (auditory fatigue), or TTS, is included in this section on sensory hearing loss, its true position is not certain. Animal experiments and even some observations in humans indicate that hair cells may not be involved in TTS at nondamaging intensities but that nerve fibers are involved. In human beings, TTS differs in many respects from PTS.

There still is no proof that the relationship is simple. For instance, the hearing of many workers who have sustained some degree of TTS daily for many years nevertheless returns to normal and remains normal. It is also known that it is not possible to predict the sensitivity of an individual to intense noise by determining TTS characteristics, such as its degree or the rapidity of its return to normal. Until more definite and valid information is available, it is safer to consider the relation between TTS and PTS as still unresolved.

The degree of TTS depends largely on the intensity and the duration of the stimulus in addition to the spectral configuration. The rate of recovery from TTS varies greatly in individuals but seems to be about the same in both ears in the same individual. There is some difference of opinion as to how long it takes for TTS to disappear after long exposure to intense noise. The estimates vary from several days to several months, but there is as yet no well-controlled study to establish the facts. **Figure 10.45** describes the recovery studies in an interesting case of TTS occurring principally in the speech frequencies.

## ACOUSTIC TRAUMA

Acoustic trauma, that is, hearing loss caused by a sudden loud noise in one ear, may be produced by firecrackers, cap guns, and firearms, and it is commonly seen in practice. Unless the noise is directed very close to only one ear, the opposite ear also shows a slight hearing loss. In most cases of acoustic trauma, the hearing loss is temporary, lasting only a few hours or days, and the hearing returns to normal. Generally, such patients do not reach the otologist, but if they do, it is interesting to watch the return of hearing by taking follow-up audiograms. In some cases of hearing impairment caused by head trauma and acoustic trauma, two types of hearing loss are present: a temporary loss and a permanent loss. As the hearing levels are

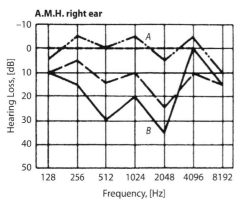
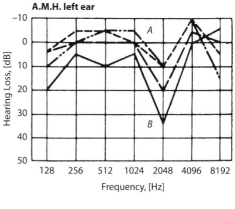
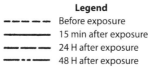

Figure 10.45 Subject was exposed to intense noise of a certain type of jet engine for a long period. The hearing loss (B) returned to its original level (A) after 2 days of rest. During this period, the subject experienced ringing tinnitus, and much distortion with reduced discrimination.

observed over several days, it is noted that the temporary hearing loss disappears, and a considerably reduced hearing loss that is permanent remains.

Usually, when the hearing loss has persisted for many weeks, it will be permanent. Some of these cases have a medicolegal aspect. When the hearing loss exceeds 70 dB and involves the speech frequencies, the auditory nerve fibers as well as the inner ear mechanism undoubtedly are involved in the permanent hearing loss.

In order to differentiate sudden hearing loss due to brief exposure to intense noise from the gradual loss caused by prolonged exposure over many months and years, the term "acoustic trauma" is restricted to the former, and the latter is called industrial or occupational hearing loss.

In acoustic trauma, the patient usually is exposed to a very intense noise of short duration like a rifle shot. This causes immediate hearing loss accompanied by fullness and ringing in the ear. If the cause is an explosion, there may also be a rupture of the eardrum and disruption of the ossicular chain. If this occurs, a conductive hearing loss is caused immediately without much serious sensory damage because the middle ear defect now serves as a protection for the inner ear.

Following acoustic trauma to the inner ear, the patient usually notes that the fullness and the ringing tinnitus subside, and hearing improves. Generally, the hearing returns to normal. Many human beings have been exposed to gunfire at one time or another and have experienced some temporary hearing loss only to have their hearing return to normal. In some cases, however, a degree of permanent hearing loss remains. The amount of loss depends on the intensity and the duration of the noise and the sensitivity of the ear. Usually, the permanent loss is very mild and consists only of a high-frequency dip. If the noise is very intense and the ear is particularly sensitive, the loss may be greater and involve a broader range of frequencies. The milder cases of hearing loss involve only one ear, usually the one closer to the gun or the source of the noise. If the noise is very intense and the hearing loss is moderate, then usually both ears are affected to an almost identical degree or perhaps one ear slightly more than the other. It is hardly possible (as a result of exposure to intense noise) to have a sensory hearing loss in one ear greater than ~50 dB in all frequencies with normal hearing in the other ear. This has important medicolegal aspects.

Because there is almost always some degree of temporary hearing loss or fatigue in acoustic trauma, the amount of permanent damage cannot be established until several months after exposure. In the interim, the individual must be free of other exposure to intense noise that might aggravate the hearing loss. The audiometric patterns in acoustic trauma are similar to those in occupational hearing loss, but the history is different, and probably the manner in which the permanent hearing loss is produced is also different. **Figure 10.46** shows a typical case of acoustic trauma. Note that recruitment is present, it is complete and continuous, and there is no evidence of abnormal tone decay.

| Right | | Left | |
|---|---|---|---|
| 2000 Hz | 4000 Hz | 2000 Hz | 4000 Hz |
| 0 | 55 | 0 | 55 |
| 15 | 65 | 15 | 70 |
| 30 | 70 | 30 | 75 |
| 45 | 75 | 45 | 80 |
| 60 | 75 | 60 | 85 |
| 75 | 80 | 75 | 85 |

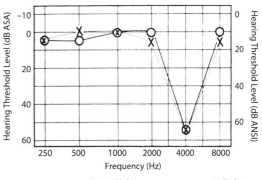

Figure 10.46 *History*: A 9-year-old boy with no clinical symptoms. The hearing defect was detected by the school nurse during routine screening. A year before detection of hearing loss, this child had been exposed to very loud cap pistol fire, immediately producing deafness and ringing tinnitus in both ears. Shortly thereafter, the ringing and the deafness subsided. *Otologic*: Normal. *Audiologic*: The audiogram shows a typical bilateral C-5 dip, characteristic of acoustic trauma. There was no abnormal tone decay. Monaural loudness balance tests show almost complete recruitment. *Abbreviations*: ANSI, American National Standards Institute; ASA, American Standards Association.

After the temporary hearing loss subsides and only permanent loss remains, the hearing level stabilizes, and according to most investigators, there is no further progression in the hearing loss, although recent research has raised questions about this long-held belief (35).

In children, comparatively little information is available concerning the sensitivity of the inner ears of children to loud noises. The infrequency of exposure to noises loud enough to produce acoustic trauma and the difficulty in testing the hearing of young children accurately may account for this paucity of information.

The example of three patients referred by a school nurse within several weeks shows that more attention should be given to the effect of loud noises on the hearing acuity in children. In all three children, permanent hearing defects were produced by inadvertent exposure to cap pistols or firecrackers. The hearing defects were of the inner ear and resembled those encountered among military personnel who have been exposed to gunfire. The loss was in higher frequencies and occurred predominantly in one frequency, the so-called C-5 dip at 4000 Hz. The hearing loss in such cases is not progressive, but once established, it is irreversible. Middle ear damage rarely accompanies this type of inner ear involvement unless the source of the noise is very close to the ear and is of a very intense low frequency (see **Figures 10.46–10.48**). Hearing loss also can be caused by toys (36).

All three patients have been studied closely, and numerous audiograms have been recorded. Repeated hearing tests demonstrated that there was no evidence of progressive hearing loss in any of the youngsters. As might be expected, only the child with substantial bilateral hearing loss presented symptoms of clinical hearing impairment. It is not uncommon to find adults, as well as children, who are completely unaware of even profound unilateral hearing losses if the defects have been present since early childhood. The hearing defects in these three patients were found during the routine testing of 800 schoolchildren.

## DIRECT HEAD TRAUMA

A direct blow to the head can produce hearing loss that may belong to almost any classification.

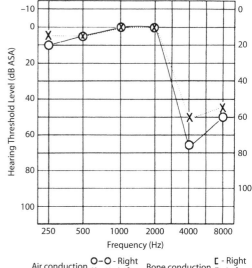

Figure 10.47 *History*: A 16-year-old boy referred because of a slight ringing tinnitus and difficulty in understanding speech in a noisy environment. This difficulty, so typical with high-frequency loss, was aggravated when several people were speaking simultaneously. He also had difficulty in hearing on the telephone. At the age of 6, he had experienced a severe exposure to a cap pistol fire quite close to his ears. Afterwards, he was aware of constant ringing tinnitus and hearing impairment. At the age of 10, his symptoms were aggravated by close exposure to the firing of a 0.22-caliber pistol. *Otologic*: Normal. *Audiologic*: Bilateral C-5 dip with reduced thresholds at 8000 Hz also. This loss is sufficient to produce difficulty in discriminating certain consonants, particularly the sibilants. The difficulty is more pronounced in the presence of ambient noise or speech, caused by the masking effect that these produce on the speech of nearby speakers. *Classification*: Sensory hearing loss. *Diagnosis*: Acoustic trauma. *Abbreviations*: ANSI, American National Standards Institute; ASA, American Standards Association.

To some extent, the type as well as the degree of hearing impairment depends on the severity and the location of the head blow. In general, the harder the blow and the more directly it hits the temporal bone, the more severe the damage and

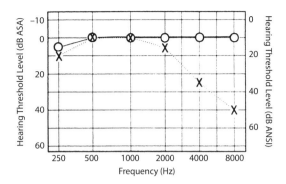

Figure 10.48 *History*: A 12-year-old boy with no clinical symptoms referable to the ears. His hearing defect was detected during the school screening program. Several years prior to his school hearing screen, he experienced sudden hearing loss and ringing tinnitus as a result of the loud report of a cap pistol fired close to his left ear. Both symptoms subsided the same day without recurrence. *Otologic*: Normal. *Audiologic*: Right ear normal. Left ear has a high-frequency loss with recruitment. *Classification*: Sensory hearing loss. *Diagnosis*: Acoustic trauma. *Abbreviations*: ANSI, American National Standards Institute; ASA, American Standards Association.

the more likely it is to involve the sensorineural mechanism. Hearing loss may be present with or without evidence of any fracture in the skull. Dizziness, tinnitus, hearing loss, and even facial paralysis may occur following trauma, often in association with headache, memory loss, lethargy, irritability, and other neurologic complaints. For many years, auditory and vestibular symptoms following trauma were considered psychogenic. However, organic causes for these complaints have been established and accepted for at least the last two decades (37, 38). Following severe head injury, the mechanisms are clear. They include localized middle- or inner ear injury from direct trauma to the ear and temporal bone, labyrinthine concussion, injury to the seventh and eighth neurovascular bundles (ipsilateral or contrecoup), and injury to the brainstem or higher pathways. In cases of severe head injury, isolated auditory and vestibular symptoms are unusual, but severe dizziness and ataxia, inability to discriminate or

process speech signals, tinnitus, and other otologic problems occur frequently in association with other signs and symptoms of neurologic injury. Vestibular symptoms associated with mild head trauma and "inner ear concussion" also are well recognized (39). When neurotologic symptoms occur following minor head trauma, they may be the most prominent posttraumatic complaints, or they may be subtle. Consequently, all patients with symptoms of hearing loss, tinnitus, dizziness, or facial nerve dysfunction following head trauma should undergo comprehensive neurotological evaluation.

Neurotological examination begins with a comprehensive history. The history must include not only information about the ear and otologic complaints but also a complete description of the injury, general medical history, and any other information that might help elucidate true causation.

**The Head Injury**. Teleologically, the ear is an extremely important structure. It is deeply embedded in the head and protected by the otic capsule, the hardest bone in the body. Hearing and balance were critical to the survival of animals and prehistoric humans. Consequently, they are well protected. In general, if the head injury is not severe enough to cause loss of consciousness, it is unlikely to cause significant, measurable hearing loss, although dips in the 3000–6000 Hz range may occur. However, other otologic complaints such as difficulty processing sentences, tinnitus, and dizziness occasionally occur with lesser injuries. The ear is more readily injured by temporal and parietal blows than by those directed at the frontal or occipital bone. Consequently, it is important to determine the exact nature of the injury, the point at which the head was struck, the force of the injury, whether there was rebound or whiplash injury, whether loss of consciousness occurred, and whether there had been any previous episodes of head trauma or otologic symptoms. As hearing loss, dizziness, and tinnitus are often not noticed until a day or more following injury, the time of onset of symptoms seems less helpful than one might expect. However, it is important to establish, especially if symptoms are noticed immediately at the time of the accident (in which case the trauma is the most likely cause) or many weeks after the accident (in which case a posttraumatic etiology is somewhat less likely).

**Longitudinal Temporal Bone Fracture**. A moderate sensorineural type of hearing loss due to direct trauma can occur even without evidence of temporal bone fracture. However, it usually accompanies a longitudinal temporal bone fracture. A sensory hearing impairment may be found in the ear on the side of the head opposite to the side that sustained the injury (contrecoup). The hearing loss has almost the same characteristics as that produced by exposure to intense noise. If the head injury is comparatively mild, only the hair cells of the basilar end of the cochlea are affected, and the effect on the hearing is like that shown in **Figure 10.49**. Note the complete recruitment, which localizes the principal site of the damage to the inner ear. If the injury is more severe, a greater area in the cochlea is affected, and even the nerve itself also may be damaged, with the classification then becoming sensorineural.

**Transverse Fracture of the Temporal Bone**. Another cause of SNHL is transverse fracture of the temporal bone. The fracture line on CT of the temporal bones is perpendicular to the superior petrosal sinus and the long axis of the temporal bone. A severe blow to the back of the head can produce this type of fracture. The accompanying hearing loss is very severe and often is total. It is caused by fracture into the vestibule of the inner ear and destruction of the cochlea. Blood fills these areas and can be seen through an intact eardrum (in contrast with the tom eardrum usually caused by longitudinal fracture).

In many cases, damage to the facial nerve causes a complete facial paralysis, including the forehead on the affected side. Cerebrospinal fluid (CSF) may fill the middle ear and drain out of the eustachian tube (leading to CSF rhinorrhea or postnasal drip), especially if the eardrum is intact. Vertigo and nystagmus invariably are present after a transverse fracture of the temporal bone, and the hearing loss generally is permanent.

A purely neural type of hearing impairment can occur occasionally with transverse fracture of the temporal bone when the fracture includes the internal meatus and crushes the auditory nerve. Generally, facial paralysis is also present but may spontaneously resolve (see **Figure 10.50**).

**Appraising Loss in Claims**. The inner ear is so well protected that a blow to the head must be quite severe to produce hearing loss. When there is evidence of fracture, there is little question about the severity of the blow. However, when there is no visible fracture and hearing loss is present, it may be difficult to determine in some cases whether the hearing loss was caused by the injury or was present previously. In such cases you should remember that if the patient did not exhibit any period of unconsciousness, it is likely that the blow was not of sufficient force to produce cochlear concussion with significant permanent hearing loss. Vertigo and tinnitus usually are associated with a head trauma severe enough to damage hearing, and both of these additional symptoms are likely to persist for a long time after the injury.

It also must be kept in mind that a portion of the conductive and the SNHL resulting from trauma may be reversible and that it is necessary to wait at least several months before appraising the degree of permanent hearing loss.

Cases have been reported in which patients did not become aware of their hearing difficulty until several weeks after the injury, and the impairment seemed to progress. This type of loss is unusual; although it is possible, it is difficult to be certain that the injury is the sole etiology.

**Audiologic Findings**. In the sensory type of hearing defect produced by trauma, audiologic findings reveal continuous and complete recruitment in the frequencies involved. If the speech frequencies are also involved, the discrimination score is reduced, and generally diplacusis is noted. If, in addition to the inner ear, the nerve endings become damaged, recruitment is not quite so prominent and may appear slightly above threshold.

There is no justification for assuming that merely because a patient sustained a head injury, any hearing loss present was caused by the injury. If the deficit is conductive, either there must be evidence of a lesion of the eardrum or the audiologic findings must indicate some ossicular chain damage. The latter can be confirmed very readily by elevating the eardrum and examining the ossicular chain. If the hearing defect is sensory or sensorineural, then the audiologic findings must fit the characteristic patterns that have been established for these types of hearing impairment.

**Figure 10.51** shows a case in which an individual claimed to have a hearing loss as the result of a

JOSEPH SATALOFF, M.D., D.Sc
ROBERT T. SATALOFF, M.D., D.M.A.
JOSEPH R. SPIEGEL, M.D.
1721 PINE STREET • PHILADELPHIA, PA. 19103

## HEARING RECORD

NAME _____ AGE _____

### AIR CONDUCTION

| | | | RIGHT | | | | | | | | LEFT | | | | | | | | |
|---|---|---|---|---|---|---|---|---|---|---|---|---|---|---|---|---|---|---|---|
| DATE | Exam | LEFT MASK | 250 | 500 | 1000 | 2000 | 3000 | 4000 | 6000 | 8000 | RIGHT MASK | 250 | 500 | 1000 | 2000 | 3000 | 4000 | 6000 | 8000 | AUD |
| 1st test | | | -5 | -10 | -5 | 0 | | -10 | | 0 | 85 | 20 | 20 | 15 | 20 | | 35 | | 40 | |
| 8 days | | | | | | | | | | | 85 | 30 | 20 | 30 | 30 | | 30 | | 35 | |
| 38 days | | | | | | | | | | | 85 | 10 | 35 | 15 | 30 | | 20 | | 50 | |
| 2 mos. | | | | | | | | | | | 85 | -5 | 10 | 10 | -10 | | 0 | | 10 | |

### BONE CONDUCTION

| | | | RIGHT | | | | | | | LEFT | | | | | | |
|---|---|---|---|---|---|---|---|---|---|---|---|---|---|---|---|---|
| DATE | Exam | LEFT MASK | 250 | 500 | 1000 | 2000 | 3000 | 4000 | RIGHT MASK | 250 | 500 | 1000 | 2000 | 3000 | 4000 | AUD |
| 1st test | | | | | | | | | 85 | 25 | 20 | 15 | 15 | | 30 | |
| 38 days | | | | | | | | | 85 | 15 | 5 | 10 | 10 | | 40 | |
| 6 mos. | | | | | | | | | 85 | 0 | 0 | 5 | 0 | | 10 | |

### SPEECH RECEPTION THRESHOLD

| DATE | RIGHT | LEFT MASK | LEFT | RIGHT MASK | FREE FIELD | DATE | RIGHT | LEFT MASK | LEFT | RIGHT MASK | FREE FIELD |
|---|---|---|---|---|---|---|---|---|---|---|---|
| | | | | | | | | | | | |

### SPEECH DISCRIMINATION

| | RIGHT | | | | LEFT | | | | | | |
|---|---|---|---|---|---|---|---|---|---|---|---|
| DATE | % SCORE | TEST LEVEL | LIST | LEFT MASK | % SCORE | TEST LEVEL | LIST | RIGHT MASK | FREE FIELD | AIDED | EXAM |
| | | | | | 94 | 50 | | 85 | | | |
| | | | | | 92 | 42 | | 85 | | | |

COMMENTS:

Figure 10.49 *History*: A 30-year-old man fell and struck head 1 week previously. No unconsciousness or vertigo. Fullness and roaring tinnitus in left ear. *Otologic*: Normal. *Audiologic*: Temporary hearing loss with complete recruitment and no tone decay.

| 2000 Hz | |
|---|---|
| R | L |
| 0 | 20 |
| 15 | 30 |
| 30 | 40 |
| 45 | 45 |

*Classification:* Temporary sensory hearing loss. *Diagnosis:* Direct trauma to head. It is difficult to predict whether such a hearing loss will return to normal levels, as in this case, but it may do so if the damage is not severe.

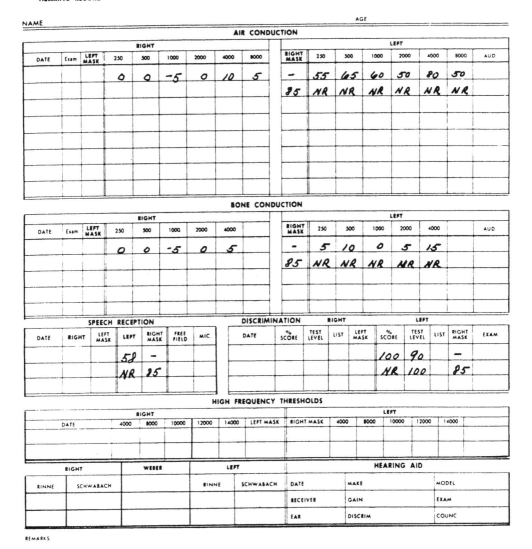

JOSEPH SATALOFF, M.D.
ROBERT THAYER SATALOFF, M.D.
1721 PINE STREET    PHILADELPHIA, PA 19103

**HEARING RECORD**

Figure 10.50 *History*: Sudden onset of hearing loss in the left ear following a fractured skull with unconsciousness coupled with left facial paralysis. X-ray demonstrated a fracture through the left internal auditory meatus. *Otologic*: Normal with no caloric responses. *Audiologic*: Without masking the right ear, there seems to be residual hearing in the left ear by air and bone as well as by speech. When masking is used, the absence of residual hearing in the left ear became apparent. *Classification*: Sensorineural hearing loss. *Diagnosis*: Injury to the left auditory nerve.

head injury. Because this was a total unilateral loss with normal hearing in the other ear, every effort was made to try to explore this case very carefully. After much investigation, it was found that the patient had mumps many years previously and that his hearing difficulty was caused by mumps labyrinthitis and was not due to the injury. After a better understanding was established with the patient, he freely admitted the situation.

Schuknecht crystallized the differential diagnosis of hearing loss due to head injuries (**Table 10.1**). Since then, improved CT techniques have greatly increased the percentage of fractures that can be detected. However, some fractures still cannot be visualized.

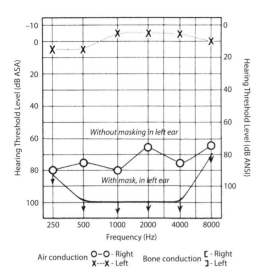

Air conduction O–O - Right / X---X - Left    Bone conduction ⊏ - Right / ⊐ - Left

Figure 10.51 *History*: A 33-year-old man who claimed his right ear went deaf after he hit his head on a pole protruding from a building. There was no head wound or unconsciousness. He denied having vertigo or tinnitus. *Otologic*: Normal with normal caloric responses. *Audiologic*: No response in the right ear with the left ear masked. *Classification*: Unilateral sensorineural hearing loss. *Diagnosis*: Deafness caused by mumps. Established by further detailed history. *Comment*: Such a severe unilateral hearing loss with normal labyrinthine responses is not produced by head injury of this type. *Abbreviations*: ANSI, American National Standards Institute; ASA, American Standards Association.

Table 10.1  Differential clinical findings in hearing loss

| | Labyrinthine concussion | Longitudinal fracture | Transverse fracture |
| --- | --- | --- | --- |
| Bleeding from ear | Never | Very common | Rare |
| Injury to external auditory canal | Never | Occasional | Never |
| Rupture of drum | Never | Very common | Rare—Commonly a hemotympanum |
| Presence of cerebrospinal fluid | Never | Occasional | Occasional |
| Hearing loss | All degrees—Partial to complete recovery | All degrees—Combined type, partial to complete recovery | Profound nerve type—No recovery |
| Vertigo | Occasional—Mild and transient | Occasional—Mild and transient | Severe—Subsides Nystagmus to opposite side |
| Depressed vestibular function | Occasional—Mild | Occasional—Mild | No response |
| Facial nerve injury | Never | 25%—Usually temporary 25%—In squamous and mastoid area | 60%—Often permanent 60%—In occiput in pyramid |

*Source:* Reference (40).

## OTOTOXIC DRUGS

With the increasing use of ototoxic drugs, it is important to ask every patient with SNHL what kind of drugs he/she has taken, particularly in relation to the onset of hearing loss. Certain drugs can produce SNHL when they are used over a long period of time. Among those drugs reported as ototoxic are streptomycin, neomycin, furosemide, gentamicin, quinine, kanamycin, and dozens of others. Sudden hearing loss from these drugs occurs principally in the presence of impaired kidney function. It may also occur from overdosage. **Figures 10.52** and **10.53** provide examples of the severe hearing damage that can result from the improper use of ototoxic drugs. These drugs are very valuable when they are properly used, and they seldom cause hearing damage under such circumstances.

It should be emphasized that the hearing damage usually occurs only after taking the drug systemically for a long period of time. In exceptional cases, such as in patients with renal failure, deafness can result after only a few doses of medication. However, generally the loss is gradual and can be followed audiometrically so that the drug can be stopped before it involves the speech ranges. Ringing tinnitus is a frequently associated symptom and sometimes precedes the hearing loss.

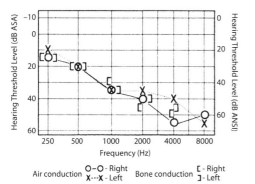

Figure 10.52 *History*: A 10-year-old boy with normal speech and otologic findings. He had a kidney infection and received kanamycin. No progressive hearing loss but has constant ringing tinnitus. *Otologic*: Normal. *Audiologic*: Bilateral downward sloping audiogram with reduced bone conduction. *Diagnosis*: Injudicious use of an ototoxic drug in the presence of kidney dysfunction. *Abbreviations*: ANSI, American National Standards Institute; ASA, American Standards Association.

Streptomycin, now used mostly for tuberculosis or for medical labyrinthectomy, is primarily "vestibulotoxic." It is particularly important to keep this drug in mind, however, because the toxicity is related to the total dose of the drug accumulated over a lifetime rather than over a short course. The early impairment results from damage to the hair

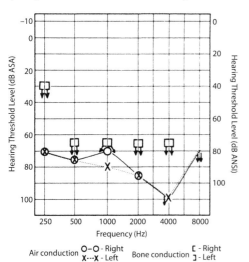

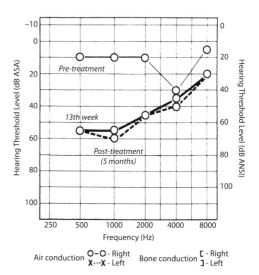

Figure 10.54 *History*: Patient received daily injections of an ototoxic drug for 3 months. His hearing was followed weekly, and in the 13th week, he developed a ringing tinnitus in the right ear, fullness, and hearing loss. The drug was stopped immediately. No vertigo. *Otologic*: Normal. *Audiologic*: Unilateral ascending hearing loss with recruitment and diplacusis. *Classification*: Sensory hearing loss. *Diagnosis*: Cochlear hearing loss from ototoxic drug exposure. *Abbreviations*: ANSI, American National Standards Institute; ASA, American Standards Association.

cells in the inner ear. A classic example of this is described in **Figure 10.54**. Most of the time, hearing loss caused by drug ototoxicity is permanent, but it is not progressive. The hearing loss can occur without any vertigo, ringing tinnitus, or other symptoms.

Numerous other drugs and agents may be ototoxic. At least 200 ototoxic agents have been reported. Some of these are listed in **Table 10.2**.

Figure 10.53 *History*: A 49-year-old man who received kanamycin injections daily for 4 weeks because of acute renal failure. Patient claims normal hearing before these injections. *Otologic*: Normal caloric responses. *Audiologic*: Severe to profound bilateral loss with no air–bone gap. No response to speech tests, except for experiencing great discomfort when speech was presented at levels >100 dB (low threshold of discomfort, an indication of recruitment). *Classification*: Sensorineural hearing loss. *Diagnosis*: Deafness caused by ototoxic effects of kanamycin. *Abbreviations*: ANSI, American National Standards Institute; ASA, American Standards Association.

# SENSORY HEARING LOSS AFTER EAR SURGERY

The increase in stapedectomies and stapedotomies for otosclerosis has focused attention on the sensorineural damage and hearing loss that may be associated with opening the vestibule of the labyrinth, as discussed earlier in this chapter.

## Mastoidectomy

Prior to the advent of stapedectomy, the oval window area and the vestibule of the inner ear were considered to be inviolable, and extreme caution was exercised to avoid disturbing the footplate during mastoid surgery. Despite this caution, surgical accidents did occur, and hearing often was lost totally in the operated ear during mastoidectomy procedures in which the oval window inadvertently was penetrated. Sometimes the deafness occurred long after surgery because of ear infection and cholesteatoma. Partial deafness from toxic labyrinthitis is still observed in chronic mastoiditis even when no surgery has been performed.

Table 10.2  Ototoxic agents

| | |
|---|---|
| Accutane capsules (D, T) | Azulfidine tablets, EN-tabs, oral suspension (T, V) |
| Acetazolamide | Bactrim DS tablets* (T, V) |
| Actifed w /Codeine cough syrup (D, T, V) | Bactrim 1-V infusion* (T, V) |
| Adipex-P tablets and caplets (D) | Bactrim* (T, V) |
| Aeroffiid inhaler syrup (D, V) | Bayer-Children's chewable aspirin (T) |
| Alcohol | Bayer-Aspirin tablets and caplets (T) |
| Aldactazide* (D, T) | Bayer Plus aspirin tablets (T) |
| Aldoclor tablets (D, T) | Therapy Bayer aspirin caplets (T) |
| Aldomet ester HCI injection (D) | 8-h Bayer timed-release aspirin, BC powder (T) |
| Aldomet oral (D) | Bleomycin |
| Aldoril tablets (D, T) | Blocarden tablets (T, V) |
| Alfenta injection* (D) | Brethaire inhaler (V) |
| Alferon-N injection (D, T) | Brerylol injection (V) |
| Altace caplets (D, T, V) | Bumetanide |
| Alurate elixir (D) | Bumex (V) |
| Arnicar syrup, tablets and injection* (D, T) | BuSpar (T) |
| Arnikacin sulfate | Butazolidin capsules and tablets (T) |
| Arnikin injection | Cama arthritis pain reliever (T) |
| Amocil* (D) | Capastat sulfate vials (~11%) (T, V) |
| Amphotericin B | Capozide (V) |
| Ampicillin | Capreomycin sulfate |
| Anafranil caplets (D, V) | Carafate tablets (V) |
| Ana-Kit Anaphylaxis Emergency Treatment Kit (D) | Carbocaine (T) |
| Anaprox/ Anaprox DST (D, T, V) | Carbon monoxide |
| Anaproxen sodium | Cardene capsules (T, V) |
| Ancobon capsules | Cardizem SR capsules* 60 mg, 90 mg, 120 mg (T) |
| Anestacon solution (D, T) | Cardura tablets (T, V) |
| Anexsia 5/500 tablets (D) | Cartrol tablets (T) |
| Anexsia 7.5/650 tabs (D) | Celestone soluspan suspension* (V) |
| Aniline dyes | Children's Advil suspension (T) |
| Ansaid tablets (D, T) | |

(Continued)

Table 10.2 (Continued) Ototoxic agents

| | |
|---|---|
| Apresazide capsules (D, V) | Chloramphenicol sodium succinate |
| Apresoline-Esidrix tablets (D, V) | Chlordiazepoxide |
| Apresoline HCl parenteral (D) | Chloroform |
| Apresoline HCl tablets (D) | Chloroquine phosphate |
| Arthritis strength bufferin analgesic capsules | Cholybar* (T, V) |
| Arthritis strength BC powder (T) | Cibalith-S (T, V) |
| Aristocort suspension (V) | Cipro 1-V (T) |
| Aristospan suspension* (V) | Cipro tablets (T) |
| Arsenic | cis-Platinum |
| Asendin tablets (D, T) | Clinoril tablets (T, V) |
| Ascriptin A/D capsules (T) | Colestid granules* (V) |
| Aspirin (T) | Colistin sulfate |
| Atgam sterile solution (D) | Coly-Mycin* (V) |
| Ativan injection (D) | Coly-Mycin M Parenteral colyte* (V) |
| Azactam for injection (T, V) | Combipres tablets (V) |
| Azo Gantanol tablets* (T, V) | Corgard tablets (T) |
| Azo Gantrisin tablets Jenest-28 tabs (D, V, T) | Cortenema* (V) |
| Cortisporin cream | Easpirin (T. V) |
| Cortisporin ointment | Ecotrin (T) |
| Cortisporin otic suspension sterile | Edecrin (T, V) |
| Cortone acetate sterile suspension (V) | E.E.S. (V) |
| Cortone acetaete tablets (V) | Elavil (T) |
| Corzide tablets (T, V) | Eldepryl (T, V) |
| Cuprimine capsules (T) | Emcyt capsules* (T) |
| Cyclosporine | Eminase* (V) |
| Cytotec (T) | Empirin with codeine phophate (T) |
| Dalaone D.P. injectable (V) | E-Mycin tablets |
| Dalgan injection (T, V) | Enalapril |
| Dapsone USP* (T, V) | Endep tablets (T) |
| Decadron elixir (V) | Enduron tablets* (V) |
| Decadron-LA sterile solution (V) | Enduronyl (V) |
| Decadron phosphate injection (V) | Engerix-B Unit-dose vials (V) |
| Decadron phosphate respihaler (V) | Enovid |
| Decadron phosphate turbinaire (V) | Equagcsic tablets (T, V) |
| Decadron phosphate w /Xylocaine injection, sterile (V) | EryPed (V) |
| | Ery-tab tablets (V) |
| Decadron tablets (V) | Erythrocin stearate filmtab (V) |
| Deconamine (T, V) | Erythromycin |
| Deferoxamine mesylate | Erythromycin base filmtab (V) |
| Deltasone tablets* (V) | Erythromycin delayed-release capsules, USP (V) |
| Depen Titratable tablets (T) | |
| Depo-Medrol sterile aqueous suspension (V) | Esidrix tablets* (V) |
| Deprol tablets (V) | Esimil tablets* (V) |
| Desferal vials (T) | Eskalith (ethmozin tablets, <2%) (T, V) |
| Desyrel and Desyrel Dividose (T, V) | Ethracrynic acid |
| Diamox parenteral (T) | Etretinate |

(Continued)

Table 10.2 (Continued)

| | |
|---|---|
| Diamox sequels (T) | Etrafon (T) |
| Diamox tablets (T) | Fansidar tablets* (T, V) |
| Dibekacin | Feldene capsules* (V. T) |
| Dihydrostreptomycin | Fenoprofen calcium |
| Dilantin w /Phenobarbital kapseals (V) | Fiorinal w /Codeine capsules (T, V) |
| Dipentum capsules* (V) | Flagry I-V (V) |
| Diptheria and tetanus toxoids and pertussis vaccine adsorbed USP (pediatric use) | Flagyl tablets (V) |
| | Flexeril tablets (T. V) |
| Diprivan injection (T) | Floxin tablets (V) |
| Disalcid (T, V) | Flucytosine |
| Ditropan | Fluorocitrate |
| Diucardin tablets* (V) | Fungizone intravenous (T. V) |
| Diulo* (V) | Furosemide |
| Diunces tablets (V) | Ganite injection (T) |
| Diuril oral suspension* (V) | Gantanol* (T. V) |
| Diuril sodium intravenous* (V) | Gantrisin ophthalmic ointment/ solution* (T. V) |
| Diuril tablets* (V) | |
| Dolobid tablets (V, T) | Ganrisin* (T. V) |
| Duragesic transdermal system (V) | Garamycin injectable (T. V) |
| Duranest injections (T) | Gentamycin |
| Dyazide capsules* (V) | Gold |
| Dyclone 0.5% and I% topical solutions, USP (T) | Halcion tablets (T) |
| Haldol deconate (V) | Kwell cream (D) |
| Haldol injection, tablets and concentrate (V) | Kwelllotion (D) |
| Habistate | Kwell shampoo (D) |
| Harmonyl tablets | Lanoxicaps (D) |
| Hexadimethrine bromide | Lanoxin injection pediatric (D) |
| Hedadin | Lanoxin tablets (D) |
| Hexalen capsules (V) | Lariam tablets (D, T, V) |
| Hibiclens antimicrobial skin cleanser | Larodopa tablets (D) |
| Hydeltrasol injection, sterile (V) | Lasix oral solution and intravenous |
| Hydeltra-T.B.A. sterile suspension (V) | Lead |
| Hydrocortone acetate sterile suspension (V) | Legain (T) |
| Hydroconone phosphate inj., sterile (V) | Leuprolide acetate |
| Hydroconone tablets (V) | Levatol (D) |
| Hydrodiuril tablets* (V) | Levien/Tri-Levlen (D) |
| Hydromox tablets (V) | Levsin/Levsinex* (D) |
| Hydromox R tablets (V) | Levo-Dromoran* (D) |
| Hydropres tablets (V) | Limbitrol (D) |
| Hylorel tablets | Lincocin* (T, V) |
| Hyperstat 1-V injection (T, V) | Lioresal tablets (D. T) |
| Hytrin tablets (T, V) | Lithane tablets (D, T, V) |
| Ibuprofen | Lithium Carbonate capsules and tablets (D. T, V) |
| Ilosone (T) | |
| Inderide tablets (V) | Lithobid tablets (D, T, V) |
| Interide LA long-acting capsules (V) | Lodine capsules (D, T) |

(Continued)

Table 10.2 (Continued) Ototoxic agents

| | |
|---|---|
| Indocin (T, V) | Loestrin (D) |
| Intal capsules* (V) | Lomotil (D) |
| Intal inhaler* (V) | Lopid capsules and tablets (D, V) |
| Interferon alfa-26 | Lopressor ampuls (D, T, V) |
| Intron A (T, V) | Lopressor HCT tablets (D, T, V) |
| Iodofonn chemicals | Lopressor tablets (D, T, V) |
| ISOMOTIC (V) | Lorazepam |
| Isoptin injectable (V) | Lorelco tablets* (D, T) |
| Jenest-28 tablets (D) | Lonab ASA tablets (D) |
| Kanamycin | Lonab (D) |
| Keftex Pulvules/Oral suspension | Lotensin tablets (D) |
| Keftab tablets (D) | Loxitane (D) |
| Kemadrin* (D) | Lozol tablets (D, V) |
| Kefurox vials, faspak and ADD-vantage (D) | Ludiomil tablets (D, T) |
| Kenalog-1 0 injections (V) | Lupron Depot 7.5 mg (D) |
| Kenalog-40 injections (V) | Lupron injection (<5%) (D) |
| Kerlone tables (>2%) (D, T) | Lysodren (D, V) |
| Ketalar | Macrodantin capsules (D. V) |
| Klonopin (V) | Mandelamine |
| Klorves effervescent tablets | Mannitol |
| Klorves effervescent granules | Marax tablets and DF syrup (V) |
| Klorves effervescent 10% liquid | Marcaine Hydrochloride 0.5% |
| K-Phos M.F. tablets (D) | w /epinephrine (D, T) |
| K-Phos neutral tablets (D) | Marcaine Hydrochloride w /epinephrine (D, T) |
| K-Phos Original Fonnula 'Sodium Free' | Marcaine spinal (D, T) |
| tablets (D) | Marinol (Dronabinol) capsules (D) |
| K-Phos No. 2 tablets (D) | Marplan tablets (D. V) |
| Matulane capsules (0) | Naprosyn (D, T, V) |
| Maxair inhaler (D) | Naprosyn suspension (D) |
| Maxzide* (D, V) | Naproxen |
| Mebaral tablets (D) | Nardil (D) |
| Meclomen capsules* (D, T) | Naturetin tablets* (D, V) |
| Medrol* (D. V) | Nebcin vials, hyporeis and ADD-vantage |
| Mefenamic acid | (D, T, V) |
| Menrium tablets (D) | NebuPent for inhalation solution (D, V) |
| Mepergan injection (D) | NegGram* (D, V) |
| Mephobamate | Nembutal sodium capsules (D, V) |
| Mercury | Nembutal sodium solution (D, V) |
| Mesantonin tablets (D) | Nembutal sodium suppositories (D, V) |
| Methadone hydrochloride diskets (D) | NeoDecadron topical cream (D) |
| Methergine* (T) | Neomycin |
| Methadone Hydrochloride oral | Neosporin cream |
| solution/tablets (D, T) | Neosporin G.U. irrigant sterile |
| Methotrexate tablets, parenteral, LPF (D) | Neptazane tablets (V) |
| Mevacor tablets (D) | Nescaine/Nescaine MPF* (D, T) |
| Mexitil capsules (D, T) | Netilmicin sulfate |

(Continued)

Table 10.2  (Continued)

| | |
|---|---|
| Micronor tablets (D) | Netromycin injection 100 mg/mL (D, T, V) |
| Midamor tablets (D, T, V) | Nicorette (D, T) |
| Miltown tablets (D, V) | Nipride I.V. infusion (D, T) |
| Minipress capsules* (D, T, V) | Nitro-Bid ointment (D) |
| Minizide capsules* (D, T, V) | Nitrogen mustard |
| Minocin intravenous* (D, V) | Nitrostat tablets* (D, V) |
| Minocin oral suspension* (D, V) | Nizoral tablets* (D, V) |
| Minocin pellet-filled capsules* (D, V) | Norethin (D) |
| Minocyline hydrochloride | Norgesic (D) |
| Mintezol (D, T) | Norinyl (D) |
| Misonidazole | Norisodrine aerotrol (V) |
| M-M-R (D) vaccine | Normodyne injection (D, V) |
| M-R-V-A-X (D) vaccine | Normodyne tablets (D, V) |
| Mobran tablets and concentrate | Normozide tablets (D, V) |
| Modicon (D) | Noroxin tablets (D) |
| Moduretic tablets (D, T, V) | Norpramin tablets (D, T) |
| Mono-Gesic tablets (T, V) | Norzine (D, T) |
| Monopril tablets (D) | Novafed A capsules (D) |
| Motofen tablets (D) | Novafed capsules (D) |
| Motrin tablets (D, T) | Novahistine DH (D) |
| Morphine sulfate Contin tablets (D) | Novahistine DMX (D) |
| MSIR (D) | Novahistine elixir (D) |
| Mumpsvax | Novahistine expectorant (D) |
| Mustargen (T, V) | Novocain hydrochloride for spinal |
| Myambutol tablets (D) | anesthesia (D) |
| Mykrox 2 mg tablets (D, T) | Nubain injection (D, V) |
| Myochrysine injection (D) | Ogen* (D) |
| Mysoline (occasional) (V) | OMIU |
| Naldecon syrup, tablets, pediatric | Omnipaque (D. T, V) |
| drops/syrup (D) | Optimine tablets (D, T, V) |
| Nalfon pulvules and tablets (D. T) | OptiPranolol sterile ophthalmic |
| Naphcon A Ophthalmic solution (D) | solution (D) |
| Oramorph SR (morphine sulfate sustained | Placidyl capsules (D) |
| release tabs) (D) | Plaquenil sulfate tablets (D, T, V) |
| Orap tablets (D) | Platinol (T) |
| Oretic tablets* (D, V) | Platinol-AQ injection (T) |
| Oreticyl* (D, V) | Plendil extended-release tablets |
| Ornade spansule capsules (D, T, V) | PMB 200 and PMB 400 (D, T) |
| Ornex* (D) | Pilocarpine |
| Opiates | Polaramine (D, T, V) |
| Orthoclone OKT3 sterile solution | Polymyxin B Bulfatel, aerosporin brand |
| Ortho novum (D) | sterile powder (D) |
| Orudis capsules (D, T, V) | Polymyxin B Sulfate |
| OSM GIYN | Pondimin tablets (D) |
| Ovcon (D) | Ponstel (D) |

Table 10.2 (Continued) Ototoxic agents

| | |
|---|---|
| P-A-C analgesic tablets* (T) | Pontocaine hydrochloride for spinal |
| Pamelor (D, T) | anesthesia (D, T) |
| Papaverine HCl vials/ampoules* (V) | Potassium bromate |
| Paradione capsules* (V) | Practolol |
| Paraplatin for injection | Prilu* (D) |
| Parlodel (D, V) | Prilosec delayed-release capsules (D, T, V) |
| Parmade tablets* (D, T) | Primaxin I.M. (D, T, V) |
| Pavabid capsules* (V) | Primaxin I.V. (D, T, V) |
| Pavabid HP capsulets* (V) | Prinivil tablets (D, V) |
| PBZ tablets and elixir (D, T, V) | Prinzide tablets (D, T, V) |
| PBZ SR tablets (D, T, V) | Pro-Banthine tablets (D) |
| PCE dispertab tablets (D, V) | Procan SR tablets (D) |
| Pediapred oral liquid* (D, V) | Procarbazine hydrochloride |
| PediaProfen suspension (D, T) | Procardia XL tablets (D, T, V) |
| Pediazole (T, V) | Procit for injection (D) |
| PediOptic suspension sterile | Pronestyl capsules/tablets* (D) |
| Pedvax HIB ampoules | Pronestyl injections* (D) |
| Peganone tablets (D) | Propagest* (D) |
| Pentam 300 injection (D) | Propylthrouracil |
| Pepcide (D, T, V) | ProSom tablets (D, T) |
| Pepto-Bismol liquid and tablets* (T) | Protopam* (D) |
| Percodan* (D) | Protostat tablets (D, V) |
| Periactin (D, T, V) | Proventil inhalation aerosol (D, T, V) |
| Permax tablets (D, T, V) | Proventil repetables tablets (D, T, V) |
| Pfizerpen-AS aqueous suspension (V) | Proventil syrup (D, V) |
| Phenergan w/Codeine (D, T) | Proventil tablets (D, V) |
| Phenergan VC w/Codeine (D, T) | Prozac pulvules (D, T, V) |
| Phenergan w /Dextromethorphan (D, T) | Quadrinal tablets (D) |
| Phenergan suppositories (D) | Quarzan capsules (D) |
| Phenergan syrup (D) | Questran light* (D, T, V) |
| Phenergan VC (D, T) | Questran powder* (D, T, V) |
| Phenergan VC w/codeine (D, T) | Quibron capsules (D) |
| Phentobarbital | Quibron-T (D) |
| Phenobarbital elixir and tablets (D, V) | Quibron-T /SR |
| Phenylbutazone | Quinaglute dura-tabs tablets (T, V) |
| Phenurone tablets* (D, V) | Quinarnm tablets (T, V) |
| Pipracil* (D) | Quinidex extentabls (D, T, V) |
| Pitressin synthetic ampoules* (V) | Quinidine |
| Quinine | Serax capsules (V) |
| Q-vel muscle relaxant pain reliever (T) | Serax tablets (V) |
| Raudixin tablets (D) | Seromycin pulvules (V) |
| Rauzide tablets (D, V) | Serpasil tablets (D, V) |
| Recombivax HB (T) | Serapsil apresoline tablets (D, V) |
| Reglan (D) | Serpasil esidrix tablets (D. V) |
| Renese (D. V) | Silvadine cream 1% |
| Renese-R tablets (D. V) | Sinemet tablets (D) |
| Restoril capsules (D) | Sinemet CR tablets (D) |

(Continued)

Table 10.2  (Continued)

| | |
|---|---|
| Retrovir capsules (D. V) | Sinequan (T) |
| Retrovir L.V. infusion (D, V) | Slo-Bid gyrocaps (D) |
| Retrovir syrup (D. V) | Solu-Cortef sterile powder* (V) |
| Rheumatrex methotrexate dose pack (D, T) | Solu-Medrol sterile power* (V) |
| Rifadin (D) | Soma compound w /codeine tablets (D. T, V) |
| Rifamate capsules (D) | Soma compound (D, T, V) |
| Rimactane capsules (D) | Soma tablets (D, V) |
| Robaxin injectable (D. V) | Stadol (V) |
| Robinul Forte tablets (D) | Streptomycin |
| Robinul injectable (D) | Stricknine |
| Robinul tablets (D) | Sulfasalazine |
| Roferon-A injection (D. V) | Sulfisoxagole/Phenazopgridine |
| Rogaine topical solution (D. V) | Sulindac |
| Rondec (D) | Surital ampoules steri-vials (D) |
| Rondec-DM (D) | Surmontil capsules (D. T) |
| Rondec-TR tablets (D) | Symmetrel capsules and syrup (D) |
| Roxanol (D) | Syntocinon nasal spray (D) |
| Roxicodone tablets, oral solution and | T-PHYL (Uniphyl) 200 mg tablets (D) |
|   intensol (D) | Tacaryl* (D. T) |
| Rufen tablets (D. T) | Talacen (T) |
| Ru-Tuss II capsules (D, T, V) | Talwin compound (D, T) |
| Ru-Tuss DE tablets (T) | Talwin injection (D. T) |
| Ru-Tuss w /Hydrocone (D, T) | Talwin Nx (D, T) |
| Rhythmol tablets (T, V) | Tambocor tablets (D, T, V) |
| Salfex (D. T, V) | Tapazole tablets (D, V) |
| Saluron* (D, V) | Tavist syrup (D, T, V) |
| Salutensin/Salutensin-Derni (D. V) | Tavist-D tablets (D, T, V) |
| Sandimmune (T, V) | Tavist tablets (D. T, V) |
| Sandostatin injection ( < 1%) (D, V) | Tegison capsules (D) |
| Scopolamine | Tegral-D (D) |
| Seconal sodium pulvules (D, V) | Tegretol chewable tablets (D, T) |
| Sectral capsules (D) | Tegretol suspension (D, T) |
| Sedapap tablets 50 mg/650 mg (D) | Tegretol suspension (D. T) |
| Salicylates | Tegretol tablets (D, T) |
| Salsalate | Temaril tablets, syrup. spansule sustained |
| Sensorcaine (D, T) |   release capsules* (D. T) |
| Sensorcaine-MPF spinal (D. T) | Tenex tablets (D. T, V) |
| Septra* (D, T, V) | Tenoretic tablets (D. V) |
| Septra I.V. infusion* (D. T, V) | Tenormin tablets and I-V injection (D, V) |
| Septra I.V. infusion ADD-Vantage viats• | Tetanus antitoxin |
|   (D. T, V) | Thalidomide |
| Ser-Ap-Es tablets (D. V) | Thalitone tablets* (D, V) |
| Thera-Gesic* (T) | Vancocin HCI, vials & ADD-Vantage |
| Thiosulfil forte tablets* (T, V) |   (D,T, V) |
| Thorazine (D) | Vancomycin hydrochloride |
| Tigan (D) | Vascor tablets (D, T, V) |

Table 10.2 (Continued) Ototoxic agents

| | |
|---|---|
| Timolide tablets (D, T, V) | Vaseretic tablets (D, T, V) |
| Timoptic in ocudose (D, T. V) | Vasotec I.V. (D, T, V) |
| Timoptic sterile ophthalmic solution (D, T, V) | Vasotec tablets (D, T) |
| Tobramycin | Velban vials (D) |
| Tocainide | Ventolin (D, V) |
| Tofranil ampuls (D, T) | Verelan capsules (D) |
| Tofranil tablets (D, T) | Versed injection (D) |
| Tofranii-PM capsules (D, T) | Vicodin tablets (D) |
| Tolectin (200, 400, 600 mg)* (D. T) | Vicodin ES tablets (D) |
| Tolinase tablets* (D. V) | Vira-A for injection (D) |
| Tonocard tablets (D. T, V) | Visken tablets (D) |
| Toradol IM injection (D, V) | Vivacil tablets (D, T) |
| Torecan (D, T) | Voltaren tablets (D, T) |
| Trancopal capsules (D) | Vontrol tablets (D) |
| Trandate tablets (D. V) | Wellbutrin tablets (D, T, V) |
| Transdern scop transdermal therapeutic system (D) | Wygesic tablets (D) |
| Tranxene (D) | Xanax tablets (D, T) |
| Trecator-SC tablets* (D, V) | Xanax injections |
| Trental (D) | Xylocaine 2% jelly (D, T) |
| Trexan tablets (D, T) | Xylocaine 5% ointment (D, T) |
| Triaminic cold tablets (D, V) | Xylocaine 10% oral spray (D, T) |
| Triaminic-DM syrup (D, V) | Xylocaine injections for ventricular arrhythmias (D, T) |
| Triaminic expectorant DH (D, T) | |
| Triaminic oral infant drops (D, T, V) | 4% Xylocaine-MPF sterile solution (D, T) |
| Triaminic repetabs tablets (D) | |
| Triaminic syrup (D) | Xylocaine 2% viscous solution (D) |
| Triaminicol multi-symptom relief (D) | Yodoxin* (V) |
| Triavil tablets (D, T) | Yohimex tablets (D) |
| Tridione* (V) | Zantac (D, V) |
| Trilifon (D) | Zantac injection/Zantac injection premixed (D, V) |
| Trilisate (D, T) | |
| Tri-Norinyl 28-days tablets (D) | Zarontin syrup (D, V) |
| Tussionex extended-release suspension (D) | Zaroxolyn tablets* (D, V) |
| Tylox capsules (D) | Zestril tablets (D, V) |
| Uricholine* (D) | Zestroetic capsules (D) |
| Urised* (D) | Zidone capsules* (D) |
| Uroqid-acid (D) | Zidovudine |
| Ursinus inlay-tabls* (D. T) | Zinacef |
| Valium injectable (V) | Zorontin capsules |
| Valium tablets (V) | Zorprin tablets (T) |
| Valpin-50 tablets Valrelease capsules (D) | Zovirax (D) |
| Vancocin HCI, oral solution and pulvules (D. T, V) | Zovirax steril powder (D) |
| | Zydone capsules (D) |
| | Zyloprim tablets (D, T, V) |

Note: All medications listed have been reported as associated with hearing impairment except those with an asterisk (*), in the table D denotes dizziness, V denotes vertigo, and T denotes tinnitus.

# SIMPLE STAPES MOBILIZATION SURGERY

SNHL is a rare complication of the procedure, but such instances occur in ~0.1% of cases (**Figure 10.55**). The cause still is not established, but the symptoms associated with the deafness typically are highly suggestive of a viral labyrinthitis. Such complications are more common after stapedectomy, and they have occurred also after fenestration surgery. Because of the relatively low complication rate and despite the approximately 50% failure rate, some surgeons still advocate offering patients the option of stapes mobilization (40).

# STAPEDECTOMY

With more frequent surgical entry into the vestibule during stapedectomy, the incidence of sensory and SNHL has increased markedly as a complication. It has been estimated that after stapedectomy ~1 or 2% of patients will experience either immediate or delayed severe SNHL in the operated ear. Some cautious observers feel that in almost every case in which the footplate is removed or fractured, some degree of temporary sensorineural damage occurs. In most cases in which the surgeon is meticulous and avoids getting blood into the vestibule or suctioning out perilymph, there are minimal sensorineural damage and few clinical symptoms. Yet even some of these patients are known to complain of mild fullness in the ear and very slight imbalance along with a minimal ringing tinnitus.

Occasionally, after stapedectomy there is measurable damage to the inner ear. Generally, the effect is temporary, but sometimes there is permanent high-frequency hearing loss associated with recruitment, impaired discrimination, and lowered threshold of discomfort for intense noise. **Figure 10.56** shows these findings.

Another disturbing complication of stapedectomy is seen in patients who had had excellent results and then suddenly, sometimes many months after the original surgery, lose practically all their hearing in the operated ear. In most cases, this loss is permanent. The causes for this and other sensorineural complications of stapedectomy surgery are not yet entirely understood. Occasionally, there is a fibrous tissue filling the entire vestibule and completely blocking off the cochlea. In other cases of this type of delayed permanent, severe deafness, the vestibule is found to have a normal appearance, and the perilymph also is normal. The cause for the cochlear damage in such cases is still unknown. In other cases, oval window granuloma or perilymph fistula may be the cause.

## Discrimination

It is apparent, however, that one should not measure the success of stapes surgery solely by threshold hearing tests. Some patients have excellent pure-tone thresholds, but their discrimination is reduced by the surgery, and their distortion can be distracting. With improving techniques and better training for stapes surgery, the incidence and the severity of sensorineural complications can be reduced steadily.

## Cases of tympanosclerosis

The dangers of surgery in these cases also are better recognized. When patients with this disease are operated on to restore hearing, and the stapes footplate is removed in the presence of tympanosclerotic changes in the middle ear, the incidence of severe sensorineural hearing impairment is very high. Many surgeons complete this procedure in two stages or even avoid doing it altogether because of the frequency of complications that occur when the oval window is opened in the presence of this disease.

# EARLY PRESBYCUSIS AND GENETIC HEARING LOSS

For want of a better explanation, a high-frequency hearing loss occasionally encountered is called early or premature presbycusis if it occurs between the ages of ~30 and 50.

Clinically, this condition is easy to overlook, but the audiogram shows a progressive hearing impairment in the high tones, which may be associated with a high-pitched tinnitus and no other symptoms. The pathological explanation generally subscribed to today is that the hair cells degenerate because of some hereditary tendency and that the syndrome is not related to metabolism or infection. In general, the loss is slowly progressive and eventually causes difficulty in discrimination as the speech frequencies become involved.

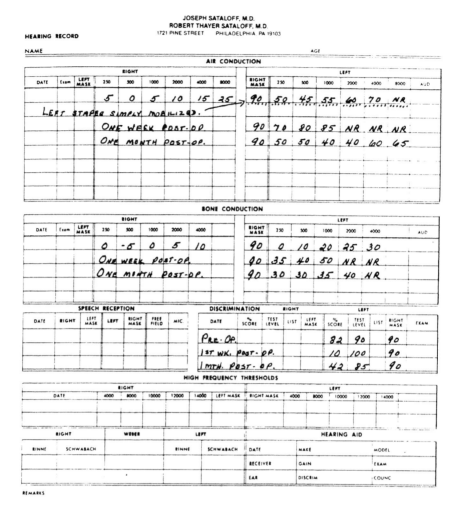

JOSEPH SATALOFF, M.D.
ROBERT THAYER SATALOFF, M.D.
1721 PINE STREET    PHILADELPHIA PA 19103

Figure 10.55 *History*: A 26-year-old women with a diagnosis of otosclerosis. Operative notes indicate that the left stapes was mobilized merely by pressure on the end of the incus. No footplate manipulation was performed. Several days postoperatively, the patient developed vertigo, roaring tinnitus, fullness, and deafness in the left ear. Loud noises bothered her left ear. *Otologic*: Healed incision. *Audiologic*: Preoperative left-ear thresholds revealed a moderate-to-severe air conduction loss. Bone thresholds were normal in the low frequencies and dropped off between 1000 and 4000 Hz. The discrimination score was 82%. Postoperative thresholds revealed a great reduction in air and bone thresholds as well as reduced discrimination. For many months postoperatively, there were hyperrecruitment, diplacusis, and lowered thresholds of discomfort. Some of these symptoms have gradually subsided. *Classification*: Conductive followed by sensorineural hearing loss. *Diagnosis*: Postoperative labyrinthosis following stapes mobilization.

| 1000 Hz | |
|---|---|
| R | L |
| 5 | 35 |
| 20 | 65 |
| 35 | 70 |
| 50 | 75 |
| 65 | 80 |
| 80 | 80 |

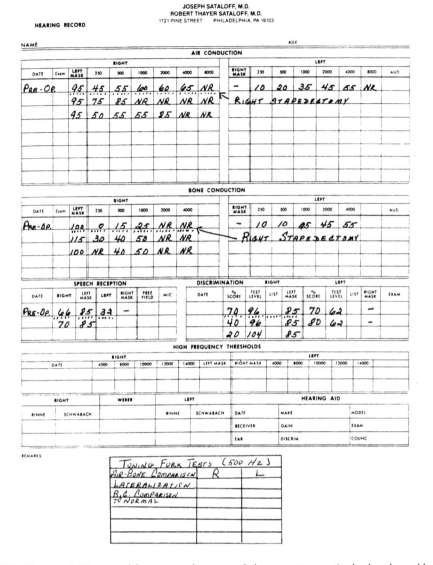

Figure 10.56 *History*: A 45-year-old woman who several days postoperatively developed hearing loss, vertigo, and nausea. There was a roaring tinnitus in the right ear. *Otologic*: Normal. *Audiologic*: Preoperative low-frequency air–bone gap in the right ear with fair discrimination. Thresholds immediately postoperatively revealed a severe reduction in air and bone conduction thresholds. Three months later, thresholds improved, but there were complete recruitment, diplacusis, distortion, and reduced discrimination. There was a lowered threshold of discomfort (loud noises were very annoying). *Classification*: Sensory hearing loss. *Diagnosis*: Postoperative labyrinthosis.

When the high-frequency losses are accompanied by recurrent attacks of rotary vertigo, especially when there is tinnitus of some sort, the diagnosis may be atypical Ménière's disease. Actually, it is not certain that this atypical picture truly is related to Ménière's disease. In some cases, especially if the hearing loss is bilateral, it may be due to so-called early presbycusis, whereas the accompanying vertigo is caused by labyrinthitis or some other labyrinthine disorder. Autoimmune inner ear conditions have been recognized recently as important, treatable causes of these symptoms.

This type of case should be distinguished from hereditary progressive SNHL, which generally starts early, progresses faster, and does not exhibit marked recruitment.

# CONGENITAL DEFECTS IN THE COCHLEA

Deafness present at birth can be caused in primarily two ways: (a) malformation of the organ of Corti and (b) toxic effects on the inner ear *in utero*. Increasing evidence suggests that toxic degeneration is far more common than congenital malformation. Even some cases previously described as hereditary congenital nerve deafness are now being recognized as having been caused actually by toxic effects in the first trimester of pregnancy. German measles infections during the mother's pregnancy are one such cause, and Rh incompatibility may be another.

Usually, the organ of Corti is affected, and the result commonly is subtotal deafness or a moderately severe hearing loss that is greater in the higher than in the lower frequencies. In both instances, the congenital defect is associated with a speech problem. If the hearing loss is severe, speech may not develop without special training. When the hearing loss is partial, speech may be defective.

Although complete proof is not available, many otologists are convinced that viral infections during the first trimester of pregnancy do cause cochlear damage and deafness in the fetus. Anoxia shortly after birth also can cause damage to the cochlea, with resultant high-frequency hearing loss.

## CAUSES OF NEURAL HEARING LOSS

Certain other causes are known to damage the auditory nerve *per se*. Abnormal tone decay becomes an important finding in some cases when there is "partial damage" to the nerve fibers, according to some investigators.

Causes of neural hearing loss include the following (among many other causes):

1. Acoustic neuroma
2. Skull fracture and nerve injury
3. Section of the auditory nerve
4. Virus infections
5. Toxicity and other neural injury

## ACOUSTIC NEUROMA

The most urgent reason for differentiating damage to the auditory nerve fibers from damage to the hair cells or the inner ear is that this distinction permits the physician to detect a tumor of the auditory nerve at the earliest possible moment. As the result of advances in hearing tests, it is now possible to diagnose most auditory nerve tumors long before other neurological symptoms or signs become apparent. **Figure 10.57** gives an example of such a case and emphasizes the need to perform discrimination testing and selected special studies in all cases of SNHL, especially if they are unilateral. A patient who comes in to have wax removed from an ear to correct a hearing loss sometimes may actually have a neoplasm of the auditory nerve (**Figure 10.58**).

## Early symptoms

The earliest symptom of many acoustic neuromas is a mild unilateral neural hearing loss. Tinnitus is common, and vertigo may or may not be present. The vertigo may be more of a constant imbalance, in contrast to Ménière's syndrome, in which rotary vertigo usually is intermittent and accompanied by a seashell-like tinnitus.

## Diagnostic criteria

In the last few decades, surgery for acoustic neuromas has improved so much that early detection is even more important than it was previously. It is now possible for the otologist to remove relatively small tumors by a middle cranial fossa or translabyrinthine approach with far less morbidity and mortality than encountered in the suboccipital craniotomy employed by neurosurgeons for larger tumors.

Unexplained dizziness, nystagmus, tinnitus, or hearing loss, especially unilateral progressive SNHL, warrants full evaluation. Even when other ear diseases are present, an undetected acoustic neuroma must be considered. The physical examination should include a complete ear, nose, and throat evaluation; assessment of the cranial nerves; cerebellar testing; and the Romberg test. Corneal sensation and ear canal sensation can be checked quickly with a wisp of cotton, and the gap reflex can be tested with a cotton swab. When the corneal reflex, gag reflex, or facial nerve is involved, the tumor is already fairly large.

Thanks to the pioneering work of William House and other neurologists, a great deal of new information about acoustic tumor diagnosis is available. Unfortunately, there is no routine test that will establish the diagnosis in all cases. Unexpectedly low discrimination scores, type III and type IV Békésy audiograms, low short increment sensitivity index (SISI) scores, and pathological tone decay each occur in only about two-thirds of patients with proven acoustic tumors. Stapedius reflex decay testing is somewhat more reliable but not as much as initially thought. Brainstem evoked-response audiometry (BERA) is the only noninvasive test that appeared to have >90% diagnostic accuracy. However, electronystagmography will show reduced vestibular response ~70% of the time. It must be remembered that this test evaluates only the lateral semicircular canal (superior vestibular nerve). Nearly 15% of acoustic neuromas arise from the inferior vestibular nerve and may show a normal ENG or VNG even in the presence of vertigo.

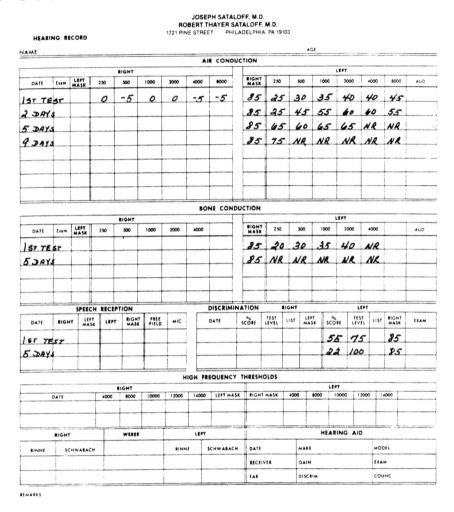

Figure 10.57 *History*: A 24-year-old man complaining of deafness, occasional buzzing, and slight vertigo. *Otologic*: Normal. No Spontaneous nystagmus. *Audiologic*: Unilateral hearing loss with reduced bone conduction. Tuning-fork tests showed lateralization to the right; A > B on left. No recruitment. Marked tone decay and poor discrimination. *Classification*: Neural hearing loss. *Diagnosis*: Acoustic neuroma. *Aids to diagnosis*: Corneal anesthesia on left, and no caloric response on left. The patient refused surgery initially because of the mildness of the symptoms. Later his hearing loss increased, and he developed significant vertigo. A large acoustic neuroma was removed.

| 1000 Hz | |
|---|---|
| L | R |
| 35 | 5 |
| 45 | 15 |
| 50 | 25 |
| 65 | 35 |

Although an acoustic nerve tumor usually occurs on one side, its presence must not be ruled out merely because a patient has bilateral SNHL. In multiple neurofibromatosis, tumors can occur on both auditory nerves and may affect only the cochlear or only the vestibular portions. Characteristics of neurofibromatosis are summarized in Appendix IV. An instance of an auditory nerve tumor causing a comparatively mild hearing loss and very marked reduction in discrimination threshold, using phonetically balanced word lists, is cited in **Figure 10.59**. In such instances, the patient may volunteer that he/she simply cannot understand anything in that ear even though he/she hears voices. This may be particularly bothersome when trying to use the telephone. This complaint should always be followed through with a thorough evaluation.

It is essential to bear in mind that the mere presence of abnormal tone decay does not necessarily mean that the patient has a tumor of the acoustic nerve. It indicates merely that nerve fibers have been damaged. Other causes also can produce damage to acoustic nerve fibers.

Acoustic neuroma is not the only retrocochlear tumor that the otologist is likely to see. Meningiomas, cholesteatomas, facial nerve neuromas, and other lesions may present a similar clinical picture.

## FRACTURED SKULL AND ACOUSTIC NERVE INJURY

A transverse fracture of the temporal bone can go through the internal auditory meatus and compress or sever the acoustic nerve. Occasionally, the seventh nerve also is damaged causing facial paralysis. Since the deafness usually is total, findings such as abnormal tone decay and disproportionately poor discrimination cannot be detected, but CT scans

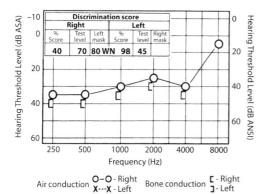

Figure 10.58 *History*: A 36-year-old man complained of having wax in his right ear, causing stuffiness for several weeks. No tinnitus or vertigo. *Otologic*: Normal ear canals and eardrums and no excess wax. No spontaneous nystagmus. *Audiologic*: Mild ascending hearing loss in the right ear with reduced bone conduction. The tuning fork lateralized to the good ear, and air was better than bone conduction in the bad ear. No diplacusis and no recruitment were present. Discrimination was remarkably poor in the right ear, especially in view of the mild hearing loss. Abnormal tone decay was present with the threshold going to 75 dB at 1000 Hz after 1 minute. *Classification*: Neural hearing loss. *Diagnosis*: Acoustic neuroma. *Aids to diagnosis*: The presence of unilateral nerve deafness with absent recruitment but abnormal tone decay and reduced discrimination indicates some pressure on the auditory nerve. In addition, there were corneal anesthesia, and no caloric responses in the right ear. An acoustic neuroma was removed surgically. *Abbreviations*: ANSI, American National Standards Institute; ASA, American Standards Association.

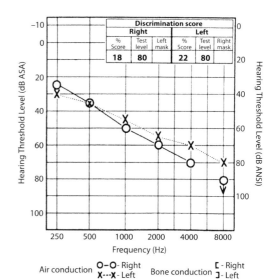

Figure 10.59 *History*: A 52-year-old man had Ménière's disease in both ears and had undergone a bilateral vestibular nerve section. According to the patient, discrimination was sharply reduced postoperatively. *Otologic*: Normal. *Audiologic*: Bilateral mild-to-moderate hearing loss with no air–bone gap. Very poor discrimination ability, which worsened in the presence of environmental noise. *Classification*: Neural hearing loss. *Diagnosis*: Surgical lesion of auditory nerves resulting from section of vestibular nerves. *Abbreviations*: ANSI, American National Standards Institute; ASA, American Standards Association.

and absent caloric responses on the involved side with normal responses on the other side help to establish the diagnosis.

## PARTIAL SECTION OF THE ACOUSTIC NERVE

Some neurosurgeons in the past have cut the vestibular portion of the auditory nerve to control severe persistent vertigo in patients with Ménière's disease. During the operation, it can be difficult for the surgeon to avoid severing at least some portion of the adjacent hearing fibers. Although the vertigo was controlled in most instances, many of the patients were left with additional hearing loss owing to section of the auditory nerve fibers. Almost invariably, the high tones were chiefly affected by the surgery. **Figure 10.59** describes a case in which both vestibular nerves were sectioned by a neurosurgeon. In this case, the low frequencies were affected also, but part or all of this may have been attributable to the preexisting Ménière's disease. Some of the high-frequency loss was present preoperatively, but this was greatly aggravated by the surgery. In addition to the change in threshold, this patient's ability to understand speech was reduced substantially after the nerve section. A hearing aid was practically useless for the individual. Neurotologists have applied microsurgical techniques with a middle-cranial fossa, retro-labyrinthine, or retrosigmoid approach and have refined vestibular nerve surgery so that hearing generally can be preserved following vestibular nerve section.

## VIRUS INFECTION

Certain viral infections, notably herpes, are supposed to cause hearing loss by affecting the acoustic nerve. In this instance, the site of injury is within the spiral ganglion. The hearing loss produced often is quite severe. **Figure 10.60** shows an interesting case.

## CONGENITAL NERVE DEAFNESS

It is common practice to call all cases of deafness present at birth "congenital nerve deafness" or "hereditary nerve deafness," especially if hearing loss is present in other members of the family. In many cases, the congenital defect is not in the

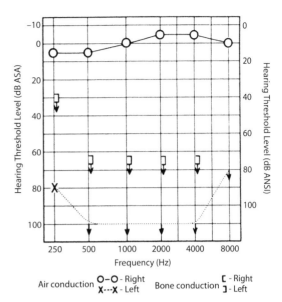

Air conduction O–O - Right, X---X - Left    Bone conduction ⊏ - Right, ⊐ - Left

Figure 10.60 *History*: A 58-year-old man who developed severe herpes with pain in the left ear. He had a left facial palsy for several weeks, and this resolved. He also had a buzzing tinnitus that cleared up. No vertigo. *Otologic*: Normal at time of examination. Caloric tests normal. *Classification*: Neural hearing loss. *Diagnosis*: Herpetic acoustic neuritis. *Abbreviations*: ANSI, American National Standards Institute; ASA, American Standards Association.

nerve itself. Because a majority of cases of congenital hearing loss have their sites of damage in the cochlea, a more accurate term would be cochlear hearing loss, but the distinction is primarily of academic interest, and such cases are classified best as "sensorineural." However, as neurotherapeutic methods become better developed and hair cell growth/regrowth becomes possible, the differentiation may become crucial.

## TOXICITY AND OTHER NERVE INJURY

The acoustic nerve can be injured by any toxin or disorder capable of injuring other nerves. Lead and other heavy metals can cause nerve deafness, for example. Many neurodegenerative diseases also can cause neural hearing loss. For a more comprehensive discussion of these subjects, the reader is referred to neurology literature.

## SURGERY AND SENSORINEURAL HEARING LOSS

Until very recently, surgical otology has concentrated on disorders of the outer ear and middle ear. The inner ear is the new frontier for the neurotologist and skull base surgeon. Although much remains to be learned, significant advancement has been made in the treatment of both vertigo and SNHL. In some cases, medical management can improve or cure symptoms or stop progression of inner ear disease. In selected instances, surgical therapy is appropriate in patients with SNHL either to improve hearing or to treat underlying disease.

A patient with SNHL needs thorough evaluation leading to a specific diagnosis before being considered a surgical candidate. Depending on the history and hearing pattern, this evaluation usually includes auditory, vestibular, neurological, metabolic, and radiological testing. In addition to routine audiometry and impedance studies, BERA is often extremely helpful even in some cases in which the hearing loss is > 80 dB at 4000 Hz. In some such patients, an unexpectedly good brainstem evoked-response audiogram is obtained, and these patients rarely have retrocochlear pathology. In other patients, we are able to obtain useful information with experimental testing using a 500-Hz stimulus rather than a click. Electronystagmograms and computerized dynamic posturography are often helpful as well. Neurological examination concentrating on the cranial nerves and cerebellum should be performed in all patients. Substantial SNHL may be associated with more generalized neurological disorders such as multiple sclerosis, neurofibromatosis, or toxic neuropathy. Blood tests are recommended in many cases. An FTA-absorption test to rule out luetic labyrinthitis is most important. When appropriate, tests for diabetes, hypoglycemia, Lyme disease, HIV, thyroid dysfunction, hyperlipoproteinemia, collagen vascular disease, polycythemia, and other disorders should also be performed. If there is any question of cerebellopontine angle (CPA) tumor, radiological examination is essential. Radiological evaluation is indicated. MRI without and with contrast should be obtained on a state-of-the-art MR scanner. The films are always reviewed by the neurotologist as well as by the radiologist. It is not rare to receive a report that say, "normal MR scan" and to find that the contents of the internal auditory canals (IACs) are not visualized on the study. Naturally, this problem can be avoided if the studies are performed regularly by a radiologist who is an expert in MR scanning of the ear. High-quality enhanced magnetic resonance imaging is very effective at detecting even small tumors. CT scans and single-photon emission computed tomography (SPECT) or positron emission tomography (PET) scans are also often essential in a neurotologic evaluation.

In most patients, it is possible to separate sensory hearing loss from neural hearing loss. Surgery may be indicated despite the presence of substantial sensory or neural hearing loss in such conditions as fistula, infection, far-advanced otosclerosis (FAO), CPA tumors, endolymphatic hydrops, profound deafness, and other entities. It is worthwhile reviewing selected situations in which the advisability of surgery is not always immediately apparent. The seven cases discussed below are examples of such situations.

## INFECTION/FISTULA

Surgical management of patients with infection or with perilymph fistula is widely recognized and will not be discussed in detail. When SNHL occurs in association with acute otitis media or mastoiditis, surgical drainage usually is indicated.

When sudden hearing loss occurs in association with barotrauma, or when fistula is suspected because of fluctuation in symptoms associated with variations of middle ear pressure, surgery for fistula repair should be considered. Although treatment with bed rest and medication may be helpful, operative repair should be considered early, particularly if the patient has previously undergone surgery in the affected ear.

## FAR-ADVANCED OTOSCLEROSIS

Otosclerosis presents infrequently in an advanced state because good therapy has been widely available for many years. Hence, we may neglect to think of it in a patient with severe sensorineural deafness or a "blank audiogram" (no response by air conduction or bone conduction). Nevertheless, it still occurs. The authors have performed stapes surgery on many such cases in the last decades, representing ~2% of stapes operations. This is similar to the experience of House and Glorig (41) and Sheehy (42), who found slightly > 1% of their stapes surgery cases were for far-advanced disease. Stapes surgery may be extremely helpful in patients with severe or profound hearing loss, especially in people who have difficulty wearing hearing aids, as illustrated by the following cases.

**Case 1** is an 88-year-old woman who is extremely vital and active but socially incapacitated by inability to communicate (**Figure 10.61**). She could not wear a hearing aid effectively because of distortion and narrow dynamic range. Following surgery, she has been able to communicate well using a behind-the-ear aid.

**Case 2** is a 58-year-old woman who had undergone prior stapedectomy in one ear and fenestration in the other ear with good results (**Figure 10.62**). She had awakened deaf after cardiac bypass surgery and had undergone two unsuccessful attempts at stapes operations before being referred. She was unable to use powerful body hearing aids effectively. Following surgery, she could communicate satisfactorily using a body aid in her left ear.

Frattali and Sataloff (43) reported nine patients and reviewed FAO in 1993. Postoperatively, seven of the nine patients (78%) used hearing aids successfully, whereas none had been aidable preoperatively. FAO generally involves air conduction levels worse than 85 dB HL and bone conduction levels beyond the limits of the audiometer. If air conduction levels exceed 85 dB HL, but bone conduction levels are measurable at some frequencies but worse than 30 dB, the condition is called advanced otosclerosis. FAO may be suspected because of clues in the history and physical examination, but definitive diagnosis requires middle ear surgery. It is not feasible to use the usual criterion (closure of air–bone gap) for assessing the results of surgery; other objective and subjective criteria should be used.

NAME _____ D.G. _____

| DATE | RIGHT EAR AIR CONDUCTION | | | | | | | LEFT EAR AIR CONDUCTION | | | | | |
|------|------|------|------|------|------|------|------|------|------|------|------|------|------|
| | 250 | 500 | 1000 | 2000 | 4000 | 8000 | | 250 | 500 | 1000 | 2000 | 4000 | 8000 |
| 8/81 | NR | 100 | 100 | NR | NR | NR | PRE | 90 | 100 | 100 | 100 | 95 | NR |
| 5/82 | 50 | 55 | 65 | 80 | 85 | 90 | POST | | | | | | |
| | | | | | | | | | | | | | |

| | | RIGHT EAR BONE CONDUCTION | | | | | | LEFT EAR BONE CONDUCTION | | | | |
|---|---|---|---|---|---|---|---|---|---|---|---|---|
| | | 65 | NR | NR | NR | | | | | | | |
| | | | | | | | | | | | | |

SPEECH RECEPTION: Right __95__ Left __90__  PRE          DISCRIMINATION: Right _____ Left _____

Figure 10.61 Preoperative and postoperative audiogram of Case 1, far-advanced otosclerosis.

NAME _____ M.B. _____

| DATE | RIGHT EAR AIR CONDUCTION | | | | | | | LEFT EAR AIR CONDUCTION | | | | | |
|------|------|------|------|------|------|------|------|------|------|------|------|------|------|
| | 250 | 500 | 1000 | 2000 | 4000 | 8000 | | 250 | 500 | 1000 | 2000 | 4000 | 8000 |
| 8/82 | NR | NR | NR | NR | NR | NR | PRE | NR | NR | NR | NR | NR | NR |
| | | | | | | | POST | 90 | 110 | 105 | 85 | NR | NR |
| | | | | | | | | | | | | | |

| | | RIGHT EAR BONE CONDUCTION | | | | | | LEFT EAR BONE CONDUCTION | | | | |
|---|---|---|---|---|---|---|---|---|---|---|---|---|
| | | | | | | | | 30 | 55 | NR | 70 | 55 |
| | | | | | | | | | | | | |

SPEECH RECEPTION: Right __XXX__ Left __XXX__          DISCRIMINATION: Right _____ Left _____

Figure 10.62 Preoperative and postoperative audiogram of Case 2, far-advanced otosclerosis.

Despite 125 cases of FAO discussed in reports written over > 30 years (44–50) (prior to the report by Frattali and Sataloff), the relationship of severe or profound cochlear hearing loss and otosclerosis is poorly understood. Histologically, the correlation between bone disease and perceptive loss remains obscure in most temporal bones described to date. Lindsay and Hemenway (51) described two types of otosclerosis. Type I is usually a conductive disturbance limited to specific areas of the oval and round windows. The second type of otosclerosis is a more aggressive form with multiple foci that form early in life. These foci involve multiple areas in the otic capsule.

Wiet et al. (49) studied the temporal bone of a 65-year-old patient with FAO who died of natural causes. There were multiple foci of otosclerosis, diffuse loss of hair cells, and loss of cochlear neurons in the basal turn. There were also areas of strial atrophy near the foci of otosclerosis. Myers and Myers (52) examined the temporal bone of a 66-year-old man who died suddenly several hours after his second stapes operation for FAO. They found atrophy of the spiral ligament with basilar membrane rupture and severe degeneration of the organ of Corti, spiral ganglion cells, and cochlea.

A convincing histologic explanation for the increased bone conduction threshold in FAO remains an issue for continued investigations. In a total of 164 temporal bones examined by Schuknecht and Barber (53), a statistical analysis failed to show any correlation between bone conduction thresholds and size of lesion, activity of lesion, involvement of the endosteum, or presence of a round-window lesion.

It is presumed that otosclerotic involvement of the cochlear endosteum causes atrophy of the spiral ligament. Basilar membrane rupture appears related to this atrophy, as two of the layers of the basilar membrane insert into the endosteum. How this is related to SNHL remains uncertain. Otosclerosis may cause atrophic changes leading to alterations of the motion mechanics in the scala media, mechanical and metabolic alterations associated with strial atrophy may be causal, or some other mechanism may be response for the sensorineural loss.

Clinically, it is extremely important to recognize FAO. Wiet et al. (49) diagnosed three cases of FAO among 175 patients who were being considered for cochlear implantation. Two of these patients underwent stapedectomy and received substantial benefit from hearing aids following surgery. Stapedectomy involves much less risk than cochlear implantation and less auditory rehabilitation. Moreover, the hearing achieved with amplification following stapedectomy is generally better than the hearing expected with a CI. When satisfactory results are not achieved, the patient can still be considered for CI surgery.

When a patient presents with acquired severe or profound hearing loss, a comprehensive neurotologic evaluation is mandatory to diagnose causes such as neoplasms, luetic labyrinthitis, autoimmune SNHL, ototoxicity, meningitis, and genetic hearing loss. However, because FAO is one of the few conditions that permits treatment capable of converting the patient's hearing from nonserviceable to serviceable with conventional hearing aids, it is especially important to be alert for this entity, and to look for residual, nonmeasurable hearing and an air–bone gap. The definitive diagnosis requires middle ear exploration. However, Sheehy (47) summarized the symptoms and signs that are generally regarded as most typical of FAO that should alert the otologist to the possible presence of this entity. They include the following:

- *History*: Gradually progressive hearing impairment in early adult life is suggestive, especially with a positive family history of otosclerosis. Eighty-six percent of Sheehy's (47) patients who had an onset of hearing impairment before age 30 years and a positive family history had oval window otosclerosis.
- *Paracusis*: The ability to hear better in noisy surroundings during an early stage of hearing impairment is highly suggestive of otosclerosis.
- *Hearing Aid Performance*: Despite the extent of the hearing loss, patients report some benefit from amplification. Word discrimination ability without lipreading is typically much better than would be predicted based on pure-tone thresholds. Eighty percent of patients with FAO wore hearing aids, as opposed to only 30% of patients with nonotosclerotic ears who had similar audiograms in Sheehy's series (47).
- *Hearing Aid History*: The patient may be wearing or in the past was wearing a hearing aid or bone conduction aid.
- *Previous Audiograms*: A prior audiogram may demonstrate an air–bone gap.

- *Voice Patterning*: The voice may not be suggestive of SNHL (modulation, pronunciation, and intensity).
- *Otoscopic Examination*: Schwartze's sign may be present.
- *Radiographic Confirmation*: Although polytomography may further support the diagnosis of FAO, preoperative confirmation with CT (with coronal views) is especially helpful. Von Glass and Philipp (54) investigated 31 patients suspected of having cochlear otosclerosis with high-resolution CT. Fourteen patients had confirmed otosclerosis associated with advanced hearing loss. In four of these patients, free otospongiotic foci were detected in the bone of the cochlear capsule.
- *Tuning Fork Test*: A Weber test lateralizing to the poorer hearing ear or a negative Rinne test in presumed SNHL may be suggestive. Because of tactile perception, tuning fork tests may sometimes be misleading. We recommend standard use of a 512-Hz tuning fork. Many patients with FAO do not hear the tuning fork well when it is placed on the forehead or nasal dorsum but hear clearly by dental bone conduction. In order to help confirm the validity of tuning fork testing, in 1980 one of the authors (R.T.S.) began asking patients to hum the pitch of the tuning fork. This is a simple task for people even with extremely modest musical ability. All the patients with FAO were able to perform this task. None of the patients with profound SNHL who subsequently went on to CI surgery was able to perform the task.
- *No Other Apparent Cause for Hearing Impairment*: When hearing loss has been of insidious onset and when all other known causes have been ruled out, the diagnosis of FAO must be considered, especially if any of the criteria listed earlier are present.

The value of surgery for this disease entity was first discussed in 1960 by House and Glorig (41). Surgical improvements are much more important to a patient with FAO than to a patient with a mild-to-moderate hearing loss because surgery can convert FAO patients from functionally deaf to easily aidable. House and Glorig were two of many investigators to conclude that opening the oval window in patients with FAO was potentially worthwhile regardless of the level of preoperative air and bone conduction thresholds. This philosophy still prevails some 30 years later.

The reported surgical experience varies (44–50). Our results support the findings of the three previous reports with the best results (44, 45, 48). The type of prosthesis and surgical technique used and involvement of the round window by otosclerosis appear to have no bearing on the success of surgery. House and Glorig (41) opened both windows in a two-stage operation. In three of five patients, the hearing was made worse. The round window should generally not be opened for this reason alone. Additionally, closure of the round window probably accounts for only 10 dB of bone conduction loss at most (41).

For routine cases of otosclerosis, we generally define surgical success as closure of the air–bone gap to within 10 dB. In experienced hands, we expect a success rate >90%. On the basis of these conventional criteria for stapedectomy surgery, results in FAO would be disappointing. However, the majority of patients with FAO clearly benefit from stapedectomy subjectively, and many have improvements in pure-tone air conduction thresholds. Some also have improvement in discrimination ability under earphones, and marked improvement in hearing aid performance is common. Patients are often able to use their amplified hearing more effectively, even when the traditional measures of discrimination do not show improvement. Careful preoperative counseling and informed consent are extremely important in patients with FAO. The patients must be aware not only of the risks of the procedure but also of the relatively limited goals. Normal hearing is not expected. Reported complications in these patients do not appear to differ statistically from those in other patients undergoing stapedectomy surgery, and most patients feel justified in accepting those risks of the potential benefit of advancing from unserviceable hearing to aidable hearing.

Controversy exists as to whether a second stapedectomy for FAO should be performed on the opposite ear. Some otologists believe that there is little justification for this in the event of a successful stapedectomy. We believe, however, that ear cases should be addressed individually, that each patient should be offered the potential benefit of binaural amplification even for a hearing loss of this severity, and that the final decision should be left to the patient after the risks have been explained fully.

If an operation for FAO has failed, many investigators suggest that an attempt at surgery on the opposite ear should also probably fail and that further surgery is not advisable. We question this anecdotal judgment and believe that the decision regarding surgery on the opposite ear should be individualized in this instance as well. When hearing loss is profound bilaterally, the patient assumes very little risk from undergoing stapes surgery, and results may be substantially different on the two ears.

In summary, the most important diagnostic aid in recognizing FAO is the tuning fork. Despite the audiogram, these patients usually can hear well by dental bone conduction. To help assure that the response is not tactile, it is sometimes useful to ask the patient to hum the tone of the tuning fork. This diagnosis should also be suspected in people who are using powerful hearing aids more effectively than expected or in people who understand loud spoken voice without lipreading. In general, discrimination remains better with FAO than with other diseases that cause this degree of hearing loss. Although most of us prefer restoring hearing to normal with stapes surgery, converting a patient from unaidable to aidable may be an equally gratifying and valuable intervention.

## CRANIAL IRRADIATION

The effects of cranial irradiation on hearing were reviewed by Sataloff and Rosen (55) in 1994. Radiotherapy has been shown to be effective in treatment regimens for a variety of tumors of the head and neck. Both clinical practice and published literature reflect contradictory opinions on the incidence, type, severity, and time of onset of hearing loss as a treatment complication. Review of relevant animal and human studies highlights the available information. References describing cranial irradiation used in conjunction with chemotherapy have been excluded because of the known ototoxic effects of the chemotherapeutic agents themselves.

## ANIMAL MODELS

Animal models have been used to study this question since 1905 when Ewald (56) placed beads containing radium in the middle ear in pigeons and noted labyrinthine symptoms.

Girden and Culler (57) subjected dogs to various doses of X-rays to evaluate the effects of radiation on hearing. His subjects demonstrated a 5.5-dB gain in acuity after a 7- to 11-day latent period but returned to baseline within a period of days to weeks. No hearing loss was noted, but the authors could not explain the mechanisms involved. Novotny (58), Kozlow (59), and Gamble et al. (60) studied the effects of ionizing radiation in guinea pigs. In Novotny's research, a hearing impairment of 8.4 dB at 4000 Hz was noted. There were no histologic changes in the inner ear. Kozlov's subjects demonstrated 3.9- to 9.1-dB diminution in the frequency ranges of 500–8000 Hz.

Gamble's study animals were radiated with doses of 500, 1000, 2000, 3000, 4000, 5000, or 6000 rads. The opposite ear was shielded and received a maximum of 500 rads of scatter radiation. Cochlear microphonics were correlated with histologic findings at 24 hours, 2 weeks, and 2 months. At 24 hours, both cochlear microphonic sensitivity and histologic examinations were normal. At 2 weeks, there was little inflammatory response in the group receiving lower doses. Animals receiving 5000 rads had mild erythema, and those with a 6000 rads dose had more erythema, some edema, and vascular changes that interfered with meaningful measures of cochlear microphonics. Inflammatory response resulted in loss of sensitivity of between 20 and 40 dB, especially at frequencies > 7000 Hz. Examination at 2 months revealed resolution of inflammatory response in all animals. The cochlear microphonics demonstrated loss of sensitivity of 30–40 dB at high frequencies. Three animals also demonstrated vestibular signs.

Using light microscopy, histologic changes were noted. There was little detectable difference between the radiated and control ears at doses of ≤ 2000 rads. At ≥ 3000 rads, the changes in cellular structure were directly dose related. The earliest changes were seen in the stria vascularis. As the dose increased, changes in hair cells were noted, with distortion and cell boundary dissolution seen at 5000 rads. Doses of 6000 rads led to shriveling of hair cells and elevation of the tectorial membrane. Additionally, at ≥ 3000 rads, 50% of temporal bones revealed distention of the endolymphatic sac and displacement of Reissner's membrane.

Temporal bones of rats examined by Keleman (61) after doses of 100–3000 rads demonstrated engorgement of middle ear membranes with extravasation. In the inner ear, damage to the cochlear duct and organ of Corti was noted.

Bohne et al. (62) report late findings in chinchillas treated with 4000–9000 rads and examined 2 years after exposure. There was dose-dependent degeneration of sensory and supporting cells and loss of eighth nerve fibers in the organ of Corti.

## RESEARCH FORMATS

Results reported in human subjects are fraught with complications of research design that mandate caution in interpretation. Older reports are affected by the magnitude of radiation voltage (kilovoltage rather than megavoltage dosing). Kilovoltage is more likely to cause radionecrosis of the temporal bone than the megavoltage equipment in current use. Megavoltage X-rays are uniformly absorbed by soft tissues and bone, and kilovoltage has increased bone absorption (63). Radiation doses administered in early studies were much higher than in current standards of care (up to 24,000 rads). Many studies were retrospective, and pretreatment audiometric measures were not available. Some studies reflect sample bias in that patients complaining of subjective hearing loss were recruited as subjects. Finally, the site of the tumor is widely variable and includes carcinoma of the ear and nasopharynx, which may have direct effects on hearing. The treatment portals often irradiated both temporal bones so intrasubject controls were impossible.

## HUMAN SUBJECTS

In 1962, Borsanyi and Blanchard (64) reported on a series of 14 patients receiving 4000–6000 rads in the region of the inner ear for treatment of a variety of head and neck cancers. Pretreatment and immediate posttreatment audiograms were obtained. "Small" shifts in hearing threshold were noted, with the greatest change at 4000 Hz and the mildest at 200 Hz. Discrimination remained within normal limits. Recruitment was present during the treatment phase but resolved spontaneously when it had not been present prior to treatment. No long-term audiologic follow-up was performed. The authors attribute the threshold shifts to a conductive loss secondary to "radiation otitis media." This is known to occur when mucosal edema impairs

eustachian tube patency and produces a middle-ear fluid collection. They hypothesized that intratreatment recruitment resulted from "temporary vasculitis of stria vascularis and arachnoid mesh in the perilymphatic space." They further observed that the late changes sometimes occurred in the temporal bone, including obliterative endarteritis resulting from edema and degeneration of collagen and smooth muscle of vessel walls impaired blood supply to the cochlea, labyrinth, and ossicles.

Leach's (65) series of 56 patients received 3000–12,000 rads for treatment of head and neck carcinoma in eight different regions. In the study, 36% of patients experienced SNHL assumed to be secondary to conductive hearing impairment. Eleven patients were evaluated prior to treatment; of these, eight patients showed immediate changes, with recovery in only two. The remaining three showed late changes. Nine additional patients were evaluated from 18 months to 10 years after their treatment. Although hearing loss was evident, there were no comparative data available. By patient reports this was noted 9 months to several years after treatment and was gradually progressive. Two of these patients had total deafness and absent ice-water caloric response in one ear. In one patient, this was a 7-year gradual progression. No correlation was found between radiation dose and the amount of hearing loss, nor were treatment duration or patient age significant. Leach also reported radiation otitis media in several cases. Significant tinnitus and vertigo were described anecdotally and preceded subject awareness of hearing loss.

One temporal bone was harvested from a patient with nasopharyngeal carcinoma who became vertiginous and profoundly deaf in a gradually progressive fashion following a 4000 rads dose. He died 1 year later. The pathology report notes the following:

> … exudate present with polymorphs and macrophages in the middle ear and mastoid bilaterally. The mucosa is congested and there is marked bone absorption by granulation tissue resulting in extensive osteoporosis. The organ of Corti is absent. A layer of red fluid covers the basilar membrane. The round window niche contains exudate. The spiral ganglion and nerve is atrophic. No maculae or cristae are seen in the vestibular apparatus.

Dias (66) reports on his series of 29 patients who presented with a variety of head and neck tumor sites. They received a range of kilovoltage radiation from 1000 to 18,000 rads. Using a location 2–3 cm deep to the external meatus, isodose curve calculations proposed a dose to the auditory apparatus of 700–10,000 rads. In this study, 19 patients had pre- and posttreatment audiograms (group I) and 10 additional patients had evaluation after treatment only (group 2). In group 1, mixed hearing loss predominated. The average decrease in acuity was 9.9 dB, and no particular frequency was more affected. Group 2 also demonstrated mixed hearing loss, with two patients evaluated at 11- and 13-years posttreatment. Their hearing remained "serviceable." One patient had undergone craniotomy for a tumor of the fourth ventricle and received 10,000 rads of radiation. He had ossicular reconstruction for dislocation necrosis of the incudostapedial joint 8 years status post craniotomy. His postoperative hearing level was 20 dB for the worse side and 13 dB for the operated ear. Dias notes that nervous tissues are among the most radiosensitive in the body and attributes most of the hearing loss to chronic tubal dysfunction secondary to the tumor and/or radiation-induced changes in soft tissue.

Schuknecht and Karmody (67) sectioned a temporal bone in a man who had received 5,200 rads over 15 days for treatment of squamous cell carcinoma of the ear canal. Hearing loss developed 8 years later. There was radionecrosis of the temporal bone; histologically, "slight atrophy of the organ of Corti was noted with atrophy of the basilar membrane, spiral ligament, and stria vascularis."

In a retrospective study by Moretti (68), 137 patients with carcinoma of the nasopharynx were reviewed. Of these, 13 had received pre- and posttreatment audiograms. Seven of the 13 had SNHL and were self-selected, owing to hearing complaints. Patients ranged in age from 17 to 74 years and received tumor radiation doses between 6000 and 24,000 rads. The onset of severe SNHL was gradual and occurred 3–6 years following radiation therapy. Profound losses had descending audiometric patterns; lesser losses had flat patterns. Although formal statistical analyses were not performed, age appeared to be correlated with hearing loss: affected patients were 42–72 years old (average 60 years); unaffected patients were 17–62 years

old (average 40 years). It should be noted that the "unaffected" group included three patients who had only 1 year of audiologic follow-up.

Thibadoux et al. (69) serially assessed the hearing sensitivity of 61 children with acute lymphocytic leukemia. It was postulated that children might be more susceptible to lower radiation doses because of their high growth rate and structural immaturity. Their treatment included combined chemotherapy, 2400 rads of cranial irradiation, and intrathecal methotrexate. Pure-tone audiometry at 500, 1000, 2000, 4000, 6000, and 8000 Hz was performed prior to irradiation and at 6, 12, and 36 months thereafter. Radiation dose was divided into 15 fractions given > 18 days to a field including the retroorbital space, C-2, both temporal bones, and all structures of the auditory system bilaterally. No statistically significant reduction in auditory sensitivity was noted for any test frequency at any test interval. This was a properly controlled prospective study with a reasonable period of follow-up that is continuing on cohort survivors. However, in spite of a theoretical increase in radiation sensitivity, the 2400-rads dose was not found to be correlated with hearing loss in this or other studies. A 3000-rads dose is the minimum with cited hearing effects.

Two case reports of delayed SNHL are provided by Coplan et al. (70) and Talmi et al. (71). Coplan et al. describe a 12-year-old girl who underwent subtotal resection of an optic glioma and received postoperative radiation: 5000 rads, total tumor radiation dose, in 25 fractions > 5 weeks. The field included the petrous portion of both temporal bones. Three years later, CT revealed residual tumor occupying the third ventricle and symmetric calcifications of the basal ganglia and both temporal lobes. Hearing loss was first suspected by the treating physicians 5 years after radiation, but the mother noted decreased hearing 2 years after initial surgery and irradiation. Pure-tone testing revealed a bilateral mixed hearing loss. The conductive component was approximately equal bilaterally, but the sensorineural component was greater on the left. Speech discrimination was moderately depressed on the left and normal on the right. There were no audiologic signs of retrocochlear pathology. The patient had temporal lobe and basal ganglia lesions compatible with radiation-induced cerebral necrosis, with more significant hearing loss lateralized to the side most affected. The pattern of delayed onset and gradual progression of hearing loss are consistent with reports in the literature.

Talmi et al. (71) reported on a 35-year-old woman evaluated for a neck mass. She had noted right blindness and right hearing loss since early childhood. She gave a history of radium treatment of a large, right-sided facial hemangioma with a total dose of 23,900 rads. Her audiogram showed SNHL on the right. The SRT was 25 dB with 90% discrimination.

Elwany (72) examined middle ear mucosa in six patients who exhibited conductive hearing loss 6–11 months after a total dose of 6,500–8,500 rads for treatment of head and neck malignancies not involving the temporal bone. Audiometry confirmed conductive hearing loss in all patients, two of whom also had a sensorineural component. Middle ear compliance and pressure were within normal limits, and tympanometry confirmed eustachian tube patency. An exploratory tympanotomy was performed, and a sample of mucosa overlying the promontory was excised. Ultrastructural changes were evaluated with electron microscopy. The author summarized as follows:

> The epithelium showed marked reduction of cytoplasmic mass, variable degrees of ciliary loss and widening of intercellular spaces with disruption of the macula adherens. The connective tissue stroma showed increased production of collagenous fibrous tissue and increased numbers of synthetically active fibroblasts. New gland formation with reduced activity was observed. The endothelial cells of capillaries were swollen, and the basal lamina duplicated. The lumina of other capillaries were completely obliterated and replaced by a fibrous cord.

In 1988, Evans et al. (63) reported on a series of 45 patients who had received postoperative radiotherapy for unilateral parotid tumors. The study comprised of 20 patients, but two were excluded for documented prior hearing loss. The remaining 18 subjects had received 5500–6000 rads, total dose, in 200–220 rads daily fractions over 5–6 weeks. The tumor and entire temporal bone received full treatment dose, and the contralateral auditory apparatus was calculated to receive <10% of the tumor dose as scatter radiation.

Pure-tone thresholds at 500, 1000, 2000, and 4000 Hz were evaluated, with the contralateral ear serving as the control. Thresholds were found to be within 10 dB of one another, and there were no statistically significant differences. The evaluation was conducted 2–16 years (mean 8 years) after irradiation. Age ranged from 27 to 75 years (mean 65 years). The authors concluded that permanent hearing loss is unlikely if the daily fraction is < 220 rads and total dose is < 6000 rads. The study included no preoperative audiometry, and additionally frequencies > 4000 Hz, associated with greater incidence and severity of hearing loss in the literature, were not evaluated. This limits the ability to rely on the data in a general population.

Chowdhury et al. (73) conducted a prospective clinical trial using Shepard grommet ventilating tubes in patients enrolled for radiation therapy of nasopharyngeal carcinoma, stages I–IV. The radiation therapy schedule consisted of 6000 rads in 24 fractions >6 weeks. Fields included the temporal bones. All cases were assigned to the tube (T) group ($n = 58$) or no tube (NOT) group ($n = 57$). Pure-tone audiograms for air and bone conduction were performed at 2000, 4000, and 6000 Hz, and ventilation tubes were inserted under local anesthesia. Tinnitus was assessed using a 3-point self-ranking score for severity.

When the pretreatment air–bone gaps were compared, there was no significant difference between the two groups. The conductive hearing loss present before treatment in the NOT group increased by 3 dB during treatment and hearing improved by 7 dB in the T group. This was significant. A decrease of 3 dB in the average sensorineural threshold also occurred at 6 months in the NOT group but was not demonstrated in the T group. These findings were statistically significant. When individual data were evaluated, five patients in the NOT group had > 10 dB loss when compared with three patients in the T group.

Tinnitus scores did not differ at the preradiation evaluation. At 6 months, the NOT group had significantly worse tinnitus, and the T group showed significantly better scores. Tinnitus may be related to negative pressure, fluid in the middle ear, or changes in the cochlea, nerve, or brain.

The mechanism of improvement is unknown. The 6-month follow-up period was insufficient to assess delayed SNHL. However, the authors have recommended placement of ventilation tubes to prevent conductive loss secondary to "radiation otitis." Radiation may increase the risk of persistent tympanic membrane perforation after the tubes come out. This may be advantageous if eustachian tube dysfunction has persisted. Otherwise, the perforations can be closed by tympanoplasty.

Directed radiation to the eighth nerve has been utilized in the treatment of acoustic neuromas. Hirsch and Noren (74) reported on 64 patients treated with stereotactic radiosurgery who had pure-tone thresholds better than 90 dB and were followed audiologically. Goals of radiosurgical treatment were eradication of the tumor, absence of complications, preservation of facial nerve function, and preservation of hearing. The size and shape of the tumor determined treatment decisions. Tumors of ≥ B18 mm could always be treated, larger tumors (up to 30 mm) had to be avoided to allow dose distribution, and tumors >33 mm were not treated. Dose planning was performed, and during treatment, the head was positioned sequentially in the focus positions. Duration of treatment was 14–20 minutes and the doses were 1800–2500 rads at tumor periphery, 2200–5000 rads at tumor center.

Patients were followed with pre- and posttreatment audiometry, stapedial reflex testing, and brainstem audiometry. Preoperatively, 51 ears had hearing thresholds (pure-tone average) <50 dB, and in 11 cases, discrimination scores were better than 80%. Retrocochlear hearing loss was found by stapedius reflex testing. BERA was abnormal in 50 of 51 cases in the ear involved with tumor.

At 1-year postradiosurgery, 26% of patients showed preserved hearing with pure-tone averages (at 500, 1000, and 2000 Hz) no > 5 dB worse than the preoperative value and discrimination scores equal to those obtained preoperatively. Severe hearing loss (pure-tone average > 90 dB) occurred in 20%, and the remaining 54% showed pronounced deterioration of thresholds and/or discrimination scores.

Gradual hearing loss was noticed in the 49 months after radiation, as permanent or fluctuant loss or a change in sound quality. Two patients experienced a verified hearing improvement, and one patient with bilateral tumors caused by neurofibromatosis suffered sudden deafness within 24 hours of treatment. Graphed data on pure-tone averages for long-term follow-up revealed a cluster between 35 and 65 dB at 2–8 years following irradiation.

Other audiologic symptoms included balance disturbances in the first year after treatment ($n = 8$). Tinnitus was unchanged. Facial weakness occurred in 15% of cases within 6–9 months after treatment and was transitory. Eighteen percent of patients experienced trigeminal dysfunction with a similar latency period. The radiation dose in these patients was 5000–10,000 rads. The authors recommended a minimum dose of 2000 rads for effective tumor shrinkage and a 3000 rads maximum for hearing preservation. However, it must be remembered that these data cannot be interpreted as reflecting the effects of radiation because radiosurgery does not cure acoustic neuromas. At best, it slows or arrests growth. Consequently, all hearing changes may be attributable to the natural progression of the underlying disease.

As part of a study supported by a grant from the National Cancer Institute, Emami et al. (75) formed a task force to update tolerance doses (TDs) for irradiation in a variety of body tissues. The goal was to provide three-dimensional treatment planning and dose delivery, including partial volumes to tissue receiving variable dose levels.

Data were collected only on conventional dose fractions (180–200 rads/day) for one-third, two-thirds, and whole-organ exposure. For each, TD 5/5 and TD 50/5 were determined: TD 5/5 reflects the probability of a 5% rate of the complication within 5 years after treatment, and TD 50/5 denotes a 50% rate of the complication probability > 5 years.

The authors offered observations regarding brain tolerance to radiation. Radionecrosis of the brain typically occurs 3 months to several years after irradiation and presents as neurologic deficits not attributable to recurrent tumor. Histologically the authors noted "pallor of white matter secondary to diffuse cerebral edema and marked changes adjacent to the tumor. These include coagulation necrosis, vascular thickening, perivascular fibrosis, calcium deposition, fibrin deposition, and chronic inflammatory infiltrates." These were thought to be attributable to radiation effects on vasculature and oligodendrocyte proliferation. The normal issue complication probability in this study cited an increase in TD 5/5 for the whole brain > 4500 rads but noted "some patients developed significant necrosis from partial brain doses as low as 5000 rads. A sharp increase exists for doses > 6000 rads."

According to these authors, there is no good evidence that the brainstem differs from the cerebrum, although traditionally the brainstem has been regarded as more radiosensitive. Because of the higher percentage of white matter in the brainstem, a 10% decrease from total brain TD was deemed advisable, and the recommendation given was a TD 5/5 of 6000 rads for one-third volume.

In the study, the sensitivity of the ear is divided into external/middle and inner ear portions. The TD 50/5 for acute radiation otitis was set at 4000 rads and, for chronic otitis, at 6500–7000 rads. The author's review of "several studies" suggested a TD 5/5 of 6000 rads and a TD 50/5 of 7000 rads for SNHL or vestibular damage. It should be noted that the studies cited are somewhat dated (see Gamble et al. [60], Leach [65], Dias [66], and Moretti [68].

Singh and Slevin (76) evaluated 28 patients irradiated for residual or recurrent parotid pleomorphic adenoma. A dosing schedule of 5000 rads in 15 daily fractions > 20 days was used. The interval between radiotherapy and assessment was at least 5 years with a median of 14 years. Pure-tone audiometry at 500, 1000, 2000, 4000, 6000, and 8000 Hz was performed, and the contralateral ear was used as a control. Significance levels of > 10 dB at 500, 1000, and 2000 Hz and > 20 dB at 4000, 6000, and 8000 Hz were selected. Bithermal caloric testing (except in cases with otitis) was also conducted.

In the study, 15 of the 28 patients had significant hearing deficit: sensorineural in 12 and mixed in 3. Seven of these had semicircular canal paresis on caloric response. The remaining 13 patients had no significant hearing loss. Losses occurred at both high and low frequencies, but losses in the 2000- to 8000-Hz range predominated. The mean difference between ears was between 52 and 63 dB at each of the four high frequencies tested. Three of the four patients who received a dose > 5250 or 5500 rads had significant hearing loss.

In their discussion, the researchers hypothesize that the differences in dose per fraction utilized in their center (330 rads as opposed to 220 rads) may account for the greater incidence and severity of hearing loss than in the study by Evans et al. (63). They suggest that the biologic dose be adjusted based on the likelihood of tumor recurrence and that patients should be informed that hearing loss may occur as a late effect of radiotherapy.

Grau et al. (77) recommend that deleterious effects of irradiation on hearing should be kept in mind in both treatment planning and follow-up after radiotherapy. They base their conclusion on a prospective assessment of 22 patients evaluated prior to and 7–84 months following radiotherapy for nasopharyngeal carcinoma. Pure-tone audiometry, SRT, discrimination scores, impedance evaluation, and BERA were performed. Bone conduction scores at 500, 1000, 2000, and 4000 Hz were considered.

The treatment protocol used external beam on laterally opposed fields with a tumor radiation dose between 6000 and 6800 rads. Eight patients received split-course treatment. One patient's inner ear fell within the penumbra of the treatment field, and dosimetric calculations reduced the inner ear dose to 75% of the central dose. Bone conduction pre- and posttreatment was compared for each frequency and ear. An absolute change in baseline was then calculated. There was no correlation between age and SNHL. Radiation dose did correlate significantly with SNHL in these patients ($p < 0.01$). A significantly higher incidence of SNHL was found for doses > 5000 rad when compared with lower doses ($p < 0.05$). The absolute hearing loss was greatest at 4000 Hz, but age correction indicated that the differences between frequencies were related to age. Frequencies > 4000 Hz were not evaluated. Latency of cochlear damage for doses > 5000 rad was evidenced by a significantly higher incidence of SNHL at observation times > 18 months. Auditory brainstem evoked-response in four patients was "severely abnormal," although the specific changes were not described. Two of the four also had "clinical signs of brainstem dysfunction and severe sensorineural hearing effects."

## TREATMENT OF BRAINSTEM TUMORS

Two reports provide useful reviews of the management and prognosis of thalamic, brainstem, and spinal cord tumors. Grigsby's (78) group provides retrospective analysis of 83 adults treated with a combination of surgery and irradiation, or irradiation alone between 1950 and 1984.

All patients received external beam radiation therapy. Orthovoltage irradiation was used, with five patients receiving a three-field approach. The remainder were treated with right and left lateral opposed portals, using megavoltage equipment. Only ten patients received whole brain radiation with a boost to the tumor site. The treated volume encompassed the entire tumor bed and a generous margin (2–3 cm). Unless cerebellar invasion was evident, no attempt was made to irradiate the whole cerebellum.

The central tumor-axis dose was 5040 ± 207 rads (SD) with a range from 75 to 6300 rads. The median daily fraction was 180 rads, five fractions per week. The majority of patients received a midplane tumor dose of 5400 rads, five fractions per week. No morbidity data were provided on survivors with regard to auditory or vestibular function, except a 9.1% incidence of eighth cranial nerve paresis.

The only factor identified by univariate analysis to be critical for survival was the primary location of the disease. Supratentorial tumors in patients were associated with a 10-year disease-free survival rate of 15.4% compared with 29.6% for those with infratentorial tumors. Grigsby et al. (79) reevaluated these data and additional pediatric data with regard to prognostic variables.

Wara et al. (80) described management of primary gliomas of the brainstem and cord. Only the recommendations for the brainstem are reviewed. Radiation has been the treatment of choice for gliomas in this site. Sagittal MRI was used to demonstrate the lesion for treatment planning. The recommended field included a margin of 1–2 cm surrounding the tumor. In the cases reported, the superior border was the top of the third ventricle; inferiorly the bottom of C-2 was used. The anterior border was generally the anterior clinoid process, and the posterior extent, 2 cm beyond the tumor, by scan. Historically, treatment regimens utilized total doses < 4500 rads, but improved survival rates have been seen with a total dose of 500 rads. Hyperfractionated irradiation allowed greater nervous system tissue tolerance. In patients with brainstem tumors with poor local control, increase in the total dose by using smaller fractions (100–120 rads) allowed doses as high as 7200 rads. This improved 2-year survival rates to 50%. According to the authors, most patients showed rapid neurologic improvement with conventional protocols but failed locally within 1–2 years. The overall 5-year survival rate cited was 30%. Adults and patients with focal lesions responded better than children and individuals with diffuse lesions.

## FUTURE RESEARCH DIRECTIONS

Available literature suffers from flaws of research design, dated conclusions, and an excessive number of confounding variables. The pathophysiologic mechanism of delayed SNHL is unknown, although vascular changes are generally assumed to be involved. A properly controlled study with pretreatment assessment of all clinically relevant audiometric and vestibular parameters, long-term audiometric follow-up, and postmortem histologic examination of temporal bones is sorely needed. Such a study should include as many *in vivo* windows on brain and auditory function as possible, possibly incorporating not only audiometry and BERA but also sequential MRI, magnetic resonance angiography (MRA), SPECT, PET, brain electrical activity mapping (BEAM), and other studies. Until this information is available, responsible clinicians are forced to extrapolate from risk data that are inadequate in many ways for definitive guidance of treatment decisions.

## SUMMARY

Despite weaknesses in the available literature, it appears reasonable to assume that radiation may be associated with hearing loss in some patients. The mechanism of hearing loss is generally believed to be attributable to radiation-induced intracochlear or vascular changes. Interestingly, most of the studies in the literature that show significant hearing change involve radiation to the nasopharynx or parotid, with direct cochlear radiation exposure. This suggests that radiation for posterior cranial fossa neoplasms may be less damaging, possibly because it is less likely to affect the inner ear directly. It is particularly important to note that none of the published studies provides confirmation of etiology in those patients believed to have radiation-related hearing loss beginning >18 months following radiation. None of the reports in the world literature has adequate, modern neurotologic assessment of patients with supposed radiation-induced hearing loss. Rather, they merely assume that if the patient was radiated prior to developing hearing loss and there is no evidence of recurrent tumor, then the hearing loss must be related to the radiation. This *post hoc, ergo propter hoc* reasoning is classically flawed logic. There are innumerable causes of SNHL that are extremely common in modern society, and many of them are unilateral. Because all patients receiving radiation have been in hospital settings, they may be at increased risk for developing many of these conditions.

Available literature supports the existence of radiation-induced otitis and radiation-induced labyrinthitis, both of which occur during or soon after treatment. However, proof is lacking for the existence of radiation-induced delayed hearing loss. Statistics suggest that it is a possibility, but in some or all cases, the hearing loss may be related not to the radiation but rather to the original tumor, the underlying disease, the body's response to tumor, unrelated disease, or to other undetected causes. When hearing loss or other neurologic complications occur at >18–36 months following radiation therapy, there is no convincing evidence that they were caused by radiation. In fact, the literature reveals an appalling failure to work-up such patients to determine the true cause of their hearing deficits. In the future, interdisciplinary collaboration among neurotologists, radiation oncologists, and other specialists should address these issues, answer many remaining questions, and substantially improve the standard of care for hearing management in patients undergoing cranial irradiation.

## ENDOLYMPHATLC SAC SURGERY

Surgery on the endolymphatic sac was first performed in January 1926, by George Portman (81) who exposed and incised the sac. In the discussion that followed his presentation of this procedure to the American Medical Association's section on Laryngology, Otology, and Rhinology, Eagleton mentioned good results in several cases of Ménière's disease after simply uncovering the posterior fossa dura. Since Portman's operation,

numerous other techniques have been developed. In 1962, William House introduced the endolymphatic-subarachnoid shunt. Reviewing House's first 50 cases, Shambaugh (82) was impressed by certain cases in which House had been unable to identify the sac and had not incised the dura. The results of these and shunted cases were often equal. Sir Terence Cawthorne reported by letter to Shambaugh a series in which he compared endolymphatic-subarachnoid shunt, incision of the endolymphatic sac, and simple decompression without opening the sac. He noted that simple decompression worked in some cases. This was felt to be due to exposure of the sac to the atmospheric pressure of the middle ear, which becomes lower than intracranial pressure anytime the patient coughs, strains, or lies down. This intermittent relative negative pressure on one wall of the sac allows it to bulge slightly and probably results in hyperemia and increased fluid resorption. Encouraged by Cawthorne's findings, Shambaugh performed a series of simple endolymphatic sac decompressions and reported a 50% cure rate for vertigo and 45% cure rate for tinnitus in his primary typical cases.

Numerous other procedures are available for Ménière's disease. These include the tack operation (now performed rarely if ever), the endolymphatic-mastoid shunt, cryosurgery, cochleosacculotomy, and others such as destructive procedures and nerve sections. Operations directed at the sac are favored because they preserve hearing in most cases. Complication rates range from 0% to 6% and include complete loss of hearing in the operated ear, CSF otorrhea, hydrocephalus, shunt tube occlusion, labyrinthitis, and meningitis (83). Most authors report improvement of vertigo in between 70% and 90%, with a median of ~80% reporting relief of vertigo and 25% reporting hearing improvement (all endolymphatic sac operations combined). Numerous endolymphatic sac series have now been reported. In 1977, Smyth et al. reported results of endolymphatic sac decompression without incision, which he updated in 1981 (84). Using sac decompression, he reported improvement or stabilization of hearing in one-third and elimination of incapacitating vertigo in three-quarters of his patients. Like other authors, he has concluded that there is no difference between surgery in which the sac is exposed and surgery in which the sac is incised and entered. Ford (85) and Graham and Kemink (86) confirmed these findings. It is noteworthy that they found the Arenberg valve implant successful in a small number of revision cases. In most series except Smyth's, the incidence of worsened hearing and complications appears to be lower in the noninvasive or less-invasive procedures. Strikingly, Thomsen and associates reported a double-blind study in which no significant difference was found between mastoidectomy without exposure of the sac (sham) and endolymphatic-subarachnoid shunt, the active group showing 80% improvement and the placebo group showing 73% improvement (87).

In light of the clinical success rate in patients selected for surgery because of intractable, incapacitating vertigo, endolymphatic sac surgery seems justified. However, because of the apparent nonspecific effects of these procedures, we favor procedures with the lowest complication rate. Procedures that violate the sac show no advantage over procedures that simply expose it. Long-term follow-up is needed to determine whether, in fact, mastoidectomy without exposure of the sac provides equally satisfactory long-term results. Consequently, at the present time, endolymphatic sac decompression is the recommended procedure.

**Case 3** is a 56-year-old man with incapacitating vertigo and a 10-year history of bilateral Ménière's disease. He had been troubled by right-sided ear fullness, tinnitus, distortion, and hearing loss (**Figure 10.63**). Three years following a right endolymphatic sac decompression, he has remained free of vertigo. Moreover, although his pure-tone thresholds remain unchanged, his discrimination is better, his tinnitus is rarely present, and he is not troubled by fullness or distortion. This case was selected to emphasize that pure-tone threshold is not the only important parameter in assessing hearing. Improvement in discrimination and relief from distortion may be extremely helpful to the patient and may make the ear much more useful even if pure-tone thresholds do not improve.

## ACOUSTIC NEUROMA

Since William House revolutionized otology by making translabyrinthine and middle fossa surgery for acoustic neuroma practical and accepted, CPA tumors have been discussed widely in the literature. Early diagnosis and treatment minimize morbidity. For this reason, most otolaryngologists look for them aggressively in selected instances. Nevertheless, misconceptions about the way in which CPA tumors present clinically may result in failure to suspect the tumor and initiate complete evaluation. The delay in diagnosis may have undesirable consequences. The following cases are selected from the author's series to illustrate particular diagnostic points.

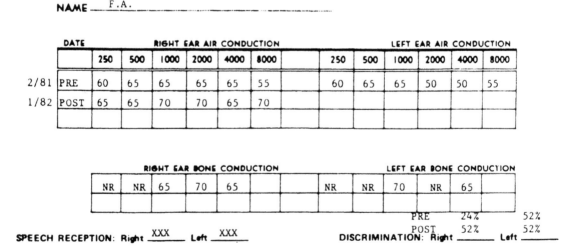

Figure 10.63 Preoperative and postoperative audiogram of Case 3, Ménière's disease.

**Case 4** is a 57-year-old white man who worked at a dye-casting company for 39 years. He was exposed to high-intensity noise from various sources. Recently, he had been operating a screw conveyor (steel on steel) at an intensity of ~84 dBA with intermittent peaks of 91 dBA lasting for ~2 s. He was aware of gradually progressive high-frequency SNHL in both ears. In October 1979, he was exposed for between 30 and 90 seconds to an extremely loud metal noise due to a defective piece of machinery. Three days later, he saw the plant nurse complaining of decreased hearing in the left ear and tinnitus. He denied vertigo. Previous audiograms confirmed that his hearing loss had been symmetrical. The audiogram following the incident showed a severe-to-profound SNHL in the left ear. He filed a legal claim for noise-induced hearing loss.

When he was referred for evaluation, his physical examination was within normal limits except for hearing acuity. There was no decreased sensation in his left ear canal. Audiogram confirmed the hearing loss (**Figure 10.64**). His discrimination score was 12%. His serological test for syphilis (MHA-TP) was negative. He had a left reduced vestibular response of 23%. BERA revealed low-amplitude responses with significantly prolonged wave I–V interval. Polytomograms of the IACs and CT scan were within normal limits. Pantopaque myelogram revealed a small filling defect within the left IAC. The right IAC appeared normal. Translabyrinthine surgery revealed an 8-mm acoustic neuroma originating from the inferior vestibular nerve. This was excised without complication.

Neither normal IAC X-rays nor a normal CT scan rules out the presence of an acoustic neuroma. In many cases, MRI with contrast is necessary. Sudden deafness is a particularly important symptom of acoustic neuroma because it deprives us of the usual symptoms and signs that allow early diagnosis, particularly progressive hearing loss. Therefore, if the tumor is missed at the time, it produces sudden deafness, it may not be diagnosed until it is large enough to cause serious neurological symptoms and signs. Some authors feel that as many as 10% (85) to 15% (88) of all acoustic neuromas may present with sudden deafness. Reviews of this subject by Sataloff and associates (89, 90) stress the need for greater awareness of this diagnostic problem.

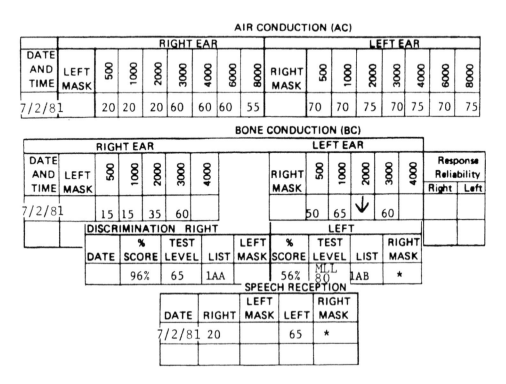

Figure 10.64 Audiogram of Case 4 illustrating severe left-sided hearing loss. This pattern is unlikely to be due to free-field noise exposure.

**Case 5** is a 78-year-old woman who had been followed for 7 years in an excellent teaching institution for bilateral hearing loss and severe left tinnitus. She had numerous cardiovascular problems and renal disease. Her work-up for acoustic neuroma had included normal polytomograms of the IACs. However, a CT scan had not been performed, and MR was not available at the time.

When she was referred, her audiogram revealed profound deafness on the left and severe hearing loss on the right with 28% discrimination (**Figure 10.65**). Her CT scan revealed a 5-cm acoustic neuroma. This was removed by a planned two-stage procedure. Translabyrinthine partial excision was used to debulk the tumor and preserve the facial nerve. Residual tumor was removed from the brainstem and lower cranial nerves ~2 weeks later.

It is important to remember that bilateral hearing loss even with "obvious" etiologies such as vascular disease and renal disease does not rule out acoustic neuroma, especially if the hearing loss is asymmetrical. Moreover, IAC bony architecture may be normal even in large tumors.

**Case 6** is a 38-year-old attorney who presented with left-sided tinnitus and progressive hearing loss worsening > 3 years (**Figure 10.66**). CT scan 3 years earlier had been negative. A recent brainstem evoked-response audiogram was normal. CT scan revealed a left IAC neoplasm (**Figure 10.67**). Because of bony erosion of the lateral portion of the IAC, no attempt was made to preserve hearing. Translabyrinthine surgery revealed a facial nerve neuroma that appeared to originate from the nervus intermedius.

Considering the findings of a basin-shaped audiogram, normal brainstem evoked-response audiogram, and previous normal CT scan, one could easily have missed this neoplasm. This case emphasizes the importance of constant suspicion and comprehensive evaluation until a definitive diagnosis is reached. Acoustic neuromas may be associated with any audiometric pattern.

NAME A.B.

| DATE | RIGHT EAR AIR CONDUCTION | | | | | | | LEFT EAR AIR CONDUCTION | | | | | |
|------|------|------|------|------|------|------|---|------|------|------|------|------|------|
| | 250 | 500 | 1000 | 2000 | 4000 | 8000 | | 250 | 500 | 1000 | 2000 | 4000 | 8000 |
| 1/84 | 65 | 70 | 65 | 55 | 70 | 70 | | NR | NR | NR | NR | NR | NR |
| | | | | | | | | | | | | | |
| | | | | | | | | | | | | | |

| | RIGHT EAR BONE CONDUCTION | | | | | | | LEFT EAR BONE CONDUCTION | | | | | |
|---|------|------|------|------|------|---|---|------|------|------|------|---|---|
| | NR | 65 | 65 | 55 | 55 | | | | | | | | |
| | | | | | | | | | | | | | |

SPEECH RECEPTION: Right XXX Left XXX          DISCRIMINATION: Right 28% Left _____

Figure 10.65 Preoperative audiogram of Case 5 showing profound hearing loss on the left and severe SNHL with poor discrimination on the right. The patient had a left acoustic neuroma.

NAME M.W.M.

| DATE | RIGHT EAR AIR CONDUCTION | | | | | | | LEFT EAR AIR CONDUCTION | | | | | |
|------|------|------|------|------|------|------|---|------|------|------|------|------|------|
| | 250 | 500 | 1000 | 2000 | 4000 | 8000 | | 250 | 500 | 1000 | 2000 | 4000 | 8000 |
| 10/81 | 10 | 20 | 20 | 15 | 15 | 25 | | 20 | 30 | 75 | 65 | 30 | 55 |
| | | | | | | | | | | | | | |
| | | | | | | | | | | | | | |

| | RIGHT EAR BONE CONDUCTION | | | | | | | LEFT EAR BONE CONDUCTION | | | | | |
|---|------|------|------|------|------|---|---|------|------|------|------|---|---|
| 3/83 | 10 | 10 | 10 | 0 | | | | 10 | 20 | 20 | 0 | | |
| | | | | | | | | | | | | | |

SPEECH RECEPTION: Right XXX Left XXX          DISCRIMINATION: Right 100% Left 60%

Figure 10.66 Basin-shaped audiogram of Case 6, left facial nerve neuroma.

**Case 7** is a 34-year-old woman whose only complaint was left-sided tinnitus. Her audiogram revealed left-sided hearing loss (**Figure 10.68**). Her physical examination showed abnormalities of cranial nerves V, VII (sensory), VIII, and IX. Her ENG revealed left reduced vestibular responses, and her brainstem evoked-response audiogram was abnormal. CT scan revealed a 6-cm acoustic neuroma (**Figure 10.69**). The tumor was removed in two stages with preservation of the facial nerve. With the patient's young age and history of occasional viral infections and "cold sores," and her other cranial nerve abnormalities, it might have been tempting to diagnose postherpetic cranial polyneuropathy.

The case is presented to emphasize the occurrence of acoustic neuromas in young people, in whom this disease is relatively common (91). In the young, it is not unusual to see large tumors with minimal symptoms and signs.

**Case 8** is a 71-year-old male with a long history of bilateral hearing loss. However, he had noted increased trouble hearing from his left ear for ~2 months. He also had had one episode of mild disequilibrium lasting 1–2 weeks, which resolved completely. He had no tinnitus. His audiogram (**Figure 10.70**) shows only mild asymmetry that could easily have been overlooked during routine testing. The patient's history of unilateral change, and his poor discrimination score on the left, resulted in additional testing. Brainstem evoked-responses were abnormal, ENG revealed left reduced vestibular response, CT scan revealed mild enlargement of the left IAC, and MRI with gadolinium-DTPA contrast showed an acoustic neuroma filling the IAC and extending into the CPA (**Figure 10.71**).

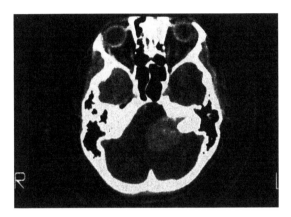

Figure 10.67 CT scan of Case 6 showing neoplasm of the left internal auditory canal, with erosion of the lateral aspect of the canal. This finding suggests a low probability of preserving hearing with total tumor removal. Patient underwent resection of a facial nerve neuroma.

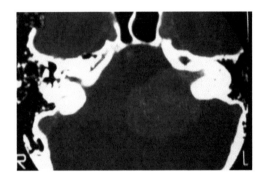

Figure 10.69 Large left acoustic neuroma of Case 7.

NAME L.T.

| DATE | RIGHT EAR AIR CONDUCTION | | | | | | | LEFT EAR AIR CONDUCTION | | | | | |
|---|---|---|---|---|---|---|---|---|---|---|---|---|---|
| | 250 | 500 | 1000 | 2000 | 4000 | 8000 | | 250 | 500 | 1000 | 2000 | 4000 | 8000 |
| 11/82 | 5 | 10 | 5 | 0 | 5 | 0 | | 15 | 20 | 20 | 50 | 50 | 65 |
| | | | | | | | | | | | | | |
| | | | | | | | | | | | | | |

| RIGHT EAR BONE CONDUCTION | | | | | | | LEFT EAR BONE CONDUCTION | | | | | |
|---|---|---|---|---|---|---|---|---|---|---|---|---|
| | | | | | | | | | | | | |
| | | | | | | | | | | | | |

SPEECH RECEPTION: Right __XXX__ Left __XXX__          DISCRIMINATION: Right __100%__ Left __64%__

Figure 10.68 Audiogram of Case 7.

JOSEPH SATALOFF, M.D.
ROBERT THAYER SATALOFF, M.D.
1721 PINE STREET    PHILADELPHIA, PA 19103

NAME _____ N. K. _____

| DATE | RIGHT EAR AIR CONDUCTION | | | | | | | LEFT EAR AIR CONDUCTION | | | | | |
| --- | --- | --- | --- | --- | --- | --- | --- | --- | --- | --- | --- | --- | --- |
| | 250 | 500 | 1000 | 2000 | 4000 | 8000 | | 250 | 500 | 1000 | 2000 | 4000 | 8000 |
| | 15 | 20 | 35 | 45 | 60 | 65 | | 20 | 30 | 45 | 65 | 70 | 85 |
| | | | | | | | | | | | | | |
| | | | | | | | | | | | | | |

| | RIGHT EAR BONE CONDUCTION | | | | | | | LEFT EAR BONE CONDUCTION | | | | | |
| --- | --- | --- | --- | --- | --- | --- | --- | --- | --- | --- | --- | --- | --- |
| | 5 | 15 | 40 | 55 | 55 | 65 | | 5 | 10 | 35 | 70 | 65 | NR |
| | | | | | | | | | | | | | |

SPEECH RECEPTION: Right __  __ Left _____          DISCRIMINATION: Right __88%__ Left __32%__

Figure 10.70 Audiogram of 71-year-old male with a long history of bilateral hearing loss. Audiogram shows only mild asymmetry.

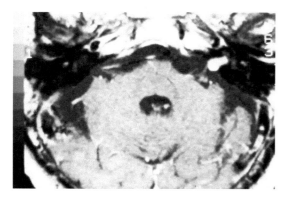

Figure 10.71 MRI with gadolinium-DTPA contrast shows an acoustic neuroma filling the internal auditory canal and extending into the cerebellopontine angle.

**Case 9** is a 50-year-old man. Fourteen years prior to his presentation, he had a 2-week episode of rotary vertigo without hearing loss or tinnitus. Thereafter, he was fine until 5 years prior to presentation when he developed sudden vertigo with no apparent etiology or antecedent precipitating event. He remained constantly off balance and had attacks of moderate-to-severe vertigo two to three times per week, thereafter. Progressive, fluctuating hearing loss began shortly after his attacks of vertigo began. He also has right tinnitus. Comprehensive metabolic and autoimmune evaluation, CT, and MRI were normal. ENG showed right reduced vestibular response, and ABR revealed a cochlear pattern on the right. Middle ear exploration for fistula revealed no evidence of perilymph leak and produced no improvement. Additional imaging studies are presented in **Figure 10.72**. Air-contrast CT showed a vascular loop (**Figure 10.72B**) at the anterior inferior cerebellar artery (straight arrow) entering the IAC and compressing the neurovascular bundle (curved arrow).

## COCHLEAR IMPLANT

In the years since the first report of electrical stimulation of the auditory nerve (92), great progress has been made (93). Primarily because of the pioneering contributions of William House and colleagues in Los Angeles, CIs now provide invaluable help to properly selected patients. Selection and rehabilitation are the essential elements of a successful CI program. The surgery is technically easy for an experienced otologist. However, selecting appropriate patients requires extensive, highly specialized testing and experience. Training a

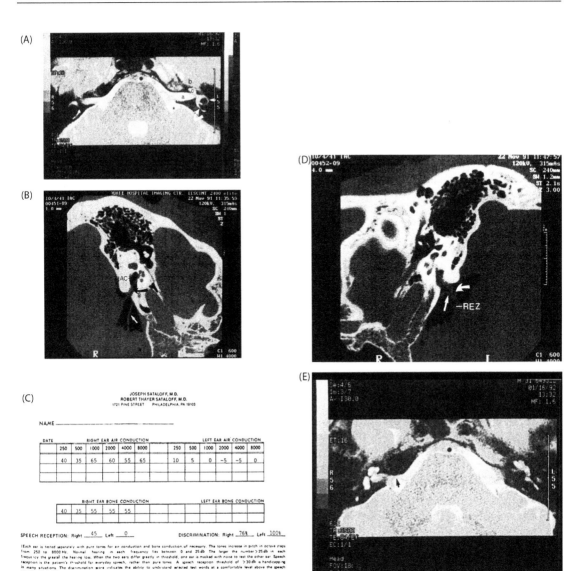

Figure 10.72 (A) Normal, high-resolution MRI presented for comparison showing the eighth cranial nerve (a), cochlear (b), and posterior semicircular canal (curved arrow). (B) Air CT reveals an anterior–inferior cerebellar artery vascular loop (straight arrow) entering the internal auditory canal (IAC) and compressing the neurovascular bundle (curve arrow). (C) Audiogram of Case 9. (D) This air-contrast CT of another ear shows another anterior–inferior cerebellar artery vascular loop (straight arrow) deflecting the eighth nerve complex (curved arrow) and causing typical thickening at the root entry zone (REZ). (E) High-resolution MRI scan of another patient showing the position of the anterior–inferior cerebellar artery (arrow). It is likely that improved MRI and MR angiogram will eventually replace air CT in the evaluation of vascular loop compression syndrome.

patient to use the implant postoperatively involves prolonged highly skilled rehabilitation. In treating appropriate patients with sensorineural deafness who cannot be helped adequately with hearing aids, CIs have proven worthwhile despite present technological limitations. Any patient with SNHL

of severe-to-profound severity deserves evaluation to determine his/her suitability for CI surgery.

In addition, criteria for cochlear implantation have changed as technology has improved. Now, even some patients with moderately severe SNHL may be appropriate candidates for cochlear implantation. In the early 2020s and a few years earlier, criteria was that if pure-tone thresholds of the better ear were greater than or equal to 60 dB HL, and if discrimination was less than or equal to 60% in the better ear (the 60/60 rule), patients were candidates for implantation. As technology advanced, criteria changed again. At present, CI can be performed for patients who meet the criteria in one ear even if contralateral hearing is normal, and insurance companies have begun to cover bilateral cochlear implantation.

## CONCLUSION

Many causes of sensorineural heating loss lend themselves to medical or surgical therapy. In addition to those discussed, vascular compression and other entities may also be managed by appropriate operative intervention. It is important for physicians to maintain a positive attitude and diligent approach toward patients with SNHL. In this way, we will not only find more patients whom we can help now but we will also find more ways to help other patients in the future.

## REFERENCES

1. Spoendlin H. The Organization of the Cochlear Receptor. Basel, Switzerland: S. Karger, 1966.
2. Lim DJ. Functional structure of the organ of Corti: a review. Hear Res 1986; 22:117–146.
3. Békésy G. Experiments in Hearing. New York, NY: McGraw-Hill, 1960.
4. Kim DO. Active and nonlinear cochlear biomechanics and the role of outer-hair-cell subsystem in the mammalian auditory system. Hear Res 1986; 22:105–114.
5. Rasmussen AT. Outlines of Neuroanatomy. Dubuque, Iowa: W.C. Brown, 1947.
6. Dallos P. Cochlear neurobiology: revolutionary developments, ASHA, Vol. June/July 1988;30: 50–55.
7. Walters JG. The effect of salicylates on the inner ear. Ann Otol 1955; 64:617.
8. Harbert F, Young IM. Threshold auditory adaptation measured by tone decay test and Békésy audiometry. Ann Otol 1964; 73:48.
9. Schuknecht HF, Gacek MR. Cochlear pathology in presbycusis. Ann Otol Rhinol Laryngol 1993; 102:1–16.
10. Pauler M, Schuknecht HF, White JA. Atrophy of the stria vascularis as a cause of sensorineural hearing loss. Laryngoscope 1988; 98(7):754–759.
11. Moscicki EK, Elkins EF, Baum HM, McNamara PM. Hearing loss in the elderly: an epidemiologic study of the Framingham Heart Study Cohort. Ear Hear 1985; 6(4): 184–190.
12. Susac JO, Hardiman JM, Selhost JB. Microangiopathy of the brain and retina. Neurology 1979; 29:313–316.
13. McCabe BF. Autoimmune sensorineural hearing loss. Ann Otol Rhinol Laryngol 1979; 88:585–589.
14. Boulassel MR, Deggouj N, Tomasi JP, Gersdorff M. Inner ear autoantibodies and their targets in patients with autoimmune inner ear diseases. Acta Otolaryngol 2001; 121:28–34.
15. Veldman JE. Immunology of hearing: experiments of nature. Am J Otol 1989; 10:183–187.
16. Hughes GB, Barna BP, Kinney SE, Calabrese LH, Nalepa NJ. Clinical diagnosis of immune inner-ear disease. Laryngoscope 1989; 98:251–253.
17. Veldman JE. Cochlear and retrocochlear immune-mediated inner ear disorders. Pathogenetic mechanisms and diagnostic tools. Ann Otol Rhinol Laryngol 1986; 95:535–540.
18. Sismanis A, Wise CM, Johnson GO. Methotrexate management of immune-mediated cochleovestibular disorders. Otolaryngol Head Neck Surg 1997; 116:146–152.
19. Hoistad DL, Schachern PA, Paparella MM. Autoimmune sensorineural hearing Joss: a human temporal bone study. Am J Otolaryngol 1998; 19:33–39.
20. Veldman JE, Roord JJ, O'Connor AF, Shea JJ. Autoimmunity and inner ear disorders: an immune-complex mediated sensorineural hearing loss. Laryngoscope 1994; 94:501–507.
21. Arnold W. Systemic autoimmune diseases associated with hearing Joss. Ann NY Acad Sci 1997; 830:187–202.

22. Harris JP. Autoimmunity of the inner ear. Am J Otol 1989; 10:193–195.
23. Ryan AF, Gloddek B. Harris JP. Lymphocyte trafficking to the inner ear. Ann NY Acad Sci 1997; 830:236–242.
24. Lasak JM, Sataloff RT, Hawkshaw M, Carey TE, Lyons KM, Spiegel JR. Autoimmune inner ear disease: steroid and cytotoxic drug therapy. ENT J 2001; 80:808–811, 815–816, 818.
25. Hirose K, Wener MH, Duckert LG. Utility of laboratory testing in autoimmune inner ear disease. Laryngoscope 1999; 109:1749–1754.
26. Carey TE, Nair TS, Cray JP et al. The search for the inner ear antigen of auto-immune sensorineural hearing loss. In: Veldman JE, Passali D, Lim OJ, eds. New Frontiers in Immunobiology. The Hague, the Netherlands: Kugler, 1999:67–74.
27. Harris JP, Ryan AF. Fundamental immune mech-anisms of the brain and inner ear. Otolaryngol Head Neck Surg 1995; 112:639–653.
28. Clements PJ. Alkylating agents. In: Dixon J, Furst DE, eds. Second Time Agents in the Treatment of Rheumatoid Diseases. New York, NY: Marcel Dekker, 1991:336–361.
29. Songsiridej N, Furst DE. Methotrexate-the rapidly acting drug. Baillieres Clin Rheumatol 1990; 4:575–593.
30. Matteson EL, Tirzaman O, Facer GW et al. Use of methotrexate for autoimmune hear-ing loss. Ann Otol Rhinol Laryngol 2000; 109:710–714.
31. Salley LH Jr, Grimm M, Sismanis A, Spencer RF, Wise CM. Methotrexate in the manage-ment of immune mediated cochleovestibu-lar disorders: clinical experience with 53 patients. J Rheumatoid 2001; 28:1037–1040.
32. Sismanis A, Thompson T, Willis HE. Methotrexate therapy for autoimmune hear-ing loss: a preliminary report. Laryngoscope 1994; 104:932–934.
33. Zavod MB, Sataloff RT, Rao VM. Frequency of cochlear enhancement on magnetic reso-nance imaging in patients with autoimmune sensorineural hearing loss. Arch Otolaryngol Head Neck Surg 2000; 126:969–971.
34. Gupta R, Sataloff RT. Noise-induced auto-immune sensorineural hearing loss. Otol Rhinol Laryngol 2003; 112(7):569–573.
35. Gates G, Schmid P, Kujawa SG, Nam B, D'Agostino R. Longitudinal threshold changes in older men with audiometric notches. Hear Res 2000; 141:220–228.
36. Yaremchuk KL, Dickson L, Burk K, Shivapuja BG. Noise level analysis of commercially available toys. JOHL 1999; 2(4):163–170.
37. Pearson BW, Barker HO. Head injury-same otoneurological sequelae. Arch Otolaryngol 1973; 97:81–84.
38. Rubin W. Whiplash and vestibular involve-ment. Arch Otolaryngol 1973; 97:85–87.
39. Tuohimaa P. Vestibular disturbances after acute mild head trauma. Acta Otol 1979; 87(suppl 359): 1–67.
40. Sataloff RT. Stapes Mobilization. In: LaRouere MJ, Babu SC, Bojrab DI, eds. Surgical Techniques in Otolaryngology – Head and Neck Surgery: Otologic and Neurotologic Surgery. New Delhi, India: Jaypee Brothers Medical Publishers, 2014:37–41.
41. House WF, Glorig A. Criteria for otoscle-rosis surgery and further experience with round window surgery. Laryngoscope 1960; 70:616–630.
42. Sheehy JL. Surgical correction of far advanced otosclerosis. Otolaryngol Clio North Am 1978; 11(1):121–123.
43. Frattali MA, Sataloff RT. Far-advanced oto-sclerosis. Ann Otol Rhinol Laryngol 1993; 102(6):433–437.
44. House WF. Oval window and round win-dow surgery in extensive otosclerosis. Laryngoscope 1959; 69:693–701.
45. Willis R. Severe otosclerosis. J Laryngol Otol 1963; 77 :250–258.
46. Myers D, Wolfson RJ, Tibbels EW Jr, Winchester RA. Apparent total deaf-ness due to advanced otosclerosis. Arch Otolaryngol 1963; 78:52–58.
47. Sheehy JL. Far-advanced otosclerosis. Diagnostic criteria and results of treatment; report of 67 cases. Arch Otolaryngol 1964; 80:244–248.
48. Sellars SL. Surgery of advanced otosclero-sis. S Afr Med J 1972; 1:434–437.
49. Wiet RJ, Morganstein SA, Zwolan TA, Pitgon SM. Far advanced otosclerosis. Cochlear implantation vs. stapedectomy. Arch Otolaryngol Head Neck Surg 1987; 113:299–302.

50. Babighian G, Smadsi M, Galavemi G, de Min G. Extreme stapedectomy. An Otorrinolaringol Ibero Am 1991; 18:239–248.

51. Lindsay JR, Hemenway WG. Occlusion of the round window by otosclerosis. Laryngoscope 1954; 164:10–14.

52. Myers EN, Myers D. Stapedectomy in advanced otosclerosis: a temporal bone report. J Laryngol Otol 1968; 82:557–564.

53. Schuknecht HF, Barber W. Histologic variants in otosclerosis. Laryngoscope 1985; 95:1307–1317.

54. Von Glass W, Philipp A. Imaging of capsule otosclerosis using computerized tomography. HNO 1988; 36:373–376.

55. Sataloff RT, Rosen DC. Effects of cranial irradiation on hearing acuity: a review of the literature. Amer J Otol 1994; 15(6):772–780.

56. Ewald CA. Die wirkung des radium auf das labyrinth. Zentralbl Physiol 1905; 10:298–299.

57. Girden E, Culler E. Auditory effects of roentgen rays in dogs. Am J Roentg 1933; 30:215–220.

58. Novotny O. Sull'azione dei raggi x sulla chioccicola della cavia. Arch Ital Otol Rhinol Laringol 1951; 62:15–19.

59. Kozlow MJ. Changes in the peripheric section of the auditory analyzer in acute radiation sickness. ORL J Otorhinolaryngeal Relat Spec 1959; 21:29–35.

60. Gamble JE, Peterson EA, Chandler JR. Radiation effects on the inner ear. Arch Otolaryngol 1968; 88:64–69.

61. Keleman G. Radiation and ear. Acta Otolaryngol Suppl 1963;184: 1–48.

62. Bohne BA, Marks JE, Glasgow GP. Delayed effects of ionizing radiation on the ear. Laryngoscope 1985; 95:818–828.

63. Evans RA, Liu KC, Azhar T, Symonds RP. Assessment of permanent hearing impairment following radical megavolt-age radiotherapy. J Laryngol Otol 1988; 102:588–589.

64. Borsanyi S, Blanchard C. Ionizing radiation and the ear. JAMA 1962; 181(11):958–961.

65. Leach W. Irradiation of the ear. J Laryngol Otol 1965; 79:870–880.

66. Dias A. Effects on the hearing of patients treated by irradiation in the head and neck area. J Laryngol Otol 1966; 80:276–287.

67. Schuknecht HF, Karmody CS. Radionecrosis of the temporal bone. Laryngoscopy 1966; 76:1416–1428.

68. Moretti JA. Sensorineural hearing loss following radiotherapy to the nasopharynx. Laryngoscope 1976; 86:598–602.

69. Thibadoux CM, Pereira WX, Hodges JM, Aur RJ. Effects of cranial radiation on hearing in children with acute lymphocytic leukemia. J Pediatr 1980; 96:405–406.

70. Coplan J, Post E, Richman R, Grimes C. Hearing loss after therapy with radiation. Am J Dis Child 1981; 135:1066–1067.

71. Talmi Y, Kalmanowitch M, Zohar Y. Thyroid carcinomas, cataract and hearing loss in a patient after irradiation for facial hemangioma. J Laryngol Otol 1988; 102:91–92.

72. Elwany S. Delayed ultrastructural radiation-induced changes in the human mesotympanic middle ear mucosa. J Laryngol Otol 1985; 99:343–353.

73. Chowdhury CR, Ho J H, Wright A, Tsao S Y, Au G K, Tung Y. Prospective study of the effects of ventilation tubes on hearing after radiotherapy for carcinomas of the nasopharynx. Ann Otol Rhinol Laryngol 1988; 97:142–145.

74. Hirsch A. Noren G. Audiological findings after stereotactic radiosurgery in acoustic neurinomas. Acta Otolaryngol 1988; 106:244–251.

75. Emami B, Lyman J, Brown A et al. Tolerance of normal tissue to therapeutic irradiation. Int J Radiat Oncol Biol Phys 1991; 21:109–122.

76. Singh IP, Slevin NJ. Late audiovestibular consequences of radical radiotherapy to the parotid. Clin Oncol (R Coli Radio) 1991; 3:217–219.

77. Grau C, Moller K, Overgaard M, Overgaard J, Elbrond O. Sensorineural hearing loss in patients treated with irradiation for nasopharyngeal carcinoma. Int J Radiat Oncol Biol Phys 1991; 21:723–728.

78. Grigsby P, Garcia D, Simpson J, Fineberg BB, Schwartz HG. Prognostic factors and results of therapy for adult thalamic and brainstem tumors. Cancer 1988; 11:2124–2129.

79. Grigsby P, Thomas P, Schwartz H. Fineberg B. Multivariate analysis of prognostic factors in pediatric and adult thalamic and brainstem tumors. Int J Radiat Oncol Biol Phys 1989; 16:649–655.

80. Wara W, Lindstadt D, Larson D. Management of primary brainstem gliomas and spinal gliomas. Sernin Radiat Oncol 1991; 1(1):50–53.

81. Portman G. Vertigo: surgical treatment by opening of the saccus endolymphaticus. Arch Otolaryngol 1927; 6:309.

82. Shambaugh GE. Surgery of the endolymphatic sac. Arch Otolaryngol 1966; 83:29–39.

83. Snow B, Kimmelman CP. Assessment of surgical procedures for Ménière's disease. Laryngoscope 1979; 89:737–747.

84. Smyth GDL, Hassard TH, Kerr AG. The surgical treatment of vertigo. Am J Otol 1981; 2(3):179–187.

85. Ford CN. Results of endolymphatic sac surgery in advanced Ménière's disease. Am J Otol 1982; 3(4):339–342.

86. Graham MD, Kemink JL. Surgical management of Ménière's disease with endolymphatic sac decompression by wide bony decompression of the posterior fossa dura: technique and results. Laryngoscope 94(5):680–683.

87. Thomsen J, Bretlau P, Tos M, Johnsen NJ. Placebo effect in surgery for Ménière's disease. Arch Otolaryngol 1981; 107:271–277.

88. Meyerhoff WL. When a person suddenly goes deaf. Med Times 1980; 108:25s–33s.

89. Sataloff RT, Davies B, Myers DL. Acoustic neuromas presenting as sudden deafness. Am J Otol 1985; 6(4):349–352.

90. Schmidt RJ, Sataloff RT, Newman J, Spiegel JR. Myers DL. The sensitivity of auditory brainstem response testing for the diagnosis of acoustic neuromas. Arch Otolaryngol Head Neck Surg 2001; 127:19–22.

91. Graham MD, Sataloff RT. Acoustic tumors in the young adult. Arch Otolaryngol 1984; 110(6):405–497.

92. Djourno A, Eyries C. Prothese auditive per excitation electrique a distance due nerf sensorial a l'aide d'um bobinage inclus a demeure. Presse Med 1957; 35:14–17.

93. House WF, Berliner Kl. Cochlear implants: progress and perspectives. Ann Otol Rhinol Laryngol 1982; 91(2, Part 3):7–24.

# 11

# Noise damage and hidden hearing loss: Cochlear synaptopathy in animals and humans

M. CHARLES LIBERMAN

## INTRODUCTION

When thinking about sensorineural hearing loss, it is important to differentiate problems with audibility, i.e., the ability to hear a sound, from problems with intelligibility, i.e., the ability to extract the meaning. It is an old concept that damage to the hair cells, the sensory transducers of the inner ear, is a primary driver of audibility issues, whereas loss of auditory nerve fibers, the electrical conduits for information transfer from the hair cells to the brain, is a key contributor to decreased intelligibility. However, for decades it was believed that hair cells were the primary target of damage in most forms of sensorineural hearing loss and that auditory nerve fibers degenerated mainly as secondary effect, i.e., if and only if the hair cells were already destroyed.

These ideas were challenged when our lab showed, in both noise-induced and age-related hearing loss in mice, that the most vulnerable elements in the inner ear were not the hair cells, but the synaptic connections between hair cells and auditory nerve fibers.[1,2] This synaptopathy could silence up to 50% of the neurons without damaging hair cells or changing thresholds (audibility), but it was hypothesized that it should have a significant effect on intelligibility, especially in difficult listening environments. It became an attractive hypothesis that such a phenomenon might underlie the condition in which a patient complaining of problems hearing in noise presents with a normal audiogram, especially if there is a history of acoustic overexposure. This audiological phenotype was given the name "hidden hearing loss".[3]

The idea that acoustic overexposure could permanently destroy neurons before it begins to elevate thresholds is concerning in a public health context, given that federal noise-exposure guidelines are designed on the premise that post-exposure threshold recovery is a sign that the inner ear structures have fully recovered. Since the discovery of synaptopathy in animal models, there has been extensive research aimed at determining whether the phenomenon is present in humans, both directly by examination of histopathology in autopsy specimens[4,5] and

DOI: 10.1201/b23379-11

indirectly by coupling non-invasive electrophysiological measures of sound-evoked neural activity with measures of hearing performance in subjects with normal audiograms.[6–9]

The purpose of this chapter is to summarize both the animal work that inspired the ideas behind "hidden hearing loss" and the human work that aims to understand the prevalence of this type of primary cochlear neural degeneration and to design procedures to diagnose it. To set the stage, we begin with an overview of normal cochlear structure and function as well as the nature of the non-invasive tests designed to differentially diagnose the extent of hair cell and neuronal damage.

## NORMAL COCHLEAR PHYSIOLOGY

### MIDDLE EAR

Sound waves in the air are funneled by the pinna, the visible part of the external ear, into the ear canal, where they ultimately reach the eardrum (tympanic membrane). The sound energy impinging on the eardrum sets up vibrations, which move the malleus, the first of the three middle ear bones. The malleus moves the incus, which connects to the stapes, which terminates in a footplate that fits snugly into the oval window of the inner ear. The sound-evoked piston-like motions of the stapes footplate set up pressure waves in the inner ear that are transduced by hair cells into electrical activity in the auditory nerve (**Figure 11.1**).

The ear can function over a remarkably wide range of sound pressure levels. As schematized in **Figure 11.2**, 0 dB sound pressure level (SPL) is at the threshold of hearing for humans for tones at 1000 Hz, or 1 kHz, which, for reference, is a little more than two octaves above middle C on the piano. Sound level is expressed in decibels (dB) because the range of levels over which we hear is so immense: each 20-dB increase in sound pressure corresponds to a factor of 10 increase in the amplitude of the pressure wave. Thus, the amplitude at the threshold of auditory pain, which is usually quoted at 140 dB, is 10,000,000 ($10^7$) times the amplitude at threshold.

A variety of pathological conditions can affect the function of the external and middle ears. This type of dysfunction is referred to as conductive hearing loss and is often surgically treatable and/or correctable with the sound amplification provided by hearing aids. In contrast, when damage to the inner ear causes hearing loss, it is called sensorineural because it typically involves either the sensory cells or the neurons found there.

### INNER EAR

The inner ear, or cochlea, is a spiraling fluid-filled tube, channeling through the hardest bone in the body, the petrous portion of the temporal bone.

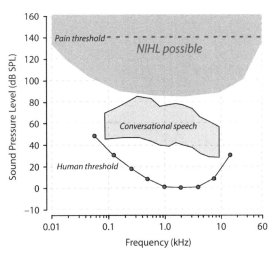

Figure 11.2 The dynamic range of human hearing ranging from threshold, near 0 dB, to the sound pressure levels for normal speech around 60 dB, to the range where noise-induced hearing loss (NIHL) can occur (above 90 dB), and the threshold of pain at 140 dB. *Abbreviation*: SPL, Sound pressure level.

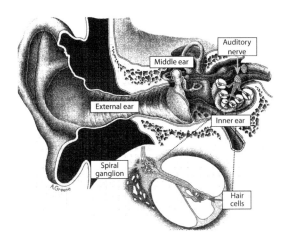

Figure 11.1 A schematic of the auditory periphery.

The fluid (pink in **Figure 11.3A**) is called perilymph, and it is much like cerebrospinal fluid and other extracellular fluids in the body (high in sodium chloride and low in potassium chloride). Stretched across this spiraling bony channel is another tube called the cochlear duct which is filled with endolymph (blue in **Figure 11.3A**), a fluid more similar to normal intracellular fluids (high in potassium and low in sodium). The cochlear duct includes a spiraling mound of cells called the organ of Corti, which houses the sensory cells (hair cells) responsible for transducing mechanical motions into electrical activity in the fibers of the auditory nerve (**Figure 11.4**).

The organ of Corti is a mechanically tuned structure. It is maximally sensitive to high frequencies (high pitches) at one end of the spiral at the base of the cochlea and to low frequencies at the apical end of the spiral (**Figure 11.3A**). This frequency tuning arises, in part, because the organ of Corti is thicker and more loosely stretched at the apex and thinner and more tightly stretched at the base of the cochlea, much like the low- vs. high-frequency strings on a guitar or piano. The frequency map of the cochlea has been experimentally measured in a number of species.[10–13] There is a logarithmic relation between best frequency and cochlear location (**Figure 11.3C**). In humans, every doubling of frequency corresponds to roughly a 5-mm increment along the

organ of Corti. Thus, there are seven octaves of best frequency (from 100 Hz to ~20,000 Hz) along the total spiral length of 35 mm in humans.[14]

The key structures of the spiraling organ of Corti are illustrated by the schematic cross-sectional view shown in **Figure 11.4**. There are three rows of outer hair cells (red) and one row of inner hair cells (blue), embedded in a matrix of supporting cells (grey), and innervated by the fibers of the auditory nerve (green). The schematic also shows the tiny tuft of hair-like extensions on top of each hair cell, which are called stereocilia. When sound-evoked motions of the middle ear bones set up vibrations in the organ of Corti, the resultant bending of the stereocilia opens submicroscopic channels in their membranes, which allows potassium ions from the endolymph to flow down an electrical gradient into the intracellular spaces within the hair cells.[16] This electrical gradient is powered by another set of cells lining the cochlear duct, called the stria vascularis (**Figure 11.5**). The membranes of the stria cells are lined with ion pumps that push potassium into the endolymph, and suck out sodium, establishing a positive resting potential inside the endolymph space that sets up an enormous driving force to push positively charged potassium ions through the hair cell stereocilia when the motion-sensitive channels are opened by sound-evoked vibrations.

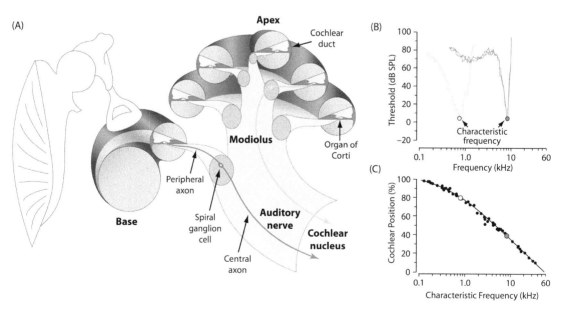

Figure 11.3 Schematic of the cochlear spiral showing two auditory nerve fibers (A), their tuning curves (B), and the cochlear frequency map for the cat (C). *Abbreviation*: SPL, Sound pressure level. (Reproduced from [15].)

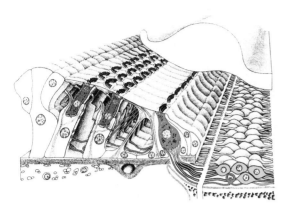

Figure 11.4 Schematic of the organ of Corti with its **outer** and **inner** hair cells and the **auditory nerve fibers** innervating them. (Modified from [17].)

This ionic current through the stereocilia changes the electrical potential inside the hair cells, which, in turn, leads to the release of chemical packets of neurotransmitter (glutamate) from the "base" of the hair cell, where it is closely contacted by the terminal endings of auditory nerve fibers.[18,19] This type of contact between the sensory cell and its primary sensory neuron is called a synapse, and the transfer of information that takes place there is called synaptic transmission. The arrival of the

neurotransmitter at the synaptic terminal opens ion channels in the auditory nerve fiber which ultimately leads to the generation of an action potential, a stereotyped rapid change in electrical potential. These action potentials are faithfully and rapidly transmitted to the brain, where they ultimately lead to the perception of sound in the auditory cortex.

The exquisitely sharp tuning of the inner ear can be seen in the "tuning curves" of single auditory nerve fibers, such as the two examples shown in **Figure 11.3B**. At low sound pressure levels near threshold, i.e. 0 dB SPL, each auditory nerve fiber responds by increasing the rate of action potentials to a very narrow range of frequencies.[20] We define a characteristic frequency as the frequency to which each fiber responds at the lowest sound pressure level: the examples in **Figure 11.3C** have characteristic frequencies near 1 and 10 kHz, and the 1-kHz fiber originates from a more apical location than the 10 kHz fiber. Auditory nerve fibers are sharply tuned because each one makes synaptic contact with only a single inner hair cell. Thus, its frequency selectivity reflects the mechanical tuning of a restricted region of the spiraling cochlear duct.[21] At higher sound pressure levels, e.g., at 80 dB, the response area of each fiber broadens to include a wider range of frequencies.

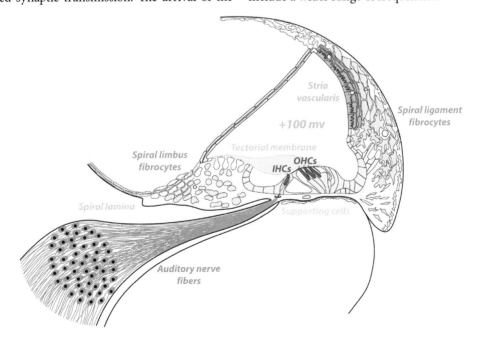

Figure 11.5 Schematic of the cochlear duct featuring the **stria vascularis**, which is the cochlea's battery. It supplies the 100-mV potential inside scala media, which is needed to drive potassium ions through the hair cells' stereocilia when sound-evoked vibrations open their ion channels. *Abbreviations*: IHCs, Inner hair cells; OHCs, Outer hair cells.

To cover the incredibly wide dynamic range of hearing, the normal population of auditory nerve fibers comprises two major subtypes, differing in their threshold sensitivity. As shown by the "tuning curves" in **Figure 11.6**, among the fibers tuned to the same frequency (and thus contacting inner hair cells in the same cochlear region), there are sensitive fibers with thresholds near the threshold of hearing (0 dB SPL) and others with thresholds 40 dB higher.[22] The scatterplot also shown in **Figure 11.6** shows that this spread of threshold sensitivities is seen across the cochlear spiral (at all regions of characteristic frequency) and that the least sensitive fibers can have thresholds 60 dB higher than the most sensitive in the same cochlear region.

This difference in sensitivity is closely correlated with differences in spontaneous discharge rate, i.e., the background rate at which a fiber fires in total silence.[22] Surprisingly, many auditory nerve fibers have spontaneous rates (SRs) as high as 100 action potentials per second while others have almost none. Fibers with low thresholds have high SRs and fibers with high thresholds have low SR. The high-threshold low-SR fibers are particularly important for hearing in a noisy environment because the low-threshold fibers are driven to their maximum rates by even a moderate-level noise and cannot respond to a signal like speech that might be embedded in the noise. By virtue of their higher thresholds, the low-SR fibers remain responsive to signals even in a high level of background noise.[23]

There are roughly 100 inner hair cells per millimeter of the organ of Corti, for a total of ~3500 inner hair cells in each human cochlea.[14] Each inner hair cell in the human ear is contacted by ~14 auditory nerve fibers (including both sensitive and insensitive ones), for a total of only about 50,000 auditory nerve fibers in each inner ear.[24,25] This is a surprisingly small number of neurons to carry all the information we receive about our acoustic environment compared to the billions of neurons in the brain and the millions in the optic nerve. The outer hair cells are contacted by a different class of auditory nerve fiber. These so-called type-II fibers comprise only 5% of the total fiber count in the auditory nerve; they are thin, and they lack the myelin sheath necessary for rapid conduction of action potentials.[26,27] It is believed that they may convey the sense of auditory pain to the central nervous system.[28,29]

Although 95% of the auditory nerve fibers contact only the inner hair cells, their responses are profoundly affected by the outer hair cells because the outer hair cells act as tiny biological motors that amplify the sound-evoked motions of the organ of Corti.[30] The membranes of these tube-shaped sensory cells are full of a molecule called prestin, which changes its conformation when the electric potential across the hair cell membrane is changed by the ionic currents that flow when the hair cell's stereocilia are vibrated. These conformational changes of the prestin molecules cause the entire cylindrical hair cell to lengthen and shorten in synchrony with the changing electrical potential. This electromotility, in turn, amplifies the sound-evoked motions of the organ of Corti and provide the exquisite frequency selectivity seen in the responses of the auditory nerve (**Figure 11.3B**).

The basic structure of the inner ear is fundamentally similar in all mammalian species including human. Although basic cellular biology of cochlear function has been worked out in experimental animals such as cat, guinea pig, gerbil, chinchilla, and mouse, it is thought that many basic mechanisms are similar to the human inner ear, i.e. (1) that the cochlea is mechanically tuned with low frequencies at the apex and high frequencies at the base, (2) that auditory nerve fibers make synaptic contact only with inner hair cells, and (3) that the sharp frequency selectivity

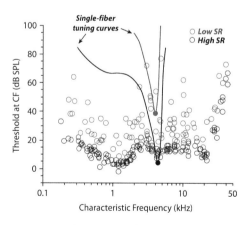

Figure 11.6 Auditory nerve fibers are of two types: low threshold (black) and high threshold (red). In the scatterplot, each point shows the threshold at characteristic frequency of a different fiber, i.e., the point at the tip of the tuning curve. Two example tuning curves are shown. Fibers with high characteristic frequencies contact inner hair cells in the base of the cochlea, whereas low-frequency fibers are from the apex. *Abbreviations*: CF, Characteristic Frequency; SPL, Sound pressure level; SR, Spontaneous rate. (Modified from [22].)

and low thresholds for these fibers rely on a cochlear amplifier powered by outer hair cells and the stria vascularis. Beyond these qualitative similarities, it is clear that there are important quantitative species differences, for example in (1) the frequency range over which the subjects hear[10] and (2) the vulnerability to acoustic injury in terms of the sound pressure levels and exposure durations required to produce temporary or permanent noise-induced damage.[31] These species differences mean that it can be difficult to extrapolate from animal tests to humans.

## MEASURES OF COCHLEAR FUNCTION

### THE AUDIOGRAM

In a clinical setting, the gold standard hearing test is the threshold audiogram, which measures the lowest sound pressure level at which tones of different frequencies can be reliably detected (**Figure 11.7**). This behavioral test requires that the subject be awake and alert. The threshold values are normalized to average values for young listeners and plotted as hearing level in dB *re* normals. The bigger the number and the lower the point on the plot, the larger the degree of threshold elevation relative to normal. In clinics, hearing levels within 20–25 dB of the average young-ear values are considered within normal limits.

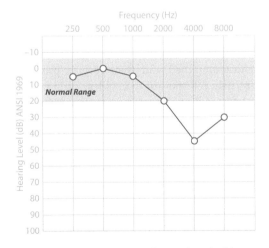

Figure 11.7 An audiogram shows thresholds at different test frequencies, expressed as the dB deviation from normal values. The pattern of hearing loss here, a 4-kHz notch, is typical of noise-induced hearing loss. *Abbreviation*: ANSI, American National Standards Institute.

Audiometric testing is standardly done in the clinic at octave frequency intervals, i.e., 125, 250, 500, 1000, 2000, 4000, and 8000 Hz, because the octave intervals correspond to roughly equal lengths along the cochlear spiral (**Figure 11.3C**). Inter-octave frequencies of 3000 and 6000 will often be tested as well because hearing loss is common in this frequency region. According to the cochlear frequency map for humans, 8000 Hz corresponds to a location about 7 mm from the base of the spiral (20% of the total 35 mm length), and the highest frequency we can hear (at least when we are young) is roughly 20 kHz.[10,14] The extended high frequencies (i.e. 8–20 kHz) are not standardly measured because (1) almost all speech sounds are at frequencies < 8000 Hz and (2) stimulus calibration at these high frequencies is more challenging.

Due to the significant time investment required to train awake animals to respond to sound in a reproducible way, most animal studies rely on two electrophysiological measures of auditory function that can be carried out in anesthetized animals: auditory evoked potentials including the auditory brainstem response (ABR), and otoacoustic emissions, particularly distortion product otoacoustic emissions (DPOAEs). Both of these tests are also applicable to awake human patients in a clinical setting.

### AUDITORY EVOKED POTENTIALS

The ABR is an electrical response that can be recorded from the skin in response to a train of short acoustic stimuli such as clicks or short bursts of a pure tone. These short acoustic stimuli evoke synchronized action potentials in different populations of neurons in the ascending auditory pathway. In animals, after anesthetization, a pair of sharp-needle electrodes is inserted through the skin: one near the external ear and one in the scalp at the midline. In awake (or sleeping) humans, small metal contacts are adhered to skin with a conductive paste: typically, one near or in the ear canal and another on the forehead. The electrical potentials evoked by sound are extremely small (microvolts), so they must be measured by averaging responses to many iterations of the stimulus (~1000). With these electrode configurations, the ABRs that result typically have five waves or peaks, as shown in **Figure 11.8**. The first wave represents the summed activity of the auditory nerve fibers, while the later waves represent activation of neuronal circuits in the brainstem and midbrain that process the sound-evoked activity on its way to the cortex.[32]

The "threshold" of the ABR response is typically defined by visual inspection of an array of waveforms stacked, as in **Figure 11.8**, in order of stimulus presentation level. In the example illustrated, the threshold would be defined as 35-dB SPL since this is the lowest level at which there appears to be a wave structure of similar morphology to that at higher levels (at least for the earlier waves). It must be noted that there can be some subjectivity in this visual selection and that these threshold values are typically higher than those that would be measured behaviorally. If there were time to average more responses, the ABR threshold could be lowered. In addition to the extraction of an ABR threshold, it can also be informative to measure the suprathreshold amplitudes and latencies of the responses. For wave 1, amplitude is often defined as the difference in voltage between the first peak (labeled "1" in **Figure 11.8**) and the subsequent trough. The latency is defined as the post-stimulus time at the peak amplitude value.

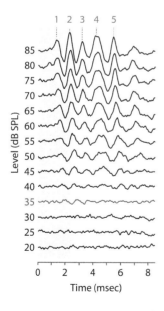

**Figure 11.8** ABR waves typically show five waves. Here, the responses measured at increasing stimulus levels are stacked to facilitate the identification of threshold (red). *Abbreviations*: ABR, Auditory brainstem response; SPL, Sound pressure level. (Modified from [33].)

A second type of auditory evoked potential, known as the envelope-following response (EFR) or the frequency-following response (FFR), has also been used in the study of cochlear synaptopathy. Our lab first introduced this test as a possible diagnostic for cochlear synaptopathy in 2015[34] because of the evidence that it might be more sensitive to the loss of auditory nerve fibers with high thresholds which we found to be most vulnerable to noise damage. Indeed, we found that EFR amplitudes were slightly more closely correlated with synaptic loss in mice with normal cochlear thresholds. However, the EFR response, which is measured in response to a continuous tone, which is amplitude-modulated in sinusoidal fashion, is more complicated to interpret because responses from the hair cells, the auditory nerve, and the brainstem and midbrain nuclei all add together rather than being separated in time into a series of waves, as they are in the ABR.

## OTOACOUSTIC EMISSIONS

Auditory evoked responses, by their nature, require functioning of the entire auditory periphery, from external ear to auditory nerve. Another minimally invasive, objective test of cochlear function is based on the measurement of otoacoustic emissions, which do not require cochlear neural function. Thus, the two tests are often applied together to aid in differential diagnosis.

Otoacoustic emissions are sounds generated in the healthy cochlea by the electromotility of the cochlea amplified and then reverse propagated from hair cell motion to cochlear fluid pressure, to stapes motion, to eardrum motion, which ultimately creates sound in the ear canal just like the motion of the diaphragm of a conventional audio speaker.[35]

One particularly useful class of otoacoustic emissions is the DPOAE, which is generated by playing two "primary" tones ($f_1$ and $f_2$) simultaneously into the ear. The mechano-electric transduction process in the hair cells distorts these tones and produces a third tone at the frequency corresponding to $(2 \times f_1) - f_2$. The amplitude of this distortion product can be measured by taking the spectrum of the sound pressure in the ear canal (**Figure 11.9A**). The amplitude of the DPOAE increases as the sound level of the primary tones is increased, and threshold can be defined as the primary tone levels required to produce a DPOAE of a criterion amplitude (**Figure 11.9B**). The suprathreshold growth of DPOAE amplitudes can also be used as a metric of cochlear health.

Given that DPOAEs are generated by the electromotile properties of the outer hair cells, they do not require inner hair cells, synaptic transmission, or auditory nerve fibers for their production.[36] As such, the presence of normal DPOAEs in the face of absent or attenuated ABRs can be used in differential diagnosis as evidence for dysfunction in the inner hair cells or auditory nerve fibers.

## MIDDLE EAR MUSCLE REFLEX

Another useful metric of peripheral auditory function is the middle ear muscle reflex. Two of the middle ear bones are connected to tiny muscles. The tensor tympani connects to the umbo of the malleus, and the stapedius muscle connects to the head of the stapes. The stapedius muscle is most relevant here because it forms the effector arm of a sound-evoked reflex that functions to minimize the effects of masking noise and also protects the ear from the damaging effects of overexposure

to continuous noise.[37] When the intensity of an acoustic stimulus, particularly a noise-type stimulus, reaches ~55-dB SPL, it can begin to elicit contractions of the stapedius muscle in both ears. These contractions stiffen the chain of three middle ear bones such that they vibrate less, especially in response to sounds below ~1 kHz.[38] The effects of this stiffening can be measured non-invasively by exciting the reflex with an elicitor tone in one ear and measuring the sound pressure of a test tone in the other ear: when the muscles contract (bilaterally), more of the energy from the test tone is reflected back into the ear canal, and that change in reflectance can be used as a measure of the threshold and suprathreshold strength of the middle ear muscle reflex.[39]

Because the reflex is normally activated at high sound pressure levels, it is less sensitive to threshold elevations in the auditory periphery. For years, it was used as the primary means of diagnosing tumors of the eighth nerve, the cranial nerve that carries both auditory and vestibular nerve fibers [14]. With advances in medical imaging that allowed direct visualization of such tumors, its clinical utility decreased; however, it has re-emerged as a possible diagnostic for the cochlear neural degeneration thought to underlie "hidden hearing loss."[40,41]

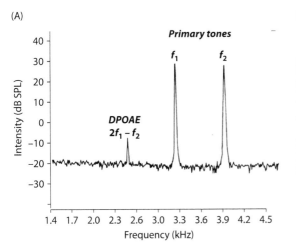

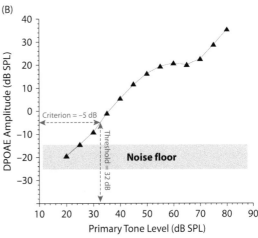

Figure 11.9 Distortion product otoacoustic emissions (DPOAEs). (A) The spectrum of the ear-canal sound pressure when two primary tones at $f_1$ and $f_2$ are presented shows the distortion product at $2f_1 - f_2$. (B) The amplitude of the $2f_1 - f_2$ distortion product increases as the sound pressure of the primary tones are increased. Threshold can be defined as the primary-tone level required to produce a DPOAE of a criterion amplitude (−5 dB SPL in this case). *Abbreviation:* SPL, Sound pressure level.

## NOISE-INDUCED HEARING LOSS

## GENERAL PRINCIPLES

It has been known for over a hundred years that overexposure to sound can cause elevation of thresholds,[42] commonly referred to as noise-induced hearing loss (NIHL). Threshold shifts can be measured in both humans and animal models by behavioral means, as well as by electrophysiological methods such as auditory evoked potentials or otoacoustic emissions, as discussed above.

NIHL can be reversible or irreversible. Threshold shifts can be measured immediately after a discrete acoustic overexposure, and thresholds will typically recover in exponential fashion, i.e., rapidly at first and subsequently with continuously decreasing speed as post-exposure time increases.[43] In animal models, an acute threshold shift (measured within minutes after overexposure) can be as large as 50 dB and yet still recover completely over the subsequent 1–2 weeks. If the acute threshold shift is larger than ~50 dB, thresholds will still recover in exponential fashion; however, they will asymptote at a level of permanent threshold shift within ~2 weeks post-exposure.

The amount of threshold shift resulting from an acoustic overexposure is a function of frequency content (i.e., spectrum of the sound), sound level, exposure duration, and intermittency.[44–46] All other things being equal, low-frequency sounds (e.g., 100–800 Hz) are less damaging than high-frequency sounds (e.g., 2000–8000 Hz). To a first approximation, the trade-off between time and intensity follows an equal-energy rule, i.e. a 100-dB exposure for 1 hour will be equally damaging as a 103-dB exposure for ½ hour, and to a 106-dB exposure for ¼ hour.[44] This basic relation underlies the Occupational Safety and Health Act (OSHA) exposure guidelines for workplace noise.[47] Intermittency, or duty cycle, is also tremendously important in determining the degree of NIHL: introducing even relatively short breaks in an otherwise continuous noise can decrease the resultant permanent threshold shifts by 20–25 dB.[48]

The relation between the spectrum of the sound exposure and the frequency pattern of hearing loss is partially governed by the mechanical tuning of the cochlea (as described above). As expected, if the spectrum of the exposure is narrow band (e.g. a pure tone), there will be a peak in threshold shift at the cochlear region tuned close to the exposure tone.[49,50] Actually, it is often offset by half an octave toward higher frequencies, but that offset is well explained by the non-linear behavior observed in cochlear mechanics at high sound pressure levels.[51]

When the noise is broadband, as is typically the case with workplace or military exposure, the maximum threshold shift is characteristically seen at mid-frequencies.[52] In humans, that maximum loss is typically seen at 4 kHz (or 6 kHz if that frequency has also been tested). This mid-frequency vulnerability likely arises because the external ear and ear canal in humans have a resonance in the mid-frequency range. Thus, the frequency components of the acoustic stimulus near 4 kHz tend to be amplified by the time they travel through the ear canal to the eardrum.

A final complexity to be considered is that the variety of acoustic overexposures that can damage the auditory periphery is immense, ranging from a daily workplace exposure to a 90-dB noise for 40 years to a single-shot exposure to a 190-dB blast wave that lasts only a few milliseconds. For practical reasons, most laboratory work in animal models has concentrated on something in the middle, i.e. 1- to 4-hour exposures to bands of noise in range of 100- to 120-dB SPL.[46] There has also been some work on impulse noise exposures at peak levels up to 180-dB SPL,[53–55] but there has been very little work on lifetime exposures even for animal models that live only a few years. Thus, the general rules summarized here and in the next section are dominated by observations on overexposures in the "middle of the range."

## STRUCTURAL CHANGES UNDERLYING PERMANENT VS. TEMPORARY NOISE-INDUCED THRESHOLD SHIFTS

### Hair cell death and damage

The inner ear cannot be biopsied, and all the key cellular structures are too small to be viewed by any non-invasive imaging techniques. Thus, the noise-induced structural changes in the inner ear can only be viewed in post-mortem specimens in which the tissue has been treated with chemical fixatives and subjected to a variety of other manipulations (e.g., embedding, sectioning staining) before viewing in the light microscope or electron microscope.

If the sound pressure is high enough and/or the duration is long enough, virtually all the cell types lining the cochlear duct can be damaged by acoustic overexposure.[46] However, the organ of Corti appears to be the most vulnerable structure, and it can be completely destroyed within small or large stretches of the cochlear spiral (**Figure 11.10C**). Of the cells within the organ of Corti, the outer hair cells are more prone to degeneration than the inner hair cells for most types of sensorineural hearing loss, including that caused by acoustic overexposure and aging.[49] In the cochlear region shown in **Figure 11.10B**, most of the outer hair cells have degenerated, while the inner hair cells and the rest of the supporting cells of the organ of Corti remain intact. In the mammalian cochlea, including in humans, hair cells do not regenerate; once they die, they are never replaced.

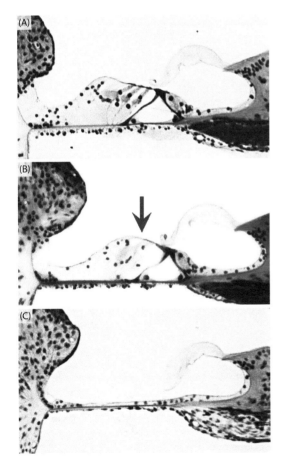

Figure 11.10 Light microscope views of the organ of Corti in a normal ear (A), and a few months after acoustic injury, showing selective loss of outer hair cells (B) and total loss of the organ of Corti (C). (Modified from [49].)

In acquired sensorineural hearing loss, inner hair cells are almost never lost without an accompanying loss of outer hair cells. However, in some unique animal models, it is possible to selectively destroy inner hair cells.[56] From these experiments, we know that threshold measures are not very sensitive to the selective destruction of inner hair cells. If diffusely spread across the spiral, the inner hair cell loss must exceed 80% before the threshold loss exceeds 25 dB, the limits typically defined for the normal hearing range.[56] The reason for this can be seen in the auditory nerve tuning curves (**Figures 11.3** and **11.6**). As sound pressure rises to 20 dB above threshold, a fiber tuned to 1 kHz begins to respond to tones an octave away at 2 kHz. Thus, even the loss of every other inner hair cell (50%) is easily compensated by slightly raising sound pressure level by a few dB, i.e., enough to recruit responses in neurons from neighboring hair cells. In a clinical or a laboratory context, a threshold shift of a few dB is not considered to be meaningful.

Not all of the hair cells that survive are functioning normally in the noise-exposed (or aging) ear. Many hair cells, both inner and outer, survive a cochlear insult with badly damaged stereocilia.[57] As shown in **Figure 11.11**, that damage can include disarray, loss, and fusion of adjacent stereocilia within the tuft on each hair cell. Given that the stereocilia are the site of the delicate cellular apparatus for mechano-electric transduction, i.e. the transformation of mechanical vibration into electrical currents, it is not surprising that the kinds of stereocilia damage shown in **Figure 11.11** lead to threshold elevations as great as 80 dB or more.[58]

All of the structural changes discussed to date are irreversible and help explain why acoustic overexposure can cause permanent elevation of thresholds. The structural changes underlying reversible threshold elevations are much more poorly understood, likely because most of them are submicroscopic. Careful evaluation of animal ears extracted during a temporary (i.e., fully reversible) threshold shift of 50–60 dB reveals no missing hair cells and no stereocilia pathology of the types described above.[59] We have seen subtle changes in the internal structure of the stereocilium,[60] and several lines of evidence suggest that there can be reversible collapse of some of the supporting cells in the organ of Corti.[61,62]

The most reproducible changes in temporary or reversible threshold shift reported are the swelling of auditory nerve terminals at their points of synaptic contact with the inner hair cells. Although severe swelling is visible in the light microscope, most studies of this phenomenon relied on electron microscopic examination which looks at much smaller regions at much higher magnifications. This terminal swelling is rampant when ears are examined within 24 hours of the exposure but are not visible at longer post-exposure times.[59,63] The disappearance of the swollen terminals along the same time course as the recovery of thresholds led many to assume (1) that the threshold shift was due to the terminal swelling *per se* and (2) that the threshold recovery indicated that all the neurons had recovered as well. As discussed below, it turns out that neither inference is true.

## Neuronal death and damage

For decades, it was assumed, for most types of sensorineural hearing loss (including age-related and noise-induced), that auditory nerve fibers degenerated if and only if the inner hair cells were first destroyed, i.e. that the hair cells were the primary targets of noise and other cochlear insults, and that auditory nerve degeneration was always a secondary event to the death of their synaptic partners.[64,65] This dogma arose because the loss of hair cells can be observed within hours or days after an acoustic injury, whereas the loss of spiral ganglion cells, the cell bodies of the auditory nerve fibers, was not detectable until months later.[49] As schematized in **Figure 11.3A**, each auditory nerve fiber is a bipolar neuron, with a cell body called a spiral ganglion cell, a peripheral axon that connects to the organ of Corti, and a central axon that projects to the cells in the brainstem.

In 2009, our group at Mass. Eye and Ear discovered that the acute swelling of synaptic terminals we and others had seen in the hours after noise exposure was not fully reversible,[2] i.e., that it could lead to the permanent loss of up to 50% of the synaptic connections between auditory nerve fibers and inner hair cells (**Figure 11.12**). To study this cochlear synaptopathy, we used antibodies to label key proteins associated with the synaptic machinery: one on the inner hair cell side (the pre-synaptic ribbon, in red), and one on the nerve fiber side (the patch of neurotransmitter receptors, in green) as illustrated in the schematic of **Figure 11.12A**. Thus, in the microscope images, each synapse between an auditory nerve fiber and an inner hair cell appears as a closely apposed pair of red and green dots (**Figure 11.12B, C**). Since each fiber contacts a single inner hair cell by a single synapse, each missing synapse indicates that one auditory nerve fiber is disconnected from any synaptic input, and is therefore completely silenced, i.e., no spontaneous discharge and no response to sound. Comparing the images in **Figures 11.12B, C** shows the obvious loss of synaptic contacts in the inner hair cells that survive after acoustic overexposure.

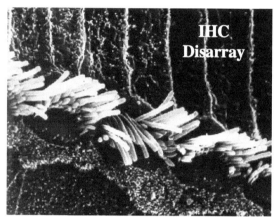

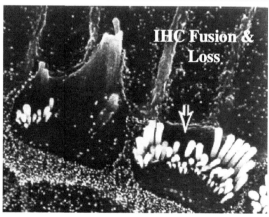

Figure 11.11 Noise-induced damage to stereocilia tufts on inner hair cells (IHCs) seen by scanning electron microscopy many months after acoustic overexposure. (Modified from [59].)

The cochlear synaptopathy manifests as an immediate swelling of the terminal that begins during the noise exposure, which in these laboratory experiments usually last from 1 to 2 hours.

The loss of synapses is obvious upon microscopic evaluation of the cochlea immediately after the termination of the exposure.[66] In this noise model, the thresholds return to normal with 1–2 weeks post-exposure, and there is never any loss of hair cells, but the synaptic loss is irreversible and is ultimately followed by the death of the entire neuron.[2] However, the loss of cell bodies in the spiral ganglion is extremely slow: it takes two years for ganglion cell loss to match the immediate 50% loss of synapses. Since spiral ganglion cell counts had always been the metric for cochlear neuronal degeneration, and since that degeneration is extremely slow, researchers had never noted neuronal degeneration in cases of temporary threshold shift: after cochlear thresholds had recovered, there was little interest in studying cochlear status at longer post-exposure times.

## THE CONCEPT OF HIDDEN HEARING LOSS IN ANIMAL MODELS

## THE PHENOMENON IN MOUSE AND ITS "DIAGNOSIS"

In our first demonstrations of noise-induced cochlear synaptopathy,[2] mice were exposed for 2 hours at 100-dB SPL to an octave band of noise in roughly the middle of their hearing range (8–16 kHz). The noise level and duration were carefully adjusted to be at the border between reversible and irreversible damage; for this noise spectrum and this duration, 100 dB was the highest level we could present and still observe complete recovery of cochlear thresholds to pre-exposure baselines. As

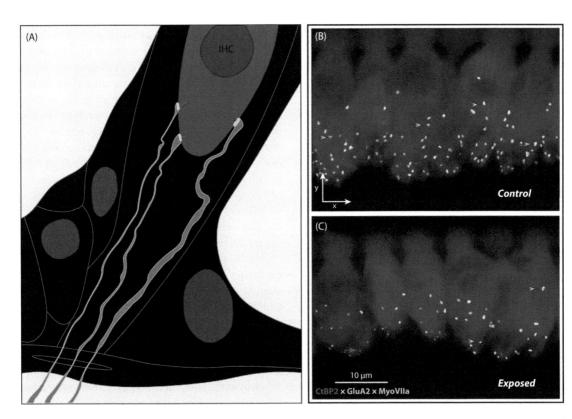

Figure 11.12 Documenting cochlear synaptopathy in the microscope. (A) Schematic showing how the synaptic contacts between auditory nerve fibers and inner hair cells (IHCs) can be visualized using antibodies against key synaptic proteins coupled to either red or green fluorescent molecules. (B, C) Microscope images of six inner hair cells from a normal and an exposed mouse ear showing the loss of ~50% of the synapses. CtBP2 is a protein in the pre-synaptic ribbon in the inner hair cell. GluA2 is one component of the receptor complex in the nerve-fiber terminals for the neurotransmitter released by the hair cell (glutamate). MyoVIIa is a protein found throughout the cytoplasm of the inner hair cell.

shown in **Figure 11.13A, B**, this threshold recovery was complete by 2 weeks post-exposure, as measured by either DPOAEs or ABRs. Despite the complete threshold recovery, the suprathreshold amplitudes of ABR wave 1 were reduced by roughly 50% (**Figure 11.13D**), i.e., in proportion to the roughly 50% loss of synapses in these animals. The recovery of the DPOAE suprathreshold amplitudes (**Figure 11.13C**) suggests that the outer hair cells, classically considered to be the most vulnerable elements to acoustic overexposure, have completely recovered.

Although a noise exposure causing a severe but ultimately reversible threshold shift can, nonetheless, cause permanent cochlear synaptopathy in some animals, not all exposures causing a temporary threshold shift also cause cochlear synaptopathy.[44,67] Indeed, the relationship between exposure parameters and the magnitude and cochlear extent of synaptopathy are far from clear, and they likely depend in a complex way on the duration, intermittency, spectrum, and intensity of the exposures and demonstrate variability based on the species under study.

In the mouse model, our group has shown that, if the thresholds have returned to normal, there is a close correlation between the fractional decline in suprathreshold ABR amplitudes and the fractional decline in the number of synapses in the cochlear region appropriate to the frequency of the tone pips used. Thus, in an animal where the synaptopathy was confined to regions above the 16 kHz place, the suprathreshold ABR amplitudes to 11 kHz remained normal, whereas those at 32 kHz were attenuated.[2,44]

These observations generated the idea that ABR suprathreshold amplitudes can be used to diagnose cochlear synaptopathy in some animals. However, the diagnostic utility in mouse depends critically on the low variance of the ABR suprathreshold amplitudes in control mice, which are genetically homogeneous and are studied in age- and sex-matched groups. The intersubject variance in suprathreshold ABR amplitudes in "normal hearing" humans is much greater for a variety of reasons, as discussed in more detail below.

Furthermore, the diagnostic utility disappears as soon as there are any threshold elevations because threshold elevations also decrease the suprathreshold amplitude of the ABR.[44] These threshold elevations compromise the diagnostic utility even if they are present only at the highest frequency regions, far from the nominal frequency region of the tone pip used to evoke responses. This is a particularly thorny problem because of the "mechanically inappropriate" threshold shifts at the extended high frequencies that are a ubiquitous aspect of NIHL, regardless of the spectrum of the acoustic overexposure.[49,68] At the stimulus intensities where suprathreshold amplitudes are measured (i.e. 80-dB SPL), most auditory nerve fibers tuned to frequencies at and above the stimulus frequency will be activated, including those at the extreme high frequencies. This can be inferred from the asymmetric shape of the tuning curves (**Figure 11.3C**): the long low-frequency "tail" means that even a fiber at the extreme base can respond to a mid-frequency tone when its level reaches 80-dB SPL. Therefore, a noise-induced lesion at the extended high frequencies (i.e., above 8000 Hz in humans) will decrease the ABR suprathreshold amplitudes to a mid-frequency tone or a click, even if the standard audiometric thresholds have returned to normal after the exposure.

The observation that in some animals there can be significant cochlear damage despite complete recovery of thresholds, the "gold standard" metric of hearing loss, suggested the catch phrase "hidden hearing loss" to describe the neuronal loss that may "hide" behind the audiogram.[3] How can ABR or behavioral thresholds recover despite a silencing of 50% of the auditory nerve fibers throughout most of the high-frequency half of the cochlea? There are two ways to resolve these at-first-paradoxical observations.

The first is to consider the same spread-of-excitation argument we considered above in the context of selective inner hair cell loss. Although auditory nerve fibers are sharply tuned, the tuning differences between adjacent inner hair cells are very small. Because there are so many inner hair cells (~500) per octave of cochlear frequency, each immediate neighbor has a characteristic frequency offset by only 1/500 of an octave. Thus, only a few dB (< 6) increase in sound pressure level is required near threshold to spread the excitation far enough on either side of one inner hair cell to double the number of responding fibers, and thereby compensate for a 50% loss of fibers. In a "hearing loss" context, 6 dB is not considered significant.

The second explanation is to that subsequent work in guinea pigs showed that it is the

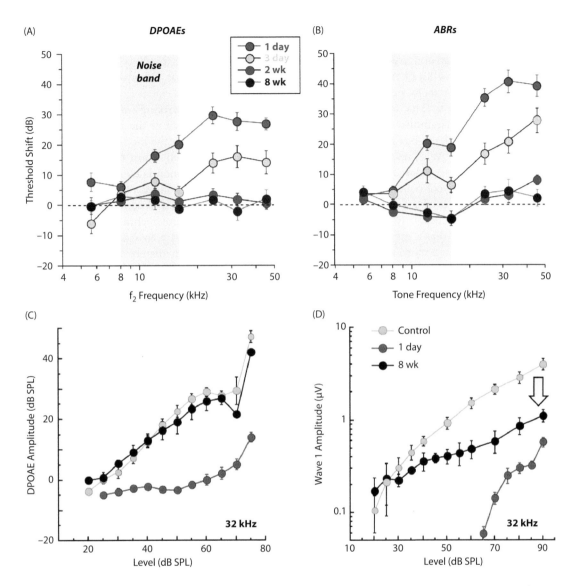

Figure 11.13 The Hidden Hearing Loss phenotype: thresholds recover after a noise exposure for both DPOAEs (A) and ABRs (B), and suprathreshold amplitudes for DPOAEs recover (C), while those for ABRs do not (D). These data are from a group of mice exposed to synaptopathic noise, as measured before (control), and then 1 day and 8 weeks post-exposure. *Abbreviations*: ABR, Auditory brainstem response; DPOAE, Distortion product otoacoustic emission; SPL, Sound pressure level. (Modified from [2].)

high-threshold auditory nerve fibers with low SRs that are most vulnerable to noise.[69] Their loss will affect the suprathreshold growth of amplitude without modifying the sound level required to achieve threshold. This explanation pertains only to the phenomenon of noise-induced synaptopathy in these animals as there is no reason to think that a partial surgical lesion would selectively target one SR group over another. However, it has also

been reported that low-SR fibers are the first to die in the process of normal aging, as seen in a gerbil model,[70] and in the aging mouse model, loss of cochlear synapses precedes the loss of hair cells, as it does after noise.[1]

The idea that low-SR fibers are more vulnerable inspired the use of the EFR and the middle ear muscle reflex as metrics of cochlear synaptopathy. With respect to the EFR, there is direct evidence that low-SR fibers can respond more vigorously than high-SR fibers to the types of amplitude-modulated tones that are used to generate an EFR,[71] whereas the low-SR fibers tend to contribute less than high-SR fibers, on a per fiber basis, to the ABR response.[72] Thus, the EFR should be more sensitive to noise-induced cochlear synaptopathy than the ABR, as has indeed been demonstrated in mouse.[34] With respect to the middle ear muscle reflex, we speculated years ago that the low-SR fibers might contribute relatively more than high-SR fibers to the neural drive for the middle ear-muscle reflex.[73] Indeed, we showed in the mouse model that a metric of middle ear muscle reflex was also a more sensitive indicator of cochlear synaptopathy than the suprathreshold amplitude of the ABR.[40,41]

## POSSIBLE SPECIES DIFFERENCES

Since the mouse differs from human with respect to the frequency range of hearing (4000–80,000 Hz vs. 100–20,000 Hz, respectively), it was important to determine if noise-induced cochlear synaptopathy was demonstrable in mammals with a hearing range more similar to humans, such as guinea pigs and chinchillas. Indeed, when noise bands were placed in the middle of the hearing range and titrated in level and duration to produce a severe but ultimately reversible threshold shift, both guinea pig and chinchilla also showed significant loss of synapses without any loss of hair cells.[74,75]

Work with non-human primates is important because they are most closely related to humans. Our group has also studied the rhesus macaque, where we have shown that a more modest amount of synaptic loss (20%) can be produced by narrow-band exposures that cause a completely reversible threshold shift and no significant loss of hair cells.[76] Importantly, the noise exposures required to produce this modest level of synaptopathy were more intense than those for mice (108 dB vs. 100 dB) and twice as long (4 hours vs. 2 hours).

Additional interspecies differences have been documented with respect to the phenomenon of cochlear synaptopathy. Firstly, having demonstrated in the guinea pig that the noise-induced loss of auditory nerve fibers was heavily biased towards those with low SRs and high thresholds,[69] we recorded from populations of auditory nerve fibers in the original mouse model of noise-induced synaptopathy and discovered no evidence for a selective loss according to SR group. In the mouse, it seems that fibers of all SR groups are equally vulnerable.[77]

An even more striking interspecies difference is in the reversibility of the cochlear synaptopathy phenomenon. In the mouse model (at least in the particular inbred strain that we used [CBA/CaJ]), the phenomenon is clearly irreversible and ultimately leads to a correspondingly large loss of spiral ganglion cells,[2] as described above. However, using exactly the same techniques in guinea pigs, we have shown that a loss of up to 60% of the synapses seen immediately after exposure can completely recover in some cochlear regions by 6 months post-exposure.[78,79] The reasons for this surprising difference in the regenerative capacities of two mammalian species even in the same family (Rodentia) are unclear, but they suggest another reason why caution must be exercised in extrapolating the mouse results on cochlear synaptopathy to humans.

## EXTRAPOLATION TO HUMANS AND CLINICAL EVALUATIONS

## HISTOPATHOLOGY OF NOISE-INDUCED HEARING LOSS IN HUMAN EARS

The inner ear cannot be biopsied and medical imaging cannot yet provide cellular-level detail about the cochlear pathology. Therefore, everything we know about the "ground truth" of the structural changes underlying sensorineural hearing loss comes from light and electron microscopic examination of inner ear tissues gathered at autopsy from tissue donors. These human studies are difficult because the (1) number of cases available for study is limited, (2) the ages of donor ears tend toward the older end of the lifespan, (3) histological preservation is variable because of the variable delay between death and tissue harvest, and (4) the medical histories of the deceased individuals tend to be complex, and it can be difficult to assign an unambiguous cause to any observed pathology.

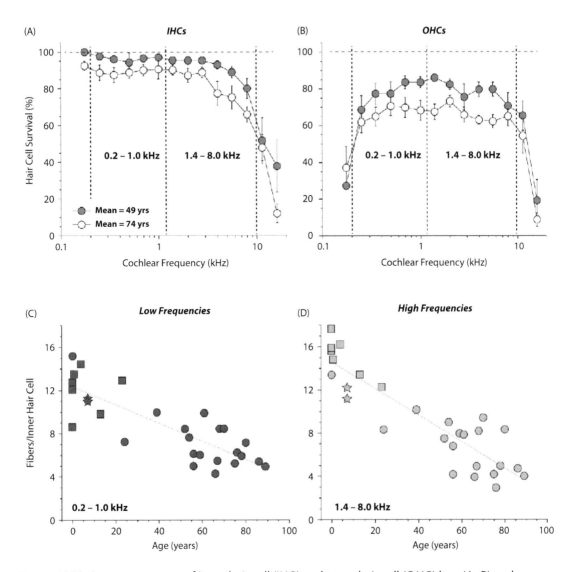

Figure 11.14 Average patterns of inner hair cell (IHC) and outer hair cell (OHC) loss (A, B) and nerve fiber loss (C, D) in "normal-aging human ears. (Modified from [4].)

Nevertheless, there are a number of conclusions about the effects of noise on the human ear that can be stated with reasonable certainty. To understand the effects of noise, one has to first document the nature of the structural changes associated with "normal aging." In **Figure 11.14**, we summarize some of the most comprehensive quantitative data on the patterns of hair cell loss and auditory nerve fiber loss in human cases in which there was no explicit history of otologic disease, either acquired or inherited.[4] Most of these cases had no associated audiometric records because they had no explicit audiometric complaint; however, we assume they had significant high-frequency hearing

loss as expected for all "normal-aging" subjects.[80] The salient point in the present context is that in the course of normal aging, there is a steady loss of auditory nerve fibers in both the low-frequency and high-frequency halves of the cochlea. By 60 years of age, all of the cases in this study had lost roughly 50% of their auditory nerve fibers, whereas there was only ~10% loss of inner hair cells, especially in the low-frequency half of the cochlea.

In our human studies, we used a different metric of cochlear neural degeneration. In the animal studies, we pioneered the use of synaptic counts as the most practical and accurate metric because the synapse degenerates first, followed within a few weeks by degeneration of the peripheral axons, and then months to years later by the loss of the cell body (spiral ganglion cell) and central axons.[49,64] Although these tiny synaptic structures could sometimes be seen in human material, the peripheral axons are more resistant to the tissue degradation that begins after death and is only stabilized when the autopsy sample is extracted and immersed in embalming solutions. Thus, in the human material, we counted peripheral axons. Their loss reflects the same process as cochlear synaptopathy, although it may slightly underestimate the extent given that its degeneration lags behind the synaptic loss by a few weeks.

The effects of noise history on the human inner ear have been reported in numerous case studies over the last few decades.[81,82]. Many of these studies noted that there was hair cell damage in the region of the cochlea appropriate to the 4-kHz region, but few were highly quantitative and none counted synapses or peripheral axons of auditory nerve fibers, which are the first neural elements to degenerate after noise damage. Recently, we examined the archival human tissue collection at the Massachusetts Eye and Ear Infirmary (MEEI) and quantified the histopathological differences between a group with a well-documented noise history ($n$ = 52) and an age-matched control group ($n$ = 51 ears).[5,83] The noise history in these cases included both an extended period of military service

or of employment in a noisy workplace (many of these cases were employed prior to the widespread application of workplace exposure controls).

In the present context, the most salient conclusions are as follows (**Figure 11.15**): 1) the patterns of hair cell loss and nerve fiber loss in the normal group are qualitatively and quantitatively similar to those we reported in our prior study,[4] although this study used a new set of cases; 2) in the 50- to 74-year-old groups, noise history exacerbated the hair cell loss especially among outer hair cells and especially in the 4-kHz region (by up to 50%) as expected from the animal work and from the 4-kHz audiometric notch observed in the noise group in this age range; and 4) the noise group showed 10%–20% more auditory nerve fiber loss throughout the cochlear spiral in the 50–74 year range, as expected from the animal studies. In the oldest groups (75–100 years), the effects of noise history disappeared in all the histopathological metrics and in the audiometric losses. In other words, although the noise clearly damaged both hair cells and neurons during the exposure years, with increasing age and increasing time after the cessation of regular acoustic overexposure, the continuing age-related degradation in the control ears brought the two groups to the same final state.

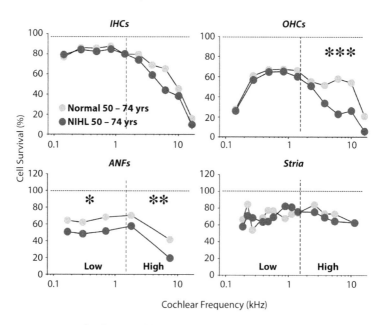

Figure 11.15 Average patterns of cell survival/loss in inner hair cells (IHCs), outer hair cells (OHCs), auditory nerve fibers (ANFs), and the stria vascularis in two groups of humans aged 50–74 years: those with vs. those without a history of noise damage. *Abbreviation*: NIHL, Noise-induced hearing loss. (Modified from [83].)

Other key caveats in the present context are (1) that cochlear neural degeneration has only been documented in humans with significant outer hair cell loss, and thus significant threshold elevations, and (2) that the additional neural degeneration associated with noise history was also associated with additional outer hair cell loss and significant additional threshold elevation. In other words, we observed a close correlation between outer hair cell loss and auditory nerve fiber loss in humans; however, there is, at present, no reliable evidence that significant neural loss can be seen in human ears with normal audiometric thresholds.

## ATTEMPTS TO DIAGNOSE COCHLEAR SYNAPTOPATHY OR "HIDDEN HEARING LOSS" IN HUMAN SUBJECTS

Since we cannot directly measure cochlear synaptopathy (or more generally cochlear neuropathy) in living subjects, research groups have attacked this issue in a number of indirect ways. Since the animal work shows that ABR (or EFR) amplitudes are correlated with cochlear synaptopathy, as long as thresholds are completely normal, many human studies have measured these auditory evoked potentials. It is easy to find a wide range of ABR (or EFR) suprathreshold amplitudes among "normal hearing subjects," but that proves nothing. Thus, the studies have either assessed the correlation (1) between ABR/EFR amplitudes and a measure of the cumulative noise history of the individual[84] or (2) between ABR/EFR amplitudes and some measure of performance on a test involving word identification in a difficult listening environment, e.g. background noise, reverberation, and/or speeding up the delivery.[85] The first strategy is based on the premise that noise exposure produces synaptopathy, and the second is based on the premise that a major effect of cochlear synaptopathy is the production of difficulties hearing in a noisy or otherwise difficult listening environment.

With respect to the first approach, some studies of normal-hearing subjects have found a statistically significant correlation, i.e. smaller evoked potentials predict greater noise exposure[86] and others have not.[84] Similarly, with respect to the second approach, some studies have found a statistically significant correlation, i.e. smaller evoked

potentials predict worse word scores[6,85] while others have not.[7,84] Among the studies that find a correlation between ABR amplitudes and word scores, some have included other tests such as EFRs and middle ear muscle reflexes and have concluded that the threshold for the middle ear-muscle reflex correlates better with word scores than any of the metrics associated with ABR wave 1.[9]

Regardless of the observed statistical correlations in some studies, none concludes that any of the physiological metrics can predict word scores or noise history on a case-by-case basis: the variability is too large, and the proportion of the variance in the outcome variable (word identification scores) that is explained by the predictor variable (ABR, EFR, or middle ear muscle metric) is too small to make any of the metrics clinically useful for diagnosis.[6,9,85] In the laboratory setting where ABR amplitudes or middle ear muscle reflexes are diagnostic of cochlear synaptopathy, that clarity exists only because of the carefully controlled nature of the laboratory experiment, where an animal with a known history free of pathogens, other diseases, or environmental toxins can be exposed to a single cochlear insult and studied at carefully calibrated times thereafter.

Any otologist or audiologist will encounter patients who complain of problems hearing in a noisy environment despite the presence of a normal or near normal audiogram. One can call this condition is "hidden hearing loss," but there is no way to identify the underlying pathology, and some of the potential causes are unrelated to cochlear damage. Before the discovery of cochlear synaptopathy, difficulty understanding speech despite a normal audiogram was diagnosed as Central Auditory Processing Disorder.[87] Such problems could originate with central auditory circuits, or because of deficits in attention and/or short-term memory,[8,88] or because of hair cell damage at the extended high frequencies unrelated to noise exposure,[89] or because of weakening of the feedback pathways to the inner ear, such as the middle ear muscle reflex, or the olivocochlear efferent reflex, both of which are known to help the peripheral auditory system control the masking effects of background noise.[37] Nevertheless, the clear correlation between ABR wave 1 amplitudes and speech recognition in noise in normal-hearing subjects makes it clear that cochlear neural degeneration is one important contributor to the phenomenon of hidden hearing loss.

## SUMMARY OF KEY POINTS

1. Permanent noise-induced threshold shifts are mainly due to loss of hair cells and irreparable stereocilia damage on surviving hair cells.
2. The mechanisms underlying reversible noise-induced threshold shifts are less well understood.
3. In animals, noise exposures that cause only reversible threshold shifts can cause permanent loss of synapses between cochlear neurons and surviving hair cells.
4. In animals, cochlear synaptopathy can be diagnosed by measuring the suprathreshold amplitude of wave 1 of the ABR, but only if thresholds have returned to normal.
5. In animals, not all exposures causing reversible threshold shifts cause synaptopathy. Since different species have different noise vulnerability, it is not possible to directly extrapolate from animal experiments to humans.
6. Aging humans lose cochlear neurons from surviving inner hair cells, and noise exposure increases this neuropathy, which likely contributes to difficulties understanding speech in noisy environments. However, in humans, this synaptopathy has only been documented histopathologically in cases where audiometric thresholds were outside the normal range.
7. In humans with normal thresholds, the correlations between evoked potentials and speech scores suggest that cochlear nerve loss is a key contributor to difficulties understanding in difficult listening environments. However, the variance in those relations is so large that diagnosing "hidden hearing loss" in an individual is not possible, and histopathological verification in normal-hearing cases is lacking at present.

## ACKNOWLEDGMENTS

Supported by grants from the National Institute on Deafness and other Communication Disorders (R01DC00188 and P50DC015857) and with the generous support of Tom and Helene Lauer.

## REFERENCES

1. Sergeyenko Y, Lall K, Liberman MC, Kujawa SG. Age-related cochlear synaptopathy: an early-onset contributor to auditory functional decline. *J Neurosci.* 2013;33(34):13686–13694.
2. Kujawa SG, Liberman MC. Adding insult to injury: cochlear nerve degeneration after "temporary" noise-induced hearing loss. *J Neurosci.* 2009;29(45):14077–14085.
3. Schaette R, McAlpine D. Tinnitus with a normal audiogram: physiological evidence for hidden hearing loss and computational model. *J Neurosci.* 2011;31(38):13452–13457.
4. Wu PZ, Liberman LD, Bennett K, de Gruttola V, O'Malley JT, Liberman MC. Primary neural degeneration in the human cochlea: evidence for hidden hearing loss in the aging ear. *Neuroscience.* 2019;407:8–20.
5. Wu PZ, O'Malley JT, de Gruttola V, Liberman MC. Primary neural degeneration in noise-exposed human cochleas: correlations with outer hair cell loss and word-discrimination scores. *J Neurosci.* 2021;41(20):4439–4447.
6. Mepani AM, Verhulst S, Hancock KE, et al. Envelope following responses predict speech-in-noise performance in normal-hearing listeners. *J Neurophysiol.* 2021;125(4):1213–1222.
7. Guest H, Munro KJ, Prendergast G, Millman RE, Plack CJ. Impaired speech perception in noise with a normal audiogram: no evidence for cochlear synaptopathy and no relation to lifetime noise exposure. *Hear Res.* 2018;364:142–151.
8. Kamerer AM, AuBuchon A, Fultz SE, Kopun JG, Neely ST, Rasetshwane DM. The role of cognition in common measures of peripheral synaptopathy and hidden hearing loss. *Am J Audiol.* 2019;28(4):843–856.
9. Mepani AM, Kirk SA, Hancock KE, et al. Middle ear muscle reflex and word recognition in "normal-hearing" adults: evidence for cochlear synaptopathy? *Ear Hear.* 2020;41(1):25–38.
10. Greenwood DD. A cochlear frequency-position function for several species–29 years later. *J Acoust Soc Am.* 1990;87(6):2592–2605.

11. Liberman MC. The cochlear frequency map for the cat: labeling auditory-nerve fibers of known characteristic frequency. *J Acoust Soc Am*. 1982;72(5):1441–1449.

12. Muller M. Frequency representation in the rat cochlea. *Hear Res*. 1991;51:247–254.

13. Tsuji J, Liberman MC. Intracellular labeling of auditory nerve fibers in guinea pig: central and peripheral projections. *J Comp Neurol*. 1997;381:188–202.

14. Schuknecht HF. *Pathology of the Ear, 2nd Edition*. Baltimore: Lea & Febiger; 1993.

15. Liberman MC. Noise-induced and age-related hearing loss: new perspectives and potential therapies. *F1000Res*. 2017;6:927.

16. Caprara GA, Peng AW. Mechanotransduction in mammalian sensory hair cells. *Mol Cell Neurosci*. 2022;120:103706.

17. Kiang NYS. Peripheral neural processing of auditory information. In: Darian-Smith I, ed. *Handbook of Physiology, sect 1: The Nervous System*. Vol 3. Bethesda: American Physiological Society; 1984:639–674.

18. Liberman MC. Single-neuron labeling in the cat auditory nerve. *Science*. 1982;216:1239–1241.

19. Liberman MC. Morphological differences among radial afferent fibers in the cat cochlea: an electron-microscopic study of serial sections. *Hear Res*. 1980;3:45–63.

20. Kiang NY, Moxon EC. Tails of tuning curves of auditory-nerve fibers. *J Acoust Soc Am*. 1974;55(3):620–630.

21. Narayan SS, Temchin AN, Recio A, Ruggero MA. Frequency tuning of basilar membrane and auditory nerve fibers in the same cochleae. *Science*. 1998;282(5395):1882–1884.

22. Liberman MC. Auditory-nerve response from cats raised in a low-noise chamber. *J Acoust Soc Am*. 1978;63(2):442–455.

23. Costalupes JA, Young ED, Gibson DJ. Effects of continuous noise backgrounds on rate response of auditory nerve fibers in cat. *J Neurophysiol*. 1984;51(6):1326–1344.

24. Makary CA, Shin J, Kujawa SG, Liberman MC, Merchant SN. Age-related primary cochlear neuronal degeneration in human temporal bones. *J Assoc Res Otolaryngol*. 2011;12(6):711–717.

25. Wu PZ, Liberman LD, Bennett K, de Gruttola V, O'Malley JT, Liberman MC. Primary neural degeneration in the human cochlea: evidence for hidden hearing loss in the aging ear. *Neuroscience*. 2019;407:8–20.

26. Ryugo DK, Dodds LW, Benson TE, Kiang NYS. Unmyelinated axons of the auditory nerve in cats. *J Comp Neurol*. 1991;308:209–223.

27. Kiang NY, Rho JM, Northrop CC, Liberman MC, Ryugo DK. Hair-cell innervation by spiral ganglion cells in adult cats. *Science*. 1982;217(4555):175–177.

28. Flores EN, Duggan A, Madathany T, et al. A non-canonical pathway from cochlea to brain signals tissue-damaging noise. *Curr Biol*. 2015;25(5):606–612.

29. Simmons DD, Liberman MC. Afferent innervation of outer hair cells in adult cats: I. Light microscopic analysis of fibers labeled with horseradish peroxidase. *J Comp Neurol*. 1988;270:132–144.

30. Dallos P. Cochlear amplification, outer hair cells and prestin. *Curr Opin Neurobiol*. 2008;18(4):370–376.

31. Dobie RA, Humes LE. Commentary on the regulatory implications of noise-induced cochlear neuropathy. *Int J Audiol*. 2017;56(sup1):74–78.

32. Melcher JR, Guinan JJ, Jr., Knudson IM, Kiang NYS. Generators of the brainstem auditory evoked potential in cat. II. Correlating lesion sites with waveform changes. *Hear Res*. 1996;93:28–51.

33. Suthakar K, Liberman MC. A simple algorithm for objective threshold determination of auditory brainstem responses. *Hear Res*. 2019;381:107782.

34. Shaheen LA, Valero MD, Liberman MC. Towards a diagnosis of cochlear neuropathy with envelope following responses. *J Assoc Res Otolaryngol*. 2015;16(6):727–745.

35. Shera CA. Mechanisms of mammalian otoacoustic emission and their implications for the clinical utility of otoacoustic emissions. *Ear Hear*. 2004;25(2):86–97.

36. Liberman MC, Chesney CP, Kujawa SG. Effects of selective inner hair cell loss on DPOAE and CAP in carboplatin-treated chinchillas. *Aud Neurosci*. 1997;3:255–268.

37. Liberman MC, Guinan JJ, Jr. Feedback control of the auditory periphery: anti-masking effects of middle ear muscles vs. olivocochlear efferents. *J Commun Disord*. 1998;31(6):471–482; quiz 483; 553.

38. Rabinowitz WM. Acoustic-reflex effects on middle-ear performance. *J Acoust Soc Am*. 1981;69 Suppl:S44.

39. Schairer KS, Feeney MP, Sanford CA. Acoustic reflex measurement. *Ear Hear*. 2013;34 Suppl 1:43S–47S.

40. Valero MD, Hancock KE, Liberman MC. The middle ear muscle reflex in the diagnosis of cochlear neuropathy. *Hear Res*. 2016;332:29–38.

41. Valero MD, Hancock KE, Maison SF, Liberman MC. Effects of cochlear synaptopathy on middle-ear muscle reflexes in unanesthetized mice. *Hear Res*. 2018;363:109–118.

42. Burns W. *Effects of Noise on Man*. London: Wm. Clowes and Sons; 1968.

43. Miller JD, Watson CS, Covell WP. Deafening effects of noise on the cat. *Acta Oto-Laryngol*. 1963;Suppl. 176.

44. Fernandez KA, Guo D, Micucci S, De Gruttola V, Liberman MC, Kujawa SG. Noise-induced cochlear synaptopathy with and without sensory cell loss. *Neuroscience*. 2020;427:43–57.

45. Clark WW, Bohne BA, Boettcher FA. Effect of periodic rest on hearing loss and cochlear damage following exposure to noise. *J Acoust Soc Am*. 1987;82(4):1253–1264.

46. Saunders JC, Dear SP, Schneider ME. The anatomical consequences of acoustic injury: a review and tutorial. *J Acoust Soc Am*. 1985;78(3):833–860.

47. Arenas JP, Suter AH. Comparison of occupational noise legislation in the Americas: an overview and analysis. *Noise Health*. 2014;16(72):306–319.

48. Sinex DG, Clark WW, Bohne BA. Effects of periodic rest on physiological measures of auditory sensitivity following exposure to noise. *J Acoust Soc Am*. 1987;82(4):1265–1273.

49. Liberman MC, Kiang NY. Acoustic trauma in cats. Cochlear pathology and auditory-nerve activity. *Acta otolaryngologica*. 1978;358:1–63.

50. Orchik DJ, Schmaier DR, Shea JJ, Jr., Emmett JR, Moretz WH, Jr., Shea JJ, 3rd. Sensorineural hearing loss in cordless telephone injury. *Otolaryngol Head Neck Surg*. 1987;96(1):30–33.

51. Ruggero MA. Responses to sound of the basilar membrane of the mammalian cochlea. *Curr Opin Neurobiol*. 1992;2(4):449–456.

52. McBride DI, Williams S. Audiometric notch as a sign of noise induced hearing loss. *Occup Environ Med*. 2001;58(1):46–51.

53. Henderson D, Spongr V, Subramaniam M, Campo P. Anatomical effects of impact noise. *Hear Res*. 1994;76(1–2):101–117.

54. Cho SI, Gao SS, Xia A, et al. Mechanisms of hearing loss after blast injury to the ear. *PLOS ONE*. 2013;8(7):e67618.

55. Hickman TT, Smalt C, Bobrow J, Quatieri T, Liberman MC. Blast-induced cochlear synaptopathy in chinchillas. *Sci Rep*. 2018;8(1):10740.

56. Takeno S, Harrison RV, Ibrahim D, Wake M, Mount RJ. Cochlear function after selective inner hair cell degeneration induced by carboplatin. *Hear Res*. 1994;75(1–2):93–102.

57. Mulroy MJ, Curley FJ. Stereociliary pathology and noise-induced threshold shift: a scanning electron microscope study. *Scan Electron Microsc*. 1982;IV:1753–1762.

58. Liberman MC, Dodds LW. Single-neuron labeling and chronic cochlear pathology. III. Stereocilia damage and alterations of threshold tuning curves. *Hear Res*. 1984;16:55–74.

59. Liberman MC, Mulroy MJ. Acute and chronic effects of acoustic trauma: Cochlear pathology and auditory nerve pathophysiology. In: Hamernik RP, Henderson D, Salvi R, eds. *New Perspectives on Noise-Induced Hearing Loss*; 1982:105–136.

60. Liberman MC, Dodds LW. Acute ultrastructural changes in acoustic trauma: serial-section reconstruction of stereocilia and cuticular plates. *Hear Res*. 1987;26(1):45–64.

61. Wang Y, Hirose K, Liberman MC. Dynamics of noise-induced cellular injury and repair in the mouse cochlea. *J Assoc Res Otolaryngol*. 2002;3(3):248–268.

62. Flock A, Flock B, Fridberger A, Scarfone E, Ulfendahl M. Supporting cells contribute to control of hearing sensitivity. *J Neurosci.* 1999;19(11):4498–4507.

63. Robertson D. Functional significance of dendritic swelling after loud sounds in the guinea pig cochlea. *Hearing Res.* 1983;9:263–278.

64. Johnsson LG. Sequence of degeneration of Corti's organ and its first-order neurons. *Ann Otol Rhinol Laryngol.* 1974;83(3):294–303.

65. Bohne BA, Harding GW. Degeneration in the cochlea after noise damage: primary versus secondary events. *Am J Otol.* 2000;21(4):505–509.

66. Liberman LD, Suzuki J, Liberman MC. Dynamics of cochlear synaptopathy after acoustic overexposure. *J Assoc Res Otolaryngol.* 2015;16(2):205–219.

67. Hickox AE, Liberman MC. Is noise-induced cochlear neuropathy key to the generation of hyperacusis or tinnitus? *J Neurophysiol.* 2014;111(3):552–564.

68. Fried MP, Dudek SE, Bohne BA. Basal turn cochlear lesions following exposure to low-frequency noise. *Trans Am Acad Ophthalmol Otolaryngol.* 1976;82:285–298.

69. Furman AC, Kujawa SG, Liberman MC. Noise-induced cochlear neuropathy is selective for fibers with low spontaneous rates. *J Neurophysiol.* 2013;110(3):577–586.

70. Schmiedt RA, Mills JH, Boettcher FA. Age-related loss of activity of auditory-nerve fibers. *J Neurophysiol.* 1996;76(4):2799–2803.

71. Joris PX, Yin TC. Responses to amplitude-modulated tones in the auditory nerve of the cat. *J Acoust Soc Am.* 1992;91(1):215–232.

72. Huet A, Batrel C, Tang Y, et al. Sound coding in the auditory nerve of gerbils. *Hear Res.* 2016;338:32–39.

73. Liberman MC, Kiang NY. Single-neuron labeling and chronic cochlear pathology. IV. Stereocilia damage and alterations in rate- and phase-level functions. *Hear Res.* 1984;16(1):75–90.

74. Lin HW, Furman AC, Kujawa SG, Liberman MC. Primary neural degeneration in the guinea pig cochlea after reversible noise-induced threshold shift. *J Assoc Res Otolaryngol.* 2011;12(5):605–616.

75. Hickox AE, Larsen E, Heinz MG, Shinobu L, Whitton JP. Translational issues in cochlear synaptopathy. *Hear Res.* 2017;349:164–171.

76. Valero MD, Burton JA, Hauser SN, Hackett TA, Ramachandran R, Liberman MC. Noise-induced cochlear synaptopathy in rhesus monkeys (*Macaca mulatta*). *Hear Res.* 2017;353:213–223.

77. Suthakar K, Liberman MC. Auditory-nerve responses in mice with noise-induced cochlear synaptopathy. *J Neurophysiol.* 2021;126(6):2027–2038.

78. Hickman TT, Hashimoto K, Liberman LD, Liberman MC. Synaptic migration and reorganization after noise exposure suggests regeneration in a mature mammalian cochlea. *Sci Rep.* 2020;10(1):19945.

79. Hickman TT, Hashimoto K, Liberman LD, Liberman MC. Cochlear synaptic degeneration and regeneration after noise: effects of age and neuronal subgroup. *Front Cell Neurosci.* 2021;15:684706.

80. Gordon-Salant S. Hearing loss and aging: new research findings and clinical implications. *J Rehabil Res Dev.* 2005;42(4 Suppl 2):9–24.

81. McGill TJ, Schuknecht HF. Human cochlear changes in noise induced hearing loss. *Laryngoscope.* 1976;86(9):1293–1302.

82. Hawkins JE, Jr., Johnsson L-G. Patterns of sensorineural degeneration in human ears exposed to noise. In: Henderson D, Hamernik RP, Dosanjh DS, Mills JH, eds. *Effects of Noise on Hearing.* New York: Raven Press; 1976:91–110.

83. Wu PZ, O'Malley JT, de Gruttola V, Liberman MC. Age-related hearing loss is dominated by damage to inner ear sensory cells, not the cellular battery that powers them. *J Neurosci.* 2020;40(33):6357–6366.

84. Prendergast G, Guest H, Munro KJ, et al. Effects of noise exposure on young adults with normal audiograms I: Electrophysiology. *Hear Res.* 2017;344:68–81.

85. Grant KJ, Mepani AM, Wu P, et al. Electrophysiological markers of cochlear function correlate with hearing-in-noise performance among audiometrically normal subjects. *J Neurophysiol*. 2020;124(2):418–431.

86. Bramhall NF, Konrad-Martin D, McMillan GP, Griest SE. Auditory brainstem response altered in humans with noise exposure despite normal outer hair cell function. *Ear Hear*. 2017;38(1):e1–e12.

87. Chowsilpa S, Bamiou DE, Koohi N. Effectiveness of the auditory temporal ordering and resolution tests to detect central auditory processing disorder in adults with evidence of brain pathology: a systematic review and meta-analysis. *Front Neurol*. 2021;12:656117.

88. Valderrama JT, Beach EF, Yeend I, Sharma M, Van Dun B, Dillon H. Effects of lifetime noise exposure on the middle-age human auditory brainstem response, tinnitus and speech-in-noise intelligibility. *Hear Res*. 2018;365:36–48.

89. Motlagh Zadeh L, Silbert NH, Sternasty K, Swanepoel W, Hunter LL, Moore DR. Extended high-frequency hearing enhances speech perception in noise. *Proc Natl Acad Sci U S A*. 2019;116(47):23753–23759.

# 12

# Regenerative therapies for sensorineural hearing loss: Current research implications for future treatment[*]

CYNTHIA L. CHOW AND SAMUEL P. GUBBELS

## INTRODUCTION

Hearing impairment is one of the most common maladies affecting older adults. Almost two-thirds of individuals 70 years of age and older have some level of hearing loss.[1] The prevalence of hearing loss increases over time and is generally associated with aging; however, it is often untreated.[2] Hearing loss can cause difficulty communicating with others, localizing sound, and perceiving warnings, all contributing to a poorer quality of life.[3] The National Institute on Deafness and Other Communication Disorders estimates there are nearly 36 million adults in the United States with some degree of hearing loss, most cases of which are caused by the loss of cochlear sensory hair cells.[4] Cochlear hair cells are highly specialized mechanosensory receptors that are responsible for

converting mechanical sound information into an electrical signal, amplifying it and transmitting it to the brain via auditory nerve fibers. In humans and other higher vertebrates, the inability of cochlear hair cells to regenerate after damage is the primary reason for the permanence of hearing loss. This chapter describes the multiple approaches being taken in pursuit of novel regenerative treatments for sensorineural hearing loss in addition to discussing the most critical challenges in the field.

## BACKGROUND

The organ of Corti is highly organized and consists of many cell types, including cochlear hair cells, supporting cells, and auditory nerve fibers

---

[*] Republished from Sataloff RT, Johns MM, Kost KM (Eds). *Geriatric Otolaryngology*. Thieme Medical Publishers and the American Academy of Otolaryngology – Head and Neck Surgery;2015:63–76; with permission from Thieme Medical Publishers, Inc.

DOI: 10.1201/b23379-12

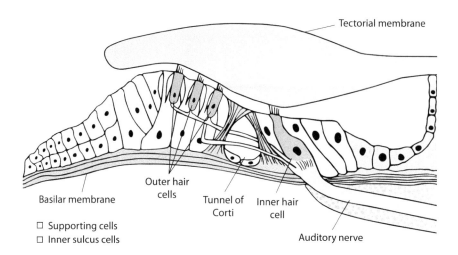

Figure 12.1 The organization of the organ of Corti. Outer hair cells and inner hair cells are arranged in a 3:1 ratio surrounded by supporting cells. Stereocilia on the apical portion of the hair cells are embedded in the tectorial membrane. Outer and inner hair cells are properly innervated at the base and attach to auditory nerve fibers, which send the auditory signal to the brain for processing.

(**Figure 12.1**). At birth, the human cochlea contains ~15,000 sensory hair cells. There are two types of sensory hair cells—inner hair cells and outer hair cells—both of which are important for hearing. Inner hair cells are responsible for converting sound information into an electrical signal, whereas outer hair cells are responsible for amplifying the signal. Auditory nerve fibers are responsible for sending sound information from cochlear hair cells to the brain for processing. Loss or damage of cochlear hair cells and auditory nerve fibers has been estimated to account for ~80% of cases of hearing loss.[5]

Currently, amplification devices and cochlear implants are the primary treatment options available for individuals with sensorineural hearing loss. Although these treatment options can return some hearing capability, the results vary between individuals. In addition, both hearing aids and cochlear implants require lifelong device usage, and they generally do not restore normal hearing qualities. As such, other approaches for restoring more normal cochlear function are actively being explored.

## HAIR CELL REGENERATION

In mammals, it is known that skin and bone marrow cells are continually replenished throughout life.[6,7] Furthermore, taste buds and olfactory bulb interneurons are constantly renewed in adult mammals[8–11]; however, such regeneration is not seen in the mammalian cochlea. It was previously thought that auditory hair cell regeneration did not occur in any context until 1988 when investigators found functional recovery of hearing due to regenerated hair cells after noise trauma in birds.[12–14] The mammalian inner ear was thought to lack this regenerative capacity to replace damaged hair cells until 1993, when investigators found evidence of hair cell regeneration in the vestibular sensory epithelia of adult mammals.[15,16] Although replacement of vestibular hair cells was observed, the newly regenerated cells occurred infrequently, and the amount of functional recovery that the regenerated cells may produce has been questioned.[17]

In the avian inner ear, hair cell regeneration begins after an auditory insult. Subsequent signaling after the insult begins a process whereby supporting cells divide and differentiate into immature hair cells and supporting cells.[18–20] Alternatively, supporting cells may transform directly into immature hair cells,[19,21,22] a process referred to as transdifferentiation. Using molecular, genetic, and environmental cues, these immature hair cells continue to become morphologically distinct as they mature over the course of several weeks.[23,24] When compared with that of birds, fish, and amphibians, the cochlear sensory epithelium in mammals appears to have lost its ability to regenerate after hair cell loss. Exactly why this loss of regenerative ability has occurred with evolution remains unclear. Regardless, many investigators have focused attention on using what is known of mammalian hair cell development to guide efforts focused on regenerating hair cells after loss.

Treatments based on regenerating lost or damaged tissue are inevitably complex, and efforts to regenerate hair cells in the mammalian cochlea are subject to unique challenges beyond those seen in other organs. First, one needs to consider the complexity of an auditory hair cell. Hair cells are morphologically distinct, with a round base and thinner apex. They contain small hair cell-like bundles called stereocilia, which extend from the apex of the cell and are embedded in the tectorial membrane. These hair cell bundles are mechanosensitive, responding to ionic flow, which transforms sound vibrations into electrical impulses. The electrical signal is then sent to the brain via auditory nerve fibers for further processing. Because of this, proper neural integration needs to be established to transmit sound information to the brain. Moreover, the cochlea has a distinct cytoarchitecture that is highly organized. This cyto-architectural organization of the cochlea is critical to its proper function. Newly generated hair cells would need to integrate in the proper location within the cochlea and furthermore within the auditory sensory epithelium (the organ of Corti) to encode sound information accurately. Last, the cochlea is a delicate, membranous, and fluid-filled structure that is surrounded by dense otic capsular bone, making surgical access to the organ of Corti challenging. Efforts to outline meaningful regenerative therapies for hearing loss in humans need to address these unique challenges, and numerous laboratories worldwide are actively engaged in this exciting area of research.

## MECHANISMS FOR AVIAN HAIR CELL REGENERATION

Currently, there are two proposed mechanisms for cochlear hair cell regeneration in the avian inner ear: supporting cell proliferation and transdifferentiation. Cell proliferation is referred to as the growth and division of cells, during which a supporting cell reenters the cell cycle giving rise to two daughter cells that differentiate into one supporting cell and one hair cell. When cochlear hair cells are destroyed, they send a signal to neighboring supporting cells to activate proliferation.[18,25] This signal prompts supporting cells to migrate through the sensory epithelium, reenter the cell cycle, and generate a daughter hair cell and a supporting cell.[15] Alternatively, hair cells may be generated via supporting cell transdifferentiation, during which a differentiated cell is transformed into another cell type without cell cycle reentry.[26] In this approach, neighboring supporting cells are converted to hair cells via nonmitotic mechanisms with consequent depletion of the supporting cell population.

As applied to the mammalian inner ear, it is not clear how these mechanisms of regeneration might affect the organization, structure, and functional integrity of the organ of Corti.[27,28] If supporting cells don't replace themselves as they transdifferentiate into hair cells, the cytoarchitecture and function of the organ of Corti might be compromised. As such, a method to regenerate hair cells in the mammalian inner ear that does not lead to depletion of the cohort of endogenous supporting cells would seem logically preferable to one that relies on transdifferentiation alone. It is possible, however, that the mammalian inner ear has some tolerance to a level of depletion of the supporting cell population if it provides a healthy, functional cohort of hair cells. Ongoing research in this area through the approaches described here will likely provide insight into these unanswered questions in the years to come.

## REGENERATIVE APPROACHES FOR THE TREATMENT OF HEARING LOSS

There are several approaches being taken in the pursuit of novel, regenerative treatments for hearing loss, each having unique potential benefits and challenges. These approaches can generally be grouped into four categories:

1. Gene transfer
2. Pharmacotherapies
3. Exogenous delivery of stem cells
4. Promotion of endogenous stem cells

# GENE TRANSFER

Gene transfer has become an attractive avenue for regenerating hair cells by introducing a gene of interest to cells. To date, several studies expressing various genes of interest have produced promising results, which are discussed next.

## Atoh1

The expression of the basic helix-loop-helix transcription factor *Atoh1* is one of the first indicators of hair cell differentiation in the cochlea.[29–32] In developing mammals, *Atoh1* is expressed in prosensory patches that give rise to the auditory sensory epithelia and is both necessary and sufficient for hair cell development and formation.[31–33] Mice without the *Atoh1* gene lack sensory hair cells in the auditory and vestibular portions of the inner ear.[29,31,32] In contrast, when *Atoh1* is overexpressed in cultured cochlear explants, supernumerary hair cells are generated.[33] Moreover, *Atoh1* has been found to be upregulated during hair cell fate specification in the adult chicken during hair cell regeneration.[34] Collectively, these findings speak to the critical role that *Atoh1* plays in determining hair cell fate specification within the inner ear.

Investigators have introduced *Atoh1*-expressing viral vectors into the organs of Corti of a variety of different rodent species. Kawamoto and colleagues showed that delivery of *Atoh1*-expressing adenoviral vectors to the organ of Corti of mature, normal-hearing guinea pigs results in expression of the gene product in the organ of Corti and in some nonsensory locations (ectopic expression in cells outside of the organ of Corti) within the cochleae.[35] Cells expressing the exogenously delivered *Atoh1* also expressed the hair cell marker myosin VIIa and displayed immature stereociliary bundles at the apex of the cell. In addition, these newly formed hair cells appeared to attract axons extended from the auditory nerve on some level. From this, the authors of this study concluded that cells in the normal-hearing adult mammalian inner ear are capable of generating new hair cells upon *Atoh1* misexpression.

Taking this a step further, Izumikawa and colleagues delivered an *Atoh1*-expressing adenovirus to the organs of Corti of deafened mature guinea pigs.[36] Animals transfected with the virus showed new hair cell formation in the organ of Corti and in some ectopic locations in the cochlea. The authors also reported a significant improvement in auditory brainstem response thresholds in the ears of animals transfected with *Atoh1*. Cross-sectional analysis revealed that some of the cells displayed a mixed phenotype, having both hair cell and supporting cell features. The source of the newly generated hair cells was unclear; however, it was hypothesized they arose from transdifferentiated and proliferated cells within the damaged regions that had been transfected with the *Atoh1*-expressing adenovirus.

In 2008, Gubbels and colleagues established a method to conduct gain-of-function studies in the developing inner ear using an *in utero* gene transfer technique.[37] Plasmids encoding *Atoh1* and green fluorescent protein (GFP) were microinjected into the otic vesicle of mice on embryonic day 11.5 and examined on embryonic day 18.5 and later time points. Ears that received *Atoh1* demonstrated supernumerary hair cell formation throughout the cochlea. Cells that formed secondary to the delivery of exogenous *Atoh1* expressed myosin VIIa and displayed stereociliary bundles. Moreover, they attracted neuronal processes and expressed the ribbon synapse marker carboxy-terminal binding protein 2. Postnatal electrophysiological analysis of the cells generated from *in utero* transfer of *Atoh1* revealed age-appropriate basolateral conductances and mechanoelectrical transduction properties. These results demonstrate that it is possible to generate cochlear hair cells by *Atoh1* misexpression after *in utero* gene transfer. Moreover, this study showed that the generated hair cells are functional on a cellular level and establish connections with the central auditory network.

Collectively, these studies suggest that a gene transfer approach using transcription factors known to be critical for hair cell development can generate hair cells in normal and deafened cochleae of both adult and developing rodents. Furthermore, these studies demonstrate that the newly generated hair cells are able to associate with the nearby auditory nerve and are functional on a cellular and possibly even an organ system level. It remains unclear if this type of approach leads to depletion of the supporting cell population and, if so, its implications. In addition, the long-term viability of hair cells generated through *Atoh1* gene transfer is similarly unclear. Regardless, *Atoh1* gene transfer–based approaches represent a promising and active area of investigation in the pursuit of novel, regenerative therapies for hearing loss.

## Cell cycle modulators

Modulating genes that have a role in cell cycle regulation is another molecular approach being pursued to achieve hair cell regeneration. Although mammalian supporting cells are generally quiescent *in vivo*, several studies have reported that these cells have the capacity to reenter the cell cycle and generate hair cell–like cells *in vitro*.[38–43] The concept of this approach is that by altering the cell cycle of residual supporting cells following hair cell loss, proliferation may ensue, with subsequent differentiation of the progeny into hair and supporting cells.

It is well established that during development, cell cycle exit continues progressively along the cochlear duct from the apex to the base, starting on embryonic day 12 and completing by embryonic day 14 in mice.[29,44–46] While this is occurring, cochlear cells begin to express hair cell markers, including *Atoh1*, myosin VI, and myosin VIIa.[29,31,32] At a similar developmental time, supporting cells begin to express the cyclin-dependent kinase inhibitor p27kip1.[44,46] The expression of p27kip1 has been shown to coincide with the cell cycle exit of hair cell and supporting cell progenitors.[29,44,47] P27kip1 is continually expressed in supporting cells, which may be responsible, to some degree, for maintaining the quiescent state of supporting cells.[46] Alternatively, hair cells rapidly downregulate p27kip1 during differentiation, expressing the cyclin-dependent kinase inhibitor p19Ink4d instead,[46,48] which is thought to maintain them in a quiescent state.

Modulation of the expression of cell cycle inhibitors, such as p27kip1, may hold promise as a potential means for promoting some level of regeneration of hair cells in the mammalian inner ear. P27kip1 appears to play a significant role in the inability of mammalian hair cells to regenerate after damage.[47,49] In the cochlea, p27kip1 is regulated at both transcriptional and posttranscriptional levels.[44] Mice deficient for p27kip1 have supernumerary hair cells and supporting cells, most of which are located in the apical region of the cochlea.[47] In addition, auditory brainstem response thresholds obtained from these mice

were significantly elevated compared with controls, suggesting severe to profound hearing loss. The significant elevation in auditory brainstem response thresholds is thought to occur from excess hair cells and supporting cells disrupting the spatial organization and mechanical properties of the basilar membrane.[47,49] In another study, White and colleagues examined the regenerative capacity of supporting cells isolated from the postnatal mouse.[41] The authors found that postmitotic supporting cells are capable of transdifferentiating into new hair cells *in vitro*. In the first experiment, the ability of postmitotic supporting cells to reenter the cell cycle was examined by isolating supporting cells expressing GFP under a p27kip1 promoter and culturing them *in vitro*. After 2 days, 60% of GFP (p27kip1) positive cells downregulated expression of p27kip1, whereas 38% of these cells incorporated BrdU, signifying that these cells had reentered the cell cycle. Additional analysis determined that these cells were then able to differentiate into hair cells. A small number of these cells expressed the hair cell marker myosin VI. These results demonstrate that postnatal supporting cells from mice have the ability to divide and differentiate into hair cells via mitotic and nonmitotic means. Collectively, these studies suggest that modulation of p27kip1 in supporting cells may establish a method, or part of a method, to regenerate hair cells following their loss.

Although p27kip1 expression coincides with cell cycle exit, it is not essential for this occurrence.[50] This suggests there are other genes that play a more central function in regulating cell cycle exit. Retinoblastoma (RB) 1 is another type of cell cycle regulator, which plays a role in holding inner ear hair cells in a state of quiescence and may represent a potential target for enabling regeneration to occur in the mammalian organ of Corti. The RB1 gene is a tumor suppressor involved in regulating cell cycle exit, differentiation, and survival. Although hair cells in the vestibular and auditory portions of the inner ear generally undergo similar processes during development and differentiation, RB1 appears to play different roles in these regions.[51,52] In 2005, Sage and colleagues found that targeted deletion of RB1 in the developing mouse utricle leads to proliferation of vestibular hair cells,[53] suggesting a potential role for alteration of RB1 as a means to achieve regeneration of hair cells in the future. More recently, inactivation of RB protein in postmitotic supporting cells resulted in cell cycle reentry, with a subsequent increase in the number of supporting cells in the neonatal mouse cochlea.[54] Moreover, some of the nuclei of proliferating supporting cells were intermittently observed in the hair cell layer above their normal position, similar to supporting cells undergoing regeneration in the avian auditory epithelium. There was no evidence of newly generated hair cells from supporting cells, suggesting that there may be a potential role involving other signaling factors to facilitate the continued differentiation of the newly generated cells into hair cells. One concern in the application of this type of strategy lies in the risk of tumor formation with manipulation of tumor suppressor genes such as RB1. As such, additional investigation will be needed to determine if efforts aimed at targeted alteration in the expression or function of genes, such as RB1, could be pursued safely as a potential therapeutic strategy for hair cell regeneration in the future.

Following hair cell formation, a mechanism to maintain the postmitotic status and continued viability of the cells is necessary to prevent their degeneration. The cyclin-dependent kinase inhibitor p19Ink4d is a factor that appears to sustain the postmitotic status of hair cells.[48] During development, mice deficient for p19Ink4d develop in a normal manner; however, hair cell loss is observed beginning on postnatal day 17.[48] In these mice, it appears that hair cells attempt to reenter the cell cycle, causing them to die by programmed cell death. As already discussed, hair cells rapidly downregulate p27kip1 during differentiation,[46] suggesting that p19Ink4d alone is responsible for maintaining the postmitotic state of the hair cells.[48] For the purpose of newly generated hair cells, continued maintenance is a constant process, and failure to regulate this accurately can have adverse effects on hearing. Accordingly, future efforts aimed at regenerating hair cells in the deafened cochlea will need to take into account the ongoing need for maintenance of the newly generated hair cells to ensure their permanence.

Collectively, studies evaluating gene transfer–based approaches for the treatment of hearing loss have produced promising results. Additional investigation is necessary to characterize key genes and cell cycle modulators that have been found to be critical for hair cell regeneration in animal and cell culture models. Furthermore, it is essential to determine if direct transdifferentiation of supporting cells into hair cells leads to a depletion of supporting cells, which might disrupt the cytoarchitecture of the organ of Corti. Moreover, the long-term viability of hair cells generated through gene transfer is similarly unclear. In addition, determining a safe and effective method to deliver genetic material into the inner ear remains a critical challenge. It is plausible that genes of interest could be introduced to the inner ear through transtympanic delivery to the middle ear with subsequent transport or diffusion through the round window membrane to the cochlea. Alternatively, direct injection of a gene of interest to the scalar fluids of the inner ear might ultimately be required for meaningful delivery within the cochlea. The ability of the gene to penetrate all areas of the cochlea would need to be determined in addition to ensuring that no further damage results from these delivery approaches to the inner ear. Beyond the challenges of gene delivery on an organ basis, genetic material needs to be transported across the cell membrane for subsequent transcription to take place. Methods to accomplish this include packaging the gene in a viral vector that has tropism for the supporting cells of the organ of Corti, usage of electrical pulsations (electroporation) to drive the genetic material through the cell membrane, or potentially packaging the genetic material in a lipid-based carrier that fuses with the cell membrane to release the gene of interest into the cytoplasm. Although these cellular delivery mechanisms are plausible approaches for gene delivery to the inner ear, a viral-based method for gene delivery appears to be the most logical candidate and the approach used in scientific studies on cochlear gene transfer to date.[35-37] Although many questions remain to be answered, gene transfer–based approaches for the treatment of hearing loss remain a promising and attractive area of investigation.

## PHARMACOTHERAPIES

Pharmacotherapeutics focuses on the use of drugs to modulate signaling pathways or gene expression in a cell. In regard to hearing loss, these drugs may target specific cellular pathways that signal supporting cells to divide or target the regulation of specific genes such as *Atoh1* in attempts to generate new hair cells. In concept, these synthetic molecules with biological activities could potentially be given systemically, transtympanically, or by intracochlear administration to affect the generation of hair cells after loss, potentially avoiding some of the challenges associated with other approaches for hair cell regeneration.

The Notch signaling pathway is one potential target for pharmacotherapeutically mediated efforts toward hair cell regeneration. This signaling pathway is responsible for establishing, at least in part, the hair cell–supporting cell mosaic of the organ of Corti during inner ear development.[55–60] During development, Notch activation in supporting cells upregulates Hes and Hey transcription factors, which inhibit *Atoh1* expression.[60–63] Thus, Notch activation suppresses hair cell differentiation in supporting cells, thereby regulating the number of hair cells and supporting cells.[60] In addition, Notch expression appears to increase during hair cell regeneration in the avian inner ear.[64] Because of this, investigators have hypothesized that disrupting the Notch signaling pathway might promote hair cell generation. During embryonic development, the absence of the Notch ligand Jagged1 resulted in a severe reduction of hair cells in both the auditory and the vestibular portions of the inner ears of mice, indicating that it is required for the prosensory inductive function of Notch.[65] Other studies that inactivated the Notch ligands Delta1 and Jagged2 reported a greater number of hair cells relative to control cochleae, in addition to an increase in the number of supporting cells, suggesting Notch signaling may also play a role in regulating hair and supporting cell proliferation.[65,66] Several other studies have also reported that during development, disruption of Notch signaling can lead to a cellular conversion from a supporting cell fate to a hair cell fate.[65–70] Collectively, these studies suggest that careful manipulation of Notch signaling in supporting cells may provide an avenue for regenerating hair cells following auditory insult.

One of the first reports of pharmacological inhibition of Notch signaling treated deafened guinea pigs using a γ-secretase inhibitor.[71] In this study, the authors reported that a small number of hair cells were generated following γ-secretase administration, with newly generated cells expressing the hair cell marker myosin VIIa. More recently, pharmacological inhibition of Notch signaling using other types of small-molecule γ-secretase inhibitors has been shown to cause partial recovery of hearing thresholds in mice exposed to noise trauma.[72] In this study, pharmacological inhibition of Notch signaling with LY411575 in deafened mice resulted in transdifferentiation of supporting cells into cochlear hair cells and partial restoration of hearing verified by auditory brainstem response testing. The supporting cells did not appear to reenter the cell cycle following γ-secretase administration, indicating that hair cells were generated through transdifferentiation. Of note, both studies used direct delivery of γ-secretase inhibitors to the scala tympani, which represents one potential advantage to a pharmaco-therapeutic approach. In contrast, other approaches for hair cell regeneration such as gene transfer and cell transplantation (to be described) are more likely to require intracochlear delivery methods, which have a higher potential risk for hearing loss. In general, for this approach to become clinically relevant, the ability of the drug to penetrate all regions of the cochlea and prevent ectopic hair cell formation needs to be explored further. In addition, generating hair cells in proper locations within the organ of Corti while avoiding depletion of the supporting cell population will need to be accomplished. Although more investigation is needed, the foregoing studies demonstrate that pharmacotherapeutic targeting of Notch signaling may enable meaningful regeneration of hair cells in the deafened cochlea in the future.

## EXOGENOUS DELIVERY OF STEM CELLS

One promising approach in regenerative therapies involves the use of stem cells as a substrate to generate mature cell types of interest with subsequent transplantation. There has been great progress with this approach for regeneration of tissue in other organ systems, with several ongoing clinical trials aimed at treating macular dystrophy and macular degeneration.[73,74] With regard to the inner ear, several laboratories are attempting to generate cochlear hair cells *in vitro* using

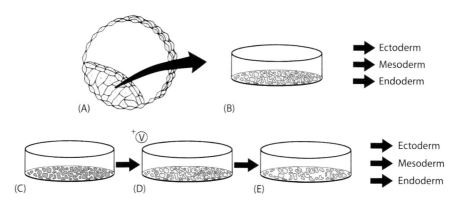

Figure 12.2 (A, B) Generation of embryonic stem cells and (C–E) induced pluripotent stem cells. In generation of human embryonic stem cells, (A) cells are isolated from the inner cell mass of a blastocyst 5–7 days after fertilization and (B) cultured *in vitro*. These cells have the potential to differentiate into all cell types in the body. In generation of human-induced pluripotent stem cells, (C) adult cells are isolated from a donor, typically fibroblasts of a skin punch biopsy, and cultured *in vitro*. (D) Genes associated with pluripotency *(Oct ¾, Sox 2, Klf4,* and *c-Myc* or *Oct ¾, Sox 2, Nanog,* and *LIN28)* are delivered into the cells via viral vectors. (E) Cells expressing markers associated with pluripotency (pink) are isolated and continually cultured. As with embryonic stem cells, these cells have the potential to differentiate into all cell types in the body.

types of pluripotent stem cells such as embryonic stem cells (ESCs) and induced pluripotent stem cells (iPSCs). Pluripotent stem cells are defined as undifferentiated, self-renewing cells that have the ability to generate mature cell types from all three germ layers. ESCs are a type of pluripotent cell derived from the inner cell mass of a blastocyst ~5–7 days after fertilization (**Figure 12.2**). iPSCs are also pluripotent; however, they are derived from fully differentiated adult cells (**Figure 12.2**), typically fibroblasts from a skin punch biopsy that have been reprogrammed into a state of pluripotency by treatment with combinations of transcription factors. During development, pluripotent cells of the inner cell mass of a blastocyst undergo sequential differentiation, becoming more specialized and tissue specific as the organism matures. The process of differentiation of pluripotent stem cells (ESCs or iPSCs) in culture to generate mature cell types recapitulates the process of development on some level. As applied to the goal of generating hair cells from pluripotent stem cells, the process of differentiating ESCs or iPSCs requires recapitulating inner ear, and subsequently hair cell development in culture (**Figure 12.3**). Several studies have reported successful differentiation of mouse pluripotent stem cells into otic progenitor cells

and hair cell-like cells, whereas reports of achieving the same goal using human stem cells are more limited.[75,76]

## Differentiation of pluripotent stem cells into hair cell-like cells

In 2010, Oshima and colleagues published a stepwise guidance protocol using mouse ESCs and iPSCs to generate mechanosensitive hair cell-like cells.[77]

The protocol uses principles of early development to direct the differentiation of pluripotent stem cells along ectoderm and otic lineages, respectively. Hair cell-like cells generated from this protocol displayed stereociliary hair bundles similar to hair cells of the postnatal mouse inner ear. Furthermore, these cells responded to mechanical stimulation and displayed electrophysiological properties similar to immature inner ear hair cells. More recently, Koehler and colleagues reported a three-dimensional *in vitro* model to generate inner ear sensory epithelia from mouse pluripotent stem cells.[78] Unlike the previous report, their model did not use mitotically inactivated chicken utricle stromal cells to guide the differentiation process; rather, they employed a

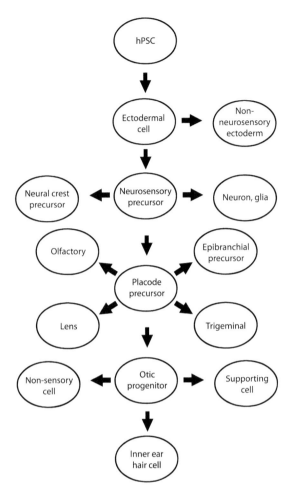

Figure 12.3 Cell fate decisions in differentiating pluripotent stem cells to an inner ear hair cell-like cell. The highlighted lineage decisions recapitulate those made by inner ear hair cells during normal development. Discrete modifications of the cell culture environment during pluripotent stem cell differentiation act to guide the cells through these fate decisions to ultimately generate an enriched population of mature inner ear hair (or supporting) cells. *Abbreviation:* hPSC, Human pluripotent stem cell.

defined, three-dimensional culture system to provide the necessary cues for hair cell differentiation. These intriguing studies provide a basis for using pluripotent stem cells to gain a deeper insight into the mechanisms underlying inner ear development, in addition to generating hair cells *in vitro* for disease modeling, molecular diagnostics, and drug discovery. Furthermore, these studies provide a method to generate populations of mouse inner

ear progenitor and hair cell-like cells to be used in the pursuit of stem cell transplantation–based treatment approaches for hearing loss. Although progress in generating hair cells from human pluripotent stem cells has been forthcoming,[75,76] additional studies will be needed to refine techniques so that the hair cell-like cells generated from human stem cells have morphological refinement and functionality comparable with those seen in the mouse ESC and iPSC studies discussed earlier.

## Cell transplantation to the organ of Corti

There have been several reports to date investigating the ability of stem cells to integrate into cochlear tissues upon inner ear transplantation.[79–88] Multiple types of stem cells and methods for transplantation have been explored using both normal-hearing and acutely deafened cochleae. One of the first reports of stem cell delivery to the inner ear of mammals was published in 2001 by investigators in Japan.[79] Neural stem cells were prepared from hippocampal tissues and injected into the scala tympani of newborn rat cochleae. Two to 4 weeks following transplantation, the authors reported grafted cell survival, with some resembling hair cells along the organ of Corti. Other studies transplanting stem cells into the damaged cochlea have described evidence of grafted cell survival and some integration into the sensory epithelia of the inner ear. In one study, investigators transplanted mouse fetal neural stem cells into the inner ears of mice following ototoxic injury.[80] Grafted cells were identified in the cochlear, vestibular, and spiral ganglion portions of the inner ear. Surprisingly, transplanted cells that integrated into the vestibular sensory epithelia expressed hair cell markers; however, this was not observed in grafted cells in the cochlear sensory epithelia. In addition, migration of transplanted cells was not observed in nondamaged control cochleae, suggesting that the molecular microenvironment of the acutely damaged mammalian cochlea may aid in the migration and integration of grafted cells. Building on this work, another group of investigators reported that neural stem cells transplanted into the sound-damaged inner ear were able to migrate throughout the cochlea.[81] The authors reported that the grafted neural stem cells in the organ of Corti expressed the hair cell markers myosin VIIa, oncomodulin, and calbindin. In addition, some of the grafted cells in the spiral ganglion exhibited a comparable phenotype to spiral ganglion neurons. In aggregate, the findings of these studies suggest that grafted stem cells can survive in the adult cochlea after transplantation for as long as 4 months in some cases. Despite the evidence of grafted cell survival,[82–87] there have been a limited number of reports demonstrating sensory integration and/or differentiation of grafted cells into hair or supporting cells after transplantation in the adult mammalian cochlea.[17,79–81,88] As such, a great deal of further investigation will be needed to identify stem cell or host-related factors that could be modified to allow for more successful integration of transplanted cells into the organ of Corti as hair cells.

Although stem cell transplantation into the adult mammalian cochlea has been met with limited success, several investigators have reported that mouse stem cells transplanted into the developing avian inner ear have the capacity to generate hair cell-like cells. In one study, investigators generated otic progenitor-like cells *in vitro* from mouse ESCs, which were subsequently transplanted into the developing inner ear of chick embryos.[89] The investigators reported that these otic progenitor cells were able to integrate into the avian auditory sensory epithelium and differentiate into cells expressing hair cell markers. More recently, another team of investigators used an alternative method to differentiate mouse ESC into hair cell-like cells.[90] Consistent with the previous report, when transplanted into the otic vesicle of developing chick embryos, these cells were found to incorporate in the correct location and function as host cells in the inner ear. Together, these studies demonstrate that mouse stem cells are capable of engraftment and differentiation under appropriate conditions when transplanted into the developing chick inner ear. This suggests that the microenvironment of the developing inner ear presents transplanted stem cells, even those from another species, with the signaling necessary to allow for engraftment and terminal differentiation as hair cells. Identification of host-related factors present in the developing inner ear that permit successful engraftment of transplanted stem cells may influence the future development of strategies whereby deafened adult mammalian cochleae may be modified or primed in some way to allow for subsequent engraftment

of transplanted stem cells. Clearly, a great deal of research will be needed to realize the potential of stem cell transplantation as a regenerative therapy for hearing loss in the future; however, steady progress continues to be made in this area.

## Cell transplantation to the auditory nerve

In 2006, Corrales and colleagues transplanted neuronal progenitor cells derived from mouse ESCs into the cochlear nerve trunk of gerbils after experimentally induced damage to the auditory nerve.[91] The transplanted cells were found to occupy substantial portions of the space previously occupied by spiral ganglion cells. Moreover, the cells were able to survive and extend processes throughout the cochlear nerve area, contacting cochlear hair cells in the organ of Corti. From this study, it appears that transplanted neuronal progenitor cells have the potential to survive, terminally differentiate, and morphologically specialize in an animal model of auditory neuronal degeneration. More recently, restoration of auditory brainstem response thresholds following lesioning of the rodent auditory nerve was reported using otic progenitor cells derived from human ESCs.[76] *In vitro*, human ESCs were directed toward an otic progenitor fate using the signaling molecules fibroblast growth factor 3 and 10. Using these growth factors, human pluripotent cells were able to differentiate into hair cell-like cells and functional auditory neurons *in vitro*. The authors transplanted the human ESC-derived neural progenitor–like cells into the spiral ganglion region of gerbils after deafening them by destroying the host auditory neurons. Analysis of the transplanted cells revealed that they were able to engraft, differentiate, and improve auditory brainstem response thresholds relative to deafened but untreated control animals. These studies demonstrate the ability of stem cell–derived neural progenitors to integrate successfully, terminally differentiate as auditory neurons, and ultimately improve auditory thresholds upon transplantation. Given these reports, the potential of stem cell transplantation for auditory nerve–related hearing loss may offer more immediate promise as a regenerative therapy when compared with stem cell transplantation into the cochlea.

Cell transplantation may be a viable treatment option in the future to replace damaged or lost cells in the inner ear; however, critical issues will need to be addressed to achieve this goal. First, an *in vitro* method to generate adequate and consistent numbers of hair cell progenitors from human pluripotent stem cells needs to be established to supply the cochlea with a sufficient number of cells to replace those that are damaged or have been lost. Because there are many types of pluripotent stem cells being used in this pursuit, the most effective cell type(s) would also need to be determined. Moreover, it is essential to identify the factors that are most critical for successful integration and terminal differentiation of grafted cells as hair cells to translate this approach to humans. Likewise, the transplanted cells also need to migrate to correct locations along the basilar membrane, avoiding the occurrence of ectopic or supernumerary hair cells to maintain the precise organization of the organ of Corti. In addition, grafted cells need to establish proper integration and neuronal circuitry for normal function. Furthermore, a safe and effective method to deliver cells to the organ of Corti must be established to ensure that it is not further damaged by the transplantation procedure itself. Last, transplanted cells face the possibility of immune responses that may ultimately lead to their rejection by the host, so immunosuppressive therapy may prove to be necessary. Although it remains to be determined if exogenous stem cells have the therapeutic potential to improve hearing ability, studies to date have provided promising results that may one day contribute to making this a viable treatment option.

## PROMOTION OF ENDOGENOUS STEM CELLS

The presence and potential of cells with stem cell–like properties in the mammalian inner ear are the topics of ongoing investigation in several laboratories. Mammalian organs with the capacity to regenerate generally contain a population of adult stem cells, which are responsible for preserving and repairing the tissue in which they are found.[92–94] These cells differ from pluripotent stem cells in that they are multipotent, meaning they are only able to differentiate into tissue-specific cell types, not all cell types. When an adult stem cell divides, one of the resulting daughter cells replaces itself as an adult stem cell, whereas the other daughter cell becomes a tissue-specific progenitor cell. Thus,

adult stem cells act as a self-repair system, repopulating themselves as adult stem cells in addition to replacing the damaged or destroyed tissue.

Adult stem cells are found in a variety of organs and tissues, including the central nervous system, skin, bone marrow, and gut. Increasing evidence suggests that the inner ear may also possess a niche of stem cells. In one study, cells with a high proliferative potential and capacity to self-renew were isolated from the vestibular portion of the adult mouse inner ear.[95] These inner ear–derived cells demonstrated the ability to form spheres, one feature of stem cells. When cultured *in vitro*, these cells showed the capacity to differentiate into cells expressing mature hair cell markers. In addition, when these sphere-derived cells were transplanted into the developing inner ear of chicken embryos, they were capable of differentiating into hair cell–like cells.

In another study evaluating the presence of adult stem cells in the mouse inner ear, investigators isolated stem cells from cochlear and vestibular tissues in mice 1–4 months of age.[96] Differences in the capacity for sphere formation were observed, with stem cells from the vestibular sensory epithelia displaying a higher capacity for sphere formation compared with those isolated from the cochlear sensory epithelia. In addition, the sphere-forming ability of the cochlear sensory epithelia rapidly decreased from the second to the third postnatal week, whereas the sphere-forming ability of the vestibular sensory epithelia declined more slowly and into adulthood. As already stated, the mammalian vestibular organ has some capacity to replace lost hair cells,[15,16] whereas the cochlea appears to lack this regenerative potential. Results from this study suggest that stem cell–like cells may be responsible for the persistence of some regenerative potential observed in the vestibular sensory epithelium. In addition, the inability of the cochlear sensory epithelium to regenerate might be due to a reduction in the number or potential of the tissue-specific stem cell population in the organ of Corti.

Although there are reports of low/undetectable progenitor cells in the adult mammalian inner ear, other lines of investigation suggest that stem cell compartments may persist within the mature cochlea. The intermediate filament protein nestin is expressed in proliferating tissues and is widely regarded as a marker of mitotically active cells and neural stem cells.[97-100] As such, nestin is commonly used to identify cells with stem cell characteristics in developing and adult tissues.[97] Several studies have reported the existence of nestin-expressing cells in the inner ears of mice; however, their presence and location differ between reports.[101-103] In the first report, nestin expression was observed in supporting cells below the inner and outer hair cells in the immature mouse cochlea, in addition to some mild expression in the outer hair cells; however, in the early adult mouse, nestin expression was downregulated and localized to only a few cells under the outer hair cell layer.[101] In another study, nestin expression was observed in supporting cells near the inner hair cell layer, with some mild expression in a few inner and outer hair cells in the immature cochlea.[102] In the mature inner ear, nestin expression was found to be limited to only the spiral ganglion. Most recently, nestin expression was found in supporting cells lateral to the outer hair cell region.[103] This expression was observed throughout the whole cochlea in newborn mice; however, the number of nestin-expressing cells decreased as the cochlea matured. Of interest, the authors reported that there appeared to be an increase in the number of nestin-expressing cells following noise trauma.[103] Collectively, the presence of nestin-expressing cells in the murine inner ear raises the possibility of the persistence of a population of stem cell-like cells within the mammalian cochlea. Further work exploring their exact presence, localization, and overall function is essential to understand any therapeutic potential that they may possess.

More recently, Lgr5, a Wnt target gene, has emerged as another area of interest for hair cell regeneration.[40,104,105] Lgr5 is a stem cell marker found in multiple proliferating adult tissues.[106-109] During embryonic development, Lgr5 is expressed in nascent hair cells and supporting cells and is later downregulated as the cells mature, with expression limited to the third row of Deiters' cells in the mature organ of Corti.[104] Analysis of these cells by other investigators revealed that they give rise to hair cell lineages *in vivo* and *in vitro*.[40] In this study, Lgr5-expressing cells were isolated and cultured *in vitro* and found to self-renew and differentiate into cells expressing the hair cell marker myosin VIIa. *In vivo*, these cells were able to give rise to hair cells. In agreement with the previous report, Lgr5 expression was downregulated to the third row of Deiters' cells; however, inner pillar cells also appeared to retain this expression as well. Additional analysis revealed these Lgr5-expressing cells proliferate and generate hair cells under certain experimental conditions in neonatal mice.[105] Evidence that these cells are able to reenter the cell cycle and proliferate offers the advantage that these cells could replenish both hair cells and supporting cells in the damaged mammalian cochlea. It remains unclear at this point how long the population of Lgr5-expressing cochlear stem cells persist into adulthood. As with nestin expression, further investigation of these cells is needed to determine their therapeutic potential as a means for regenerating cochlear hair cells.

In summary, the presence of endogenous stem cells in the mammalian inner ear presents the possibility of local therapy aimed at recruiting and directing these cells to repopulate the organ of Corti with functional cochlear hair cells after the native population of hair cells has been lost or damaged. Some studies on the topic have reported that, over time, the number and/or viability of multipotent stem cells in the cochlea decreases.[96,101-104] Consequently, there exists the possibility that, by the time these cells are needed for most patients with acquired causes of hearing loss, they no longer exist. Accordingly, further research is warranted to determine the function, location, and persistence into adulthood of cochlear stem cells to better define their potential as the basis for a novel therapeutic approach for hearing loss.

## CONCLUSION

The past 30 years of research have provided a better understanding of the mechanisms underlying inner ear development, avian cochlear hair cell regeneration, pluripotent stem cell differentiation, cell transplantation, the presence of endogenous stem cells, and the potential therapeutic application of gene transfer and pharmacotherapies for hearing loss. Although much has been learned about the use of exogenous stem cells, inner ear stem cells, gene transfer, and pharmacotherapies for the replacement of damaged cells, these approaches for the treatment of hearing loss are still in experimental stages. There are many intricate components, and therefore challenges, involved in the process of auditory nerve and cochlear hair cell regeneration. As such, it is possible that a combination of the approaches described here or others not yet evident will yield novel, clinically meaningful treatments for hearing loss in the future. Although there are no clinical trials in this field to date for adults with hearing loss, several recent discoveries using cell culture and animal models give hope that otolaryngologists will have novel, regenerative therapeutic options for the management of sensorineural hearing loss in the future.

## CHALLENGES OF REGENERATIVE THERAPY

- Challenges facing all approaches
  - Identifying the safest and most efficient method to access the cochlea.
  - Repopulating the cochlea with an adequate amount of cells.
  - Avoidance of generating hair cells outside of the organ of Corti.
  - Maintenance of newly generated cells.
  - Reestablishment of neuronal circuitry.
- Gene-based treatment and pharmacotherapies
  - Generation of replacement hair cells without significantly compromising the supporting cell population.
  - Ensuring that treatment does not compromise the cytoarchitecture of the organ of Corti.
  - Unregulated cell proliferation carries the risk of tumor formation.
- Exogenous stem cells
  - Determine the timing of transplantation relative to damage for optimal success.
  - Proper migration, integration, and terminal differentiation of transplanted cells into the organ of Corti as hair cells.
  - Immune rejection of transplanted cells.
- Endogenous stem cells
  - Identifying if endogenous cochlear stem cells persist into adulthood and maintain potency to become hair cells.
  - Determining the spatial and temporal organization of adult stem cells in the cochlea.
  - Identifying a method for allowing cochlear stem cells, if present, to enter the cell cycle, proliferate, and replace lost hair cells.

## KEY POINTS

- Multiple approaches such as the following are being taken in pursuit of regenerative treatments for sensorineural hearing loss:
  - Gene transfer
  - Pharmacotherapies
  - Exogenous delivery of stem cells
  - Promotion of endogenous stem cells
- All approaches are still in experimental stages with no clinical trials to date in adults.
- Each approach has its own unique advantages and disadvantages.
- A combination of these approaches may be necessary for successful treatment of sensorineural hearing loss in the future.

## ACKNOWLEDGMENTS

Samuel Gubbels receives support (KL2 award and Type I pilot) from the Clinical and Translational Science Award (CTSA) program, previously through the National Center for Research Resources (NCRR) grant 1UL1RR025011, and now by the National Center for Advancing Translational Sciences (NCATS), grant 9U54TR000021. The content is solely the responsibility of the authors and does not necessarily represent the official views of the NIH. SG also receives support from NIH/NIDCD 1 R03 DC012432–01, 1 R01 DC013912–01, as well as P30 HD003352.

## REFERENCES

1. Lin FR, Thorpe R, Gordon-Salant S, Ferrucci L. Hearing loss prevalence and risk factors among older adults in the United States. J Gerontol A Biol Sci Med Sci 2011;66(5):582–590
2. Dillon CF, Gu Q, Hoffman HJ, Ko CW. Vision, hearing, balance, and sensory impairment in Americans aged 70 years and over: United States, 1999-2006. NCHS Data Brief 2010;31(31):1–8
3. Arlinger S. Negative consequences of uncorrected hearing loss—a review. Int J Audiol 2003;42(Suppl 2):S17–S20

4. National Institute on Deafness and Other Communication Disorders. Quick Statistics. 2010. http://www.nidcd.nih.gov/health/statistics/Pages/quick.aspx. Accessed December 16, 2013

5. Davis AC. Hearing disorders in the population: first phase findings of the MRC National Study of Hearing. In: Lutman ME, Haggard MP, eds. Hearing Science and Hearing Disorders. New York, NY: Academic Press 1983;35–60

6. Morrison SJ, Spradling AC. Stem cells and niches: mechanisms that promote stem cell maintenance throughout life. Cell 2008;132(4):598–611

7. Watt FM, Lo Celso C, Silva-Vargas V. Epidermal stem cells: an update. Curr Opin Genet Dev 2006;16(5):518–524

8. Miura H, Kusakabe Y, Harada S. Cell lineage and differentiation in taste buds. Arch Histol Cytol 2006;69(4):209–225

9. Altman J. Autoradiographic and histological studies of postnatal neurogenesis. IV. Cell proliferation and migration in the anterior forebrain, with special reference to persisting neurogenesis in the olfactory bulb. J Comp Neurol 1969;137(4):433–457

10. Lois C, Alvarez-Buylla A. Long-distance neuronal migration in the adult mammalian brain. Science 1994;264(5162): 1145–1148

11. Kornack DR, Rakic P. The generation, migration, and differentiation of olfactory neurons in the adult primate brain. Proc Natl Acad Sci USA 2001;98(8):4752–4757

12. Corwin JT, Cotanche DA. Regeneration of sensory hair cells after acoustic trauma. Science 1988;240(4860):1772–1774

13. Ryals BM, Rubel EW. Hair cell regeneration after acoustic trauma in adult Coturnix quail. Science 1988;240(4860): 1774–1776

14. Smolders JW. Functional recovery in the avian ear after hair cell regeneration. Audiol Neurootol 1999;4(6):286–302

15. Warchol ME, Lambert PR, Goldstein BJ, Forge A, Corwin JT. Regenerative proliferation in inner ear sensory epithelia from adult guinea pigs and humans. Science 1993;259(5101):1619–1622

16. Forge A, Li L, Corwin JT, Nevill G. Ultrastructural evidence for hair cell regeneration in the mammalian inner ear. Science 1993;259(5101):1616–1619

17. Groves AK. The challenge of hair cell regeneration. Exp Biol Med 2010;235(4):434–446

18. Bhave SA, Stone JS, Rubel EW, Coltrera MD. Cell cycle progression in gentamicin-damaged avian cochleas. J Neurosci 1995;15(6):4618–4628

19. Duncan LJ, Mangiardi DA, Matsui JI, Anderson JK, McLaughlin-Williamson K, Cotanche DA. Differential expression of unconventional myosins in apoptotic and regenerating chick hair cells confirms two regeneration mechanisms. J Comp Neurol 2006;499(5):691–701

20. Stone JS, Choi YS, Woolley SM, Yamashita H, Rubel EW. Progenitor cell cycling during hair cell regeneration in the vestibular and auditory epithelia of the chick. J Neurocytol 1999;28(10–11):863–876

21. Roberson DW, Alosi JA, Cotanche DA. Direct transdifferentiation gives rise to the earliest new hair cells in regenerating avian auditory epithelium. J Neurosci Res 2004;78(4):461–471

22. Adler HJ, Raphael Y. New hair cells arise from supporting cell conversion in the acoustically damaged chick inner ear. Neurosci Lett 1996;205(1):17–20

23. Duckert LG, Rubel EW. Ultrastructural observations on regenerating hair cells in the chick basilar papilla. Hear Res 1990;48(1–2):161–182

24. Duckert LG, Rubel EW. Morphological correlates of functional recovery in the chicken inner ear after gentamycin treatment. J Comp Neurol 1993;331(1):75–96

25. Warchol ME. Cell density and N-cadherin interactions regulate cell proliferation in the sensory epithelia of the inner ear. J Neurosci 2002;22(7):2607–2616

26. Beresford WA. Direct transdifferentiation: can cells change their phenotype without dividing? Cell Differ Dev 1990; 29(2):81–93

27. Colvin JS, Bohne BA, Harding GW, McEwen DG, Ornitz DM. Skeletal overgrowth and deafness in mice lacking fibroblast growth factor receptor 3. Nat Genet 1996;12(4):390–397

28. Fritzsch B, Beisel KW, Hansen LA. The molecular basis of neurosensory cell formation in ear development: a blueprint for hair cell and sensory neuron regeneration? BioEssays 2006;28(12):1181–1193

29. Chen P, Johnson JE, Zoghbi HY, Segil N. The role of Math1 in inner ear development: Uncoupling the establishment of the sensory primordium from hair cell fate determination. Development 2002;129(10):2495–2505

30. Lumpkin EA, Collisson T, Parab P, et al. Math1-driven GFP expression in the developing nervous system of transgenic mice. Gene Expr Patterns 2003;3(4):389–395

31. Woods C, Montcouquiol M, Kelley MW. Math1 regulates development of the sensory epithelium in the mammalian cochlea. Nat Neurosci 2004;7(12):1310–1318

32. Bermingham NA, Hassan BA, Price SD, et al. Math1: an essential gene for the generation of inner ear hair cells. Science 1999;284(5421):1837–1841

33. Zheng JL, Gao WQ. Overexpression of Math1 induces robust production of extra hair cells in postnatal rat inner ears. Nat Neurosci 2000;3(6):580–586

34. Cafaro J, Lee GS, Stone JS. *Atoh1* expression defines activated progenitors and differentiating hair cells during avian hair cell regeneration. Dev Dyn 2007;236(1):156–170

35. Kawamoto K, Ishimoto S, Minoda R, Brough DE, Raphael Y. Math1 gene transfer generates new cochlear hair cells in mature guinea pigs *in vivo*. J Neurosci 2003;23(11): 4395–4400

36. Izumikawa M, Minoda R, Kawamoto K, et al. Auditory hair cell replacement and hearing improvement by *Atoh1* gene therapy in deaf mammals. Nat Med 2005;11(3):271–276

37. Gubbels SP, Woessner DW, Mitchell JC, Ricci AJ, Brigande JV. Functional auditory hair cells produced in the mammalian cochlea by *in utero* gene transfer. Nature 2008;455(7212): 537–541

38. Chai R, Kuo B, Wang T, et al. Wnt signaling induces proliferation of sensory precursors in the postnatal mouse cochlea. Proc Natl Acad Sci USA 2012;109(21):8167–8172

39. Doetzlhofer A, White P, Lee YS, Groves A, Segil N. Prospective identification and purification of hair cell and supporting cell progenitors from the embryonic cochlea. Brain Res 2006;1091(1):282–288

40. Shi F, Kempfle JS, Edge AS. Wnt-responsive Lgr5-expressing stem cells are hair cell progenitors in the cochlea. J Neurosci 2012;32(28):9639–9648

41. White PM, Doetzlhofer A, Lee YS, Groves AK, Segil N. Mammalian cochlear supporting cells can divide and trans-differentiate into hair cells. Nature 2006;441(7096):984–987

42. Savary E, Hugnot JP, Chassigneux Y, et al. Distinct population of hair cell progenitors can be isolated from the postnatal mouse cochlea using side population analysis. Stem Cells 2007;25(2):332–339

43. Sinkkonen ST, Chai R, Jan TA, et al. Intrinsic regenerative potential of murine cochlear supporting cells. Sci Rep 2011; 1:26

44. Lee YS, Liu F, Segil N. A morphogenetic wave of p27Kip1 transcription directs cell cycle exit during organ of Corti development. Development 2006;133(15):2817–2826

45. Ruben RJ. Development of the inner ear of the mouse: a radioautographic study of terminal mitoses. Acta Otolaryngol 1967;Suppl 220:1–44

46. Chen P, Segil N. p27(Kip1) links cell proliferation to morphogenesis in the developing organ of Corti. Development 1999;126(8):1581–1590

47. Löwenheim H, Furness DN, Kil J, et al. Gene disruption of p27(Kip1) allows cell proliferation in the postnatal and adult organ of Corti. Proc Natl Acad Sci USA 1999;96(7):4084–4088

48. Chen P, Zindy F, Abdala C, et al. Progressive hearing loss in mice lacking the cyclin-dependent kinase inhibitor Ink4d. Nat Cell Biol 2003;5(5):422–426

49. Kanzaki S, Beyer LA, Swiderski DL, et al. p27(Kip1) deficiency causes organ of Corti pathology and hearing loss. Hear Res 2006;214(1–2):28–36

50. Chen ZY. Cell cycle, differentiation and regeneration: where to begin? Cell Cycle 2006;5(22):2609–2612

51. Huang M, Sage C, Tang Y, et al. Overlapping and distinct pRb pathways in the mammalian auditory and vestibular organs. Cell Cycle 2011;10(2):337–351

52. Sage C, Huang M, Vollrath MA, et al. Essential role of retinoblastoma protein in mammalian hair cell development and hearing. Proc Natl Acad Sci USA 2006;103(19):7345–7350

53. Sage C, Huang M, Karimi K, et al. Proliferation of functional hair cells *in vivo* in the absence of the retinoblastoma protein. Science 2005;307(5712):1114–1118

54. Yu Y, Weber T, Yamashita T, et al. *In vivo* proliferation of post-mitotic cochlear supporting cells by acute ablation of the retinoblastoma protein in neonatal mice. J Neurosci 2010;30(17):5927–5936

55. Kimble J, Simpson P. The LIN-12/Notch signaling pathway and its regulation. Annu Rev Cell Dev Biol 1997;13:333–361

56. Louvi A, Artavanis-Tsakonas S. Notch signaling in vertebrate neural development. Nat Rev Neurosci 2006;7(2):93–102

57. Lanford PJ, Lan Y, Jiang R, et al. Notch signaling pathway mediates hair cell development in mammalian cochlea. Nat Genet 1999;21(3):289–292

58. Eddison M, Le Roux I, Lewis J. Notch signaling in the development of the inner ear: lessons from Drosophila. Proc Natl Acad Sci USA 2000;97(22):11692–11699

59. Lewis J. Rules for the production of sensory cells. Ciba Found Symp 1991;160:25–39, discussion 40–53

60. Kiernan AE. Notch signaling during cell fate determination in the inner ear. Semin Cell Dev Biol 2013;24(5):470–479

61. Zine A, Aubert A, Qiu J, et al. Hes1 and Hes5 activities are required for the normal development of the hair cells in the mammalian inner ear. J Neurosci 2001;21(13):4712–4720

62. Li S, Mark S, Radde-Gallwitz K, Schlisner R, Chin MT, Chen P. Hey2 functions in parallel with Hes1 and Hes5 for mammalian auditory sensory organ development. BMC Dev Biol 2008;8:20 [Database]

63. Lanford PJ, Shailam R, Norton CR, Gridley T, Kelley MW. Expression of Math1 and HES5 in the cochleae of wildtype and Jag2 mutant mice. J Assoc Res Otolaryngol 2000;1(2):161–171

64. Stone JS, Rubel EW. Delta1 expression during avian hair cell regeneration. Development 1999;126(5):961–973

65. Brooker R, Hozumi K, Lewis J. Notch ligands with contrasting functions: Jagged1 and Delta1 in the mouse inner ear. Development 2006;133(7):1277–1286

66. Kiernan AE, Cordes R, Kopan R, Gossler A, Gridley T. The Notch ligands DLL1 and JAG2 act synergistically to regulate hair cell development in the mammalian inner ear. Development 2005;132(19):4353–4362

67. Doetzlhofer A, Basch ML, Ohyama T, Gessler M, Groves AK, Segil N. Hey2 regulation by FGF provides a Notch-independent mechanism for maintaining pillar cell fate in the organ of Corti. Dev Cell 2009;16(1):58–69

68. Hayashi T, Kokubo H, Hartman BH, Ray CA, Reh TA, Bermingham-McDonogh O. Hesr1 and Hesr2 may act as early effectors of Notch signaling in the developing cochlea. Dev Biol 2008;316(1):87–99

69. Takebayashi S, Yamamoto N, Yabe D, et al. Multiple roles of Notch signaling in cochlear development. Dev Biol 2007;307(1):165–178

70. Yamamoto N, Tanigaki K, Tsuji M, Yabe D, Ito J, Honjo T. Inhibition of Notch/RBP-J signaling induces hair cell formation in neonate mouse cochleas. J Mol Med 2006;84(1):37–45

71. Hori R, Nakagawa T, Sakamoto T, Matsuoka Y, Takebayashi S, Ito J. Pharmacological inhibition of Notch signaling in the mature guinea pig cochlea. Neuroreport 2007;18(18): 1911–1914

72. Mizutari K, Fujioka M, Hosoya M, et al. Notch inhibition induces cochlear hair cell regeneration and recovery of hearing after acoustic trauma. Neuron 2013;77(1):58–69

73. Picanço-Castro V, Moreira LF, Kashima S. Covas DT. Can pluripotent stem cells be used in cell-based therapy? Cell Reprogram 2014;16(2):98–107

74. Pan CK, Heilweil G, Lanza R, Schwartz SD. Embryonic stem cells as a treatment for macular degeneration. Expert Opin Biol Ther 2013;13(8):1125–1133

75. Ronaghi M, Nasr M, Ealy M, et al. Inner ear hair cell-like cells from human embryonic stem cells. Stem Cells Dev 2014; 23(11):1275–1284

76. Chen W, Jongkamonwiwat N, Abbas L, et al. Restoration of auditory evoked responses by human ES-cell-derived otic progenitors. Nature 2012;490(7419):278–282

77. Oshima K, Shin K, Diensthuber M, Peng AW, Ricci AJ, Heller S. Mechanosensitive hair cell-like cells from embryonic and induced pluripotent stem cells. Cell 2010;141(4):704–716

78. Koehler KR, Mikosz AM, Molosh AI, Patel D, Hashino E. Generation of inner ear sensory epithelia from pluripotent stem cells in 3D culture. Nature 2013;500(7461):217–221

79. Ito J, Kojima K, Kawaguchi S. Survival of neural stem cells in the cochlea. Acta Otolaryngol 2001;121(2):140–142

80. Tateya I, Nakagawa T, Iguchi F, et al. Fate of neural stem cells grafted into injured inner ears of mice. Neuroreport 2003;14(13):1677–1681

81. Parker MA, Corliss DA, Gray B, et al. Neural stem cells injected into the sound-damaged cochlea migrate throughout the cochlea and express markers of hair cells, supporting cells, and spiral ganglion cells. Hear Res 2007;232(1–2):29–43

82. Coleman B, Hardman J, Coco A, et al. Fate of embryonic stem cells transplanted into the deafened mammalian cochlea. Cell Transplant 2006;15(5):369–380

83. Hildebrand MS, Dahl HH, Hardman J, Coleman B, Shepherd RK, de Silva MG. Survival of partially differentiated mouse embryonic stem cells in the scala media of the guinea pig cochlea. J Assoc Res Otolaryngol 2005;6(4):341–354

84. Hu Z, Wei D, Johansson CB, et al. Survival and neural differentiation of adult neural stem cells transplanted into the mature inner ear. Exp Cell Res 2005;302(1):40–47

85. Naito Y, Nakamura T, Nakagawa T, et al. Transplantation of bone marrow stromal cells into the cochlea of chinchillas. Neuroreport 2004;15(1):1–4

86. Sakamoto T, Nakagawa T, Endo T, et al. Fates of mouse embryonic stem cells transplanted into the inner ears of adult mice and embryonic chickens. Acta Otolaryngologica 2004;Supplement 551:48–52

87. Tamura T, Nakagawa T, Iguchi F, et al. Transplantation of neural stem cells into the modiolus of mouse cochleae injured by cisplatin. Acta Otolaryngologica 2004;Supplement 551:65–68

88. Han Z, Yang JM, Chi FL, et al. Survival and fate of transplanted embryonic neural stem cells by *Atoh1* gene transfer in guinea pigs cochlea. Neuroreport 2010;21(7):490–496

89. Li H, Roblin G, Liu H, Heller S. Generation of hair cells by step-wise differentiation of embryonic stem cells. Proc Natl Acad Sci USA 2003;100(23):13495–13500

90. Ouji Y, Ishizaka S, Nakamura-Uchiyama F, Yoshikawa M. *In vitro* differentiation of mouse embryonic stem cells into inner ear hair cell-like cells using stromal cell conditioned medium. Cell Death Dis 2012;3:e314

91. Corrales CE, Pan L, Li H, Liberman MC, Heller S, Edge AS. Engraftment and differentiation of embryonic stem cell-derived neural progenitor cells in the cochlear nerve trunk: growth of processes into the organ of Corti. J Neurobiol 2006;66(13):1489–1500

92. Leblond CP, Clermont Y, Nadler NJ. The pattern of stem cell renewal in three epithelia (esophagus, intestine and testis). Proc Can Cancer Conf 1967;7:3–30

93. Shihabuddin LS, Ray J, Gage FH. Stem cell technology for basic science and clinical applications. Arch Neurol 1999;56(1): 29–32

94. Weissman IL. Stem cells: units of development, units of regeneration, and units in evolution. Cell 2000;100(1): 157–168

95. Li H, Liu H, Heller S. Pluripotent stem cells from the adult mouse inner ear. Nat Med 2003;9(10):1293–1299

96. Oshima K, Grimm CM, Corrales CE, et al. Differential distribution of stem cells in the auditory and vestibular organs of the inner ear. J Assoc Res Otolaryngol 2007;8(1):18–31

97. Lendahl U, Zimmerman LB, McKay RD. CNS stem cells express a new class of intermediate filament protein. Cell 1990;60(4):585–595

98. Sejersen T, Lendahl U. Transient expression of the intermediate filament nestin during skeletal muscle development. J Cell Sci 1993;106(Pt 4):1291–1300

99. Kachinsky AM, Dominov JA, Miller JB. Intermediate filaments in cardiac myogenesis: nestin in the developing mouse heart. J Histochem Cytochem 1995;43(8):843–847

100. Suzuki S, Namiki J, Shibata S, Mastuzaki Y, Okano H. The neural stem/progenitor cell marker nestin is expressed in proliferative endothelial cells, but not in mature vasculature. J Histochem Cytochem 2010;58(8):721–730

101. Lopez IA, Zhao PM, Yamaguchi M, de Vellis J, Espinosa-Jeffrey A. Stem/progenitor cells in the postnatal inner ear of the GFP-nestin transgenic mouse. Int J Dev Neurosci 2004;22(4): 205–213

102. Smeti I, Savary E, Capelle V, Hugnot JP, Uziel A, Zine A. Expression of candidate markers for stem/progenitor cells in the inner ears of developing and adult GFAP and nestin promoter-GFP transgenic mice. Gene Expr Patterns 2011; 11(1–2):22–32

103. Watanabe R, Morell MH, Miller JM, et al. Nestin-expressing cells in the developing, mature and noise-exposed cochlear epithelium. Mol Cell Neurosci 2012;49(2):104–109

104. Chai R, Xia A, Wang T, et al. Dynamic expression of Lgr5, a Wnt target gene, in the developing and mature mouse cochlea. J Assoc Res Otolaryngol 2011;12(4):455–469

105. Shi F, Hu L, Edge AS. Generation of hair cells in neonatal mice by b-catenin over-expression in Lgr5-positive cochlear progenitors. Proc Natl Acad Sci USA 2013;110(34):13851–13856

106. Barker N, van Es JH, Kuipers J, et al. Identification of stem cells in small intestine and colon by marker gene Lgr5. Nature 2007;449(7165):1003–1007

107. Barker N, Huch M, Kujala P, et al. Lgr5(+ve) stem cells drive self-renewal in the stomach and build long-lived gastric units in vitro. Cell Stem Cell 2010;6(1):25–36

108. Jaks V, Barker N, Kasper M, et al. Lgr5 marks cycling, yet long-lived, hair follicle stem cells. Nat Genet 2008;40(11):1291–1299

109. Ootani A, Li X, Sangiorgi E, et al. Sustained in vitro intestinal epithelial culture within a Wnt-dependent stem cell niche. Nat Med 2009;15(6):701–706

# 13

# Sudden sensorineural hearing loss

ROBERT THAYER SATALOFF, KEVIN L. LI, AND PAMELA C. ROEHM

The term sudden sensorineural hearing loss (SSNHL) was introduced in 1944 by DeKleyn (1). A variety of definitions ensued and continue to exist in the literature today. However, most authorities would agree that SSNHL refers to a sensorineural hearing loss (SNHL) of ~30 dB over three contiguous audiometric frequencies occurring within a 3-day period or less. The condition affects ~4000 Americans yearly and accounts for ~1% of all cases of SNHL (2). All ages are affected; however, the incidence increases with age with a peak in the 50–60-year range (3). There is no sexual or geographic predominance and no laterality.

The proposed etiologies of sudden hearing loss can be categorized as follows: infectious, vascular, traumatic, neoplastic, immunologic, neurologic, metabolic, and toxic. In the overwhelming majority of patients, there remains no identifiable etiology for SSNHL despite the fact that over the years more than 100 possible causes have been suggested (3). In fact, a cause can be found in only 10%–15% of patients with the remainder labeled "idiopathic" (4–6).

In addition to the conditions discussed in this chapter, additional causes, treatments, and examples of SSNHL are discussed in Chapter 10.

## INFECTIOUS

Bacteria, viruses, and fungi have all been implicated in SSNHL. Of these infectious agents, viruses are believed, by some, to be the most common culprit, causing viral cochleitis or viral neuritis. The most convincing evidence of virus-induced sudden hearing loss is the presence of viruses and/or viral particles in the cochlea. Westmore et al. (7) was able to isolate mumps virus from the inner ear of a patient with sudden hearing loss, and Davis et al. (8) isolated cytomegalovirus (CMV) from the perilymph of an infant with congenital CMV. Davis and Johnson (9) were able to induce a mumps labyrinthitis in hamsters by inoculating the animals' subarachnoid space. Seroconversion and increased viral titers suggest a viral etiology in selected patients with SSNHL. Studies have demonstrated an increased incidence of seroconversion to various viruses including herpes simplex, herpes zoster, CMV, influenza, parainfluenza, mumps, measles, and adenovirus but fail to demonstrate a relationship between titer results, severity of hearing loss, and prognosis (10–12). Further evidence for a viral etiology is the finding of temporal bone histopathologic changes consistent

DOI: 10.1201/b23379-13

with viral infection. Schuknecht and Donovan (13) demonstrated atrophy of the organ of Corti, tectorial membrane, stria vascularis, cochlear nerve, and vestibular organs in cases of known viral labyrinthitis, and multiple authors have demonstrated similar findings in patients with a history of sudden hearing loss (14–16).

Recently, there have been reports of COVID-19-related SSNHL, but the data is conflicting as these are often single institution studies from around the world. For example, Chern et al. have reported a case of bilateral SSNHL and vertigo due to intralabyrinthine hemorrhage in a COVID-19-positive patient (17). In an Italian study of 42 patients, Parrino et al. noted a significantly higher rate of SSNHL with acute cochleovestibular symptoms during the COVID pandemic compared to previous years. Moreover, they noted an average worse presenting hearing loss on pure-tone audiometry (18). In contrast, Chari et. al noted a decline in the total number of SSNHL patients presenting to their institution during the COVID pandemic; however, the overall proportion of patients presenting with SSNHL remained similar to prior years (19). There have been a handful of systematic reviews in the past few years that have looked at the effects of SARS-CoV-2 on the auditory and vestibular systems, with no clear causative link to SSNHL (19–22).

Evaluation of SSNHL should rule out common causes that are treatable or that can lead to other medical issues and should include laboratory evaluation for syphilis, Lyme disease, autoimmune inner ear disease and other disorders, and imaging studies to rule out acoustic neuroma and other brain tumors. A comprehensive evaluation for etiologies can include an extensive search for direct or indirect proof of an infection but is rarely useful (23). Extensive laboratory work-up includes a CBC with differential to evaluate for an increase in the white blood cell count in addition to an evaluation of viral titers. At the time of presentation, titers may be drawn for herpes, influenza A and B, coxsackie virus, toxoplasmosis, and CMV. A repeat set may be drawn ideally several weeks later, to evaluate during convalescence for a change in titer suggesting recent infection. Evaluation for Lyme disease can be performed, and syphilis should be ruled out with a fluorescent treponemal antibody absorption (FTA-ABS) or microhemagglutination assay-*Treponema palladium* (MHA-TP) which is to be run regardless of a negative VDRL or RPR result, as luetic labyrinthitis is typically a form of late, tertiary syphilis.

Patients with SSNHL may be treated with acyclovir (400 mg po 5X/day × 10 days) in patients presenting with sudden hearing loss because of the high suspicion of a viral etiology, but this has not been found to be useful in most patients. In addition, many physicians elect to prophylactically treat patients with doxycycline 100 mg po bid against *Borrelia burgdorferi* infection while awaiting Lyme titers.

## VASCULAR

Given the cochlea's dependence upon a single terminal branch of the labyrinthine artery, the idea of a vascular etiology for sudden hearing loss is very attractive. The cochlea has been shown to be highly intolerant of ischemic insult as demonstrated by the loss of cochlear action potentials after as little as 60 seconds of interrupted blood supply in animal models (24) and by the permanent loss of cochlear function following 30 minutes of labyrinthine artery occlusion (25). Histopathologic studies of the inner ear have been performed demonstrating characteristic changes following experimental interruption of the labyrinthine artery in animals (23, 25). Complete occlusion of the artery results in severe degeneration of the membranous labyrinth whereas microembolization causes patchy areas of necrosis (26).

Multiple mechanisms of vascular occlusion exist including embolism, thrombosis, vasospasm, and hypercoagulable states. The association of sudden hearing loss with migraine, sickle cell disease, macroglobulinemia, thromboangiitis obliterans (Buerger's disease), and cardiopulmonary bypass supports the vascular theory (27, 28). A recent meta-analysis also noted a higher risk for stroke in patients with SSNHL with a hazard ratio up to 4.08. In this study, the authors note that hypertension, diabetes, a history of myocardial infarction, elevated LDL, and total cholesterol appear to be independent risk factors for SSNHL. However, the authors note the data was very heterogenous. (29). The high incidence of spontaneous recovery, losses frequently limited to few frequencies, paucity of vertigo in most cases, and a large number of patients without vascular risk factors argue against ischemia as a *predominant* cause of sudden hearing loss. These phenomena may be explained in part because the cochlea is more vulnerable to ischemia than the vestibular labyrinth and sensory cells of the basal turn are more vulnerable than those at the cochlear apex. Nonetheless, in cases with no identifiable cause, the vascular theory influences management strongly.

Vascular evaluation includes CBC, PT/PTT, bleeding time, and lipid profile (30). Prophylactic therapy with vasodilators and/or volume expanders is advocated by some. Intravenous histamine can be administered to promote blood flow and eliminate vasospasm and is delivered intravenously at a rate adequate to cause facial flushing. Carbogen is a mix of 5% carbon dioxide and 95% oxygen which has been demonstrated to increase perilymphatic oxygen tension (31). Several short-term inhalations were performed over the course of a day with this mixture (usually 30-minute inhalations every 3 hours around the clock), and any improvement in subjective hearing is noted. Diatrizoate sodium (Hypaque) was noted by Morimitsu to reverse a patient's sudden hearing loss (32) prompting further study of 60 patients in which a 37% recovery rate was reported (33). Hypaque was used due to its volume expanding properties and its possible mechanical effect on injuries to the stria vascularis.

A number of different vascular-directed therapies have been described in the literature and continue to be employed including hyperbaric oxygen therapy, stellate ganglion block, papaverine, pentoxifylline, dextran, and nicotinic acid (34, 35).

## IMMUNOLOGIC

The immune system protects us from nonself at a cost. In fighting infection, the immune system initiates an inflammatory response. In the nonforgiving environment of the inner ear, this inflammatory response can be detrimental resulting in cochleovestibular symptoms. Harris et al. (36) demonstrated that, in an animal model infected with CMV, immunosuppression resulted in a lesser degree of hearing loss than in immunocompetent controls. Furthermore, the positive response often seen with corticosteroid administration lends support to the notion that the inflammatory response can be detrimental in sudden hearing loss.

Autoimmunity refers to the process by which the body recognizes its own antigens as "foreign" resulting in an immune response directed against itself. Autoimmune inner ear disease can occur both in isolation and in the context of systemic disease. History, clinical findings, response to immunosuppressive (e.g., steroids) medication, and immunologic evaluation of the patient's serum are all important in the diagnosis of autoimmune sensorineural hearing loss (AISNHL). Although autoimmune inner ear disease is characterized most often by a bilateral or unilateral progressive SNHL that occurs over a period of weeks to months, sudden SNHL may be the presenting complaint in as many as one-quarter of patients with AISNHL (37).

In addition to the history, laboratory findings may indicate an autoimmune etiology in the patient with sudden hearing loss. Nonspecific markers of immune system up-regulation include a complement panel and ESR in addition to rheumatoid factor, antinuclear antibody, antimicrosomal antibody, and anticardiolipin antibody. The presence or absence of four specific antigens has been associated with AISNHL: the *presence* of B35, CW4, and CW7 and the *absence* of DR4 (38, 39). In addition to these markers, Western blot analysis for antibodies against an inner ear 68-kD protein has been demonstrated by Harris and Sharp (39). Disher et al. (40) found this protein to be present in ~50% of patients with possible AISNHL. The antibody in question may be the monoclonal antibody KHRI-3 which binds to an inner ear-supporting cell antigen and has been demonstrated to precipitate a 68- to 70-kD antigen. The presence of antibodies to inner ear antigens supports the concept that an autoimmune process is responsible for inner ear disease in these patients.

One of the major criteria in determining hearing loss of autoimmune origin is response to steroid therapy. Therefore, patients should be started on high-dose prednisone (1 mg/kg per day) immediately upon presentation following initial laboratory testing. Close monitoring of hearing response, both subjective and objective, is necessary, and any drop in hearing during prednisone taper should alert the physician to increase the steroid dose. In 2001, Gianoli and Li (41) treated patients who had failed to respond or who could not tolerate systemic steroids. They reported a 44% hearing salvage in patients who underwent transtympanic steroid administration on four separate occasions over the course of 10–14 days and concluded that transtympanic steroid therapy may be an alternative treatment for those failing or unable to tolerate systemic therapy. For patients who are unable to tolerate steroid therapy or continue to relapse while on the taper, some recommend that cytotoxic therapy be added. In 2001, Lasak et al. (37) noted that 59% of patients with AISNHL demonstrated a positive response to this regimen with steroid-only responders demonstrating a greater improvement in pure-tone average (14.8 vs. 4.5 dB) whereas cytotoxic-agent responders demonstrated improvements in speech discrimination scores (26.2 vs. 6.9%). Methotrexate (MTX) 7.5–15 mg po weekly is often the first cytotoxic medication chosen due to its lower incidence of side effects when compared with other agents. While on MTX, patients may be placed on folic acid and must have baseline laboratory tests before initiating therapy. Monitoring of their complete blood count as well as renal and hepatic function must be continued at regular intervals throughout the entire course of treatment. Cyclophosphamide is often chosen as a second-line agent, and patients should be kept well hydrated to help prevent hemorrhagic cystitis when receiving this drug. Traditionally, cyclophosphamide has been given orally on a daily basis. However, intravenous pulsed therapy has been used with excellent results and far fewer side effects.

Other unusual causes of SSNHL are the result of immune-regulated conditions, including multiple sclerosis and neurosarcoidosis. Ozunlu et al. (42) described a case of sudden hearing loss that was the presenting symptom in a patient with multiple sclerosis. The patient improved with steroid therapy but never reversed her initial ABR findings of absent waves II–V. Sarcoidosis is a chronic, idiopathic granulomatous disease with frequent pulmonary, ocular, and lymphatic system manifestations. Neurosarcoidosis affects 1%–5% of all cases of sarcoidosis patients and rarely results in cranial neuropathies. Souliere et al. (43) presented two cases of steroid responsive neurosarcoidosis presenting with SSNHL. Neurosarcoidosis rarely occurs in the absence of systemic symptoms, and a review of the literature demonstrates that eighth nerve neurosarcoidosis invariably presents with ocular symptoms. The treatment for these patients involves high-dose steroids with an extended taper.

## TRAUMATIC

Traumatic disruption of the integrity of the otic capsule is a well-accepted etiology for sudden hearing loss. The mechanism of trauma may be obvious, as in the event of temporal bone fracture with resulting disruption of the cochlea or its nerve. However, trauma may also result from relatively innocuous activities associated with straining or by exposure to a loud noise.

Cochlear membrane breaks may occur in either an intracochlear fashion or via fistulization through the round or oval windows. For this reason, it is important that the otolaryngologist inquire about the events surrounding the onset of hearing loss. Certain patients are theoretically at increased risk for a traumatic etiology for their hearing loss including those with prior ear surgery or those with inner ear anomalies. Hughes et al. (44) assert that in order to entertain the diagnosis of perilymph fistula (PLF), the hearing loss must be "closely associated with a well-defined event of trauma, exertion, or barotrauma." Although this assertion is not accepted universally, the diagnosis of perilymphatic fistula can be made with certainty only following the intraoperative observation of perilymph leakage.

A CT scan of the temporal bones should be obtained to rule out mastoid pathology or abnormalities. These abnormalities may be obvious, as in the event of temporal bone fracture or more subtle as in the event of a patent cochlear aqueduct. Treatment for endolymphatic hydrops with membrane rupture includes complete bedrest with a low-sodium diet and diuretics. Management of perilymphatic fistula is controversial. However, with an adequate history, exploration with packing of the round and oval windows can be justified.

## NEOPLASTIC

Cushing (45) first described a case of sudden hearing loss as the presenting complaint in a patient with vestibular schwannoma (VS) in 1917. The typical presentation of a VS is progressive, asymmetric hearing loss. Traditionally, the rate of sudden hearing loss in VS has been reported to be between 5% and 20%. However, one outlying study reported VS in 19 of 40 patients presenting with sudden deafness (46). Berenholz et al. (47) listed seven theories regarding the pathogenesis of SSNHL in VS. Of these, nerve compression and vascular compression by the tumor are the two theories that continue to receive the most attention.

Most otologists would agree that VS should be ruled out in patients presenting with sudden hearing loss. Gadolinium-enhanced MRI is the study of choice to detect VS owing to its sensitivity—detecting tumors as small as 2 mm—and a specificity which allows it to differentiate VSs from other cerebellopontine angle (CPA) lesions.

Reversal of SSNHL occurring both spontaneously and with steroid therapy has been described. Friedman et al. (48) presented a retrospective study examining the effect of a history of sudden hearing loss on hearing preservation in 45 patients undergoing surgery at the House Ear Clinic between 1990 and 1998. They concluded that patients with SSNHL who remain hearing preservation candidates have the same rate of hearing preservation when compared with those demonstrating a pattern of progressive hearing loss. Negative prognostic factors included preoperative tinnitus, advanced age, longer auditory brainstem response (ABR) latencies, and poorer speech discrimination scores.

Meiteles et al. (49) presented an interesting case of sudden hearing loss in an only hearing ear. The patient initially failed high-dose steroid therapy and underwent subsequent emergency decompression and resection of his VS with a rapid improvement and restoration of hearing. The authors concluded that a therapeutic window may exist during which sudden hearing loss caused by intracanalicular tumors is reversible and that in select patients emergency resection and nerve decompression should be considered.

Gadolinium-enhanced MRI obtained at the onset of symptoms should include the brainstem and cerebral hemispheres, in addition to the internal auditory canals. In this way, abnormalities such as demyelinating plaques and focal areas of ischemia can be evaluated. ABR may be performed for site-of-lesion information, in addition to electroencephalography and single-photon emission computed tomography (SPECT) scan to evaluate for any electrophysiological, metabolic, or vascular disturbances not picked up with other forms of imaging. In addition, a consultation with a neurologist is beneficial for comprehensive evaluation.

## TOXIC

Ototoxicity as a result of exposure to certain medications is a well-accepted mechanism of hearing loss, both progressive and sudden. Aminoglycosides and loop diuretics are the most commonly cited medications and produce irreversible hearing loss whereas salicylates can cause reversible hearing loss.

Every patient presenting with hearing loss should be questioned about all medications and exposure to environmental toxins. Those agents known to cause hearing loss should be stopped immediately, and hearing change should be monitored closely.

## METABOLIC

Electrolyte and hormonal imbalance may play a role in SSNHL as it has been reported in association with conditions such as hyperlipidemia, hypothyroidism, diabetes mellitus, and pregnancy (13, 16, 30, 35, 50). Because of the low incidence of SSNHL, it is difficult to link sudden hearing loss with such conditions definitively. Nonetheless, a complete metabolic panel should be considered at the time of presentation, and many otologists recommend lipid profiling, thyroid function tests, and glucose testing.

## MANAGEMENT

The management of SSNHL is highly controversial due to the condition's uncertain etiology in the vast majority of cases. Techniques vary from simple observation to a comprehensive "shotgun" approach in which multiple treatment modalities are implemented simultaneously and then progressively withdrawn (16, 35).

Identification of a cause for the patient's hearing loss and subsequent directed therapy may improve the likelihood of hearing recovery. Therefore, every attempt should be made by the evaluating physician to find a causative factor. A thorough history is mandatory and should focus on the events surrounding the onset of hearing loss as well as any associated otologic symptoms including vertigo, tinnitus, or aural fullness. A history of trauma should be elucidated and should include questioning regarding episodes of increased straining associated with coughing, choking, or vomiting. Past medical history should be reviewed with particular attention paid to previous otologic disease and/or surgery as well as the presence of autoimmune disease in the patient or immediate family members. All medications should be listed, and ototoxic agents should be discontinued immediately.

Physical examination in patients with sudden hearing loss is often normal except for hearing assessment but should be performed with care in hopes of detecting abnormalities suggestive of a cause for the patient's symptoms. A thorough evaluation of the external auditory canal and tympanic membrane can help rule out obvious conditions such as cerumen impaction, herpes zoster, and otitis media. Decreased sensation of the lateral, posterosuperior aspect of the ear canal (i.e., Hitselberger's sign) can suggest the presence of a VS and should be documented. Tuning-fork evaluation helps to confirm laterality and to determine the nature of hearing loss, and it should correlate with audiologic findings. A comprehensive vestibular evaluation should be performed to determine the involvement of the vestibular system. Neurologic evaluation follows with complete cranial and peripheral nerve examination, and consultation with a neurologist may be an important adjunct.

Audiologic studies are an indispensable component of the work-up of sudden hearing loss. An audiogram with tympanometry must be performed immediately upon presentation to quantify the degree of hearing loss and to establish a reference point for the patient. Subsequent frequent audiometry should be performed to monitor changes in hearing and response to therapy. Electronystagmography can detect vestibular impairment and is helpful in quantifying the degree of impairment in the vestibulocochlear apparatus and differentiating conditions that usually involve only hearing (such as mumps) from those that may affect hearing and balance (such as VS and AISNHL).

Imaging of the temporal bone with computed tomography evaluates for bony disease and integrity of the otic capsule, whereas MRI and MRA of the IAC's, brainstem, and cerebral hemispheres evaluate for the presence of acoustic neuroma, skull base lesions, ischemia, demyelination, or other central pathology. A chest radiograph may also be ordered to rule out mediastinal lymphadenopathy associated with sarcoidosis.

A number of serologic tests are ordered by the senior author (R.T.S.) in nearly all cases to complete the evaluation. A complete blood count with differential can detect early changes associated with hematologic diseases such as leukemia and multiple myeloma. Chemistries can demonstrate electrolyte imbalances, and a lipid profile will often detect those at increased risk for vascular disease. Immune system involvement is evaluated with antigen-nonspecific serologic tests, acute phase reactants, Western blot immunoassay, and HLA typing for the markers B35, CW4, CW7, and DR4. The association of syphilis with hearing loss is well known and treponemal disease is evaluated with either FTA-ABS or MHA-TP tests. These tests should be run regardless of RPR or VDRL results. Lyme titers should be drawn according to geography and season. Acute and convalescent viral titers may be drawn for herpes simplex, herpes zoster, CMV, parainfluenza, mumps, measles, and adenovirus, and other tests for thyroid function and collagen vascular diseases also may be appropriate, in addition to coagulation studies discussed previously (see Vascular Etiology in Chapters 10 and 15).

The management of cause-specific SSNHL is relatively straightforward. Unfortunately, 85%–90% of cases remain idiopathic. The probable multifactorial pathogenesis of idiopathic SSNHL makes the management of this condition extremely difficult. While few advocate simple observation, those who do cite improvement in approximately two-thirds of patients who receive no intervention (51). Others, including the senior author (R.T.S.), advocate a multifaceted approach with therapy directed at all hypothesized etiologic factors in patients who fail to respond to an initial trial of steroid therapy and other oral medicines.

Most patients are directed to adhere to a low-sodium (2 gram) diet and are placed on diuretic therapy to address endolymphatic hydrops. Systemic steroid therapy is begun immediately at a dose of 1 mg/kg per day of prednisone to address inflammatory and autoimmune factors. This dose is tapered slowly after ~1 week, any change in hearing is noted, and adjustments in dose are made accordingly while following audiograms at least weekly. Patients in whom systemic steroids are contraindicated, or in who are unable to tolerate such therapy, may benefit from transtympanic steroid administration as outlined by Gianoli and Li (41). Because a high degree of suspicion surrounds viral involvement in SSNHL, we advocate immediate implementation of acyclovir 1–2 g divided five times daily for at least 10 days (52), or Valacyclovir 1 g bid for 10 days. Doxycycline is also started as prophylaxis against *Borrelia burgdorferi* while awaiting acute and convalescent Lyme titers.

To address possible vascular causes, a combination of vasodilators and volume expanders can be used to treat patients with SSNHL. During the initial outpatient trial, an oral vasodilator is used. Carbogen (5% carbon dioxide and 95% oxygen) inhalations have been demonstrated to increase partial pressure of arterial oxygen and increase perilymphatic oxygen tension (31). Carbogen therapy is administered as 10-min inhalations, 8 × daily for 3–7 days, and improvements in symptoms during treatment are noted. Diatrizoate meglumine (Hypaque) acts as a volume expander, although the exact mechanism in SSNHL is unknown. This agent, in addition to a continuous histamine infusion—at a rate that causes facial flushing—is used by the senior author to promote cochlear blood flow and helps eliminate vasospasm.

Despite earlier literature indicating that a "shotgun" approach to treatment is no better than spontaneous recovery (35), the experience of the senior author and numerous other otologists of recovery following the addition of each of the aforementioned agents has sometimes led to multiagent therapy in patients who have failed an outpatient steroid trial or have SSNHL in a better-hearing-ear to be comprehensive. Each agent is removed sequentially based upon subjective and objective responses. Adjustments in therapy are made based on hearing outcomes and side effects for the individual patient.

A study in 1984 outlined prognostic indicators for patients presenting with SSNHL (51). In 225 consecutive patients treated over 8 years, Byl reported 69% of patients had a meaningful improvement in hearing. Severity of initial hearing loss, severity of vertigo, and time from onset to initial visit were determined to be the most important factors in predicting hearing recovery. Also important, but more variable, were patient age, audiogram pattern, erythrocyte sedimentation rate, and the state of the opposite ear. Byl determined that extremes of age (> 60 or < 15) decreased the patient's chances of recovery by 50%. Patients with upsloping or mid-frequency losses were found to be more likely to recover hearing, as were those with an elevated ESR. Finally, a below-normal pure-tone average in the contralateral ear was found to be a negative predictor for recovery.

## CONCLUSION

SSNHL presents a diagnostic dilemma in the overwhelming majority of cases. The condition should be treated as an otologic emergency and efforts should be made by the evaluating physician to identify a cause for hearing loss. When no cause is demonstrated, the treatment remains controversial. Therefore, until a more complete understanding of SSNHL comes to fruition, we recommend a therapeutic regimen which is comprehensive in nature, and which addresses simultaneously all hypothesized etiologies of the disease.

## ACKNOWLEDGMENT

The authors are grateful to Drs. Jeffrey M. Zimmerman, Heidi Mandel, and Steven Mandel for their contributions to the chapter on this topic in the previous edition.

## REFERENCES

1. DeKleyn A. Sudden complete or partial loss of function of the octavus system in apparently normal persons. Acta Otolaryngol 1944; 32:407–429.
2. Jaffe BF. Clinical studies in sudden deafness. Adv Otorhinolaryngol 1973; 20:221–228.
3. Byl FM. 76 cases of presumed sudden hearing loss occurring in 1973: prognosis and incidence. Laryngoscope 1977; 87:817–825.
4. Jaffe BF, Maassab HF. Sudden deafness associated with adenovirus infection. New Engl J Med 1967; 276:1406–1409.
5. Mattox DE. Medical management of sudden sensorineural hearing loss. Otolaryngol Head Neck Surg 1980; 88:111–113.

6. Saeki N, Kitahara M. Assessment of prognosis in sudden deafness. Acta Otolaryngol Suppl 1994; 51:56–61.

7. Westmore GA, Pickard BH, Stem H. Isolation of mumps virus from the inner ear after sudden deafness. Br Med J 1979; 1:14–15.

8. Davis LE, James CG, Fiber F, McLauren LC. Cytomegalovirus infection from a human inner ear. Annals Otol Rhinol Laryngol 1979; 88:424–426.

9. Davis LE, Johnson RT. Experimental viral infections of the inner ear. I. Acute infections of the newborn hamster labyrinth. Lab Invest 1976; 34:349–356.

10. Koide J, Yanagita N, Hondo R, Kurata T. Serological and clinical study of herpes simplex virus infection in patients with sudden deafness. Acta Otolaryngol Suppl 1988; 456:21–26.

11. Wilson WR. The relationship of the herpesvirus family to sudden hearing loss: A prospective clinical study and literature review. Laryngoscope 1986; 96:870–877.

12. Wilson WR, Veltri RW, Laird N, Sprinkle PM. Viral and epidemiologic studies of idiopathic sudden hearing loss. Otolaryngol Head Neck Surg 1983; 91:653–658.

13. Schuknecht HF, Donovan ED. The pathology of idiopathic sudden sensorineural hearing loss. Arch Otorhinolaryngol 1986; 243:1–15.

14. Khetarpal U, Nadol JB, Glynn RJ. Idiopathic sudden sensorineural hearing loss and postnatal viral labyrinthitis: a statistical comparison of temporal bone findings. Ann Otol Rhinol Laryngol 1990; 99:969–976.

15. Lindsay J, Davey P, Ward P. Inner ear pathology in deafness due to mumps. Ann Otol Rhinol Laryngol 1960; 69:918.

16. Kuhn M, Heman-Ackah SE, Shaikh JA, Roehm PC. Sudden sensorineural hearing loss: a review of diagnosis, treatment, and prognosis. Trends Amplif 2011; 15(3):91–105.

17. Chern A, Famuyide AO, Moonis G, Lalwani AK. Bilateral sudden sensorineural hearing loss and intralabyrinthine hemorrhage in a patient with COVID-19. Otol Neurotol 2021;42(1):e10–e14.

18. Parrino D, Frosolini A, Toninato D, Matarazzo A, Marioni G, de Filippis C. Sudden hearing loss and vestibular disorders during and before COVID-19 pandemic: An audiology tertiary referral centre experience. Am J Otolaryngol 2022; 43(1):103241.

19. Chari DA, Parikh A, Kozin ED, Reed M, Jung DH. Impact of COVID-19 on presentation of sudden sensorineural hearing loss at a single institution. Otolaryngol Head Neck Surg 2021; 165(1):163–165.

20. McIntyre KM, Favre NM, Kuo CC, Carr MM. Systematic review of sensorineural hearing loss associated with COVID-19 infection. Cureus 2021; 13(11)e19757.

21. Men X, Wang J, Sun J, Zhu K. COVID-19 and sudden sensorineural hearing loss: A systematic review. Front Neurol 2022; 13:883749.

22. Frosolini A, Franz L, Daloiso A, de Fillippis C, Marioni G. Sudden sensorineural hearing loss in the COVID-19 pandemic: A systematic review and meta-analysis. Diagnostics 2022:12(12):3139.

23. Yoon TH, Paparella MM, Scharchem PA. Systemic vasculitis: temporal bone histopathologic study. Laryngoscope 1990; 99:600–609.

24. Suga F, Preston J, Snow JB. Experimental microembolization of cochlear vessels. Arch Otolaryngol 1970; 92:213–220.

25. Kimura R, Perlman HB. Arterial obstruction of the labyrinth. Part I. Cochlear changes. Ann Otol Rhinol Laryngol 1958; 67:5–40.

26. Kim JS, Lopez I, DiPatre PL, Liu F, Ishiyama A, Baloh RW. Internal auditory artery infarction: clinicopathologic correlation. Neurology 1999; 52:40–44.

27. Arenberg IK, Allen GN, Deboer A. Sudden hearing loss immediately following cardiopulmonary bypass. J Laryngol Otol 1972; 86:73.

28. O'Keeffe LJ, Maw AR. Sudden total deafness in sickle cell disease. J Laryngol Otol 1991; 105:653–655.

29. Oussoren FK, Schermer TR, van Leeuwen RB, Bruintjes TD. Cardiovascular risk factors, cerebral small vessel disease, and subsequent risk of stroke in patients with idiopathic sudden sensorineural hearing loss: systematic review and meta-analyses of the current literature. Audiol Neurootol 2023; 9:1–29.

30. Ullrich D, Aurbach G, Drobik C. A prospective study of hyperlipidemia as a pathogenic factor in sudden hearing loss. Eur Arch Otorhinolaryngol 1992; 249:273–276.

31. Fisch U. Management of sudden deafness. Otolaryngol Head Neck Surg 1983; 91:3–8.

32. Morimitsu T. New theory and therapy of sudden deafness. In: Shambaugh GE, Shea JJ, eds. Proceeding of the Shambaugh Fifth International Workshop on Middle Ear Microsurgery and Fluctuant Hearing Loss. Huntsville, AL, USA: Strode Publishers, Inc., 1977:312–421.

33. Emmett JR, Shea JJ. Diatrizoate meglumine (Hypaque) treatment for sudden hearing loss. Laryngoscope 1979;89:1229–1238.

34. Probst R, Tschopp K, Lüdin E, Kellerhals B, Podvinec M, Pfaltz CR. A randomized, double-blind, placebo-controlled study of dextran/pentoxifylline medication in acute acoustic trauma and sudden hearing loss. Acta Otolaryngol 1992; 112:435–443.

35. Wilkins SA, Mattox DE, Lyles A. Evaluation of a "shotgun" regimen for sudden hearing loss. Otolaryngol Head Neck Surg 1987; 97:474–480.

36. Harris JP, Fan JT, Keithley EM. Immunologic responses in experimental cytomegalovirus labyrinthitis. Am J Otol 1990; 11:304–308.

37. Lasak JM, Sataloff RT, Hawkshaw M, Carey TE, Lyons KM, Spiegel JR. Autoimmune inner ear disease: steroid and cytotoxic drug therapy. Ear Nose Throat J 2001; 80:808–822.

38. Bowman CA, Nelson RA. Human leukocytic antigens in autoimmune sensorineural hearing loss. Laryngoscope 1987; 97:7–9.

39. Harris JP, Sharp PA. Inner ear autoantibodies in patients with rapidly progressive sensorineural hearing loss. Laryngoscope 1990; 100:516–524.

40. Disher MJ, Ramakrishnan, Nair TS et al. Human autoantibodies and monoclonal antibody KHRI-3 bind to a phylogenetically conserved inner-ear-supporting cell antigen. Ann NY Acad Sci 1997; 830:253–265.

41. Gianoli GJ, Li JC. Transtympanic steroids for treatment of sudden hearing loss. Otolaryngol Head Neck Surg 2001; 125:142–146.

42. Ozunlu A, Mus N, Gulhan M. Multiple sclerosis: a cause of sudden hearing loss. Audiology 1998; 37:52–58.

43. Souliere CR, Kava CR, Barrs DM, Bell AF. Sudden hearing loss as the sole manifestation of neurosarcoidosis. Otolaryngol Head Neck Surg 1991; 105:376–381.

44. Hughes GB, Freedman MA, Haberkamp TJ, Guay ME. Sudden sensorineural hearing loss. Otolaryngol Clin North Am 1996; 29:393–405.

45. Cushing H. Tumors of the Nervus Acusticus and the Syndrome of the Cerebellopontine Angle. Philadelphia, PA: WB Saunders, 1917.

46. Chaimoff M, Nageris BI, Sulkes J, Spitzer T, Kalmanowitz M. Sudden hearing loss as a presenting symptom of acoustic neuroma. Am J Otolaryngol 1999; 20:157–160.

47. Berenholz LP, Eriksen C, Hirsh FA. Recovery from repeated sudden hearing loss with corticosteroid use in the presence of an acoustic neuroma. Ann Otol Rhinol Laryngol 1992; 101:827–831.

48. Friedman RA, Kesser BW, Slattery WH 3rd, Brackmann DE, Hitselberger WE. Hearing preservation in patients with vestibular schwannomas with sudden sensorineural hearing loss. Otolaryngol Head Neck Surg 2001; 125:544–551.

49. Meiteles LZ, Liu JK, Couldwell WT. Hearing restoration after resection of an intracanalicular vestibular schwannoma: a role for emergency surgery? Case report and review of the literature. J Neurosurg 2002; 96:796–800.

50. Wilson WR, Laird N, Young FM, Soeldner JS, Kavesh DA, MacMeel JW. The relationship of idiopathic sudden hearing loss to diabetes mellitus. Laryngoscope 1982; 92:155–160.

51. Byl FM. Sudden hearing loss: eight years' experience and suggested prognostic table. Laryngoscope 1984; 94:647–661.

52. Tucci DL, Fanner JC, Kitch RD, Witsell DL. Treatment of sudden sensorineural hearing loss with systemic steroids and valacyclovir. Otol Neurotol 2002; 23:301–308.

# 14

# Mixed, central, and functional hearing loss

ROBERT THAYER SATALOFF AND PAMELA C. ROEHM

## MIXED HEARING LOSS

Whenever the hearing loss of a patient includes a mixture of both conductive and sensorineural characteristics, he/she is said to have a mixed hearing loss. The hearing deficiency may have started originally as a conductive failure, such as otosclerosis, and later developed a superimposed sensorineural component, or the difficulty may have been sensorineural in the beginning, such as presbycusis, and a conductive defect, perhaps resulting from middle ear infection, may have developed subsequently. In some cases, the conductive and the sensorineural elements may have started simultaneously, as in a severe head injury affecting both the inner ear and the middle ear.

In clinical practice, most cases with an original sensorineural etiology remain in that classification without an added conductive element. In contrast, most cases that start as conductive hearing impairment later develop some sensorineural involvement. Familiar examples are otosclerosis with presbycusis or cochlear otosclerosis and chronic otitis media with labyrinthitis.

## SENSORINEURAL INVOLVEMENT

Otosclerosis was at one time thought to retain its purely conductive character for years; today, it is recognized that this condition develops sensorineural impairment in the same cases. **Figures 9.5** and **14.1** show examples of sensorineural features in otosclerosis.

Similar evidence of sensorineural involvement often is seen in chronic otitis media. According to one hypothesis, some toxic inflammatory metabolites produce a cochleitis or labyrinthitis (**Figure 14.2**).

Mixed hearing loss is becoming more common also in otosclerosis after stapedectomy. The sensorineural deficit may be caused by penetration of the oval window with exposure of the perilymph. Despite meticulous surgical care, the inner ear also can be traumatized readily and made more susceptible to infection by this procedure. In surgical trauma to the inner ear, high-frequency hearing loss often falls below the preoperative level, and the patient may complain of reduced discrimination though the pure-tone threshold is improved. Other symptoms suggestive of sensory damage, such as recruitment, distortion, and a lower threshold of discomfort, may be noted.

**Figure 14.3** illustrates an important aspect of mixed hearing loss. The patient attributed his hearing loss to wax in his ears, but when the wax was removed, we noted an underlying sensorineural hearing loss of which the patient had not been aware. This example serves as a warning to physicians to avoid assuring any patient that his/her

DOI: 10.1201/b23379-14

**JOSEPH SATALOFF, M.D.**
**ROBERT THAYER SATALOFF, M.D.**
1721 PINE STREET     PHILADELPHIA, PA 19103

NAME _____

| DATE | RIGHT EAR AIR CONDUCTION | | | | | | | LEFT EAR AIR CONDUCTION | | | | | |
|---|---|---|---|---|---|---|---|---|---|---|---|---|---|
| | 250 | 500 | 1000 | 2000 | 4000 | 8000 | | 250 | 500 | 1000 | 2000 | 4000 | 8000 |
| | 70 | 80 | 70 | 75 | 90 | NR | PRE-OP. | | | | | | |
| | 30 | 35 | 45 | 45 | 65 | 70 | POST-OP. | | | | | | |
| | | | | | | | | | | | | | |

| | RIGHT EAR BONE CONDUCTION | | | | | | | LEFT EAR BONE CONDUCTION | | | | | |
|---|---|---|---|---|---|---|---|---|---|---|---|---|---|
| | NR | 50 | 50 | 60 | NR | | PRE-OP. | | | | | | |
| | 30 | 30 | 35 | 40 | NR | | POST-OP. | | | | | | |

**SPEECH RECEPTION: Right _____ Left _____**          **DISCRIMINATION: Right _____ Left _____**

Figure 14.1 *History:* A 67-year-old man with insidious deafness for 25 years. No tinnitus or vertigo. Wears a hearing aid on the right ear. *Otologic:* Normal. Complete stapes fixation confirmed at surgery. *Audiologic:* Bilateral reduced air and bone conduction thresholds with some air–bone gap in the right ear. The left ear was not as severely involved as the right but did not exhibit any air–bone gap. Tuning-fork tests showed bone conduction better than air in the right, with lateralization to the right ear. The tuning fork sounded louder on the teeth than on the mastoid. *Classification:* Mixed hearing loss. *Diagnosis:* Otosclerosis with secondary sensorineural involvement. *Aids to diagnosis:* The presence of an air–bone gap, good tuning-fork responses, especially by teeth, and satisfactory hearing aid usage in conjunction with negative otoscopic findings are important in making the diagnosis. In this case, the air–bone gap was closed. The apparent improvement in postoperative bone conduction is seen commonly, but it does not mean that the sensorineural hearing loss has improved.

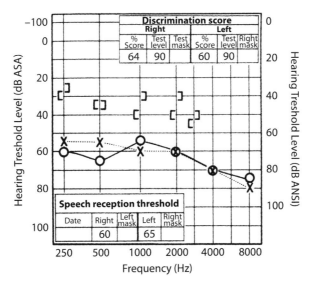

Figure 14.2 *History.* A 60-year-old man with bilateral chronic otorrhea for 40 years. Insidious hearing loss for many years, which is now stable. No tinnitus or vertigo. *Otologic:* Putrid discharge with evidence of cholesteatoma. *Audiologic:* Moderate-to-severe bilateral flat loss. Bone conduction is reduced at all frequencies, but a 20- to 30-dB air–bone gap remains. Discrimination is reduced bilaterally. *Classification:* Mixed hearing loss. *Diagnosis:* Chronic otitis media with neural or cochlear involvement.

hearing loss can be corrected merely by removing cerumen because mixed hearing loss may be found subsequently.

## EVALUATING CONDUCTIVE AND SENSORINEURAL COMPONENTS

On the other hand, pure conductive hearing loss may be misdiagnosed as mixed hearing loss because the high frequencies and the bone conduction are somewhat reduced.

In the case cited, hearing returned to normal when the fluid was removed from the middle ear; actually, there was no sensorineural damage (see **Figure 9.20**). Whenever there is any possibility of fluid in the middle ear, a diagnostic myringotomy should be considered to avoid an erroneous diagnosis of sensorineural hearing loss. A high-frequency hearing loss with reduced bone conduction may create a mistaken impression on sensorineural damage.

The bone conduction test as now performed is not a completely reliable measure of sensorineural hearing thresholds. Excessive reliance on this test may mislead the physician. **Figure 14.4** illustrates a case in which the bone conduction was almost undetectable audiometrically with a vibrating tuning fork on the patient's mastoid bone or forehead. Yet, when the instrument was placed directly on the patient's teeth, a good bone conduction response was obtained. This was a case of mixed hearing loss followed by a satisfactory surgical result.

In every case of mixed hearing loss, one should determine how much of the deficit is conductive and how much is sensorineural. The prognosis depends largely on this estimate. For instance, a patient's

JOSEPH SATALOFF, M.D.
ROBERT THAYER SATALOFF, M.D.
1721 PINE STREET     PHILADELPHIA, PA 19103

HEARING RECORD

NAME                                                                                          AGE

### AIR CONDUCTION

| | | | RIGHT | | | | | | | LEFT | | | | | |
|------|------|-------------|-----|-----|------|------|------|------|---------------|-----|-----|------|------|------|------|-----|
| DATE | Exam | LEFT MASK | 250 | 500 | 1000 | 2000 | 4000 | 8000 | RIGHT MASK | 250 | 500 | 1000 | 2000 | 4000 | 8000 | AUD |
| | | | *IMPACTED CERUMEN* | | | | | | | *IMPACTED CERUMEN* | | | | | | |
| | | | 25 | 30 | 35 | 45 | 50 | 50 | | 25 | 30 | 35 | 45 | 55 | 55 | |
| | | | *CERUMEN REMOVED* | | | | | | | *CERUMEN REMOVED* | | | | | | |
| | | | 5 | 10 | 15 | 30 | 50 | 50 | | 5 | 10 | 15 | 30 | 50 | 55 | |

### BONE CONDUCTION

| | | | RIGHT | | | | | | | LEFT | | | | | |
|------|------|-------------|-----|-----|------|------|------|--|---------------|-----|-----|------|------|------|-----|
| DATE | Exam | LEFT MASK | 250 | 500 | 1000 | 2000 | 4000 | | RIGHT MASK | 250 | 500 | 1000 | 2000 | 4000 | AUD |
| | | | 5 | 5 | 10 | 25 | 30 | | | 5 | 10 | 15 | 30 | 50 | |

Figure 14.3 *History:* A 45-year-old man with fullness in both ears and hearing loss for one week. No tinnitus or vertigo. No history of ear infections. He wanted the wax removed to restore his hearing. *Otologic:* Bilateral impacted cerumen. Removed, and eardrums normal. *Audiologic:* Bilateral reduced air conduction thresholds with greater loss in high frequencies. No bone thresholds were obtained before removal of cerumen, but tuning-fork tests showed bone better than air, bilaterally. After cerumen was removed, air conduction thresholds improved, but a high-frequency loss remained. Bone conduction thresholds approximated the air conduction thresholds. Tuning-fork tests showed air better than bone after removal of wax. *Classification:* Mixed hearing loss before removal of cerumen. Sensorineural loss after removal of cerumen. *Diagnosis:* Impacted cerumen with progressive nerve deafness. *Aids to diagnosis:* It is always advisable to do audiometric studies before and after removing impacted cerumen and before reaching a diagnosis.

JOSEPH SATALOFF, M.D.
ROBERT THAYER SATALOFF, M.D.
1721 PINE STREET    PHILADELPHIA, PA 19103

**HEARING RECORD**

NAME

AGE

| | | | AIR CONDUCTION | | | | | | | | | | | | | |
|---|---|---|---|---|---|---|---|---|---|---|---|---|---|---|---|---|
| | | | RIGHT | | | | | | LEFT | | | | | | | |
| DATE | Exam | LEFT MASK | 250 | 500 | 1000 | 2000 | 4000 | 8000 | RIGHT MASK | 250 | 500 | 1000 | 2000 | 4000 | 8000 | AUD |
| 1ST TEST | | | 80 | 95 | NR | NR | NR | NR | | 75 | 75 | 85 | 95 | 95 | NR | |
| 2 mos. | | | 40 | 45 | 65 | 70 | 75 | NR | | | | | | | | |
| 1 YR. | | | | | | | | | | 45 | 55 | 65 | 65 | 75 | NR | |
| | | | | | | | | | | | | | | | | |
| | | | | | | | | | | | | | | | | |
| | | | | | | | | | | | | | | | | |
| | | | | | | | | | | | | | | | | |
| | | | | | | | | | | | | | | | | |

Figure 14.4 *History:* A 62-year-old woman with severe deafness. Using a powerful aid for many years. Voice is normal. No tinnitus or vertigo. Several aunts also use hearing aids. *Otologic:* Normal. *Audiologic:* Bone conduction is better than air, but patient denied hearing the tuning fork on the mastoid or the forehead but heard it fairly well on the teeth. *Classification:* Mixed hearing loss. *Diagnosis:* Otosclerosis with sensorineural hearing loss. *Comment:* Both oval windows were overgrown with otosclerosis which required drilling. Note the good hearing improvement in spite of poor response to tuning fork. The surgery was done only because she did well with a hearing aid and had a good air–bone gap. A 1-year interval was allowed between operations on the two ears.

chronic otitis media have resolved and leave a 65-dB hearing loss. The tentative conclusion that a tympanoplasty is likely to restore the patient's hearing must be revised when bone conduction and discrimination studies show substantial sensorineural involvement so that the chances of restoring hearing are poor. On the other hand, in some cases of otosclerosis with air conduction levels almost above the measurable limits of the audiometer, the prognosis for restoring hearing to the bone conduction hearing level by stapes surgery may be very good.

The best way to approximate the conductive and the sensorineural components of a hearing loss is to perform all possible tests for estimating the patient's sensorineural potential or "cochlear reserve." In addition to routine bone conduction, speech discrimination scores are essential. A good rule to follow is as follows: If the patient hears and discriminates well when speech is made louder, then the conductive element probably is a major cause of the hearing difficulty, and there is a good chance that surgery will improve the hearing. If, on the other hand, the patient does not understand any better with a hearing aid or when the voice is raised, then the outlook for improved hearing is not as favorable even if the conductive portion of the mixed hearing loss is corrected. For example, the patient described

in **Figure 14.4** heard reasonably well with a hearing aid in the right ear, though there seemed to be no useful residual hearing. Successful stapes surgery confirmed the preoperative evaluation. Because of the severe hearing loss in the right ear, it was not possible under office conditions to amplify speech sufficiently to test the patient's discrimination. However, the results with a hearing aid indicated fairly good discrimination. In another patient with mixed hearing loss and almost as much neural involvement, the discrimination was not good. Consequently, after a successful stapes mobilization, the hearing level was improved, but the discrimination was not helped, and so, that patient was not as pleased with the result.

## Range of conditions

Mixed hearing loss usually includes the following range of features: (a) visible pathology in the external ear canal or in the middle ear, associated with reduced bone conduction and other findings of sensorineural hearing loss; (b) normal otologic observations, somewhat reduced bone conduction, but a significant air–bone gap; (c) reduced speech discrimination, though usually of a mild degree, with improved discrimination as the intensity of speech is raised; and (d) unilateral hearing loss with the conductive element predominating and the tuning fork lateralizing to the more severely impaired ear. In such cases, there is always an air–bone gap.

## PROGNOSIS

In mixed hearing loss, the prognosis depends on the relative proportion of conductive and sensorineural pathology. If the sensorineural component is slight, the surgical prognosis is good, and under favorable circumstances, the hearing may approximate the level of the bone conduction. However, the discrimination is not improved much even after correction of the conductive defect.

## CENTRAL HEARING LOSS

For the purpose of this book, a hearing loss is classified as "central" if it is caused by a lesion that affects primarily the central nervous system from the auditory nuclei to the cortex. The process of verbal communication is complex. The auditory pathway consists of a series of transducers that repeatedly change the speech stimulus so that it can be handled effectively by the cortex. The eardrum and the ossicular chain modify the amplitude of the sound waves, and the cochlea analyzes these waves into fundamentals that then are reflected as impulses to the cortex. The chief function of the auditory cortex is to interpret and to integrate these impulses and to provide the listener with the exact meaningful information intended by the speaker or to permit the listener to react appropriately to the actual implication of the sound.

## REACTION TO TESTS IN DIAGNOSIS

It appears, then, that interference with the neural impulse pattern traveling up the central pathways to the cortex would manifest itself not so much by a lowering of the hearing threshold for pure tones as by reduced ability to interpret information. On the strength of this reasoning, otologic authorities have suggested various techniques to diagnose central hearing impairment. Since damage to the central auditory pathway causes little or no change in the pure-tone threshold, the tests are designed to measure more complex function. For example, one test involves filtering out the higher frequencies of certain speech samples and then comparing the ability of persons with normal hearing to understand such speech sequences with that of patients with central hearing loss. It has been found that when this test is given to patients with unilateral central hearing loss (due to a brain tumor, for example), the *opposite* ear, which presumably hears normally, may have much poorer discrimination than the ear of a person who has normal hearing. This means that in unilateral central hearing loss, the contralateral ear can be affected. A similar adverse effect is noted in the ear opposite the tumor when certain words are interrupted periodically or accelerated. Interestingly enough, the patient with central hearing impairment has no difficulty perceiving high-frequency sounds such as the letter *s* and *f* that are affected so characteristically in peripheral sensorineural lesions, but he/she has difficulty interpreting what is heard.

## CHARACTERISTIC FEATURES

The principal characteristics of central hearing loss are as follows: (a) hearing tests do not indicate peripheral hearing impairment; (b) the pure-tone threshold is relatively good compared with the ability of the patient to discriminate, and especially to interpret, what he/she hears; (c) the patient has difficulty interpreting complex information; (d) there is usually an accompanying shortened attention span due to other processing or memory problems, and other neurological findings; and (e) apart from unusual cases with unilateral vascular lesions or neoplasms, hearing loss of this type resembles a bilateral perceptive disorder without any evidence of recruitment.

Some authors include sensory aphasia in the classification of central hearing loss, but most otologists consider this condition to be beyond the scope of their specialty.

The prognosis for central hearing impairment is poor, but reeducation seems to offer a useful approach. There is no characteristic audiometric pattern, except that the disparity between the hearing level and the speech interpretation is quite marked.

Present knowledge of central hearing loss is rather meager. There can be extensive brain damage without apparent hearing abnormality. When symptoms do occur, they usually are associated with some general disease such as encephalitis (**Figure 14.5**), vascular accident, or neoplasm. Other causes include brain tumors and infections.

In certain cases, central hearing loss may mimic peripheral causes of deafness, including occupational deafness. This is particularly true of impairment associated with pathology in the cochlear nucleus. In particular, the spheroid cells of the superior ventral cochlear nucleus (SVCN) show an anatomical frequency gradient, low ventral to high dorsal (1, 2). For example, erythroblastosis typically causes hearing loss that centers around 3000–4000 Hz. This may be caused by injury to SVCN spheroid cells, the second-order neurons of the ascending auditory pathway, even in the presence of normal hair cells in the organ of Corti (2). Central pathology must be included in the differential diagnosis of the hearing loss producing a 4000-cycle dip on the audiogram.

**JOSEPH SATALOFF, M.D.**
**ROBERT THAYER SATALOFF, M.D.**
1721 PINE STREET    PHILADELPHIA, PA 19103

**HEARING RECORD**

NAME _____    AGE ___

### AIR CONDUCTION

| DATE | Exam | LEFT MASK | RIGHT 250 | 500 | 1000 | 2000 | 4000 | 8000 | RIGHT MASK | LEFT 250 | 500 | 1000 | 2000 | 4000 | 8000 | AUD |
|------|------|-----------|-----------|-----|------|------|------|------|-----------|----------|-----|------|------|------|------|-----|
| 1ST TEST | | | 55 | 55 | 50 | 35 | 25 | 25 | | 45 | 45 | 40 | 30 | 20 | 20 | |
| 2 YRS. | | | 60 | 45 | 50 | 20 | 20 | | | 20 | 25 | 0 | 15 | 15 | | |
| 3 YRS. | | | 50 | 40 | 45 | 15 | 20 | | | 35 | 30 | 10 | 10 | 15 | | |
| 5 YRS. | | | 35 | 25 | 45 | 15 | 15 | 15 | | 15 | 15 | 0 | 10 | 10 | 15 | |

### BONE CONDUCTION

| DATE | Exam | LEFT MASK | RIGHT 250 | 500 | 1000 | 2000 | 4000 | RIGHT MASK | LEFT 250 | 500 | 1000 | 2000 | 4000 | AUD |
|------|------|-----------|-----------|-----|------|------|------|-----------|----------|-----|------|------|------|-----|
| 1ST TEST | | | NR | 50 | 40 | 30 | 30 | | NR | 45 | 20 | 20 | 15 | |
| 2 YRS. | | | NR | 45 | 55 | 25 | 20 | | | 25 | 40 | 15 | 30 | 30 | |

### SPEECH RECEPTION

| DATE | RIGHT | LEFT MASK | LEFT | RIGHT MASK | FREE FIELD | MIC. |
|------|-------|-----------|------|-----------|------------|------|
| | | | | | | |

### DISCRIMINATION

| DATE | RIGHT % SCORE | TEST LEVEL | LIST | LEFT MASK | LEFT % SCORE | TEST LEVEL | LIST | RIGHT MASK | EXAM. |
|------|---------------|------------|------|-----------|--------------|------------|------|-----------|-------|
| 1ST TEST | 18 | 95 | | 80 | 56 | 80 | | | – |
| 3 YRS. | 56 | 65 | | 60 | 40 | | | | – |

### HIGH FREQUENCY THRESHOLDS

| DATE | RIGHT 4000 | 8000 | 10000 | 12000 | 14000 | LEFT MASK | RIGHT MASK | LEFT 4000 | 8000 | 10000 | 12000 | 14000 |
|------|------------|------|-------|-------|-------|-----------|-----------|-----------|------|-------|-------|-------|
| | | | | | | | | | | | | |

| | RIGHT | WEBER | LEFT | | HEARING AID | | |
|---|-------|-------|------|---|-------------|---|---|
| | RINNE | SCHWABACH | | RINNE | SCHWABACH | DATE | MAKE | MODEL |
| | | | | | | RECEIVER | GAIN | EXAM. |
| | | | | | | EAR | DISCRIM | COUNC. |

REMARKS

Figure 14.5 *History.* At age 8, this patient had to be helped to walk because of muscular incoordination and vestibular imbalance resulting from varicella encephalitis at age 18 months. Her eyesight and walking were affected, and hearing loss started 3 days after the encephalitis was diagnosed. Her hearing gradually improved, and her speech is very good with only a slight voice defect. Prior to the initial visit, she had another encephalitis attack, and hearing was depressed but gradually improved. *Otologic:* Normal, and caloric test was normal. *Audiologic:* The very poor discrimination score in the right ear was confirmed on several subsequent studies. The improvement in discrimination scores is not uncommon in such cases. There was no tone decay, and recruitment was not significant. *Classification:* Central hearing loss. *Diagnosis:* Encephalitis.

## CENTRAL AUDITORY PROCESSING DISORDERS (CAPD)

CAPD are common, relatively minor abnormalities usually characterized by decreased understanding of speech in the presence of background noise. Most of the research in this area has concentrated on school-aged children where these difficulties are now often recognized first. Children with severe CAPD may appear immature in the classroom or may even seem to have a hearing handicap. The entity has become recognized only relatively recently. Consequently, many adults have this problem undiagnosed. Common complaints include inability to study or read in the presence of noise, slowing of reading speed caused by noise from vacuum cleaners or air conditioners, and suspicion by family members and friends that the patient has a hearing loss. If people talk to a person with CAPD while he or she is involved in auditory concentration such as listening to a television program, the person will often "not hear." However, if one gets the person's attention by calling his or her name before speaking, the first sentence will not be missed, and hearing is normal.

Various test batteries have been developed to assess specific areas of auditory behaviors. These include selective attention, auditory closure, rate of perception, and sequencing ability. If those tests are not readily available, testing speech discrimination at different levels can suggest this diagnosis, particularly in the setting of normal or near-normal patient hearing thresholds in quiet. Once a person has been diagnosed as having CAPD, treatment involves altering the listening environment to obtain the best possible signal-to-noise ratio as well as counseling the patient and family members. Good listening and visual behaviors are also stressed. Compensation for, and tolerance of, CAPD may diminish somewhat in the presence of advancing age or deteriorating hearing. Evaluation and treatment by a neuropsychologist can be extremely helpful, especially if other cognitive problems are present or suspected.

## FUNCTIONAL HEARING LOSS

Functional or psychogenic hearing loss is the customary diagnosis when there is no organic basis for the patient's apparent deafness. The inability to hear results entirely or mainly from psychological or emotional factors, and the peripheral hearing mechanism may be essentially normal. If there is some slight damage to the peripheral end-organ, the observed hearing loss is disproportionate to the organic lesion.

## CAUSE AND CHARACTERISTIC FEATURES

The basis for functional hearing loss in most patients is psychogenic, the product of emotional conflict. For example, anxiety is to the emotions what pain is in the physical realm. *Normal* anxiety is the natural reaction to an actual threat to one's welfare; it is recognized as such and recedes when the cause is removed or with the passage of time. In contrast, *neurotic* anxiety is an excessive reaction and may exist even in the absence of an external threat. Seldom is the true cause recognized consciously by the patient, and the anxiety persists beyond any recognizable need.

When anxiety is converted in part to a somatic symptom such as deafness, there generally is other evidence of emotional disturbance, such as insomnia. Tinnitus is a characteristic feature of "hysterical deafness," and patients often claim that the noise is unbearable. Hearing acuity usually varies, depending on the patient's emotional state at the time of testing. Patients may appear to be overly concerned about their auditory symptoms when in reality some or all of the tinnitus and the deafness are caused by anxiety, the origin of which lies elsewhere.

When all or nearly all of the anxiety is transferred to the ear, the case is one of true conversion or hysteria. The patient then usually is indifferent to the symptoms despite their apparent severity and may delay seeking medical advice until persuaded to do so by his/her associates. The patient underreacts emotionally; the reason is that he/she has partially solved an emotional conflict by permitting it to assume a somatic form. This illusion is incomplete, and careful scrutiny will show residual emotional symptoms. Psychiatric evaluation is indicated.

### A product of both military and civilian life

Functional hearing loss, then, can be an unconscious device by which the patient seeks to escape from an intolerable problem that he/she cannot face consciously. Hysterical blindness and paralysis are other examples of the same type of somatization or "conversion reaction." Often seen in military life during wartime, such situations occur also in civilian life. For example, the patient may go with his wife to consult the physician. The physician asks the patient about his problem, but before he can answer, his wife says, "He just doesn't hear me, doctor." When hearing tests indicate no hearing impairment, the physician talks to the patient alone. It then may become apparent (though the process of interrogation may take considerable time) that the patient subconsciously does not want to listen to his wife and therefore has developed a psychogenic hearing loss as a defense mechanism. Probably the classic example of psychogenic deafness is the young soldier in battle, too frightened to charge and yet ashamed of retreating while his/her buddies bravely go forward. In the absence of a rational way out, his/her unconscious mind conjures up the concept of deafness.

The chief statistics of functional hearing loss originate in the Armed Forces and the Veterans Administration hearing centers. Twenty-five percent of hearing-impaired patients are reported to have significant functional hearing losses. Strangely enough, a large percentage of such patients during World War II had little or no combat service. Disruption of family life and subjection to military discipline produced sufficient trauma to bring on psychogenic hearing loss.

The complexities of civilian society also have produced an abundance of emotional conflict and insecurity—sufficient to account for a complete spectrum of emotional disturbance, including psychogenic hearing loss. Too often, such cases escape medical attention or diagnosis.

## FUNCTIONAL OVERLAY

It is, of course, entirely possible for hearing loss of functional origin to be superimposed on true organic hearing impairment, in which case the term "functional overlay" is used. The problem then is to recognize the two components in the patient's hearing impairment.

The history and the otologic examination often provide important clues such as the unrealistic attempts of a patient to account for the difficulty. For example, the patient may claim that his/her hearing was excellent until a physician cleaned out his/her ears with such force that he/she suddenly went completely deaf. Another patient may carry on a normal conversation with the physician and hear everything said, while repeated hearing tests consistently suggest a severe deafness which is inconsistent with the patient's conversational accomplishments.

## DIAGNOSIS BY SPECIFIC FEATURES

The diagnosis of functional hearing loss should not be made solely by exclusion or merely because tests performed reveal no organic evidence of abnormality. There are specific features that characterize functional hearing impairment which should be required for the diagnosis.

A critical appraisal of routine hearing tests usually will justify a diagnosis of functional hearing loss if this is present. For an organic hearing loss, all tests must not only give fairly consistent results when they are repeated but they also must correlate with one another. It is a mistake to attribute well-marked discrepancies to individual variations. Several authors have suggested critical observations that should alert physicians to the possible presence of a functional hearing impairment. These leads have been found useful:

1. A medical history that could not possibly explain the patient's condition, such as the sudden onset of profound deafness following instillation of drops into the ears. Care must be taken to exclude all organic causes and not simply to disprove the patient's explanation.
2. Too spectacular an improvement with a hearing aid, especially when the patient has set the controls at minimal amplification, or a sudden disproportionate improvement in hearing after a simple procedure such as drum massage or insufflating the eustachian tube. In such cases, the power of suggestion rather than the mechanical procedure probably should receive the credit.
3. Large fluctuations in hearing acuity as determined by any single test.

The importance of repeated tests cannot be overemphasized. They are needed especially to establish basic hearing against which to evaluate the results of any treatment to be undertaken.

4. Inconsistency in the results of two or more tests. For example, the patient may hear everything when spoken to, and yet his/her audiogram may show a very severe hearing loss, such as 80 dB or more. In functional hearing loss of the psychogenic type, these inconsistencies usually are constant and repeatable, whereas in malingering they usually are inconstant, and the results of the tests vary considerably when they are repeated.

5. Inconsistency within a complete audiogram, particularly comparing pure-tone thresholds with speech tests of hearing. Speech reception thresholds should be within 7 dB of pure-tone averages of speech frequencies (500, 1000, and 2000 Hz). Speech discrimination should be less than 60%–70% for severe-profound or worse hearing thresholds. Patients with inorganic hearing loss are often unable to suppress their responses on speech testing and so will have speech reception thresholds or speech discrimination which is too good for the degree of hearing loss indicated by their pure-tone testing.

6. Positive Stenger testing. This test is based on the principle that if sounds are presented to both ears simultaneously, only the louder of the two sounds will be detected and the patient will indicate that they hear only in the ear that the sound is presented more loudly. For this test, the sound is presented louder than thresholds in the "good" ear and simultaneously presented lower than thresholds in the "bad" ear (3). Patients with organic unilateral hearing loss will acknowledge hearing the sound in their better ear during this test. Patients with unilateral nonorganic hearing loss will typically not acknowledge hearing these sounds at all, despite hearing them, because they recognize the signal in the "poor" ear as being higher than their previously tested hearing "threshold" in that ear. Patients with nonorganic hearing loss consciously or unconsciously feel that hearing those sounds will demonstrate that their unilateral hearing loss is fictitious.

7. In alleged complete deafness, the presence of cochlear nerve reflexes with loud noises indicates either malingering or hysteria. Psychogalvanic skin resistance tests, impedance audiometry, delayed auditory feedback tests, otoacoustic emissions testing, and evoked-response audiometry also are used to establish true hearing when subjective responses are unreliable or appear invalid.

Psychogenically induced hearing loss usually is a uniform flat-tone loss in all frequencies, suggestive of conductive hearing impairment. However, in these patients, the bone conduction is practically absent. In a patient with unilateral functional deafness, there may be complete absence of bone conduction on the side of the bad ear, though the good ear has normal acuity. Such a patient even may deny hearing shouting directed at the bad ear in spite of the good hearing in the opposite ear.

## AUDIOMETRIC PATTERNS IN FUNCTIONAL HEARING LOSS

There is no characteristic audiometric pattern in functional hearing loss, but the consistent inconsistencies serve to alert the physician. Usually, the hearing impairment is bilateral, and the bone conduction level is the same as the air conduction level. **Figure 14.6** shows a hearing loss due to a functional overlay. Here the patient has some organic hearing loss caused by otosclerosis, but she does not use her residual hearing effectively and actually hears much less than she should. This is not rare in otosclerosis.

## SHOULD THE PHYSICIAN UNDERTAKE PSYCHOTHERAPY?

The general practitioner or otologist must decide whether psychiatric involvement in patients with functional hearing loss is or is not too profound and complex to handle personally. The physician is more likely to assume the responsibility

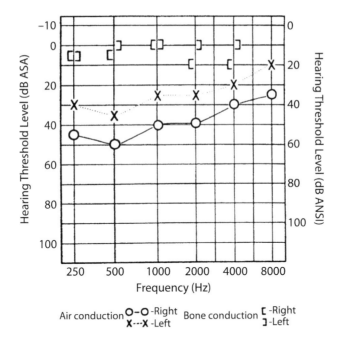

Air conduction O—O -Right   Bone conduction Ϲ -Right
           X---X -Left                    Ϡ -Left

Figure 14.6 *History:* A 34-year-old woman with otosclerosis and hearing loss for over 10 years. Mother and aunt have the same difficulty, but all refuse to use hearing aids. Patient reluctantly admits having some hearing loss. She often says, "What?" even when addressed loudly and habitually asks for repetition even though she evidently hears. She often repeats a question before answering and obviously has much better hearing than her responses indicate. The patient appears to be frustrated and emotionally disturbed and does not use her residual hearing effectively. Her associates have been led to believe that her hearing loss is worse than it actually is. This is a functional overlay on an organic otosclerosis. After positive suggestion, this patient acquired a hearing aid and is doing much better. She refuses ear surgery. *Abbreviations*: ANSI, American National Standards Institute; ASA, American Standards Association.

of limited psychotherapy if any of the following favorable factors are present: (a) the duration of the functional disturbance is short, and there is a history of previous stability, (b) the history shows that an important emotional crisis is now past, and (c) the physician is reasonably sure of his/her ability to win the patient's confidence and resolve the problem quickly. However, if the patient shows evidence of chronic or repeated emotional disturbances, psychiatric attention is essential, and it is advisable in nearly all patients with significant functional hearing loss.

## MALINGERING

Malingering is the deliberate fabrication of symptoms that the patient knows do not exist. The patient is motivated by the desire to seek some advantage: financial compensation, escape from military service, or evasion of responsibility for failure. Malingering has become increasingly common in school children, frequently in response to emotional disturbances resulting from home or school conflict.

Characteristically, the malingerer abandons the symptoms when he/she thinks he/she is no longer being observed. By contrast, a psychogenic patient with a functional hearing loss believes in the symptoms, and they interfere with pleasures as well as work.

A minor form of malingering, pleading a headache to forego a dull social affair, generally is tolerated as a "white lie." However, to fake a disability as severe as deafness transcends normal behavior.

JOSEPH SATALOFF, M.D.
ROBERT THAYER SATALOFF, M.D.
1721 PINE STREET     PHILADELPHIA, PA 19103

**HEARING RECORD**

NAME _____     AGE _____

**AIR CONDUCTION**

| | | RIGHT | | | | | | | | LEFT | | | | | | |
|---|---|---|---|---|---|---|---|---|---|---|---|---|---|---|---|---|
| DATE | Exam | LEFT MASK | 250 | 500 | 1000 | 2000 | 4000 | 8000 | RIGHT MASK | 250 | 500 | 1000 | 2000 | 4000 | 8000 | AUD |
| | | - | 25 | 15 | 15 | 20 | 30 | 35 | - | 45 | 50 | 55 | 55 | 60 | 75 | |
| | | | | | | | | | 80 | 65 | 70 | 75 | 70 | 70 | NR | |
| | | | | | | | | | - | 70 | 75 | 75 | 80 | 85 | NR | |
| RUDMOSE AUDIOMETRY | | 15 | 15 | 25 | 15 | 15 | 15 | - | 40 | 40 | 40 | 40 | 50 | 60 | |
| PGSR | | | | | | | | | - | 10 | 15 | 15 | 20 | 25 | 35 | |
| | | | | | | | | | | | | | | | | |
| | | | | | | | | | | | | | | | | |

**BONE CONDUCTION**

| | | RIGHT | | | | | | LEFT | | | | | | |
|---|---|---|---|---|---|---|---|---|---|---|---|---|---|---|
| DATE | Exam | LEFT MASK | 250 | 500 | 1000 | 2000 | 4000 | RIGHT MASK | 250 | 500 | 1000 | 2000 | 4000 | AUD |
| | | - | 15 | 20 | 25 | 25 | 25 | - | 45 | 55 | 55 | 45 | 45 | |
| | | | | | | | | 80 | NR | 55 | NR | NR | NR | |
| | | | | | | | | | | | | | | |
| | | | | | | | | | | | | | | |

Figure 14.7 *History:* A 37-year-old construction worker knocked to ground by a beam. No unconsciousness, but the left ear required sutures. Noted some hearing loss in left ear after accident, which has progressively worsened. Denies ever having tinnitus or vertigo. This is a medicolegal problem, and he is suing for compensation for deafness. *Otologic:* Normal. Normal caloric findings. *Audiologic:* Note varying and inconsistent hearing levels during repeated audiograms. It is difficult to determine how much of the hearing loss is organic and how much functional. Psychogalvanic skin resistance testing confirmed a marked functional overlay, with only a 15-dB loss in all frequencies. *Classification:* Functional hearing loss. *Etiology:* Malingering.

Unlike the individual who believes the symptoms are real, the malingerer who pretends deafness usually has no "pattern" in the alleged impairment. The hearing tests are replete with inconsistencies. When subjected to tests that the patient does not understand, for example, a malingerer suspects he/she may be uncovered by the doctor and his/her testing machine. He/she wishes to preserve the fabrication that he/she is deaf, but when he/she is asked whether a signal of a given strength is heard, he/she does not know when to say "yes" and when to say "no" and falters in his answers. Yesterday's audiogram may have shown a 70-dB hearing level for pure tones but a loss of only 10 dB for speech reception. When the tests are repeated, his/her answers may vary by as much as 30–40 dB.

If the patient claims he/she has one "good" and one "bad" ear, and the examiner obstructs the "good ear" with a finger, then shouts into it loudly enough to be heard easily by bone conduction alone, the malingerer claims he/she hears nothing.

When a patient malingers by exaggerating a true organic hearing loss, the task of learning the truth becomes more difficult. Such a problem may assume considerable importance in medicolegal cases, particularly if they involve compensation claims for occupational deafness. **Figures 14.7–14.11** show audiograms of several patients with false hearing impairments; the legends explain the motivating factors.

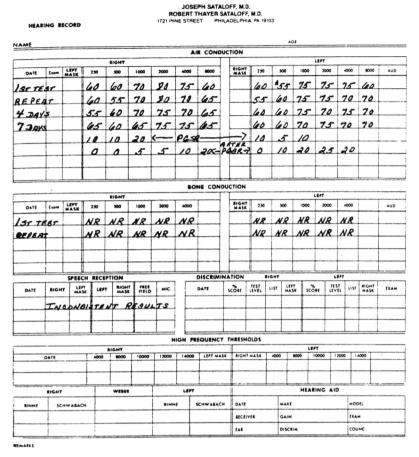

JOSEPH SATALOFF, M.D.
ROBERT THAYER SATALOFF, M.D.
1721 PINE STREET    PHILADELPHIA, PA 19103

HEARING RECORD

Figure 14.8 *History:* A 21-year-old woman with a series of emotional conflicts including breakup with her boyfriend, flunking out of college, and pending divorce of her parents. She now claims she cannot hear what goes on around her and for that reason flunked out of school. Her responses are generally delayed, and she seems to be "distant." *Otologic:* Normal. *Audiologic:* Even though she gave consistent pure-tone thresholds which showed a severe hearing loss, she often seemed able to hear soft voices behind her back. She denied hearing by bone conduction with a tuning fork. Psychogalvanic skin response (PGSR) showed normal hearing. *Classification:* Functional. *Etiology:* Emotional disturbance. Her hearing returned to normal after psychotherapy.

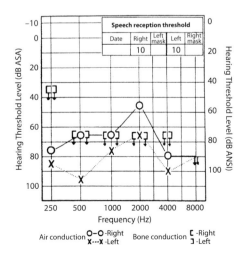

Figure 14.9 *History:* An 11-year-old girl who is doing poorly at school, and parents are concerned because she does not seem to hear them. No history of otologic disturbance, but an aunt uses a hearing aid. *Otologic:* Normal. *Audiologic:* In spite of an apparent severe bilateral hearing loss, the girl responds to speech at 10 dB. *Classification:* Functional. *Diagnosis:* Emotional conflict. This child was using a hearing loss device (on the basis of her aunt's handicap) to solve her school and home difficulties. She was helped by several discussions in the office. *Abbreviations:* ANSI, American National Standards Institute; ASA, American Standards Association.

JOSEPH SATALOFF, M.D.
ROBERT THAYER SATALOFF, M.D.
1721 PINE STREET     PHILADELPHIA, PA 19103

**HEARING RECORD**

NAME _____ AGE _____

### AIR CONDUCTION

| | | | RIGHT | | | | | | | LEFT | | | | | | |
|---|---|---|---|---|---|---|---|---|---|---|---|---|---|---|---|---|
| DATE | Exam | LEFT MASK | 250 | 500 | 1000 | 2000 | 4000 | 8000 | RIGHT MASK | 250 | 500 | 1000 | 2000 | 4000 | 8000 | AUD |
| | | | 50 | 45 | 45 | 35 | 30 | 35 | | 5 | 5 | 5 | 0 | 0 | 5 | |

### BONE CONDUCTION

| | | | RIGHT | | | | | | LEFT | | | | | |
|---|---|---|---|---|---|---|---|---|---|---|---|---|---|---|
| DATE | Exam | LEFT MASK | 250 | 500 | 1000 | 2000 | 4000 | RIGHT MASK | 250 | 500 | 1000 | 2000 | 4000 | AUD |
| | | | 50 | 45 | 55 | 45 | | | | | | | | |

### SPEECH RECEPTION

| DATE | RIGHT | LEFT MASK | LEFT | RIGHT MASK | FREE FIELD | MIC. |
|---|---|---|---|---|---|---|
| | | | | | | |

### DISCRIMINATION

| | RIGHT | | | LEFT | | | | |
|---|---|---|---|---|---|---|---|---|
| DATE | % SCORE | TEST LEVEL | LIST | LEFT MASK | % SCORE | TEST LEVEL | LIST | RIGHT MASK | EXAM. |
| | 88 | 40 | | | 90 | 5 | | | |

Figure 14.10 Audiogram of a 13-year-old boy with moderate sensorineural hearing loss on first evaluation. *History:* The boy was an in-patient on an adolescent medical service when he came to the attention of the author. He had been admitted with paralysis and anesthesia of his right leg. After full evaluation, he had been found to have conversion disorder. During the process of his work-up, he was found to have a right-sided hearing loss. Before his otologic evaluation, he had been evaluated by the neurology service and found to be normal except for a right-sided hearing loss. An ophthalmologist has found a mild refractive error and a peculiar, functional visual defect. Psychiatric consultation had confirmed the diagnosis of conversion reaction. He had had a normal lumbar puncture, electromyogram, electroencephalogram, skull series, internal auditory canal X-rays, CT scan, and multiple normal blood studies, including a full evaluation for collagen vascular disease. Otoscopic examination at the time of his admission had been reported to be normal. Audiometry revealed a right-sided sensorineural hearing loss with a 40-dB speech reception threshold and 88% speech discrimination score. Tympanometry was normal. However, he showed Metz recruitment and reflex decay at 500 Hz and 1000 Hz in the right ear. A brainstem evoked-response audiogram was performed and revealed a normal pattern in the left ear and no normal waves including wave 1 in the right ear. His primary physicians were considering scheduling him for myelogram and arteriogram at the time he was sent for otologic consultation. At the time of examination, the patient admitted to having noticed a hearing loss approximately 2 weeks earlier. He denied tinnitus. He had some fainting feeling, but no spinning, vertigo, or sensation of motion. He admitted to mild right otalgia within the last few days. He denied any prior history of ear disease, trauma to his ear, or any special concern about his ears. Except for his psychogenic paralysis and anesthesia, he appeared to be in good health. The physical examination was entirely normal except for a massive amount of tissue paper completely blocking the right ear canal and pressed against the eardrum. The child denied having put the tissue paper in his ear. After removal of the paper, his ear appeared to be normal except for a very mild external otitis. Repeated audiometric testing showed an inconsistent right sensorineural hearing loss. A Stenger test was performed and was positive. Hearing was estimated to be within the normal range. A repeat brainstem evoked-response audiogram was scheduled. At the time this was performed, the right ear was again found to be filled with tissue paper which he had inserted since his recent otoscopic examination. Without the foreign-body occlusion, he was found to have a normal evoked-response audiogram. *Summary:* This 13-year-old patient managed to document his functional hearing loss with an initially normal otoscopic examination, a right-sided sensorineural hearing loss, stapedius reflex decay, and an abnormal brainstem evoked-response audiogram. Only through repeated otoscopic examinations and careful special testing was his normal hearing documented before he was subjected to myelography.

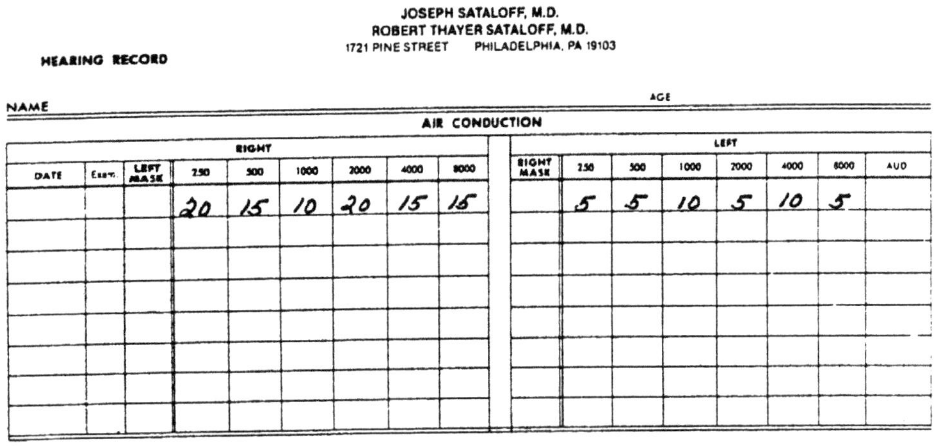

JOSEPH SATALOFF, M.D.
ROBERT THAYER SATALOFF, M.D.
1721 PINE STREET    PHILADELPHIA, PA 19103

HEARING RECORD

NAME _____    AGE ___

| | | | AIR CONDUCTION | | | | | | | | | | | | | |
|---|---|---|---|---|---|---|---|---|---|---|---|---|---|---|---|---|---|
| | | | RIGHT | | | | | | | | LEFT | | | | | | |
| DATE | Exam. | LEFT MASK | 250 | 500 | 1000 | 2000 | 4000 | 8000 | RIGHT MASK | 250 | 500 | 1000 | 2000 | 4000 | 8000 | AUD |
| | | | 20 | 15 | 10 | 20 | 15 | 15 | | 5 | 5 | 10 | 5 | 10 | 5 | |
| | | | | | | | | | | | | | | | | |
| | | | | | | | | | | | | | | | | |
| | | | | | | | | | | | | | | | | |
| | | | | | | | | | | | | | | | | |
| | | | | | | | | | | | | | | | | |
| | | | | | | | | | | | | | | | | |
| | | | | | | | | | | | | | | | | |

Figure 14.11 Audiogram of the 13-year-old boy after tissue paper was removed from right ear.

# REFERENCES

1. Dublin WB. The cochlear nuclei revisited. Otolaryngol Head Neck Surg 1982; 90:744–760.
2. Dublin WB. The cochlear nuclei—Pathology. Otolaryngol Head Neck Surg 1985; 93:447–462.
3. Kinstler DB, Phelna JG, Lavender TW. The Stenger and speech Stenger tests in functional hearing loss. Audiology 1972;11:187–193.

# 15

# Systemic causes of hearing loss

ROBERT THAYER SATALOFF, ALEXANDER J. BARNA, AND PAMELA C. ROEHM

## HEARING LOSS ASSOCIATED WITH NONHEREDITARY SYSTEMIC DISEASE

Although a great deal of attention has been paid to hereditary diseases associated with hearing loss, relatively little emphasis has been placed on recognizing the many nonhereditary diseases that are linked with deafness. Consequently, even some otolaryngologists may overlook important diagnostic information. Awareness of these illnesses is essential in distinguishing them from the many hereditary conditions they may mimic. Moreover, this knowledge often allows the physician to make important systemic diagnoses or to diagnose hearing loss early.

For example, the alert pediatrician always screens a child for hearing loss following an episode of meningitis. Similarly, internists and family practitioners should be aware of hearing problems in patients with syphilis, hypothyroidism, renal disease, and many other conditions. This chapter summarizes the more common and more serious systemic diseases associated with loss of hearing.

## Rh INCOMPATIBILITY

Differences in blood type between mother and child may produce deafness. If the father's blood type is Rh positive and the mother's is Rh negative, the fetus may carry the Rh factor on its blood cells. When fetal and maternal circulations mix, the mother will form antibodies directed at the Rh antigen on her child's red blood cells. The consequent immunologic attack on the infant's erythrocytes produces hemolysis and may occur in the inner ear to produce profound congenital deafness. The hearing loss is usually bilateral and most severe in the high frequencies (1). Genetically, the infant born of a woman's first pregnancy is not affected because the mixing of fetal and maternal blood that initiates the immunologic process usually occurs at the time of delivery of the first child. Subsequent Rh-positive children may then suffer severe hemolysis during fetal development because of the persistence of maternal antibodies to the Rh factor which recognize antigenic fetal red blood cells.

Modern developments have made this type of hearing loss preventable in most patients. Rh screening should be done routinely before parenthood. When Rh incompatibility exists, the mother should be treated in the immediate postpartum period with a drug such as RhoGAM (Kedrion Biopharma). This immunoglobulin effectively suppresses the formation of maternal antibodies to the Rh factor. The drug also should be given following miscarriage, abortion, or ectopic pregnancy because these events may initiate the immunologic mechanism by introducing a

DOI: 10.1201/b23379-15

small number of Rh-positive red blood cells into the maternal circulation.

## HYPOXIA

Oxygen deprivation in the neonatal period may produce sensorineural hearing loss. This connection may explain the increased incidence of deafness associated with traumatic, cyanotic, or premature birth, although the causal relationship has not been proven (2). Children who have suffered a complicated delivery should be screened.

## NEONATAL JAUNDICE

Chronic bilirubin encephalopathy/kernicterus has long been known to cause sensorineural hearing loss (3). The elevated bilirubin level first impacts the auditory brainstem center followed by the cochlear nerve (4). The audiogram usually reveals mild sensorineural hearing loss in the lower frequencies, gradually falling off to a severe hearing loss from 2000 Hz and above (**Figure 15.1**). Auditory neuropathy also can occur from hyperbilirubinemia causing abnormal processing of sound leading to disrupted sound localization and speech discrimination (4). Rh or ABO blood-group incompatibility between mother and child is one of the most common causes, although several others, such as hepatic and biliary dysfunction, can be responsible. Acute bilirubin encephalopathy is most likely to cause damage between 3 and 7 days of life, but damage may occur at older ages, even in adolescence (5). Regardless of the cause, hyperbilirubinemia should arouse suspicion of hearing loss. Hearing screening is recommended.

## RUBELLA

*German measles* is the classic example of *in utero* disease producing severe sensorineural hearing loss, although other viruses may produce similar deafness. Rubella is caused by an RNA virus which is present in the throat secretions, blood, and stool of infected persons. It probably enters the body by penetrating the upper respiratory mucosa (6). Congenital rubella is caused by transplacental transmission of the virus to the fetus. The disease is most common in children between 5 and 9 years of age, but many cases occur in younger children, adolescents, and young adults.

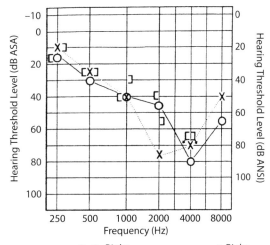

Air conduction O–O· Right   Bone conduction ⸤·Right
            X--X· Left                     ⸥·Left

Figure 15.1 Bilateral sloping sensorineural hearing loss with some recovery at 8000 Hz in a child with a history of neonatal jaundice but no history of noise exposure. There was no recruitment of abnormal tone decay. *Abbreviations*: ANSI, American National Standards Institute; ASA, American Standards Association.

The incubation time between exposure and appearance of the rash of rubella is from 14 to 21 days. Headache, fever, malaise, lymphadenopathy, and mild conjunctivitis may precede the rash by as much as a week, particularly in adults. The exanthem often is the first sign of the disease in children. Rubella may cause lymph node enlargement alone, without skin lesions, and it may be unrecognized until serologic studies are performed. Respiratory symptoms are not prominent. Forchheimer spots are small red lesions on the soft palate. These spots may be present but are not pathognomonic.

The rash of German measles is characterized by small, maculopapular, pink lesions, which are usually discrete. Sometimes they coalesce to form a diffuse erythematous exanthem. The rash starts on the forehead and face and spreads to the trunk and extremities. Usually, it is present for ~3 days and is preceded by tender lymphadenopathy which persists for several days after resolution of the rash. Postauricular and suboccipital nodes are most dramatically involved. Arthralgias and swelling of small joints may accompany the exanthematous period and may persist longer than other signs and symptoms. Purpura, hemorrhage, and encephalomyelitis also may occur.

Congenital rubella typically includes corneal clouding, chorioretinitis, cataracts, microphthalmia, microcephaly, intellectual impairment, patent ductus arteriosus, intraventricular septal defeat, pulmonic stenosis, and deafness. The *expanded rubella syndrome* described after the American epidemic of 1964 also includes thrombocytopenia, purpura, hepatosplenomegaly, interstitial pneumonia, metaphyseal bone lesions, and intrauterine growth delay. In the 1964 epidemic, ~10% of women with rubella discovered during the first trimester delivered infants with the rubella syndrome. However, asymptomatic maternal rubella may also produce the disease.

Rubella deafness is characterized by sensorineural hearing loss with a flat audiometric pattern. The severity of hearing loss may differ substantially between the two ears (7). Severe to profound deafness has been found in 4%–8% of children with histories of maternal rubella, and it has also been recognized following asymptomatic maternal infections (2). Histopathological studies reveal cochleosaccular aplasia and occasional middle ear anomalies (**Figure 15.2**).

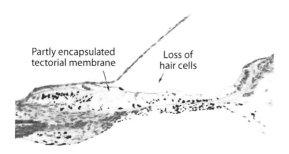

Figure 15.2 Maternal rubella producing temporal bone pathology. The organ of Corti is slightly flattened, and the hair cells are missing. The tectorial membrane is rounded, retracted into the inner sulcus, and partially encapsulated. (From Schuknecht [2], p. 180. Courtesy Harvard University Press.)

Rubella may be confused with infectious mononucleosis and viral disease, such as erythema infectiosum and enteroviral exanthems, which do not have the same teratogenic potential. The diagnosis of rubella may be confirmed by isolating viruses

or documenting changes in antibody titer. The antibodies generally are present by the second day of the exanthem, and titers rise for 2 or 3 weeks. The initial determination of antibody titer should be performed as soon after exposure as possible to help distinguish rising titers of acute infection from persistent elevation secondary to prior immunity. Lymphocytosis and atypical lymphocytes may be present but are nonspecific. In congenital rubella, serologic testing may revert to negative by the age of 3–4 years (6). Hence, a negative serologic test in an older child does not exclude a diagnosis of congenital rubella. Attenuated live viral vaccines have been given to young children in the United States since 1969. Although the attenuated virus can be detected for up to a month after immunization, transmission to other people is rare. The purpose of the vaccination program is to decrease the incidence of the disease, thereby decreasing the probability of pregnant women encountering the infection. Adult women who are shown to be susceptible to rubella by serologic testing may be vaccinated also. Arthralgias and joint swelling occur in ~25% of immunized adult women, sometimes beginning as long as 2 months after vaccination (6). Subclinical rubella may develop following immunization, but viremia and fetal infection generally do not ensue. However, the attenuated virus vaccine itself can produce fetal damage (6). Therefore, it must never be given to pregnant women or those who may become pregnant within 2 months following immunization.

Gamma globulin may be given to patients following exposure to the disease and may prevent clinical rubella. Despite this intervention, serologic titers may rise, and fetal infection still may occur (6, 8). Amniocentesis and culture of amniotic fluid may confirm fetal infection by recovery of the virus. However, negative cultures do not rule out infection. Because of the high incidence of birth defects, abortion should be considered seriously in any case of rubella found during the first 3–4 months of pregnancy, when infection is most likely to result in congenital anomalies.

## MUMPS

Mumps appears to be the most common cause for unilateral hearing loss in the United States (9). Interestingly, the vestibular system is only rarely affected by mumps. Because the disease often occurs in childhood and because children are so adaptable, deafness may not be recognized for many years if hearing in the unaffected ear is normal. The deafness is almost always total and unilateral. When these patients are tested, the ear that has normal hearing must be masked carefully to avoid crossover and the false impression that patients have residual hearing in the affected ear.

## RUBEOLA AND OTHER INFECTIONS

Measles (rubeola), cytomegalic inclusion disease, herpes, roseola, infectious mononucleosis, varicella, *mycoplasma* pneumonia, typhoid fever, scarlet fever, influenza, and other infections have also been associated with sensorineural hearing losses (10–12). The hearing loss may be severe or profound and may be sudden or gradually progressive. So far, only symptomatic and preventive therapy is available. These diseases may occur in adults, in children, and *in utero*. Particular effort should be made to protect pregnant mothers from exposure to these infectious agents. Measles and scarlet fever are also notorious for their destruction of the eardrum and middle ear.

## UPPER RESPIRATORY INFECTIONS AND FLU

The "common cold" often has an associated earache which may result from referred pain caused by pharyngeal inflammation or from otitis media. When the illness is bacterial, otalgia may be due to an otitis media secondary to pneumococcus, *Haemophilus* (especially, but not exclusively, in children), *Streptococcus*, or *Staphylococcus*. Anaerobic organisms also may be involved (13). In newborns, Gram-negative organisms such as *Escherichia coli* are common pathogens. When the illness is viral, viruses often can be cultured from middle ear fluid, although this is rarely necessary. Otitis media is especially common following epidemic influenza. In addition to the conductive hearing loss caused by otitis media, both bacterial and viral infections can lead to labyrinthitis with sensorineural hearing loss, tinnitus, and vertigo. One of the key symptoms of the labyrinthine involvement is a feeling of fullness in the ear; consequently, this symptom should not always be attributed to middle ear fluid.

## ZIKA VIRUS

Zika virus is another infectious disease that can lead to hearing loss after infection. Moderate-to-severe sensorineural hearing loss has been reported in cases of Zika infection (14). *In utero* infection also can occur and leads to a condition termed Congenital Zika Syndrome that is characterized by microcephaly, decreased brain tissue, retinal damage, clubfoot, and hypertonia. Microcephaly also may be a risk factor for the development of hearing loss, and more research is needed in this area to determine whether viral infection itself or resultant anatomic abnormalities lead to hearing loss. Audiologic assessment is warranted for any infant with known Zika virus exposure *in utero*.

## CORONAVIRUS DISEASE 2019 (COVID-19)

SARS-CoV-2 emerged as a novel infectious pathogen that led to widespread international concern as a global pandemic. Symptoms range from completely asymptomatic to mild upper respiratory tract infection symptoms to severe pneumonia and death. The virus can invade neurons and is known to cause sensory dysfunction such as anosmia and ageusia. There have been reports of patients with sudden sensorineural hearing loss, either unilateral or bilateral, after infection (15, 16). Patients also reported tinnitus. Currently treatment strategies include either systemic or intratympanic corticosteroid therapy within 2 weeks of symptoms beginning. Both treatments provide similar clinical benefits to treat the sudden sensorineural hearing loss. However, intratympanic administration resulted in fewer side effects of systemic corticosteroid use (17, 18). Further research is needed to understand the long-term sequalae of COVID-19 and its impact on otologic function.

## FUNGAL DISEASES

Fungal infections may invade the ear and produce conductive or even profound sensorineural hearing losses. This reaction is most common in immune-compromised or seriously ill patients, or in severe diabetics. Aspergillosis, candidiasis, blastomycosis, cryptococcosis, and other fungal infections occur. Mucormycosis is a particularly devastating infection. The ear involvement can occur with or without fungal meningitis.

## LASSA FEVER

Lassa fever is an acute febrile illness caused by infection with an arenavirus endemic in West Africa but reported in the United States (19, 20). Symptoms include malaise, weakness, arthralgia, and low back pain initially. In the ensuing several days, cough, sore throat, headache, epigastric pain, and chest discomfort are common. Vomiting, diarrhea, and fever usually occur by day 5. As the illness worsens, respiratory distress and bleeding, head and neck edema, pleural and pericardial effusions, shock, and death may be seen. Most patients begin recovering within ~10 days. Sudden sensorineural hearing loss occurs in approximately 33% of patients who recover (21). In an endemic area, 81% of local inhabitants with sudden deafness were found to have antibodies to Lassa virus (20).

## LYME DISEASE

Lyme disease is caused by *Borrelia burgdorferi*, a spirochete transmitted by *Ixodes* ticks. A red papule appears 3–20 days following a tick bite and expands to a large annular red lesion associated with fever, backache, malaise, stiff neck, arthritis (particularly in the knees), lymphadenopathy, a complete heart block (in 8%), and neurological abnormalities. Neurologic disorders associated with Lyme disease may include encephalitis, radiculoneuritis, and neuropathies of any cranial nerve. Unilateral and bilateral facial paralysis has been reported. Hearing loss may occur in association with Lyme disease (22, 23). Previous studies have shown an association between sudden sensorineural hearing loss and serological diagnosis of Lyme disease (24–26). Hearing loss has been identified in a patient with nonluetic interstitial keratitis, vestibuloauditory dysfunction, and bilateral recurrent facial paralysis previously thought to have been Cogan syndrome. Occasionally the audiovestibular manifestations of this infection can mimic Ménière's syndrome. Lyme should be considered in patients with hearing loss in combination with vertigo and/or facial paralysis. In rare cases, it may also cause retrocochlear hearing loss similar to that caused by acoustic neuroma due to expansive granulomatous lesions in the posterior cranial fossa (27). Testing patients with sudden sensorineural hearing loss for Lyme disease may be warranted, especially if patients were in an area that would increase their exposure and overall risk. Treatment includes antibiotics and steroids in selected cases.

## HIV/AIDS

The AIDS clinical syndrome is characterized by immunodeficiency, frequently complicated by opportunistic infection and neoplasia. AIDS-related diseases may affect every body system, including the head and neck. Patients with AIDS are particularly susceptible to infectious agents including viruses, bacteria, and fungi. *Pneumocystis jirovecii* infection has been found in the external and middle ear (28, 29). These infections are associated with mixed conductive and sensorineural hearing loss.

Viral infections of the head and neck are common in AIDS patients, particularly those caused by cytomegalovirus (CMV), Epstein–Barr virus (EBV), human papilloma virus (HPV), and herpes viruses, both simplex and zoster. All cranial nerves may be affected. Herpes zoster is particularly likely to involve the eighth cranial nerve, causing hearing loss, vertigo, and often severe pain and facial paresis or paralysis. HIV-associated syphilis may also be responsible for sensorineural hearing loss (30).

Hearing loss may be caused not only by the great number of opportunistic otologic infections associated with AIDS but also with drug-induced ototoxicity, central nervous system toxoplasmosis, and meningitis (especially that caused by tuberculosis or cryptococcus). The HIV-I virus itself is known to be neurotropic and may be itself capable of causing eighth nerve dysfunction including hearing loss.

## MENINGITIS

Meningitis is still a relatively common severe infection in adults and children. When it causes hearing loss in an adult, the patient usually reports it; however, it may go unrecognized in children. The incidence of associated deafness is impressively high: ~40% in fungal meningitis and between 6% and 35% in bacterial meningitis. Hearing loss is uncommon in aseptic (viral) meningitis (31, 32). The hearing loss is bilateral in ~80% of cases and partial in ~70%. Many patients suffering partial hearing loss recover to some extent. However, any patient with meningitis—especially a child—should have a hearing evaluation upon recovery.

## TUBERCULOSIS

Although tuberculosis affecting the ear is relatively uncommon today, it is still encountered. Most commonly, it occurs as a chronic ear infection resistant to treatment. Multiple perforations of the tympanic membrane and watery otorrhea are typical. Complications, such as meningitis and facial paralysis, may ensue (33). Usually, because the diagnosis is not suspected, patients undergo numerous courses of various antibiotics, and occasionally even surgery, without improvement. Ear disease may be the first sign of tuberculosis. Once the diagnosis is made (by acid-fast staining of aural drainage or granulation tissue, or appropriate culture), a careful evaluation for systemic involvement is required, and antituberculosis therapy should be instituted. Drug-resistant tuberculosis has continued to emerge and may require the use of ototoxic drugs such as aminoglycoside antibiotics that can cause hearing loss. Previous studies have shown that approximately 41% of patients with drug-resistant tuberculosis have hearing loss (34). Because of this finding, patients with tuberculosis should be started on aminoglycoside antibiotics only when absolutely necessary, and ototoxicity monitoring should be implemented to decrease the incidence and severity of hearing loss from use of these medications.

## SARCOIDOSIS

Sarcoidosis is a chronic inflammatory disease that leads to the formation of non-caseating granulomas. The condition most commonly affects young, female, black patients and is generally diagnosed by clinical suspicion, biopsy results showing non-caseating granulomas, and characteristic chest X-ray results (**Figure 15.3**) (35). It can occur in virtually any organ, however, including the ear (36). It has unknown etiology and may cause sensorineural hearing loss which may be sudden or fluctuant or both. A case of middle ear sarcoidosis has also been reported, with soft tissue masses found on CT and audiogram demonstrating mixed hearing loss (37). Sarcoidosis should be suspected, particularly in people who are known to have the systemic disease. It also must be in the differential in patients with chronic ear disease resistant to therapy, however, particularly when associated with uveitis, facial nerve paralysis, other neuropathy, diabetes insipidus, or meningitis.

## GRANULOMATOSIS WITH POLYANGIITIS (WEGENER'S GRANULOMATOSIS)

This disease is characterized by necrotizing vasculitis and granulomatous lesions of the nose, paranasal sinuses, lungs, and kidneys. It may occur as a granulomatous otitis resistant to conventional antibiotic therapy (38, 39). Bleeding from the ear has even been the initial symptom in some cases. Conductive hearing loss is associated with serous otitis media or middle ear granulomas, and sensorineural hearing loss may infrequently result from inner ear granulomas or vascular causes. Other unusual granulomatous diseases must also be considered in any case of persistent middle ear disease that does not respond as expected to routine therapy. The occurrence of *lethal midline granuloma* in the ear has also been reported but is quite unusual and may represent an incorrect diagnosis. Treatment is now available for both these previously fatal diseases: Wegener granulomatosis is currently best treated with immunosuppressants (particularly, corticosteroids and cyclophosphamide, with newer biologic agents available for treatment failures), and midline granuloma is responsive to orthovoltage irradiation.

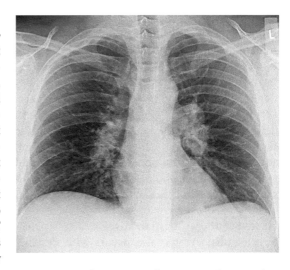

Figure 15.3 Chest X-ray of patient with sarcoidosis shows typical hilar adenopathy.

## VASCULITIS

*Rheumatoid arthritis, giant-cell arteritis, polyarteritis nodosa, leukocytoclastic vasculitis, Behçet's disease* (40, 41), and various other vasculitides have been associated with hearing loss. Sensorineural hearing loss is common, and middle ear fluid with conductive hearing loss also may occur. Occasionally, middle ear disease may precede other manifestations of a vasculitis syndrome, or it may persist following otherwise successful therapy with steroids or other medications. In patients with known systemic vasculitis and conductive hearing loss that does not respond to conventional therapy, exploratory tympanotomy and middle-ear biopsy may be indicated. This combination may be performed as a diagnostic measure early in the course of the disease if primary vasculitis is suspected. Early detection and prompt treatment are the mainstays of therapy.

In fact, any systemic disease which affects blood vessels adversely may be associated with hearing loss. Such entities include diabetes, atherosclerosis and other vascular diseases, and syphilis which are discussed elsewhere in this chapter as well as collagen vascular diseases including rheumatoid arthritis, lupus, and Sjögren disease.

## LANGHERHANS CELL HISTIOCYTOSIS

**Langerhans cell histiocytosis** is caused from uncontrolled proliferation of Langerhans cells and can be classified into the subtypes of: *Letterer–Siwe disease, Hand–Schüller–Christian disease,* and *eosinophilic granuloma.* These conditions are similar to congenital lipid-storage diseases such as *Gaucher disease* and *Neimann–Pick disease,* but there is no familial tendency, and the accumulation of lipid appears to be a secondary occurrence. *Letterer–Siwe disease* (**Figure 15.4**) occurs with destructive skeletal lesions (particularly in the skull), anemia, purpura, hepatosplenomegaly, and adenopathy. Temporal bone lesions may be found (42) but are usually not isolated lesions. Death supervenes generally before the age of 2.

**Hand–Schüller–Christian disease**, a less severe form of histiocytosis, also occurs with destructive skull lesions that often involve the temporal bone (**Figure 15.5**). Classically, diabetes insipidus, exophthalmos, and defects in the calvarium

are present. Apparent chronic ear infection with otorrhea is common, so mastoidectomy often is performed before the correct diagnosis is made (2, 43, 44). However, preferred treatment is radiation therapy rather than surgery in most cases. Early childhood death is not as prominent as it is with *Letterer–Siwe* disease, and the disease may even arise as late as the second or third decade of life. Delayed growth, anemia, hypogenitalism, and pathological fractures may be other features.

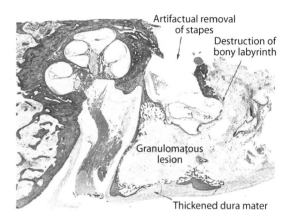

Figure 15.4 Letterer–Siwe disease with an extensive destructive lesion involving the posterior right temporal bone. The mastoid bone and the bony labyrinth surrounding the canal have been destroyed and replaced by viable vascular granulation tissue. The perilymphatic and endolymphatic spaces contain fibrinous precipitate. (From Schuknecht [2], p. 387. Courtesy Harvard University Press.)

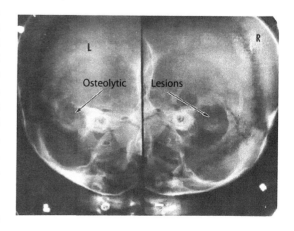

Figure 15.5 Bilateral destructive lesions of the mastoid in Hand–Schüller–Christian disease. (From Schuknecht [2], p. 387. Courtesy Harvard University Press.)

**Eosinophilic granuloma** is the mildest form of histiocytosis. It occurs with one or two lytic lesions of the skull, without systemic involvement. The disease usually becomes apparent in childhood or young adulthood, with 80% of patients > 30 years of age. The long bones, ribs, and vertebrae may be involved, rather than the skull, and localized pain is the most common symptom. A draining ear also may be a feature.

## HYPOPARATHYROIDISM

Hypoparathyroidism is one of the metabolic diseases related to calcium metabolism. The disease causes vitamin D deficiency and subsequent hypocalcemia. Long-standing untreated hypoparathyroidism appears to be associated with a high incidence of sensorineural hearing loss (33). Hearing loss is much less common in well-treated hypoparathyroidism. It is unclear whether hearing loss associated with hypoparathyroidism is reversible (45).

## ALLERGY

It has long been recognized that allergy can be associated with conductive hearing loss, especially serous otitis media in children. Eustachian-tube congestion and dysfunction may be the mechanism of action, but an allergic response within the middle ear mucosa itself may also play a role. More recently, an association between allergy and sensorineural hearing loss, particularly Ménière's syndrome, has been suggested (46).

## HYPERLIPOPROTEINEMIA

A significant percentage of patients with inner ear disease have been found to have hyperlipoproteinemia (47). Frequently, these patients have symptoms similar to those of Ménière's disease, particularly fluctuating sensorineural hearing loss in the low frequencies. However, the hearing loss may follow any sensorineural pattern. Hyperlipoproteinemia may be associated with dietary habits, pregnancy, and a number of diseases, including diabetes, hypothyroidism, myeloma, biliary obstruction, nephrotic syndrome, obesity, pancreatitis, and dysgammaglobulinemia. Oral contraceptives may cause a type 4 hyperlipoproteinemia pattern on lipoprotein electrophoresis. Vestibular abnormalities also may be prominent. High suspicion and early detection are essential not only to help manage otologic disease but also to prevent the development of atherosclerotic cardiovascular disease.

## HYPERTENSION

Hypertension is common and associated with numerous diseases. Several studies have suggested a correlation between noise-induced hearing loss and high blood pressure (48–66). Some studies have shown a high correlation between hypertension and noise exposure, others have shown no correlation. Some have suggested that noise exposure may increase stress and blood pressure (although it has not been shown that this response is abnormal or damaging), and others have suggested that the tendency toward hypertension is associated with greater risk of hearing impairment. Talbott et al. (67) has even suggested that noise-induced hearing loss may be a marker of hypertension in older noise-exposed populations. It is certainly recognized that some conditions such as hyperlipoproteinemia are associated with increased risks of both hypertension and hearing loss. At present, it appears that people with hypertension have a higher incidence of hearing loss (with or without noise exposure). There is no compelling evidence to indicate that these people are at greater risk of sustaining noise-induced hearing loss than others, nor that noise is capable of causing significant, prolonged hypertension in humans. Past studies have shown that hypertension is associated with high-frequency sensorineural hearing loss (68, 69). It is thought that hypertensive changes in the blood vessels of the cochlea may disrupt blood flow and lead to hearing loss in these patients (70, 71). Additional research in this area is still needed.

## SYPHILIS

At the present time, secondary syphilis is still a relatively rare cause of otologic problems. The classic forms of late (or tertiary) syphilitic disease, such as gumma formation, which may involve the ear and produce hearing loss, are also uncommon. However, *inner ear syphilis* may occur more frequently (72). It is a specialized form of tertiary syphilis. Diagnosis requires a fluorescent treponemal antibody (FTA)-absorption test, microhemagglutination assay-*Treponema palladium* (MHA-TP), or other sophisticated assay. RPR and VDRL tests are generally negative. Even following treatment for congenital syphilis or in the presence of uninfected cerebrospinal fluid, live spirochetes can be sequestered in the fluid within the ear (73, 74).

Spirochetes show unusual resistance to antibiotic therapy in the ear, in the anterior chamber of the eye, and in joint spaces. Of special importance in treatment rationale is their dividing time of 90 days (75), when compared with 33 hours in early syphilis.

Symptoms may be Ménière-like with fluctuating hearing loss, vertigo, and tinnitus, or there may be a sensorineural hearing loss of any pattern. As many as 6%–7% of adults with Ménière-like syndrome or with sensorineural hearing loss of unknown etiology may have this entity (46, 72) although the percentage is much lower in most practices. Rapidly progressive sensorineural hearing loss, worse on one side than the other and with poor discrimination, is particularly characteristic (**Figure 15.6**).

JOSEPH SATALOFF, M.D.
ROBERT THAYER SATALOFF, M.D.
1721 PINE STREET    PHILADELPHIA, PA 19103

**HEARING RECORD**

NAME _____    AGE _____

**AIR CONDUCTION**

| DATE | Exam | LEFT MASK | 250 | 500 | 1000 | 2000 | 4000 | 8000 | RIGHT MASK | 250 | 500 | 1000 | 2000 | 4000 | 8000 | AUD |
|------|------|-----------|-----|-----|------|------|------|------|------------|-----|-----|------|------|------|------|-----|
| 10/77 | | | 30 | 40 | 55 | 70 | 70 | 60 | | 10 | 30 | 55 | 70 | 70 | 50 | |
| 11/77 | | | 15 | 20 | 35 | 55 | 55 | 35 | | 15 | 20 | 45 | 65 | 55 | 50 | |
| 1/78 | | | 15 | 20 | 30 | 55 | 45 | 30 | | 10 | 20 | 20 | 65 | 60 | 50 | |
| 3/79 | | | 15 | 20 | 30 | 55 | 45 | 30 | | 10 | 15 | 20 | 55 | 55 | 50 | |

**BONE CONDUCTION**

| DATE | Exam | LEFT MASK | 250 | 500 | 1000 | 2000 | 4000 | | RIGHT MASK | 250 | 500 | 1000 | 2000 | 4000 | | AUD |
|------|------|-----------|-----|-----|------|------|------|--|------------|-----|-----|------|------|------|--|-----|
| 10/77 | | | 25 | 30 | 50 | ↓ | ↓ | | | 10 | 25 | 55 | 60 | ↓ | | |
| 11/77 | | | 15 | 15 | 35 | 55 | 50 | | | 10 | 20 | 45 | 55 | 55 | | |
| 3/79 | | | 15 | 20 | 30 | 55 | 40 | | | 10 | 10 | 20 | 55 | 50 | | |

| SPEECH RECEPTION | | | | | | | | DISCRIMINATION | RIGHT | | | | LEFT | | | |
|------|-------|-----------|------|------------|------------|-----|--|------|------------|------------|------|------------|------------|------------|------------|------|
| DATE | RIGHT | LEFT MASK | LEFT | RIGHT MASK | FREE FIELD | MIC | | DATE | % SCORE | TEST LEVEL | LIST | LEFT MASK | % SCORE | TEST LEVEL | LIST | RIGHT MASK | EXAM |
| 10/77 | 45 | | 30 | | | | | 10/77 | 74 | | | | 60 | | | | |
| 11/77 | 30 | | 25 | | | | | 11/77 | 84 | | | | 70 | | | | |
| 3/79 | 20 | | 20 | | | | | 3/79 | 96 | | | | 78 | | | | |

Figure 15.6 *History:* A 50-year-old man with ringing tinnitus and rapidly progressive hearing loss within the last 3 months, worse on the right. Sounds are muffled and "garbled." No history of noise exposure, infection, ototoxic drugs, or trauma. No family history of deafness. Firmly denied exposure to gonorrhea or syphilis. *Otologic:* Normal. *Audiologic:* Bilateral asymmetrical sensorineural hearing loss with somewhat depressed discrimination. Diplacusis present. Tone decay absent. *Laboratory:* VDRL negative, FTA-ABS, and MHA-TP strongly positive. Thyroid function tests, glucose-tolerance test, cholesterol, triglycerides, and internal auditory canal X-ray films normal. *Diagnosis:* Syphilitic hearing loss. *Course:* The patient was treated initially with steroids while waiting for the serological tests because of the rapidly progressive hearing loss and the strong suspicion of syphilis. Hearing improved within 3 weeks. Subsequently, antibiotics were started after the 11/77 audiogram. He received 2.4 million units of Bicillin i.m. weekly for 6 months, and steroids were tapered. His hearing remained good a year later. *Abbreviations:* FTA-ABS, Fluorescent treponemal antibody absorption; MHA-TP, Microhemagglutination assay-*Treponema palladium*.

Syphilis should be investigated in all cases of sudden deafness because it is one of the few causes that responds well to therapy, and, if it is untreated, deafness in the remaining ear may follow. As such, some otologists advocate the use of high-dose steroids while the results of the FTA-absorption test are pending.

Syphilis otopathology shows endolymphatic hydrops, as in Ménière's disease, and osteitis of the otic capsule (**Figure 15.7**) (2). Often, vestibular function is reduced bilaterally. The question of optimum treatment remains unanswered, although steroids and intensive antibiotic therapy are advocated most widely. However, it is clear that the usual antibiotic regimens for tertiary syphilis or neurosyphilis are not sufficient to eradicate infection of the inner ear. Prolonged treatment (a year or more) is recommended.

## HYPOTHYROIDISM

Congenital hypothyroidism typically presents asymptomatically at birth, making newborn screening vitally important so that prompt treatment can begin. If treatment is not started, clinical features including abnormally long persistence of neonatal jaundice, poor feeding, hoarse crying, lethargy, delayed development, short stature, coarse features with protruding tongue, broad at nose, sparse hair, dry skin, and delayed bone age can develop over the first 6 weeks of life. Auditory pathways require adequate levels of thyroid hormone for proper development of the inner ear (76). The auditory defect experienced in these children is generally a sensorineural hearing loss, although it may be mixed (77).

About 50% of adult patients with myxedema have hearing losses, which may be conductive, sensorineural, or mixed (78, 79). The sensorineural hearing loss is typified by a low discrimination score, which may respond well to thyroid therapy. There may not be any change in puretone threshold, although threshold improvement may occur as well. Patients with hypothyroidism may also develop other otologic symptoms, such as tinnitus (80). Hypothyroidism is found in up to 3% of patients with symptoms of Ménière's disease and is believed to produce endolymphatic hydrops (46). Thyroid replacement also appears to be effective in eliminating Ménière's symptoms in patients with this etiology. Pendred syndrome,

Hashimoto thyroiditis, and other causes of thyroid dysfunction must be included in the differential diagnosis.

## HYPOADRENALISM AND HYPOPITUITARISM

Pituitary or adrenal hypofunction may be associated with symptoms of Ménière's disease (46). A 5-hour glucose-tolerance test curve should alert the clinician to this possibility. The otologic symptoms are usually bilateral. Insulin stimulation test, or ACTH plasma cortisol stimulation test, can aid in the diagnosis. Hormone replacement therapy should be instituted as soon as the diagnosis is made.

## AUTOIMMUNE SENSORINEURAL HEARING LOSS

Autoimmune sensorineural hearing loss was originally described as an entity of young adults characterized by bilateral, asymmetric, rapidly progressive sensorineural hearing loss with marked vestibular dysfunction (81). It is often associated with tissue destruction of the mastoid, middle ear, or eardrum. There is more some indication that minor trauma such as a myringotomy to evacuate middle ear fluid may rarely trigger this disease process.

More recently, it has become apparent that autoimmune sensorineural hearing loss may occur in any age group and may produce almost any audiometric pattern. This disease entity may cause bilateral total deafness with or without substantial dizziness. Various laboratory tests may be helpful in establishing the diagnosis including tests of the humoral and cell-mediated immune systems, complement tests, haplotype, and others. Current test protocol includes quantitative serum immunoglobins by group, C-3, C-4, CH-50, C-1Q, T-cell subsets; HLA-A, B, C typing; HLA-DR typing, Western blot for cochlear antibodies and other tests. This evaluation is ordered only in patients in whom there is a reasonably high clinical suspicion of autoimmune disease, and other diagnoses that cause sudden sensorineural hearing loss are excluded. Bowman and Nelson (82) have shown that increased Cw7 correlates positively with immune hearing loss or possibly with steroid responsiveness. Absence of DR4 suggests an increased disease susceptibility, and the presence of Cw4 and B35 are associated more weakly with autoimmune sensorineural hearing loss. Treatment includes steroids and cytotoxic drugs such as methotrexate or cyclophosphamide. Rarely plasmapheresis may be necessary.

A special type of autoimmune sensorineural hearing loss called sympathetic cochleitis involves bilateral hearing loss following injury or surgery to one ear. It is believed to be due to exposure of inner ear protein to the immune system. It is also treated with steroids and cytotoxic agents.

## RENAL FAILURE

High-frequency sensorineural hearing may be found in patients with severe renal disease. Dialysis patients have been studied in particular. Their audiograms show a dip at 6000 Hz, with some depression at 4000 and 8000 Hz as well. The loss usually does not go < 2000 Hz, and wide fluctuations in threshold may occur during a single dialysis period (83). The pathogenesis of this otopathology is unclear. Hyperlipidemia has been evaluated and does not seem to be the cause. Prior exposure to ototoxic drugs frequently complicates evaluation, and its significance is unclear. Nevertheless, patients with renal failure require monitoring of auditory function.

## AGING

The general aging process affects all parts of the body, and the ear is no exception (84). Presbycusis begins in childhood as a progressive loss of hair cells and nerve fibers within the inner ear. This process starts in the highest frequency regions and gradually progresses to the speech range. When bilateral, symmetrical, sloping, high-frequency sensorineural hearing loss is identified in elderly persons, presbycusis is likely. Caution must be exercised because of the tendency to assign all such patients to this category without proper evaluation. Actually, a number of such patients have hereditary forms of hearing loss. These forms are sometimes associated with other manifestations which should be diagnosed properly. Others may have a variety of nonhereditary causes, such as syphilis or acoustic neuroma. The tendency to ascribe an "obvious" diagnosis to a given hearing loss must be

restrained unless a thorough evaluation has been performed.

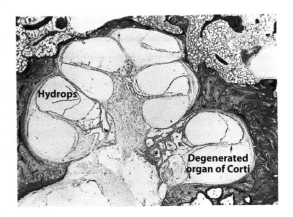

**Figure 15.7** Congenital syphilitic labyrinthitis in a 70-year-old woman. Severe endolymphatic hydrops can be seen, as well as coalesced areas of bone destruction, severe degeneration of the organ of Corti, and absence of the organ of Corti in the basal 10 mm. Absence of cochlear neurons in the lower basal turn and ~50% degeneration of cochlear neurons elsewhere can be seen. (From Schuknecht [2], p. 265, Courtesy Harvard University Press.)

## PSYCHOSIS

The presence of hearing loss has been studied in adult patients with paranoid and affective psychosis (85). Sensorineural hearing loss was found in ~60% of patients with paranoid psychosis and >70% of patients with affective psychosis. Conductive hearing loss was found in ~20% of the paranoid group and <2% of people with affective psychosis. It has also been suggested that the duration of hearing loss is longer in the paranoid group and frequently may precede the onset of psychosis. The effect of hearing loss on psychological development in early childhood is well recognized. The proclivity for relatively mild paranoid tendencies, neurosis, and other psychological disturbances in older hard-of-hearing patients has been well established also. However, the association with frank psychosis is an interesting subject where further research is still needed.

## MALIGNANCY

Primary carcinomas and sarcomas of the ear occur (86–88) and are discussed in separate chapters, but tumors from distant sites also may metastasize to the temporal bone. This fact is frequently unrecognized but should be considered if otitis develops in a patient with a known cancer. It also emphasizes the need to look for a primary tumor elsewhere when a carcinoma of the ear is found. Metastatic carcinoma to the ear has been reported from breast, kidney, lung, stomach, larynx, prostate, thyroid, nasopharynx, uterus, meninges, scalp, rectum, the parotid gland, intestine, brain, carotid chemodectoma, spinal cord, and other sites (89). Tumors of the *skull base* also can produce hearing loss by direct involvement of the ear or by interference with eustachian tube function, leading to fluid in the middle ear and conductive hearing loss. Direct extension from adjacent basal cell carcinomas, melanomas, meningiomas, benign, or malignant neural tumors of nearby cranial nerves, glomus tumors, hemangiomas (which may be multiple), and a variety of other neoplasms also may be implicated. Nasopharyngeal cancers classically occur with unilateral serous otitis media in an adult, secondary to eustachian tube occlusion. This malignancy is more common among people of Asian descent but must be searched for in any patient with unexplained serous otitis.

Malignancies such as Hodgkin disease, leukemia, lymphoma, and myeloma, which produce defects in the immunologic system, increase the incidence of ear infection and resultant hearing loss and serious otologic complications. The importance of this possibility may be overlooked in patients with dramatic systemic disease. Untreated otitis media can lead not only to a progressive hearing loss but also to meningitis and death, particularly in an immunocompromised patient.

Treatment for malignancy may involve *radiation therapy*, with its complications including hearing loss. Dryness and scaling of the skin of the external auditory canal may lead to buildup of debris and conductive hearing loss. *Osteoradionecrosis* of the temporal bone may produce chronic infection and may result in conductive or even severe sensorineural hearing deficit years after the initial treatment and radiation exposure (2, 90, 91). Management of osteoradionecrosis is variable with the goal of treating specific symptoms.

## COAGULOPATHIES

A few conditions such as cochlear artery occlusion may be associated with vascular dysfunction of the inner ear. Hypercoagulable states such as those associated with certain tumors, polycythemia, Buerger's disease, macroglobulinemia, and some viral infections have been implicated as etiological factors in certain cases of sudden hearing loss (92). Coagulation defects coincident with primary coagulopathies or secondary to diseases such as leukemia can cause inner ear hemorrhage and consequent deafness (2). Such hearing losses are not reversible but may be prevented by appropriate management of the underlying disease. Therapy is especially critical if hearing has been lost in one ear already.

## GLOMUS JUGULARE AND GLOMUS TYMPANICUM

Glomus jugulare tumors are rare, but when they occur, hearing loss and tinnitus are frequently the only symptoms. This peculiar neoplasm (paraganglioma) arises from cells around the jugular bulb and expands to involve neighboring structures (2). In doing so, the neoplasm most frequently extends to the floor of the middle ear, causing conductive hearing loss and pulsating tinnitus. As the disease progresses, it may appear as chronic otitis media and may even extend through the eardrum and appear to be granulation tissue in the ear canal. Unsuspecting biopsy of this apparent granulation tissue may cause profuse bleeding because of the marked vascularity of the tumor. As the disease extends, it may destroy portions of the temporal bone and jugular bulb and can extend intracranially.

Glomus tumors may also arise from cells along the medial wall of the middle ear. These are called glomus tympanicum tumors and are generally easier to manage surgically. It is essential to distinguish between glomus tympanicum and glomus jugulare before attempting surgical intervention.

As in any expanding neoplasm, early diagnosis of a glomus tumor facilitates surgical cure. Since conductive hearing loss may be the only symptom in many patients, the physician is obligated to establish a cause for every case of unilateral conductive hearing loss.

Physical examination may disclose a pinkish mass in the middle ear. Positive pressure on the eardrum may reveal blanching of the mass. Pulsating tinnitus may be audible to the examiner by using a Toynbee tube or a stethoscope placed over the ear. The finding of objective tinnitus may occur not only with glomus tumors but also with carotid artery aneurysms, intracranial arteriovenous malformations, carotid artery stenosis, and other conditions. Glomus tumors must be distinguished from other masses, such as carotid artery aneurysms, high jugular bulbs, meningiomas, and adenomas, that may appear in the middle ear.

Radiological evaluation is now the mainstay of glomus tumor diagnosis. Biopsy is rarely indicated. CT scans of the temporal bone are used to assess bone erosion, and MRI, MR angiography, traditional arteriography, and retrograde jugular venography are used to identify the extent of the neoplasm (**Figure 15.8**). Four-vessel arteriograms are now being recommended by some otologists because of the high incidence of associated tumors. Up to 10% of patients with glomus tumors will have associated bilateral glomus tumors, glomus vagale, carotid body tumor, or thyroid carcinoma (93). The vast majority of glomus patients are female, and the tumor is extremely rare in children. For this reason, biopsy is appropriate to rule out other lesions if the diagnosis is considered seriously in a child. Biopsy is also used in patients who are not surgical candidates prior to instituting palliative radiation therapy. However, such biopsies must be carefully performed in the operating room, and with blood available for replacement if necessary.

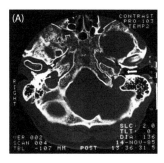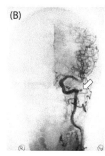

Figure 15.8 CT of the temporal bones without contrast (A) and angiogram (B) demonstrating a glomus tympanicum tumor.

## INTERNAL CAROTID ARTERY ANEURYSM

Although aneurysmal presentations in the temporal bone are rare (94), they require accurate diagnosis and well-planned surgical management

when they occur. Symptoms of hearing loss, vertigo, tinnitus, a feeling of fullness in the ear, and even facial nerve paralysis may be found. Central symptoms include headache, nausea, vomiting, and convulsions and may occur as the disease progresses. Early ear involvement may suggest *glomus tumors* symptomatically. Carotid artery aneurysm must be kept in the differential diagnosis whenever a middle ear mass is found, especially if it is pulsatile or associated with pulsating tinnitus.

## VASCULAR DISEASE

Patients with advanced atherosclerosis, particularly those who have suffered myocardial infarctions, have a higher incidence than the normal population of high-frequency sensorineural hearing loss. The pathogenesis is undetermined, but it is believed to be related to vascular changes within the inner ear (95). The *subclavian steal syndrome* involves collateral circulation from the vertebral artery in the presence of proximal left subclavian artery stenosis. Hearing loss occurs in ~10% of patients (96) and results from compromise of the vertebrobasilar system, which provides blood to the inner ear. Other otologic symptoms, such as tinnitus, vertigo, and facial paralysis, also may occur with this syndrome because the vertebral artery supplies the pons, medulla, cerebellum, vestibular and cochlear labyrinth, and portions of the temporal bone, as well as the upper spinal cord, thalamus, and occipital cortex. Similar symptoms may occur with more limited dysfunction of the vertebral system, such as the *lateral medullary infarction syndrome*. Surgical treatment is available but is beyond the scope of this chapter.

Sudden hearing loss is often ascribed to "vascular causes." Although this explanation is tempting, histological confirmation is scarce, although the phenomenon certainly exists—at least in association with larger cerebrovascular occlusive events. Many diseases which may cause anoxia of tissues may be responsible for sensorineural hearing loss, but more research is needed to prove the relationship. Such conditions include chronic hypotension, anemia, vasovagal abnormalities, and other similar maladies.

## STROKE

Hemorrhage into the ear produces deafness, as noted in the discussion of coagulopathies. Similar findings occur following spontaneous *subarachnoid hemorrhage*, which produces blood in the internal auditory canal and cochlea. Major cerebrovascular occlusions may produce severe hearing deficits. *Occlusion of the vertebral* or *posterior–inferior cerebellar artery* produces lateral medullary syndrome or *Wallenberg syndrome*. This syndrome is characterized by ipsilateral ptosis and miosis; enophthalmos; facial hypesthesia; palatal, pharyngeal, and laryngeal paralysis; contralateral hypesthesia and decreased thermal sensation in the trunk and extremities; as well as occasional involvement of the sixth, seventh, and eighth cranial nerves (97, 98). Sensorineural hearing loss occurs, and vestibular function is abnormal (99).

**Occlusion of the anterior vestibular artery** alone produces vestibular symptoms without hearing loss (2). *Occlusion of the anterior–inferior cerebellar artery* generally produces sudden vertigo with nausea and vomiting, hearing loss, facial paralysis, and cerebellar and sensory disturbances. Degeneration of the membranous labyrinth and brainstem auditory and vestibular nuclei occurs. Ipsilateral loss of pain and temperature sensation on the face are common, associated with decreased pain and temperature sensation on the opposite side of the body. Patients who survive usually improve slowly.

**Vertebrobasilar ischemia** may have similar, but transient symptoms, of which vertigo is the most prominent. Other associated findings may be hearing loss, diplopia, headaches, and speech difficulties. Although atherosclerotic vascular disease is the usual etiology, arthritis, syphilis, aneurysms, and subclavian steal syndrome also must be kept in mind.

**Lateral venous sinus thrombosis** and *thrombophlebitis of the jugular bulb* or the *internal jugular vein* may cause mastoid infection, brain abscess, or septicemia and meningitis due to septic emboli, and they may lead to hearing loss. In the past, these diseases generally have been seen as complications of ear surgery. Recently, however, jugular thrombophlebitis and its complications (including retrograde extensions) have been seen in individuals with substance use disorder who use the subclavian or internal jugular veins as access routes.

## OBSTRUCTIVE SLEEP APNEA

Obstructive sleep apnea (OSA) is a very common condition that may be found in up to 1 billion people across the world (100). Risk factors for developing OSA include obesity, cigarette/tobacco use, and alcohol consumption. It is characterized by repeated pauses in breathing often due to narrowing or collapse of the airway during sleep that leads to hypoxia and a pro-inflammatory state. Recent studies have shown an association between OSA and sensorineural hearing loss, especially in high frequencies (101, 102). One theory for these findings is that decreased oxygen saturation damages the cochlea and leads to hearing loss (101). Other theories include noise-induced sensorineural hearing loss from chronic exposure to loud snoring, although that is a very controversial hypothesis (103). Further research is needed.

## MULTIPLE SCLEROSIS

Diffuse demyelinating disease, such as multiple sclerosis, may involve all parts of the nervous system. The first symptoms often are transient episodes of blurred vision, vertigo, clumsiness, or transient cranial nerve palsy. Later in the disease, intention tremor, scanning speech, diffuse neurological weakness, and nystagmus may develop. Sensorineural hearing loss and tinnitus may occur in approximately 1.1% of patients (104). The disease usually occurs in the third or fourth decade of life; it is progressive and may be fatal. Most commonly, the hearing loss is high frequency, progressive, and bilateral (105), but it may be sudden, unilateral, and profound (2). Some recovery frequently occurs. The hearing loss often fluctuates and may even return to normal after severe depression. Often, abnormal tone decay may persist even when hearing is nearly normal (13). Brainstem evoked-response audiometry may be useful in establishing the diagnosis.

## INFESTATIONS

A variety of tropical diseases can produce hearing loss, although these are rarely seen in the United States (106). *Halzoun*, caused by *Fasciola hepatica*, may be found anywhere where sheep and goats are raised, but it is especially common in South America, Latin America, and Poland. The disease has also been found in Africa, Asia, Europe, and North America. Infection usually occurs by eating raw aquatic plants, such as watercress, and causes hepatic distomiasis. Symptoms include dyspnea, dysphagia, deafness, and occasionally asphyxiation.

*Myiasis*, caused by infestation of human tissue by fly larvae, may produce ear infection or more serious disease by penetration of the body through the ear. *Cochliomyia hominivorax*, or primary screwworm flies, are found in the American tropics and throughout the southern United States. They infect humans by laying eggs in open wounds or discharging orifices. They create deep malodorous wounds and may occur as an otitis or mastoiditis. Infestation is fatal in ~10% of cases. Other forms of myiasis affecting the ears may be found elsewhere in the world and should be suspected in known travelers. Parasitic infections of the external auditory canal are common in the tropics, in warmer portions of the United States, and may also be found sporadically throughout the country, especially in swimmers.

## CONCLUSION

The great many diseases that may be associated with hearing loss highlight the need for a thorough history and physical examination in each patient with hearing impairment. Moreover, they remind us to search for unsuspected hearing loss early in patients with these maladies. Much more information is needed to clarify the nature of hearing loss associated with systemic diseases. Of particular importance is the need for temporal bone specimens for further research. Only through constant clinical attention and diligent investigation can we hope to diagnose, understand, and prevent hearing loss of all causes.

## SUMMARY

Hearing loss may accompany many systemic diseases. Familiarity with the otologic manifestations of these conditions facilitates early diagnosis and treatment of hearing impairment. Moreover, attention to these relationships often leads to the diagnosis of otherwise unsuspected, potentially serious systemic diseases in patients who complain of hearing loss.

## HEARING LOSS ASSOCIATED WITH HEREDITARY DISEASES AND SYNDROMES

Most diseases can be classified as hereditary or nonhereditary. Either type may be present at birth or may manifest later in life. Hereditary problems are frequently classified according to the mode for inheritance. An autosomal dominant disease will be apparent in the person who carries the gene; the chance that it will be transmitted to any given offspring is 50%. In autosomal recessive inheritance, neither parent may show a trait, but both are carriers. The chance that they will pass the trait to any given offspring is 25%.

Each person carries a great many genes for recessive traits, but these may be expressed only if mating occurs with someone with the same traits. The chances of this occurring are greatly increased in consanguinity. The chances are one in two that a carrier mother will pass an X-linked trait to any of her sons. An affected male transmits the carrier state to all of his daughters but none of his sons.

Understanding these patterns and the diseases with which they are associated allows us to predict the birth of affected children and helps us to counsel the parents of an afflicted child about the likelihood of having a second abnormal birth. Thus, this knowledge is critical not only in minimizing the occurrence of hereditary deafness but also in reassuring parents of children whose deafness or malformation resulted from other causes that the chance of having a second affected child is very small.

A nationwide survey found that approximately 37.5 million people in the United States admit to having a significant hearing loss (107). Three out of every 1000 children in the United States are born with some degree of hearing loss, and genetic factors may account for as many as 50% of all cases of hearing loss, although that assertion is controversial (108). Therefore, it is important to consider genetic or hereditary hearing loss in the differential diagnosis of all cases of hearing impairment. These conditions may produce hearing loss of any audiometric pattern, including bilateral dips that are indistinguishable from audiograms from patients with noise-induced hearing loss. Such conditions may occur in young men or women with no history of noise exposure. When inheritance is recessive rather than dominant, there may be no family history of hearing loss. So, care must be exercised in order to avoid missing the diagnosis.

## DIABETES MELLITUS

Diabetes is one of the fastest growing chronic diseases across the world. Currently, at least 28.5 million people in the United States have been diagnosed with diabetes, and 96 million adults have prediabetes (109). Two distinct types of diabetes exist. Type 1 occurs from an autoimmune destruction of insulin producing pancreatic β-cells, and type 2 occurs from the development of insulin resistance in which cells no longer respond to insulin. Studies have shown that patients with diabetes are 2 times more likely to have hearing loss compared to those without diabetes (110). The hearing loss generally is sensorineural, progressive, bilateral, and most severe in the high frequencies (2) and tends to be worse in the elderly diabetic (111). A syndrome similar to Ménière's disease may be associated with diabetes and presents symptoms of fluctuating sensorineural hearing loss, episodic vertigo, tinnitus, and a feeling of fullness in the ear (112). Sudden, profound hearing loss may occur in diabetic patients also, but the causal relationship has not been proven (111, 113).

Pathological examination has revealed small blood vessel changes in the inner ear similar to those found in the kidney and elsewhere (114). In addition, atherosclerosis of large blood vessels, possibly associated with elevated serum cholesterol and triglyceride levels, develops prematurely. Laboratory research also supports an association of diabetes and hearing loss (115).

Because of the significant incidence of diabetes, any person over age 18 with an unexplained sensorineural hearing loss or Ménière-like symptom complex should have a fasting blood sugar and a 2-hour postprandial blood sugar determination. If these tests are abnormal, a glucose-tolerance test should be carried out. Even if the tests are normal, it often is worthwhile to repeat them periodically. If this is done, it is not uncommon for the otologist to be the first clinician to diagnose diabetes. In addition, annual audiometric screening is recommended for all known diabetics.

## MALIGNANT OTITIS EXTERNA

This disease is life-threatening and invariably found in diabetic or immunocompromised patients. Pain, rather than hearing loss, is usually the most prominent sign. It is a noncancerous infection, usually caused by *Pseudomonas aeruginosa*, extending to the temporal bone and the skull base (**Figure 15.9**). Treatment often requires hospitalization and high-dose intravenous antibiotics, although the advent

of fluoroquinolones has made outpatient treatment possible. Sometimes extensive surgical debridement of the temporal bone is required. The keystones of prevention are vigorous treatment of any diabetic with otitis externa and early recognition of referral for infections that do not resolve.

## HYPOGLYCEMIA

Hearing losses may also be found in patients with hypoglycemia and can be seen with symptoms comparable to Ménière's disease (116, 117). Glucose intolerance is another finding in a high percentage of patients with fluctuant hearing.

## FAMILIAL HYPERLIPOPROTEINEMIA

This condition affects around 1 in every 250 people and is commonly associated with hearing loss (47, 118). Generally, it is transmitted in an autosomal dominant pattern, although occasionally it appears to be recessive. It can be classified into one of three groups (familial hypercholesterolemia, familial combined hyperlipidemia, or familial hypertriglyceridemia) or subclassified as one of six types (types I, IIa, IIb, III, IV, and V).

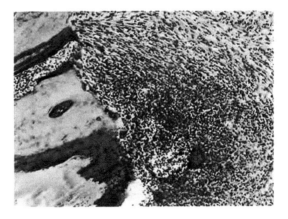

Figure 15.9 Malignant otitis externa with an abscess in the area of the cochlear aqueduct. The infection destroyed the bone beneath the cochlea and entered the posterior fossa. (From Linthicum and Schwartzman [119], p. 43. Courtesy W.B. Saunders.)

It is important to distinguish between the hereditary hyperlipoproteinemias and acquired disease secondary to diet, nephrotic syndrome, hypothyroidism, or other disease states. Types IIa,

IIb, and IV are particularly important because of their association with sensorineural hearing loss. The pathology and implications can be similar to those seen in diabetic patients. Screening laboratory studies include fasting serum cholesterol and serum triglyceride determination and should be repeated at defined intervals. If either test is abnormal, a lipoprotein electrophoresis should be obtained after a 14-hour fast. These tests should be done in children with sensorineural hearing loss also, especially in children of hyperlipidemic parents.

Treatment is available for many patients with hyperlipoproteinemia and includes diet control and medications such as statins, cholestyramine, nicotinic acid, clofibrate, or PCSK9 inhibitors.

## CLEFT PALATE

Cleft lip, with or without cleft palate, occurs about once in every 1000 births in the American population (120, 121). Isolated cleft palate occurs about once in every 1700 births (121). Overall Asian and American indigenous populations have the highest risk of developing cleft lip or palate, followed by white populations with intermediate risk, and Black populations with the lowest risk (122). Although clefts have a familial tendency, they do not follow a classic pattern of inheritance. Moreover, there seems to be interaction between genetic and *in utero* hormonal or substance use factors, such as maternal smoking. Clefts also may be associated with numerous other congenital malformations (123). If parents of an affected child are normal, their chances of having another affected child are ~2%. If one of the parents is affected or if both a parent and child are affected, the incidence is considerably higher.

Nearly all cleft palate patients have abnormal eustachian tube function and a high incidence of serous otitis media (124, 125). If untreated, this problem will produce conductive hearing loss and may lead to suppurative or adhesive otitis media. Similar problems may even occur with a submucous cleft palate, which an examiner may feel but not see. This disorder should be suspected and searched for in the presence of the bifid uvula. Treatment includes decongestants with or without antibiotics and the placement of tympanotomy tubes when middle ear ventilation fails to improve.

## RETINITIS PIGMENTOSA

*Usher syndrome* is a combination of retinitis pigmentosa and congenital sensorineural hearing loss and is usually recessive (126). The hearing loss is congenital, although it frequently is not discovered until the child is 1 or 2 years of age and sometimes even older. It is cochlear, bilateral, and more severe in the high frequencies (126–129). This syndrome can be classified into three types. Type 1 is characterized by severe hearing loss and vestibular dysfunction and retinitis pigmentosa that is diagnosed in childhood. Type 2 is characterized by moderate hearing loss with normal vestibular function and retinitis pigmentosa that occurs after childhood. Type 3 is characterized by progressive hearing loss and vestibular dysfunction and retinitis pigmentosa that can occur at any time (130). A decreased sense of smell is also often present (131). Retinitis pigmentosa and hearing loss may be combined with a number of other maladies. *Refsum syndrome* (132) is an autosomal recessive disease that is associated with progressive peripheral neuropathy, intellectual deficits, and elevated serum phytanic acid. Hearing loss associated with this syndrome is typically mild-to-moderate high-frequency loss (133). The lipid-storage defect may be treated with dietary restriction of phytanic acid and limiting foods such as beef, lamb, fish, and dairy products (134). The *Bardet–Biedl syndrome* combines retinitis pigmentosa and hearing loss with hypogonadism, polydactyly, obesity, and intellectual impairment (135). Patients with *Laurence–Moon syndrome* have intellectual impairment, hypogenitalism, and spastic paraplegia (135). In *Alström syndrome*, obesity and diabetes mellitus are combined with hearing loss and retinitis pigmentosa (136). In *Cockayne syndrome*, they are combined with retinal atrophy, intellectual impairment, dwarfism, and a cachectic prematurely aged face. These patients usually die in their 20s (137). *Kearns–Sayre syndrome* combines retinitis pigmentosa and mixed hearing loss with progressive external ophthalmoplegia and cardiac conduction defects (135).

In general, all patients with these syndromes are functionally blind by the time they reach age 50, and often earlier. They comprise ~10% of people with hereditary deafness. Some can be helped with hearing aids, but often the hearing loss is too severe even though it generally is not progressive.

As such, any deaf child should have a careful ophthalmological evaluation. Conversely, any person with retinitis pigmentosa should have a hearing test.

## GLAUCOMA

A familial tendency is associated with glaucoma, especially of an open-angle type. Children and siblings of patients with glaucoma may have higher ocular pressures than normal and may have anatomical features that predispose them to glaucoma (138).

The relationship between glaucoma and hearing loss has been controversial. Data suggest a very high incidence of auditory vestibular dysfunction in glaucoma patients (139). Combined cochlear and vestibular hypofunction has been found in up to 60% of cases; pure cochlear hearing loss has been found in ~25%. Only ~25% of glaucoma patients with otologic dysfunction were symptomatic, their most common complaint being loss of hearing. The usual audiologic picture is bilateral cochlear hearing loss, although this may be found coincidentally in the older patient. In acute congestive glaucoma, nearly all patients tested have had bilateral hearing losses, and about one-third have had vestibular dysfunction as well.

Additionally, the majority of patients who have had glaucoma for >2 years have been found to have hearing losses; the severity of this loss appears to correlate with the severity of the glaucoma. Because of the frequently delayed recognition of hypoacusis, routine audiograms in patients with glaucoma may be useful until the relationship is better understood.

Exfoliation syndrome (EFS) is similar to glaucoma and arises due to extracellular fibrillar deposition throughout the body. EFS is considered one of the most common causes of open-angle glaucoma (140). Previous studies have shown that patients with EFS have more severe hearing loss compared to control patients, especially with hearing loss in high frequencies (140, 141). Overall, there are mixed results regarding the association of EFS with hearing loss, as the condition arises at the same age range as presbycusis. More research is needed to confirm or refute a causal link between EFS syndrome and hearing loss. Similar to glaucoma patients, it may be useful to screen patients with EFS for hearing loss.

## OTHER OPHTHALMOLOGICAL ABNORMALITIES

At least 20 other syndromes manifest combinations of eye and ear disease. They include foveal dystrophy and sensorineural hearing loss, which may involve as many as 5% of children with hereditary deafness (142); optic atrophy and deafness (*Leber disease*) (143); intellectual impairment, retinal pseudotumor, and deafness (*Norrie disease*) (144); nonsyphilitic keratitis and auditory vestibular abnormalities (*Cogan syndrome*) (145); vestibular dysfunction, uveitis, alopecia, white eyelashes and hair, and elevated cerebrospinal fluid pressure in the early stage (*Vogt–Koyanagi syndrome*) (146); saddle nose, myopia, cataract, and hearing loss (*Marshall syndrome*); and vestibulocerebellar ataxia, retinitis pigmentosa, and nerve deafness (*Hallgren syndrome*) (127).

*Hallgren syndrome* is particularly interesting because it accounts for ~5% of all hereditary deafness (142). Ninety percent of these patients are profoundly deaf, apparently at birth; 90% have ataxia and 10% have nystagmus. Twenty-five percent appear to be mentally deficient, usually schizophrenic.

## ALPORT SYNDROME

This partially sex-linked, autosomally transmitted syndrome (146, 147) may be detected during the first week of life by the presence of hematuria and albuminuria. Hypertension, renal failure, and death usually occur before the age of 30 in males. Females demonstrate a much less severe form of the disease. Hearing loss occurs in 50% of cases and is progressive, bilateral, and cochlear (130). It generally is first detected when the patient is ~10 years old. This syndrome is estimated to account for ~1% of hereditary deafness (142). Treatment consists primarily of controlling urinary tract infections and renal failure. Frequently, the need for ototoxic drugs for urinary tract infection complicates the hearing loss.

*Muckle–Wells syndromes*, a variant of Alport, includes urticaria, amyloidosis, and relative infertility (148, 149). This disease usually begins during adolescence. *Herman syndrome* combines hereditary nephritis and autosomal dominant nerve deafness with intellectual impairment, epilepsy, and diabetes mellitus (150).

Approximately 10 other recognized syndromes combine hearing loss with renal disease. This frequent association warrants a routine urinalysis in the evaluation of sensorineural hearing loss, particularly in children and young adults. A number of these syndromes are associated with hypertension as well, so blood pressure also should be checked.

## WAARDENBURG SYNDROME

This dominant syndrome (**Figure 15.10**) includes partial albinism (classically seen as a white forelock of hair), laterally positioned medial canthi, different colored irises, and congenital nonprogressive sensorineural hearing loss (150). Vestibular abnormalities and temporal bone radiological abnormalities may occur (147). The deafness may be total, with only slight residual hearing in the low frequencies; moderate, with near-normal hearing in the higher frequencies and severe loss in the low frequencies; or unilateral, with near-normal hearing on one side (2). Only 20% of patients with Waardenburg syndrome demonstrate hearing loss; however, Waardenburg syndrome accounts for ~1% of all hereditary deafness (142). At present, no treatment exists other than sound amplification when applicable. Genetic counseling is relevant in these cases.

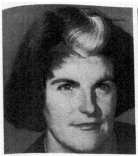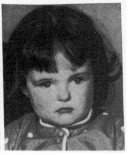

Figure 15.10 Mother and daughter with Waardenburg syndrome showing white forelock and isochromic light iris. (From Smith [151], p. 143. Courtesy W.B. Saunders.)

## ALBINISM AND NERVE DEAFNESS

Generalized albinism and nerve deafness (as opposed to the localized albinism of Waardenburg syndrome) usually is recessive (118), although dominant forms (*Tietze syndrome*) have been described (152). In contrast to Waardenburg syndrome, with its localized areas of albinism, this syndrome is characterized by totally white skin, white hair, as well as absence of pigment in the iris, the sclera, and the fundus of the eye (153). Nystagmus and progressive high-tone, bilateral, sensorineural hearing loss also usually begin from ages 6 to 12 years. The disease is caused by the absence of the copper-containing enzyme tyrosinase. Thus far, no treatment is available other than symptomatic measures (inclusive of a hearing aid).

## NOONAN SYNDROME WITH MULTIPLE LENTIGINES (LEOPARD SYNDROME)

Leopard is an acronym for: *lentigines, electrocardiographic defect, ocular hypertelorism, pulmonary stenosis, abnormalities of genitalia, retardation of growth*, and *sensorineural deafness* (154). The syndrome is transmitted as an autosomal dominant. The lentigines usually are absent at birth but develop progressively (**Figure 15.11**). Sensorineural hearing loss occurs in ~25% of cases and is usually mild. Treatment includes hearing aids where applicable, surgical correction of pulmonary stenosis, dermabrasion of the lentigines, and correction of other associated abnormalities as necessary.

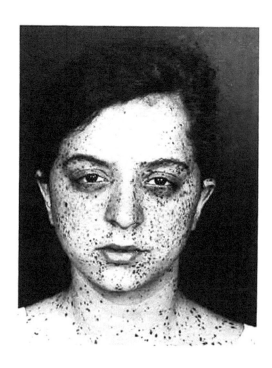

Figure 15.11 Noonan syndrome with multiple lentigines (Leopard) syndrome. (From Konigsmark and Gorlin [135], p. 239. Courtesy W.B. Saunders.)

# NEUROFIBROMATOSIS TYPE 1

Among the other syndromes that combine abnormalities of skin and hearing, generalized von Recklinghausen disease, now termed neurofibromatosis type 1, (**Figure 15.12**) has been well recognized since 1882. Multiple neurofibromas and café-au-lait spots are the most common features. Epilepsy frequently accompanies the syndrome; intellectual impairment occurs in some cases. Neurofibromas may occur anywhere, including the eighth cranial nerve, sometimes bilaterally. Malignant degeneration of the neurofibromas has also been reported (155). Inheritance is as an autosomal dominant. A localized form of neurofibromatosis type 1 exists and may arise as bilateral acoustic neurofibromas (156). These behave somewhat differently from acoustic neuromas unassociated with neurofibromatosis type 1 and may be quite large at the time of discovery (119). Vestibular testing may show decreased or absent caloric response. Treatment requires resection of the acoustic tumors if feasible. Patients with neurofibromatosis 1 experiencing hearing loss should undergo magnetic resonance imaging to determine whether a neurofibroma is causing the issue.

# PAGET DISEASE

Osteitis deformans, Paget disease of bone, is found at autopsy in ~3% of people > 40 years of age and may occur in as much as 10% of the population > 80 (135). In general, Paget disease is an autosomal dominant syndrome. Bone pain is the most frequent symptom. The pathology involves a combination of abnormal deposition and resorption of bone in a mosaic pattern (**Figure 15.13**) and manifests itself with bony deformation, particularly of the weight-bearing portions of the skeleton. Enlargement of the cranium is classic. Sarcomatous changes have been found in 1%–2% of cases (157).

Various neurological changes have been reported. The hearing loss, which is not a constant feature of Paget disease, may be conductive (caused by malformation of the ossicles or oval window area) or sensorineural (2, 158). One mechanism for sensorineural hearing loss is narrowing of the internal auditory canal, producing pressure on the auditory nerve. However, this does not seem to occur as commonly as does the cochlear hearing loss. The diagnosis is made by X-ray films and detection of elevated serum alkaline phosphatase and urinary hydroxyproline levels. Treatment may include reconstructive middle ear surgery, although this procedure is often unrewarding because of the progression and unpredictability of the disease. The current mainstay of treatment is the use of bisphosphonates to decrease the overall amount of bone resorption, or calcitonin also may be an option (158).

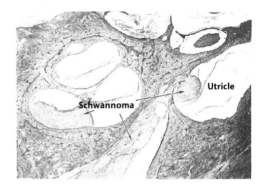

Figure 15.12 Neurofibromatosis type 1 (von Recklinghausen disease) with bilateral vestibular schwannomas. In this photomicrograph, the neoplasm extends from the internal auditory canal into the basal turn of the cochlea and into the vestibule. (From Schuknecht [2], p. 376. Courtesy Harvard University Press.)

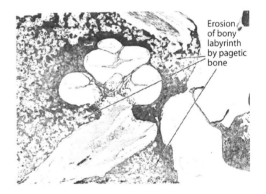

Figure 15.13 Paget disease with extensive involvement of the bony labyrinth but with a normal-appearing membranous labyrinth. (From Schuknecht [86]. Courtesy Harvard University Press.)

# FIBROUS DYSPLASIA

Fibrous dysplasia of the temporal bone is commonly associated with hearing loss (159). The process may be monostotic or polyostotic. Disseminated fibrous dysplasia is usually a feature of McCune–Albright syndrome, in which fibrous dysplasia, skin pigmentation, and various endocrine disturbances occur, almost always in females. The monostotic and polyostotic forms occur in males and females, and both may be associated with hyperparathyroidism. Fibrous dysplasia may occur in the temporal bone and be associated with hearing loss (**Figure 15.14**). Conductive hearing loss is the most common and occurs from crowding of the ossicular chain (160). Hearing may be improved by surgery in selected cases.

## OSTEOGENESIS IMPERFECTA

This autosomal dominant disease (**Figure 15.15**) occurs in varying severity in two forms (2). *Osteogenesis imperfecta congenita* is present at birth, is more severe, and leads to multiple fractures and, frequently, early death. *Osteogenesis imperfecta tarda*, much less severe, becomes evident later in life and is more localized. Blue sclera, bone fragility, and hearing loss are the principal features (Van der Hoeve–de Kleijn's syndrome [161] or Lobstein disease), but other systems, particularly the teeth, may be involved. Marked hearing impairment is found in 30–60% of patients with the tarda type (162, 163). The hearing loss usually is conductive and bilateral, although mixed and purely sensorineural hearing losses have been reported. The tympanic membrane may be bluish and quite thin. At one time, osteogenesis imperfecta and otosclerosis were thought to be the same disease since stapes fixation occurs in both, but this does not appear to be the case (2, 119). The surgical treatment (stapedectomy) is the same, however, with possible technical modifications (164).

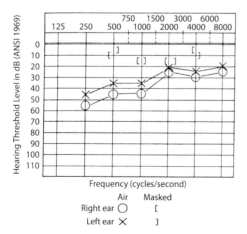

Figure 15.14 Fibrous dysplasia of the temporal bone in a 14-year-old girl. Her bilateral conductive hearing loss was due to involvement of the ear canal impinging on the malleus and incus. *Abbreviation*: ANSI, American National Standards Institute.

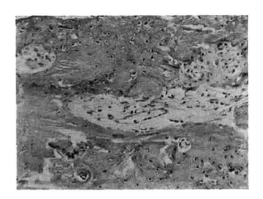

Figure 15.15 Osteogenesis imperfecta. The calcium and phosphorus content of this temporal bone is below normal, and the bone matrix appears immature. (From Linthicum and Schwartzman [119]. Courtesy W.B. Saunders.)

## SYNDROMIC CRANIOSYNOSTOSIS

Craniosynostosis is characterized by the closure of one or more of the calvarial sutures and leads to distinctive anatomical characteristics (**Figure 15.16**). The shape of the cranium varies, depending on the sutures involved. Ocular hypertelorism, exophthalmos, shallow orbits, beaked nose, and maxillary hypoplasia are common. This group of disorders affects approximately 1 out of every 3000 births (165). Mutations in the fibroblast growth factor receptor (FGFR) genes are most common, and inheritance is autosomal dominant. Various combinations of FGFR mutations lead to distinct syndromic craniosynostoses such as Apert syndrome, Pfeiffer syndrome, Crouzon syndrome, Beare–Stevenson syndrome, Crouzon-dermo-skeletal, and Jackson–Weiss syndrome. These syndromes also are characterized mainly by conductive hearing loss that is associated with ossicular deformity or stapes fixation, although mixed or sensorineural hearing loss can occur (166). Muenke syndrome is unique in that it is characterized by mild-to-moderate sensorineural hearing loss at low frequencies (166). The treatment is surgical in most cases. Craniotomy is performed in infancy to decrease cerebral compression, with cosmetic maxillofacial reconstruction becoming more and more satisfactory (167).

## CLEIDOCRANIAL DYSOSTOSIS

This dominant syndrome is occasionally associated with conductive or mixed progressive hearing loss and concentric narrowing of the external auditory canals (135). It occurs with hypoplasia or aplasia of one or both clavicles or with pseudoarthrosis. Abnormal eruption of teeth and incomplete ossification of the skull are further manifestations of this ossification defect of membranous bone. On physical examination, patients often can bring their shoulders together in front of their sternum. Facial bones are underdeveloped, the palate is high and arched, and the frontal sinuses do not develop.

## TREACHER COLLINS AND FRANCESCHETTI–KLEIN SYNDROMES

Mandibulofacial dysostosis was first described in the 1840s, and the facial appearance is classic (**Figure 15.17**) [168]: Hypoplastic zygomas produce downward-sloping palpebral fissures. Cheekbones are depressed, the chin recedes, the mouth has a large "fishlike" appearance, the mandible is hypoplastic, and coloboma of the lower eyelids with lack of cilia is common. Auricular malformations occur in ~85% of such patients (169). About one-third have external auditory canal atresia or an ossicular defect. Conductive hearing loss is most common and occurs in 55% of cases, although sensorineural

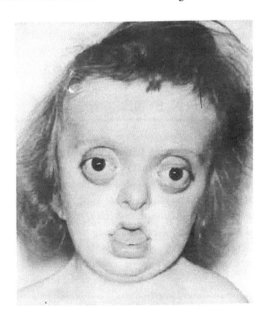

Figure 15.16 Crouzon syndrome showing exophthalmos, hypertelorism, and underdeveloped maxillae. The patient had a 60-dB conductive hearing loss and an IQ of 110. (From Schuknecht [2], p. 176. Courtesy Harvard University Press.)

deafness at high frequencies has also been reported (130, 170). Surgical treatment is rewarding in carefully selected patients, but early amplification should be used in patients with bilateral hearing losses. The inheritance pattern is autosomal dominant.

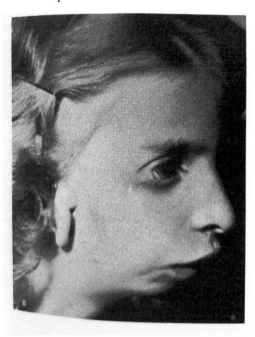

Figure 15.17 Treacher Collins syndrome with auricular dysplasia, malar hypoplasia, and defect of the lower eyelid. (From Smith [171], p. 111. Courtesy W.B. Saunders.)

## PIERRE ROBIN SEQUENCE

The striking facies in this apparently autosomal dominant syndrome is characterized by an "Andy Gump" appearance (**Figure 15.18**). A receding mandible and relatively large protruding tongue may produce respiratory obstruction. Cleft palate, cardiac, skeletal, and ophthalmological anomalies are also associated. The patients have low-set ears with auricular malformations and conductive hearing loss (2, 172). Genetic counseling is required. Management of the hearing loss may involve hearing aids or surgical intervention.

## OSTEOPETROSIS

This disease, known also as Albers–Schönberg disease and "marble bone" disease, may be transmitted as an autosomal dominant or an autosomal recessive disorder, but hearing loss has been associated primarily with the recessive form (135). It is estimated that approximately 78% of patients with the recessive form have hearing loss (173). The disease produces increased density of the entire bony skeleton (**Figure 15.19**). Cranial enlargement may occur, and mild hypertelorism has been noted. Patients have short stature due to impaired longitudinal bone growth. Fractures are common. Foramina of the cranial nerves may be narrowed, intracranial pressure may be increased, and visual loss occurs in 80% of cases. Facial paralysis is also common.

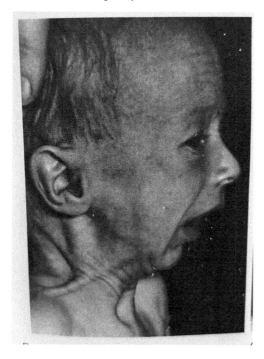

Figure 15.18 The classic "Andy Gump" appearance in the Pierre Robin syndrome. (From Smith [171], p. 8. Courtesy W.B. Saunders.)

Intellectual impairment is seen in ~20% of cases. Hemolytic anemia, thrombocytopenia, lymphadenopathy, hepatosplenomegaly, and osteomyelitis (frequently following dental extraction) occur. Patients tend to have a conductive hearing loss; however, between 25% and 50% of patients have a moderate mixed hearing loss beginning in childhood (170, 174–176). The incidence of otitis media is increased in this disease due to bone marrow suppression. The diagnosis is made by radiographic evaluation, and treatment is symptomatic. Frequent examination for otitis media should be performed in children with this disease. Hearing aids may prove helpful in some cases.

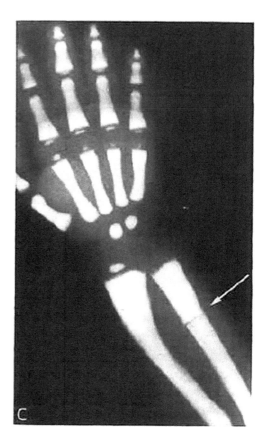

Figure 15.19 Markedly increase bony density with fractures of the radius and ulna in a patient with Albers–Schönberg disease. (From Konigsmark and Gorlin [135], p. 157. Courtesy W.B. Saunders.)

## KLIPPEL–FEIL SYNDROME

This well-known syndrome of cervical–vertebral fusion, often associated with spina bifida, cervical ribs, neurological abnormalities, strabismus, and other features, may be associated with hearing loss (2). When the Klippel–Feil anomalies are combined with abducens nerve paralysis, a retracted ocular bulb, and hearing loss, the condition is called *Wildervanck syndrome* (135, 177, 178). A cleft palate or torticollis may be associated as well, and inheritance probably is multifactorial. Hearing loss may be unilateral or bilateral, moderate to severe. Both conductive deafness and sensorineural deafness have been described, and vestibular studies are usually abnormal. Incomplete expression of the disease is common. The hearing loss is congenital and does not generally progress. Treatment may be surgical or may require a hearing aid.

# DWARFISM

A great many musculoskeletal anomalies are associated with hearing loss. As with all congenital anomalies, the presence of short stature or other obvious physical malformations should alert the clinician to look early for a hearing defect.

# CORNELIA DE LANGE SYNDROME

Cornelia de Lange syndrome (CDLS) is characterized by multiple congenital malformations and intellectual impairment (**Figure 15.20**). Sataloff et al. (179) examined 45 patients with this rare disease and found numerous otolaryngologic abnormalities. Virtually all had hearing loss, and most had impaired language development. Importantly, there was a direct correlation between the severity of hearing loss and the severity of language and other problems. While the predominant form of hearing loss in CDLS is sensorineural, conductive hearing loss secondary to persistent otitis media with effusion also may be present (180, 181). It appeared that unrecognized or untreated hearing loss may have exacerbated the difficulties experienced by these patients.

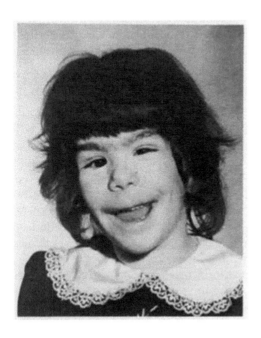

Figure 15.20 A 4-year-old girl with typical appearance of Cornelia de Lange syndrome: Small nose, prominent philtrum, convergent eyebrows, and long, curly eyelashes. (Republished from Sataloff et al. [179] with permission.)

# HUNTINGTON CHOREA

This autosomal dominant degenerative disease has its onset at ~35 years of age. Death generally ensues within 10–15 years. Emotional disturbance is followed by the onset of choreiform movements, seizures, dementia, and death. Cranial nerve deficits, including auditory nerve dysfunction, occur later in the disease (142).

# FRIEDREICH ATAXIA

An autosomal recessive degenerative disease, this entity usually appears in childhood and culminates in death in the midteen years. Early symptoms include ataxia, clumsiness, tremor, ataxic gait, and slurring of speech. Neurological deficits become more severe as the disease progresses. Optic atrophy and, rarely, retinitis pigmentosa occur. Hearing loss is sensorineural, mild, and progressive. These are several other closely related syndromes in which hearing loss is more prominent. Vestibular function testing may show central or peripheral abnormalities (182).

# BASSEN–KORNZWEIG SYNDROME

Abetalipoproteinemia may occur as progressive ataxia in childhood, much like Friedreich ataxia (119, 183). This syndrome is recessive and is associated with sensorineural hearing loss and progressive central nervous system demyelination secondary to the inability to transport triglycerides in the blood. Affected children have fatty stools, weakness, sensory losses, and atypical retinitis pigmentosa. Treatment is dietary modification supplemented with and includes taking high doses of fat-soluble vitamins and linoleic acid but cannot always prevent progression of symptoms.

# UNVERRICHT–LUNDBORG DISEASE

Sensorineural hearing loss may be associated with this recessive syndrome (184). The disease usually develops in childhood and starts as a seizure disorder. Intellectual impairment, cerebellar ataxia, choreoathetosis, and extrapyramidal signs develop along with massive myoclonic epilepsy. Treatment consists of anticonvulsant drug therapy.

## SCHILDER DISEASE

This syndrome probably is recessive (142). It is thought to be a type of multiple sclerosis and involves massive disruption of nerve myelin, especially in the cerebral hemispheres. The onset generally happens in childhood and is always fatal. It manifests as a gait disorder, along with increased intracranial pressure, papilledema, abducens nerve paralysis, and optic neuritis (185). Deafness and cortical blindness may be initial symptoms. The deafness is progressive, and in some cases, it appears to be cortical (186). As yet, no treatment exists. The disease is also known as *encephalitis periaxialis diffusa*, and it is one of a group of diffuse cerebral scleroses.

## NEUROLOGICAL DEFICIENCY

In at least 20 additional syndromes, hearing loss is associated with other neurological deficits. The intimate relationship between the ear and the central nervous system makes this association natural. Despite this, it is tempting to omit a thorough neurological evaluation in patients with hearing loss, particularly in children, who are difficult to test. However, the abundance and gravity of these diseases should encourage diligent attention to a thorough, complete evaluation.

## PENDRED SYNDROME

Nearly 10% of hereditary sensorineural hearing loss is associated with this recessive syndrome of nonendemic goiter and deafness (142). The disease involves abnormal iodine metabolism and appears to be caused by absence of the enzyme iodine peroxidase. The thyroid enlargement usually appears ~8 years of age, but in some cases, it may be present at birth. Later in life, the goiter frequently becomes nodular.

Although patients generally are euthyroid, some may be mildly hypothyroid. Intellectual impairment is noted in some, but not all, cases of Pendred syndrome. The hearing loss usually is congenital, bilateral, sensorineural, and moderate to profound, and it usually is worse in the high frequencies. There may be slow progression during childhood. More than 50% of these patients have a severe hearing deficit (135). Vestibular function frequently is abnormal, although vertigo is uncommon. Inheritance is autosomal recessive. CT of the temporal bones may reveal a Mondini malformation of the cochlea (130, 187, 188).

The disease must be differentiated from *congenital hypothyroidism with deafness*, which may be found in areas where iodine is missing from the diet. However, cretinoid features are absent in Pendred syndrome.

Several laboratory tests, including the perchloride test and the fluorescent thyroid-image test, aid in establishing the diagnosis of this syndrome. Genetic testing can be done to assess the presence of pathogenic genetic mutations. Therapy should include thyroid replacement, and the hearing loss must be treated symptomatically.

## HYPERPROLINEMIA

This autosomal recessive disease is characterized by elevated plasma proline and hyperprolinuria (iminoglycinuria). There are two types (189). In *type 1*, activity of the enzyme proline oxidase is decreased. In *type 2*, proline-5-carboxylate dehydrogenase is deficient. Sensorineural hearing loss is seen in some patients who have *type 1* disease. Prolinemia with intellectual impairment and hearing loss constitutes *Shaffer syndrome*. However, much more work is needed to clarify the nature of this disease and to establish therapy.

## HOMOCYSTINURIA

This autosomal recessive disease is caused by deficiency of the enzyme cystathionine synthase (171). Nearly 60% of patients have intellectual impairment (190). The syndrome is characterized by ectopia lentis (occurring by the age of 10 years), tall stature, long extremities, medial degeneration of the aorta and elastic arteries, malar flush, glaucoma, high-arched palate, cataracts, hepatomegaly, and other anomalies.

Sensorineural hearing loss occurs (118). Homocystinuria is now being treated with a low-methionine diet, cystine supplements, and massive doses of vitamin $B_6$ (189, 191).

## MARFAN SYNDROME

Arachnodactyly, ectopia lentis, and an appearance similar to that of the homocystinuria patient characterize this disease. However, intellectual impairment is not present. Marfan syndrome is inherited in an autosomal dominant fashion and is associated with a mutation in the gene encoding fibrillin-1 (192). Previously, the life expectancy for these patients was 45 years of age due to cardiovascular complications. However, increased screening and treatment of these patients has increased the life expectancy to 72 years (193). Conductive hearing loss may be present, secondary to collapse of the external auditory canals and auricles, caused by cartilaginous abnormalities and inadequate support (2). Persistent otitis media and eustachian tube dysfunction also may lead to conductive hearing loss (192). A few reports of associated sensorineural hearing loss exist.

## MUCOPOLYSACCHARIDOSES

Mucopolysaccharidoses (MPSs) are a group of lysosomal storage disorders that occur due to inability to degrade glycosaminoglycans (GAGs). Currently, there are seven subtypes that are differentiated based on deficiency of 1 of 11 enzymes that are responsible for metabolism of GAGs (151, 194).

**Hurler syndrome** (MPS Type I) is characterized by cloudy corneas, developmental delays, small stature, stiff joints, gargoyle-like facies (**Figure 15.21**), claw-like hand deformities, and death before the age of 10 years without treatment but can be extended into the early 20s and 30s with treatment with alpha L-iduronidase injections and hematopoietic stem cell transplants. The condition usually is recognized during the first year of life through clinical evaluation and with screening for urinary GAGs. The inheritance is autosomal recessive. The nasopharynx is deformed, and lymphoid tissue is markedly increased, leading to nasal obstruction and chronic nasal discharge. This discharge may cause eustachian tube obstruction, compounding middle ear disease. Primary pathology may also be found within the middle ear, however, apparently resulting from the presence of the disease *in utero*. Hurler syndrome can be diagnosed by amniocentesis or chorionic villus sampling. Sensorineural hearing loss may occur in this disease, but it is usually mild (2, 135).

**Scheie syndrome** is an allelic form of Hurler syndrome. The broad mouth and full lips characteristic of gargoylism are present by the age

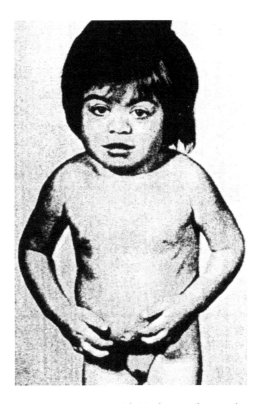

Figure 15.21 Patient with Hurler syndrome showing scaphocephalic cranial enlargement, coarse facies with full lips, flared nostrils, low nasal bridge, and hypertelorism. (From Smith [151], p. 245. Courtesy W.B. Saunders.)

of 8 years. Corneal clouding occurs, as do retinal pigmentation, hirsutism, and aortic valvular defects, which also may be found in the other MPSs. Psychoses and intellectual impairment may occur but are not as striking as in the related syndromes. The lifespan is long, and the inheritance is autosomal recessive. Although documentation is inadequate, it is suspected that mixed hearing loss develops in 10%–20% of these patients, usually in middle age (135).

*Hunter syndrome* (MPS Type II) has a similar habitus but does not show corneal clouding. It is X-linked, so the disease is expressed only in males. The onset of signs and symptoms usually occurs around age 2, and most patients die by the age of 20. However, some patients with the milder form of the syndrome have lived into their 60s. Similar to Hurler syndrome, Hunter syndrome is treated with enzyme replacement therapy (in this case, with idursulfase) and hematopoietic stem cell transplant. About 50% of these cases are accompanied by progressive hearing loss. The loss usually is not severe (195) and is most commonly mixed or sensorineural.

In **Sanfilippo syndrome** (MPS Type III), an autosomal recessive anomaly, hearing loss is uncommon (135). When present, it appears around the age of 6 or 7, and then it progresses. These patients live into mid-adulthood and develop their symptoms early in childhood. They show progressive intellectual impairment, mild coarsening of the facial features, and stiffening of joints.

In **Morquio syndrome** (MPS Type IV), which is also autosomal recessive, mixed hearing loss is common and usually begins in the teen years (196, 197). Recurrent otitis media is also common (194). Onset of symptoms is between ages 1 and 3, and the features are very similar to those of Hurler syndrome, including the corneal clouding. The coarsening of facial features is milder, however. Severe kyphosis and knock knees are characteristic. Treatments include weekly enzyme replacement therapy (with elosulfase alfa) and hematopoietic stem cell transplantation.

Patients with *Maroteaux–Lamy syndrome* (MPS Type VI) show features similar to those of Hurler syndrome, but they do not have progressive intellectual impairment. They usually develop their symptoms and signs somewhat later than in Hurler syndrome, and deformities are generally less severe. By about the age of 8 years, ~25% will exhibit hearing loss (probably conductive), apparently associated with recurrent otitis media (135, 194). The conductive hearing loss can be treated with tympanotomy tube placement or other surgical interventions.

**Sly syndrome** (MPS Type VII) is an autosomal recessive condition characterized by intellectual impairment, skeletal dysplasia, coarse facial features, cardiac abnormalities, and hearing loss. Conductive hearing loss has been seen secondary to recurrent otitis media or cerumen impaction and sensorineural may also occur (194). Due to the rareness of this condition, more research is needed.

**Natowicz syndrome** (MPS Type IX) is an autosomal recessive condition that is extremely rare with only a handful of cases seen. It occurs due to a deficiency of hyaluronidase and leads to accumulation of tissue masses and short stature (194). Hearing loss has not been reported, but

more research is needed to confirm or refute this finding.

Diagnosis of the MPSs is confirmed by detecting stored or excreted specific mucopolysaccharides. Treatment options for these conditions include enzyme replacement therapy that depends on the specific MPS subtype and hematopoietic stem cell transplantation. Currently, it is unknown whether these treatments will have any impact on audiological function. (194).

**Pseudo-Hurler polydystrophy** is an autosomal recessive generalized gangliosidosis rather than a MPS (191). The defects are severe, similar to those of Hurler syndrome, and they include a cherry-red spot in the macula of the eye in about half of the patients. Patients will have characteristic absence of fingers and metacarpals giving a cleft appearance of the hand. Death generally occurs by 2 years of age. Information regarding hearing loss is lacking and will not be truly relevant until some effective therapy is found for the underlying disease.

## ERRORS OF METABOLISM

Most of these diseases are autosomal recessive. *Tay–Sachs disease* is a sphingolipidosis caused by absence of hexosaminidase A (198). This enzyme is now available for treatment of this disease. In addition, a blood test is available to detect carriers. In some areas, the test is performed routinely prior to marriage between Jewish people, among whom the disease is most common in the United States (118). In the infantile form of the disease, flaccidity, motor regression, blindness with a macular cherry-red spot, and apathy begin at ~6 months of age. The disease progresses to spasticity and death by age 3 or 4. In the juvenile form, loss of vision usually is the symptom; the course is slower, and death usually occurs in the 20s. High-frequency sensorineural hearing loss is felt to result from the basic metabolic anomaly (137, 199). Otitis media also is frequent, resulting in a possible mixed hearing loss (200).

**Wilson disease**, or hepatolenticular degeneration, affects the brain, liver, and kidney and may result in deafness (201). The Kayser–Fleischer ring, involving Descemet's membrane of the cornea, is pathognomonic. The disease is caused by deficiency of plasma ceruloplasmin, the primary copper-containing plasma protein. This deficiency produces excess serum copper. The inheritance pattern is autosomal recessive, and a test to detect carriers is available (202). Treatment with fair results relies on low-copper diets and attempts to remove serum copper with chelating agents such as penicillamine and dimercaprol (BAL) (142).

**Fabry Anderson syndrome**, a lipid-storage disease, produces mild sensorineural hearing loss in ~50% of patients (135). The disease is known also as *cardiovasorenal syndrome of Ruiter-Pompen and diffuse angiokeratomas*. It is characterized by elevated blood pressure, heart enlargement, angiokeratomas of the skin, pain in the extremities, abnormalities of sweat secretion, and albuminuria. Frontal bossing and a prominent mandible and lips are common. Corneal clouding may occur, and macular purplish spots on lips and near skin mucosal junctions are common. Death frequently is caused by myocardial infarction or renal failure (203).

Other inborn errors of metabolism, including mannosidosis, other mucolipidoses, and other diseases, may be associated with hearing loss. Some of these diseases may be relatively mild and are easily overlooked unless they are in the differential diagnosis.

## JERVELL AND LANGE–NIELSEN SYNDROME

This syndrome accounts for ~1% of hereditary deafness (142). It is autosomal recessive and is associated with sudden death (204–206). It is known also as *cardioauditory syndrome* and *surdo cardic syndrome*. It is characterized by profound congenital hearing loss and electrocardiographic abnormalities, particularly a prolonged Q–T interval and large T waves, but it also can occur in patients with less severe hearing loss (**Figure 15.22**). No evidence of organic heart disease is found. Often, the disease is first suspected after an episode of fainting early in childhood. Such episodes are probably caused by a Stokes–Adams attack, similar to that seen in adult cardiac patients. This condition should be considered in patients with hearing loss and a family history of sudden death and in any patient with sensorineural hearing loss and a history of fainting (130). Once the diagnosis has been made by electrocardiography, appropriate treatment measures can be taken. In patients with this disease, a high index of suspicion may be lifesaving.

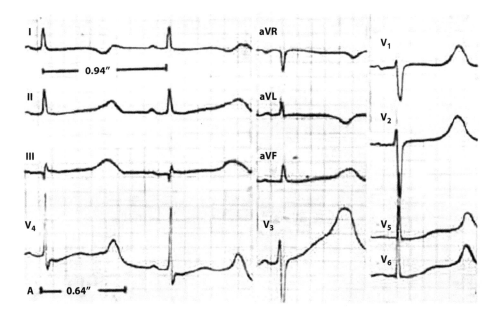

Figure 15.22 Electrocardiogram from a patient with Jervell and Lange–Nielsen syndrome showing prolonged QT intervals of 0.64 second, with 0.41 second begin the upper limit of normal. (From Konigsmark and Gorlin [135], p. 360. Courtesy W.B. Saunders.)

*Noonan syndrome with multiple lentigines* and *Kearns–Sayre* syndrome, already discussed, and a few other diseases, such as Refsum syndrome, may also combine hearing loss with electrocardiographic or cardiac anomalies. This association also occurs in MPSs. In these severe diseases, however, gross pathology is obvious.

## FAMILIAL STREPTOMYCIN OTOTOXICITY

In several families, even low doses of streptomycin have produced severe ototoxicity with impairment of vestibular function (135). Inheritance appears to be autosomal dominant but may be multifactorial. Before prescribing any ototoxic drugs especially streptomycin, a careful history of prior exposure to ototoxic drugs, as well as familial sensitivity to such drugs, is required.

## SICKLE CELL DISEASE

One in every 365 African Americans and 100,000 Americans overall are affected by sickle cell disease (207). This autosomal recessive disease is characterized by anemia, splenomegaly, and attacks of abdominal pain, jaundice, weakness, and anorexia develop. Sensorineural hearing loss occurs in ~20%–25% of patients with the disease (208, 209). Pathology in the inner ear is consistent with ischemic changes and is believed to be due to thromboembolic disease secondary to sickling (210). Sudden total deafness has also been reported and is believed to be caused by a vascular occlusion. In some cases, severe sensorineural hearing loss associated with sickle cell crisis has spontaneously returned to normalcy (211). Treatment is generally symptomatic.

## CYSTIC FIBROSIS

Cystic fibrosis is an autosomal recessive disease and is known also as *mucoviscidosis* or *fibrocystic disease of the pancreas* and occurs with mutations in the CFTR gene that leads to abnormalities in chloride channels of cells that produce mucus and sweat. It affects more than 30,000 people in the United States each year and 1 in every 2500 live births in people of European descent (212).

Currently, newborns are screened for cystic fibrosis in all US states. Mutations to the CFTR gene can lead to pancreatic enzyme deficiency which produces malabsorption and steatorrhea. Children with cystic fibrosis fail to gain weight despite increased appetite. Recurrent respiratory tract infection may be followed by respiratory failure, other organ-system involvement, and death. Improvements in therapy have led to a better prognosis, with the median age of survival being about 50 years. Since patients are living with cystic fibrosis longer, patients are more likely to develop pulmonary exacerbations from bacterial infections that result in decreased lung function. *Pseudomonas aeruginosa* is one of the main culprits that leads to these exacerbations, and patients typically are given an IV course of a combination of antibiotics for treatment (213). Aminoglycosides are used often as a part of combination therapy, and their usage can lead to hearing loss. Adult patients are likely to receive one course of aminoglycosides per year, which can lead to decrease in hearing thresholds (214). When possible, treatment plans that avoid aminoglycosides and other ototoxic drugs should be used to decrease the risk of further hearing loss.

## PRIMARY CILIARY DYSKINESIA

Primary ciliary dyskinesias are autosomal recessive disorders that lead to defects in and impairment of motile cilia (215). The association of situs inversus, bronchiectasis, and sinusitis has been recognized as an entity since 1933 by Kartagener, leading to the name Kartagener syndrome (216), although earlier reports exist in the literature (217). Kartagener syndrome is the most common subtype of primary ciliary dyskinesia and accounts for 50% of cases. In addition to the classic findings (**Figure 15.23**), poor pneumatization of the mastoid air cells and bilateral conductive hearing loss in the 30- to 40-dB range are common (216). The conductive hearing loss is usually due to middle ear fluid, implicating eustachian tube obstruction. Middle ear mucosal biopsy has shown chronic inflammatory changes. All patients with this disease need to be screened for hearing loss and to have their hearing restored medically, surgically, or, if needed, through use of a hearing aid.

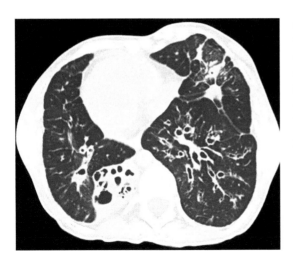

Figure 15.23 Typical bronchiectasis in a patient with Kartagener syndrome.

# IMMUNE DEFICIENCY SYNDROMES

The numerous syndromes that involve hypofunction of the immune system, such as *Wiskott–Aldrich syndrome, ataxia telangiectasia, Bruton agammaglobulinemia, hypogammaglobulinemias, and thymic dysplasia*, are associated with an increased incidence of infection. The ear is frequently involved, and the physician should check for otitis media. This examination is particularly important because in cases of severely depressed immune response, the signs of ear infection may be absent. Nevertheless, the presence of fluid may cause substantial hearing loss and may even lead to more serious otopathology.

# CHROMOSOME ANOMALIES

**Turner syndrome** is characterized by sexual infantilism, streak gonads, short stature, webbed neck (**Figure 15.24**), coarctation of the aorta in 70% of cases, and other stigmata. It is associated with an XO karyotype, and patients are phenotypic females. However, other chromosome anomalies with Turner-like syndromes have been found. About one- to two-thirds of patients exhibit a hearing loss (135). Sensorineural impairment with a bilateral symmetrical dip centered ~2000 Hz is common (218). The underlying etiology of

sensorineural hearing loss is unknown but may be due to the vascular anomalies found in *Turner syndrome* that led to alteration of the vascular supply of the cochlea (219). Conductive hearing loss also is common, and bouts of otitis media or recurring cholesteatoma may occur frequently due to structural abnormalities of the skull and decreased middle ear ventilation (219). Severe deafness can be found in ~10% of cases.

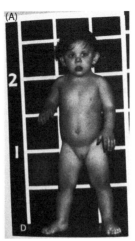
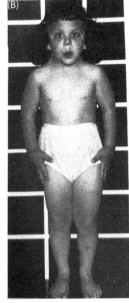

Figure 15.24 A patient with Turner syndrome at age 2 years (A) and 4 years (B), with height ages of 17 months and 3 years, respectively. Note prominent ears, lateral neck web, and hyperconvex deep-set fingernails. (From Smith [151], p. 59. Courtesy W.B. Saunders.)

Similar otologic findings occur in *Klinefelter's syndrome* (XXY karyotype), which is characterized by male phenotypes, medullary gonadal dysgenesis, gynecomastia, and often intellectual impairment (220). Other genotypes have also been reported. *Noonan syndrome* is an autosomal dominant disorder known also as male Turner syndrome without chromosome abnormality. The features are similar, except that in Noonan syndrome (191), intellectual impairment is more likely. Congenital heart disease is also more common and usually consists of pulmonic stenosis. External ear anomalies in these patients also have been described (221). Conductive hearing loss due to otitis media with effusion is the most common hearing loss seen in *Noonan syndrome*. However, sensorineural hearing loss also has been reported (221). Patients with *XX gonadal dysgenesis* are tall females with sexual infantilism. As in Turner syndrome, they have streak gonads. Deafness has been noted in some cases and may be of a severe congenital variety (135).

**Down syndrome**, or **trisomy 21**, is the most common chromosomal condition diagnosed in the United States and occurs in approximately 1 in every 700 live births (121). The more familiar features (**Figure 15.25**) include the mongoloid slanted and widespread eyes, epicanthus, nystagmus, abnormal earlobes, intellectual impairment, short stature, gap between the great and second toe, broad, at hand, and protuberant abdomen. Up to 78% of patients with *Down* syndrome report conductive hearing loss, although sensorineural, and mixed hearing loss may also occur (222–225).

*Trisomy 13, trisomy 18, chromosome 18 long-arm deletion syndrome, chromosome 4 short-arm deletion syndrome,* and *cri-du-chat syndrome (chromosome 5 short-arm deletion syndrome)* are other major chromosome anomalies that may be associated with hearing loss.

## NO ASSOCIATED ANOMALIES

Recessive sensorineural hearing loss without associated defects is the most common form of hereditary hearing loss (2). It usually is not progressive and generally is congenital, bilateral, and may vary from mild to severe. Certain audiometric patterns, such as the sloping type (**Figure 15.26**) and basin-shaped curve (**Figure 15.27**), are particularly characteristic of hereditary hearing loss, but nearly any pattern may occur. Vestibular function is typically normal. X-linked inheritance may also occur (135, 226) (**Figures 15.28** and **15.29**). Dominant sensorineural hearing loss first occurs between the ages of 6 and 12 years. The hearing loss is most commonly bilateral, progressive, and high frequency (147). As in recessive and X-linked hearing loss, however, any pattern may occur.

**Hereditary progressive sensorineural hearing loss** is also quite common and may be dominant or recessive. Colloquially, this condition is often

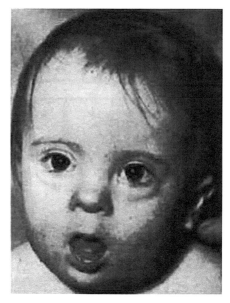

Figure 15.25 Infant with Down syndrome showing at facies, straight hair, protrusion of tongue, inner canthal folds, small auricles, and speckling of iris with lack of peripheral patterning. (From Smith [151], p. 35. Courtesy W.B. Saunders.)

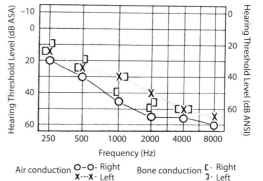

Figure 15.26 *History*: A 7-year-old boy whose mother noted poor hearing when the child was 2. Speech development was slow. He had difficulty pronouncing sibilants, and *s* was slurred. An older brother had a similar hearing loss. The hearing problem was nonprogressive in both children. *Otologic*: Ears normal. *Audiologic*: Pure-tone air and bone conduction thresholds indicate a bilateral, gradually sloping loss with no air–bone gap. *Speech reception threshold*: Right, 38 dB; left, 38 dB. *Discrimination score*: Right, 78%; left, 80%. There was no abnormal tone decay. *Classification*: Sensorineural hearing loss. *Diagnosis*: Menasse-type congenital hereditary hearing loss. *Abbreviations*: ANSI, American National Standards Institute; ASA, American Standards Association.

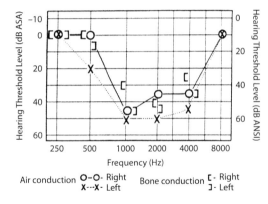

Air conduction **O–O**- Right    Bone conduction **⊏**- Right
               **X···X**- Left                    **⊐**- Left

**Figure 15.27** *History*: This child's father had a similarly shaped audiogram and a deep monotonous voice, which was apparent also in the child. Enunciation was good. *Otologic*: Ears normal. *Audiologic*: Air and bone conduction thresholds reveal a bilateral, basin-shaped curve with no air–bone gap. Right ear discrimination was 80% at 70 dB. *Classification*: Sensorineural. *Diagnosis*: Congenital and inherited. *Abbreviations*: ANSI, American National Standards Institute; ASA, American Standards Association.

referred to as *genetic deafness*. This condition is characterized by sensorineural hearing loss that gets gradually worse over time. It is most commonly worse in the higher frequencies, but patterns resembling a 4000-Hz dip are not rare. The audiogram pattern frequently resembles that of presbycusis, but the condition usually becomes apparent in the second, third, fourth, or fifth decades. When similar hearing loss has occurred in previous generations of the same family, dominant hereditary progressive hearing loss may be diagnosed. However, absence of a positive family history does not rule out this condition. A recessive inheritance pattern is common.

**Hereditary Ménière's syndrome** is a dominant disorder but is rare (227). Like sporadic Ménière's disease, it is characterized by fluctuating hearing loss, episodic vertigo, and tinnitus.

**Otosclerosis** is found histologically at autopsy in ~10% of white people and in ~20% of patients >60 years (**Figure 15.30**) (2, 228). The incidence is much lower in black patients. Inheritance follows

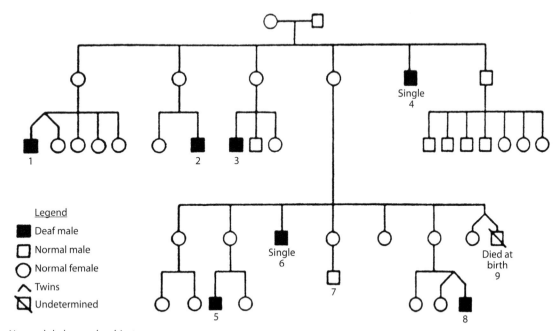

**Figure 15.28** This family tree indicates some interesting genetic aspects of sex-linked hereditary deafness. Audiograms were available for this family for all the living persons with profound congenital nerve deafness. Not all the members of this family have been given hearing tests, but those reported as not deaf have normal speech and clinically normal hearing as reported by close relatives. (From Sataloff et al. [226].)

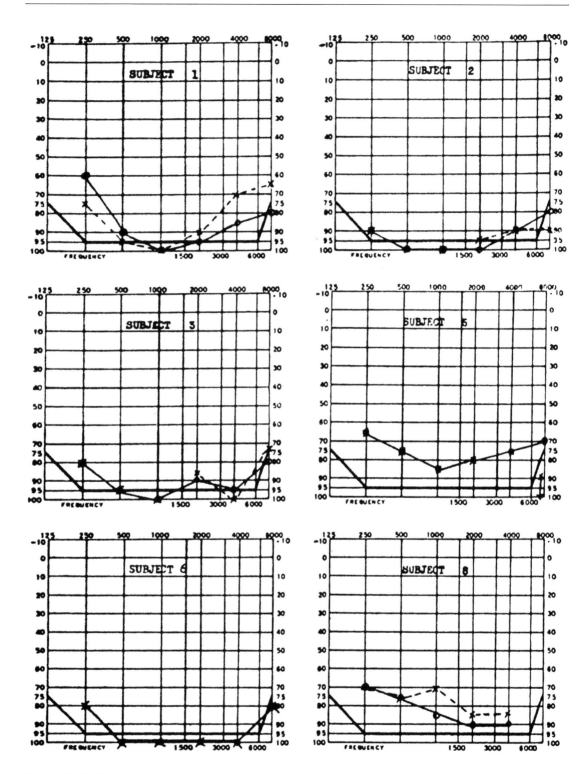

Figure 15.29 The audiogram obtained on six of the seven deaf individuals in the family referred to in **Figure 15.28** (Subjects 4, 7, and 9 are not shown.) *Subject 1* (in **Figures 15.28** and **15.29**) was 53 years of age and had little intelligible speech. He was the first-born and only male child in his family and had a twin sister. *Subject 2* was a 44-year-old deaf-mute. He was the first-born and only male. *Subject 3* was a 37-year-old first-born man who received his education at a school for the deaf. *Subject 4*

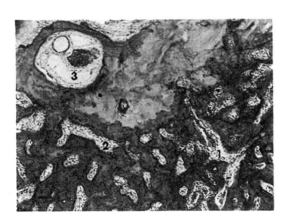

Figure 15.30 Otosclerotic bone showing a focus of otospongiosis (1), otosclerosis (2), and adjacent normal bone. Jacobson's nerve is seen on the promontory (3). (From Linthicum and Schwartzman [119], p. 49. Courtesy W.B. Saunders.)

an autosomal dominant pattern with variable penetrance and female predilection. It can occur as conductive or mixed hearing loss. Although controversial, there is reason to believe that otosclerosis can occur purely as sensorineural hearing loss with cochlear involvement alone.

In general, the hearing loss in otosclerosis is slowly progressive and usually occurs in early adult life. Vestibular function is usually normal. Frequently, otosclerosis is accelerated by pregnancy. The conductive component of the hearing loss can be treated by stapedectomy or with a hearing aid. Sodium fluoride may be helpful in selected cases (229).

Numerous other patterns of isolated hereditary hearing loss or hereditary hearing loss associated with malformations of the ears occur.

## SUMMARY

Fortunately, many of the hereditary causes of hearing loss are preventable or treatable. Most of the syndromes involve known inheritance patterns, which makes genetic counseling useful in their management. Recessive syndromes can be minimized by avoiding consanguineous marriages. Screening programs, such as for sickle cell trait and Tay–Sachs disease, are also helpful.

Many of the inborn errors of metabolism and chromosome anomalies can be detected *in utero* by amniocentesis, chorionic villus sampling, or blood tests. The effects of maternal and paternal advanced age and other factors associated with increased appearance of congenital anomalies can be minimized as physician and patient populations become more familiar with these diseases and their causes.

disappeared >40 years ago at the age of 7. At that time, he was known to be deaf and unable to speak. *Subject 5* was a 16-year-old attending a school for the deaf. He was the first-born son and had a sister, whose hearing is normal. He used a hearing aid with fair results and had fairly intelligible speech. The usefulness of early amplification and adequate training is evident in this subject. *Subject 6* was a 37-year-old bachelor classified as a deaf-mute with little intelligible speech. *Subject 7* was a 5-year-old first-born male child with normal hearing and speech. He was conceived after a 5-year period of apparent sterility requiring dilatation and curettage (D and C). The mother denied any miscarriages or abortions prior to the subject's birth. *Subject 8* was a 3-year-old first-born male and had a twin sister. He had no speech and had profound nerve deafness. Both his twin sister and older sister had normal hearing and speech development. The hearing threshold on this youngster was obtained with repeatedly consistent psychogalvanic skin resistance tests. *Subject 9* was a male twin who died at birth. There are three sets of twins in the pedigree. In each set, there is a male and female, and the male was the first-born son and demonstrated deaf mutism in two of the three sets. It is apparent from this pedigree that deafness is manifest only in males and is transmitted through the maternal side. There are seven first-born males with profound congenital nerve deafness, a condition not present in subsequently born males or found in any females. There are insufficient subsequent males to establish statistically that deafness is restricted to the first-born males. Deafness did not exist in the children of the normal male member of the pedigree. The family pedigree exhibited demonstrates clearly that profound congenital nerve deafness can be hereditary and sex-linked. Early recognition and adequate educational measures are essential in such instances. (From Sataloff et al. [226].)

# REFERENCES

1. Asher P. A study of 63 cases of athetosis with special reference to hearing defects. Arch Dis Child 1952; 27:475–477.
2. Schuknecht H. Pathology of the Ear. Cambridge, MA: Harvard University Press, 1974; 168–184, 262–266, 311–330, 374–379, 383–388, 420–424, 444–446, 488.
3. Coquette M. Les sequelles neurologiques tardives de l'ictere nucleaire. Ann Pediatr 1944; 163:83–104.
4. Olds C, Oghalai JS. Audiologic impairment associated with bilirubin-induced neurologic damage. Semin Fetal Neonatal Med 2015; 20(1):42–46.
5. Barnett HL, Einhorn AH. Pediatrics. 15th ed. New York, NY: Appleton-Century-Crofts, 1972:1676–1682.
6. Wintrobe MM, Thorn GW, Adams RD et al. Harrison's Principles of Internal Medicine. 7th ed. New York, NY: McGraw-Hill, 1974:964–966.
7. Barr B, Lundstrom R. Deafness following maternal rubella. Acta Otolaryngol 1961; 53:413–423.
8. Vaughan VC, McKay RJ, Nelson WE. Textbook of Pediatrics. 10th ed. Philadelphia: Saunders, 1969:659–663.
9. Sataloff J. Hearing Loss. Philadelphia: Lippincott, 1966:142, 379–381.
10. Paparella MM. Otologic manifestations of viral disease. Adv Otorhinolaryngol 1973; 20:144–154.
11. Linday JR. Histopathology of deafness due to postnatal viral disease. Arch Otolaryngol 1973; 98:218–227.
12. Hardy JB. Fetal consequences of maternal viral infections in pregnancy. Arch Otolaryngol 1973; 98:218–227.
13. Brook I. The role of anaerobic bacteria in otitis media: Microbiology, pathogenesis, and implications on therapy Infect Dis 1987; 8:109–117.
14. Ficenec SC, Schieffelin JS, Emmett SD. A review of hearing loss associated with Zika, Ebola, and Lassa fever. Am J Trop Med Hyg Sep 2019; 101(3):484–490.
15. Meng X, Wang J, Sun J, Zhu K. COVID-19 and sudden sensorineural hearing loss: a systematic review. Front Neurol 2022; 13:883749.
16. Mehraeen E, Afzalian A, Afsahi AM, et al. Hearing loss and COVID-19: an umbrella review. Eur Arch Otorhinolaryngol Aug 2023; 280(8):3515–3528.
17. Chandrasekhar SS, Tsai Do BS, Schwartz SR, et al. Clinical practice guideline: sudden hearing loss (update). Otolaryngol Head Neck Surg Aug 2019; 161(1_suppl):S1–s45.
18. Tsuda T, Hanada Y, Wada K, Fujiwara E, Takeda K, Nishimura H. Efficacy of intratympanic glucocorticoid steroid administration therapy as an initial treatment for idiopathic sudden sensorineural hearing loss during the COVID-19 pandemic. Ear Nose Throat J Jul 12 2021; 100:1455613211032534
19. Holmes GP, McCormick JB, Trock SC, et al. Lassa fever in the United States. N Engl J Med 1990; 323(16):1120–1123.
20. Ryback LP. Deafness associated with Lassa fever. JAMA 1990; 264(16):2119.
21. Mateer EJ, Huang C, Shehu NY, Paessler S. Lassa fever-induced sensorineural hearing loss: A neglected public health and social burden. PLoS Negl Trop Dis Feb 2018; 12(2):e0006187.
22. Hanner P, Rosenhall U, Edstrom S, Kaijser B. Hearing impairment in patients with antibody production against Borrelia burgdoferi antigen. Lancet 1989; 1(8628):13–15.
23. Fox GM, Heilskov T, Smith JL. Cogan's syndrome and seroreactivity to Lyme borreliosis. J Clin Neuro Ophthalmol 1990; 10(2):83–87.
24. Sowula K, Szaleniec J, Stolcman K, Ceranowicz P, Kocoń S, Tomik J. Association between sudden sensorineural hearing loss and Lyme disease. J Clin Med Mar 8 2021; 10(5):1130.
25. Peeters N, van der Kolk BY, Thijsen SF, Colnot DR. Lyme disease associated with sudden sensorineural hearing loss: case report and literature review. Otol Neurotol Jul 2013; 34(5):832–837.
26. Espiney Amaro C, Montalvão P, Huins C, Saraiva J. Lyme disease: sudden hearing loss as the sole presentation. J Laryngol Otol Feb 2015; 129(2):183–186.
27. Mokry M, Flaschka G, Kleinert G, Kleinert R, Fazekas F, Kopp W. Chronic Lyme disease with an expansive granulomatous lesion in the cerebellopontine angle. Neurosurgery 1990; 27(3):446–451.

28. Coleman CU, Green I, Archibold RAK. Cutaneous pneumocystosis. Ann Inter Med 1987; 106:396–398.

29. Sandler ED, Sandler JM, Leboit PE, Wening BM, Mortensen N. Pneumocystis carnii otitis media in AIDS: A case report and review of the literature regarding extrapulmonary pneumocystosis. Otolaryngol Head Neck Surg 1990; 103(5)Part 1:817–821.

30. Witt LS, Wendy Fujita A, Ho J, Shin YM, Kobaidze K, Workowski K. Otosyphilis. Open Forum Infect Dis Feb 2023; 10(2):ofac685.

31. Nadol JB. Hearing loss as a sequela of meningitis. Laryngoscope 1978; 88:739–755.

32. Keane WM, Potsic WP, Rowe LD et al. Meningitis and hearing loss in children. Arch Otolaryngol 1979; 105:39–44.

33. Paparella MM, Shumrick PA. Otolaryngology. Vol. 2. Philadelphia: W.B. Saunders, 1973:161–167.

34. Dillard LK, Martinez RX, Perez LL, Fullerton AM, Chadha S, McMahon CM. Prevalence of aminoglycoside-induced hearing loss in drug-resistant tuberculosis patients: A systematic review. J Infect Jul 2021; 83(1):27–36.

35. Crouser ED, Maier LA, Wilson KC, et al. Diagnosis and detection of sarcoidosis. An official American Thoracic Society clinical practice guideline. Am J Respir Crit Care Med Apr 15 2020; 201(8):e26–e51.

36. Hybels RL, Rice DH. Neuro-otologic manifestations of sarcoidosis. Laryngoscope 1976; 86:1873–1878.

37. Arsovic N, Babic B, Dimitrijevic M, Bukurov B, Vucinic V. Otitis media and facial paralysis as presenting symptoms of a primary middle ear sarcoidosis. Otol Neurotol Oct 2013; 34(8):e121–e122.

38. Blarr IM, Lawrence M. Otologic manifestations of fatal granulomatosis of the respiratory tract. Arch Otolaryngol 1961; 73:639–643.

39. Karmody CS. Wegener's granulomatosis: presentation as an otologic problem. Otorhinolaryngol 1978; 86:574–584.

40. Hill JH, Graham MD, Gikas PW. Obliterative fibrotic middle ear disease in systemic vasculitis. Ann Otol Rhinol Laryngol 1980; 89:162–164.

41. Rahne T, Plontke S, Keyßer G. Vasculitis and the ear: a literature review. Curr Opin Rheumatol Jan 2020; 32(1):47–52.

42. Keleman G. Histiocytosis involving the temporal bone (Letterer-Siew, Hand-Schuller-Christian). Laryngoscope 1960; 70:1284–1304.

43. Schwartzman JA, Pulec JL, Linthicum FH. Uncommon granulomatous disease of the ear. Ann Otol Rhinol Laryngol 1972; 81:389–393.

44. Schuknecht NF Perlman HB. Hand-Schuller-Christian disease of the skull. Ann Otol Rhinol Laryngol 1948; 57:643–676.

45. Ikeda K, Kobayashi T, Kusakari J, Takasaka T, Yumita S, Furukawa T. Sensorineural hearing loss associated with hypoparathyroidism. Laryngoscope 1987; 97:1075–1979.

46. Pulec J. Symposium on Ménière's disease. Laryngoscope 1972; 82:1703–1715.

47. Spencer JT Jr. Hyperlipoproteinemia in the etiology of inner ear disease. Laryngoscope 1973; 83:639–678.

48. Kent SJ, von Gierke HE, Tolan GD. Analysis of the potential association between noise-induced hearing loss and cardiovascular disease in USAF aircrew members. Aviation Space Environ Med April 1986; 57(4):348–361.

49. Takala J, Varke S, Vaheri E, Sievers K. Noise and blood pressure. Lancet November 1977; 2(8045): 974–975.

50. Hedstrand H, Drettner B, Klockhoff I, Svedberg A. Noise and blood-pressure. Lancet December 1977; 2(8045): 1291.

51. Manninen O, Aro S. Noise-induced hearing loss and blood pressure. Int Arch Occup Environ Health 1979; 42:251–256.

52. Manninen O. Cardiovascular changes and hearing threshold shifts in men under complex exposures to noise, whole body vibrations, temperatures, and competition-type psychic load. Int Arch Occup Environ Health 1985; 56:251–274.

53. Pillsbury HC. Hypertension, hyperlipoproteinemia, chronic noise exposure: is there synergism in cochlear pathology? Laryngoscope 1986; 96:1112–1138.

54. Colletti V, Fiorino FG. Myocardial activity during noise exposure. Acta Otolaryngol, 1987; 104:217–224.

55. Verbeek JHAM, van Dijk FJH, de Vries FF. Non-auditory effects of noise in industry. Int Arch Occup Environ Health 1987; 59:51–54.

56. Carter NL, Beh HC. The effect of intermittent noise on cardiovascular functioning during vigilance task performance. Psychophysiology 1989; 26(5):548–559.

57. Andriukin AA. Influence of sound stimulation on the development of hypertension. Cor VASA 1961; 3(4):285–293.

58. Carter NL. Heart-rate and blood-pressure response in medium-artillery gun crews. Med J Aust 1988; 149:185–189.

59. Cavatorta A, Falzoi M, Romanelli A, et al. Adrenal response in the pathogenesis of arterial hypertension in workers exposed to high noise levels. J Hypertension 1987; 5(suppl. 5):S463–S466.

60. Wu TN, Ko YC, Chang PY. Study of noise exposure and high blood pressure in shipyard workers. Am J Industr Med 1987; 12:431–438.

61. Flynn AJ, Dengerink HA, Wright JW. Blood pressure in resting, anesthetized and noise exposed guinea pigs. Hear Res 1988; 34:201–206.

62. Gold S, Haran I, Attias J, Shapira I, Shahar A. Biochemical and cardiovascular measures in subjects with noise-induced hearing loss. J Occup Med 1989; 31(11):933–937.

63. Michalak R, Ising H, Rebentisch E. Acute circulatory effects of military low-altitude flight noise. Int Arch Occup Environ Health 1990; 62:365–372.

64. Theorell T. Family history of hypertension—an individual trait interacting with spontaneously occurring job stressors. Scand J Work Environ Health 1990; 16(suppl. 1):74–79.

65. Milkovic-Kraus S. Noise-induced hearing loss and blood pressure. Int Arch Occup Environ Health 1990; 62:259–260.

66. Tarter SK, Robins TG. Chronic noise exposure, high-frequency hearing loss, and hypertension among automotive assembly workers. J Occup Med 1990; 32(8):685–689.

67. Talbott EO, Findlay RC, Kuller LH, et al. Noise-induced hearing loss: a possible marker for high blood pressure in older noise-exposed populations. J Occup Med 1990; 32(8):690–697.

68. Tan TY, Rahmat O, Prepageran N, Fauzi A, Noran NH, Raman R. Hypertensive retinopathy and sensorineural hearing loss. Indian J Otolaryngol Head Neck Surg Dec 2009; 61(4):275–279.

69. Esparza CM, Jáuregui-Renaud K, Morelos CMC, et al. Systemic high blood pressure and inner ear dysfunction: a preliminary study. Clinical Otolaryngology 2007; 32(3):173–178.

70. Reed NS, Huddle MG, Betz J, et al. Association of Midlife Hypertension with Late-Life Hearing Loss. *Otolaryngol Head Neck Surg.* Dec 2019; 161(6):996–1003.

71. Gates GA, Mills JH. Presbycusis. The Lancet (British edition) 2005; 366(9491):1111–1120.

72. Zoller M, Nadol JB, Girard KF. Detection of syphilitic hearing loss. Arch Otolaryngol 1978; 104:63–65.

73. Wiet RJ, Milko DA. Isolation of spirochetes in the perilymph despite prior antisyphilitic therapy. Arch Otolaryngol 1975; 101:104–106.

74. Mach LW, Smith JL, Walter EK, Montenegro E N, Nicol W G. Temporal bone treponemes. Arch Otolaryngol 1969; 90:11–14.

75. Smith JL. Spirochetes in late seronegative syphilis, despite penicillin therapy. Med Times 1968; 96:621–623.

76. Andrade CLO, Alves CAD, Ramos HE. Congenital hypothyroidism and the deleterious effects on auditory function and language skills: a narrative review. Front Endocrinol 2021; 12:671784.

77. Meyerhoff WL. Hearing loss and thyroid disorders. Minn Med 1974; 57(11):987–998.

78. Trotter WR. The association of deafness with thyroid dysfunction. Br Med Bull 1960; 16:92–98.

79. Bataskis JG, Nishiyama RH. Deafness with sporadic goiter. Pendred's syndrome. Arch Otolaryngol 1962; 76:401–406.

80. Hsu A, Tsou YA, Wang TC, Chang WD, Lin CL, Tyler RS. Hypothyroidism and related comorbidities on the risks of developing tinnitus. Sci Rep. Mar 1 2022; 12(1):3401.

81. McCabe B. Autoimmune sensorineural hearing loss. American Neurotological Society Meeting. Los Angeles, 1979: 30–31.

82. Bowman CA, Nelson RA. Human leukocytic antigens in autoimmune sensorineural hearing loss. Laryngoscope 1987; 97:7–9.

83. Johnson DW, Mathog RH. Hearing function and chronic renal failure. Ann Otol Rhinol Laryngol 1976; 85:43–49.

84. Johnson LG, Hawkins JE. Sensory and neural degeneration with aging as seen in microdissections of the human ear. Ann Otol Rhinol Laryngol 1972; 81:179–183.

85. Cooper AF, Curry AR. The pathology of deafness in the affective and paranoid psychoses of later life. J Psychosom Res 1976; 20:97–105.

86. Naufal PM. Primary sarcomas of the temporal bone. Arch Otolaryngol 1973; 98:44–50.

87. Conley JJ. Cancer of the middle ear and temporal bone. NY State J Med 1974; 74:1575–1579.

88. Clairmont AA, Conley JJ. Primary carcinoma of the mastoid bone. Ann Otol Rhinol Laryngol 1977; 86:306–309.

89. Schuknecht HF, Allan AF, Murakami Y. Pathology of secondary malignant tumors of the temporal bone. Ann Otol Rhinol Laryngol 1968; 77:5–22.

90. Ramsden RT, Bulman CH, Lorigan BP. Osteoradionecrosis of the temporal bone. J Laryngol Otol 1975; 8(9):941–955.

91. Yuhan BT, Nguyen BK, Svider PF, et al. Osteoradionecrosis of the temporal bone: an evidence-based approach. Otol Neurotol Oct 2018; 39(9):1172–1183.

92. Jaffe BF, Penner JA. Sudden deafness associated with hypercoagulation. Trans Am Acad Ophthalmol Otol 1968; 72:774–778.

93. Glasscock ME. Surgery of glomus tumors of the temporal bone. Middle Section Meeting, American Laryngological, Rhinological, and Otological Society, Inc., Indianapolis, IN, Jan 1979:19–21.

94. Conley J, Hildyard V. Aneurysm of the internal carotid artery presenting in the middle ear. Arch Otolaryngol 1969; 90:61–64.

95. Podoshin L, Fradis M, Pillar T, Zisman D. Senso-neural hearing loss as an expression of arteriosclerosis in young people. Eye Ear Noise Throat Monthly 1975; 54:18–23.

96. Shapiro SLP. Otologic aspects of the subclavian steal syndrome. Eye Ear Nose Throat Monthly 1971; 50:28–31.

97. Hiller F. The vascular syndromes of basilar and vertebral arteries and their branches. J Nerv Ment Dis 1952; 116:988–1016.

98. Vick NA. Grinker's Neurology, 7th ed. Charles C Thomas, Springfield, IL, 1976: 486–492.

99. Hallpike C. Clinical otoneurology and its contributions to theory and practice. Proc R Soc Med 1965; 58:185–196.

100. Malhotra A, Ayappa I, Ayas N, et al. Metrics of sleep apnea severity: beyond the apnea-hypopnea index. Sleep Jul 9 2021; 44(7):zsab030.

101. Kasemsuk N, Chayopasakul V, Banhiran W, et al. Obstructive sleep apnea and sensorineural hearing loss: a systematic review and meta-analysis. Otolaryngol Head Neck Surg. 2023; 169(2):201–209.

102. Wang C, Xu F, Chen M, et al. Association of obstructive sleep apnea-hypopnea syndrome with hearing loss: a systematic review and meta-analysis. Front Neurol 2022; 13:1017982.

103. Sardesai MG, Tan AK, Fitzpatrick M. Noise-induced hearing loss in snorers and their bed partners. J Otolaryngol Jun 2003; 32(3):141–145.

104. Mirmosayyeb O, Naderi M, Raeisi S, et al. Hearing loss among patients with multiple sclerosis (PwMS): a systematic review and meta-analysis. Mult Scler Relat Disord Jun 2022; 62:103754.

105. von Leden H, Horton B. Auditory nerve in multiple sclerosis. Arch Otolaryngol 1948; 48:51–57.

106. Imperato PJ. Tropical diseases of the ear, nose and throat. In: English GM, ed. Otolaryngology. Vol. 5. Philadelphia: Harper & Row, 1979:32–41.

107. Blackwell DL, Lucas JW, Clarke TC. Summary health statistics for U.S. adults: National Health Interview Survey, 2012 (PDF). National Center for Health Statistics. Vital Health Stat 10(260). 2014.

108. Young A, Ng M. Genetic Hearing Loss. [Updated 2023 Apr 17]. In: StatPearls [Internet]. Treasure Island (FL): StatPearls Publishing; 2024 Jan-. Available from: https://www.ncbi.nlm.nih.gov/books/NBK580517/

109. National Diabetes Statistics Report (no date) Centers for Disease Control and Prevention. Available from: https://www.cdc.gov/diabetes/php/data-research/index.html#:~:text=29.7%20million%20people%20of%20all,304%2C000%20with%20type%201%20diabetes. (Accessed: 29 June 2022).

110. Horikawa C, Kodama S, Tanaka S, et al. Diabetes and risk of hearing impairment in adults: a meta-analysis. J Clin Endocrinol Metab 2013; 98(1):51–58.

111. Axelsson A, Fagerberg SE. Auditory function in diabetes. Acta Otolaryngol 1988; 66:49–64.

112. Kitabchi AE, Shea JJ, Duckworth WC, Adams F. High incidence of diabetes and glucose intolerance in fluctuant hearing loss. J Lab Clin Med 1971; 78(6):995–996.

113. Jorgensen MB. Sudden loss of inner ear function in the course of long standing diabetes mellitus. Acta Otolaryngol 1960; 51:579–584.

114. Rosen Z, Davis E. Microangiopathy in diabetics with hearing disorders. Eye Ear Nose Throat Monthly 1971; 50:31–35.

115. Triana RJ, Suits GW, Garrison S, et al. Inner ear damage secondary to diabetes mellitus. Arch Otolaryngol Head Neck Surg 1991; 117:635–640.

116. Weille F. Hypoglycemia in Ménière's disease. Arch Otolaryngol 1968; 87:555–557.

117. Parkin JL, Tice R. Hypoglycemia and fluctuating hearing loss. Ann Otol Rhinol Laryngol 1970; 79:992–997.

118. Proctor C. Diagnosis, prevention and treatment of hereditary sensorineural hearing loss. Laryngoscope 1977; 87:1–60.

119. Linthicum FH, Schwartzman JA. An Atlas of Micropathology of the Temporal Bone. Philadelphia: W.B. Saunders, 1974:58–60, 70–72, 74–75.

120. Grace LG. Frequency of occurrence of cleft palates and harelips. J Dent Res 1943; 22:495–497.

121. Mai CT, Isenburg JL, Canfield MA, et al. National population-based estimates for major birth defects, 2010-2014. Birth Defects Res Nov 1 2019; 111(18):1420–1435.

122. Dixon MJ, Marazita ML, Beaty TH, Murray JC. Cleft lip and palate: understanding genetic and environmental influences. Nat Rev Genet Mar 2011; 12(3):167–178.

123. Gorlin RJ, Cervenka J, Pruzansky S. Facial clefting and its syndromes. Birth defects. Original Article Series 1971; 7:3–49.

124. Sataloff J, Fraser M. Hearing loss in children with cleft palates. AMA Arch Otolaryng 1952; 55(1):61–64.

125. Goudy S, Lott D, Canady J, Smith RJ. Conductive hearing loss and otopathology in cleft palate patients. Otolaryngol Head Neck Surg Jun 2006; 134(6):946–948.

126. Kloepfer H, Lagvaite J. The hereditary syndrome of congenital deafness and retinitis pigmentosa (Usher's syndrome). Laryngoscope 1966; 76:850–862.

127. Hallgren V. Retinitis pigmentosa combined with congenital deafness; with vestibulo-cerebellar ataxia and mental abnormality in a proportion of cases. A clinical and genetico-statistical study. Acta Psychiatr Scand Suppl 1959; 138:1–101.

128. McLeod AC, McConnel FE, Sweeney A, Cooper MC, Nance WE. Clinical variation in Usher's syndrome. Arch Otolaryngol 1971; 94:321–334.

129. Landau J, Feinmesser M. Audiometric and vestibular examination in retinitis pigmentosa. Br J Ophthalmol 1956; 40:40–44.

130. Bayazit YA, Yilmaz M. An overview of hereditary hearing loss. ORL J Otorhinolaryngol Relat Spec 2006; 68(2):57–63.

131. Davenport SLH, Omenn GS. The heterogeneity of Usher syndrome [abstract 215]. Fifth International Conference on Birth Defects, Montreal, 1977:21–27.

132. Refsum S. Heredopathia atactia polyneuritiformis. Acta Psychiatr Scand 1946; 38(suppl.):1–303.

133. Bamiou D-E, Spraggs PRD, Gibberd FB, Sidey MC, Luxon LM. Hearing loss in adult Refsum's disease. Clin Otolaryngol Allied Sci 2003; 28(3):227–230.

134. Steinberg D, Mize CE, Herndon JH Jr., Fales HM, Engel WK, Vroom FQ. Phytanic acid in patients with Refsum's syndrome and response to treatment. Arch Intern Med 1970; 125:75–87.

135. Konigsmark BW, Gorlin RJ. Genetic and Metabolic Deafness. Philadelphia: W.B. Saunders, 1976:40–41, 76, 98–100, 156–159, 164–168, 188–191, 221–222, 311–312, 330–335, 345–351, 355, 364–370.

136. Alstrom CH, Hallgren B, Nilsson LBN, Asander H. Retinal degeneration combined with obesity, diabetes mellitus and neurogenous deafness. Acta Psychiatr Neurol Scand Suppl 1959; 129:1–35.

137. Paddison RM, Moossy J, Derbes VJ, Kloepfer W. Cockayne's syndrome. Derm Trop Ecol Geogr 1963; 2:195–203.

138. Newell PW, Ernest JT. Ophthalmology. 3rd ed. Mosby, St. Louis, MO, 1974:332.

139. Seth RRS, Dayal D. Inner ear involvement in primary glaucoma. Ear Nose Throat J 1978; 57:69–75.

140. Shih MC, Gordis TM, Lambert PR, Nguyen SA, Meyer TA. Hearing loss in exfoliation syndrome: systematic review and meta-analysis. Laryngoscope May 2023; 133(5):1025–1035.

141. Papadopoulos TA, Naxakis SS, Charalabopoulou M, Vathylakis I, Goumas PD, Gartaganis SP. Exfoliation syndrome related to sensorineural hearing loss. Clin Exp Ophthalmol Jul 2010; 38(5):456–461.

142. Proctor C. Hereditary deafness. American Academy of Ophthalmology and Otolaryngology, 1975 Instructional Section, Course 543; 2–4, 14.

143. Wilson J. Leber's hereditary optic atrophy: some clinical and aetiological considerations. Brain 1963; 86:347–362.

144. Warburg M. Norie's disease (atrofia bulborum hereditaria). Acta Ophthalmol 1963; 41:134–146.

145. Cogan DG. Syndrome of non-syphilitic interstitial keratitis and vestibulo-auditory symptoms. Arch Ophthalmol 1945; 33:144–149.

146. Alport AC. Hereditary familial congenital hemorrhagic nephritis. Br Med J 1927; 1:504–506.

147. Proctor C. Hereditary Sensorineural Hearing Loss, American Academy of Ophthalmology and Otolaryngology. Rochester, MN, 1978:5–24.

148. Muckle TJ, Well M. Urticaria, deafness and amyloidosis: a new heredo-familial syndrome. Q J Med 1962; 31:235–248.

149. Proctor C. Hereditary deafness, American Academy of Ophthalmology and Otolaryngology, 1971, Instructional Section, Course 516, 6.

150. Herrman C Jr, Aquilar MJ, Sacks OW. Hereditary photomyoclonus associated with diabetes mellitus, deafness, nephropathy, and cerebral dysfunction. Neurology 1964; 14:212–221.

151. Smith DW. Recognizable Patterns of Human Malformation. Philadelphia: W.B. Saunders, 1970:60–61, 242–255.

152. Tietz W. A syndrome of deaf-mutism associated with albinism showing dominant autosomal inheritance. Am J Hum Genet 1963; 15:259–264.

153. Waardenburg PJ. A new syndrome combining developmental anomalies of the eyelids, eyebrows and nose root with pigmentary defects of the iris and head hair and with congenital deafness. Am J Hum Genet 1951; 3:195–253.

154. Gorlin RJ, Anderson RD, Moller JH. The LEOPARD (multiple lentigines) syndrome revisited. Birth Defects 1971; 7(4):110–115.

155. Batsakis JG. Tumors of the Head and Neck. Baltimore: Williams & Wilkins, 1974:231–235.

156. Kongismark BW. Hereditary deafness in man, part 2. N Engl J Med 1969; 281(14):776–777.

157. Poretta CA, Dahlin DC, James JM. Sarcoma in Paget's disease of bone. J Bone Joint Surg 1957; 39A:1314–1329.

158. Kravets I. Paget's disease of bone: diagnosis and treatment. Am J Med Nov 2018; 131(11):1298–1303.

159. Sataloff RT, Graham MD, Roberts BR. Middle ear surgery in fibrous dysplasia of the temporal bone. Am J Otol 1985; 6(2):153–156.

160. Boyce AM, Brewer C, DeKlotz TR, et al. Association of Hearing Loss and Otologic Outcomes With Fibrous Dysplasia. JAMA Otolaryngol Head Neck Surg. Feb 1 2018; 144(2):102–107.

161. Van der Hoeve J, de Kleijn A. Blaue Sclera, Knochenbruchigkeit und Schwerhorigkeit. Arch Ophthalmol 1918; 95:81–93.

162. Dessoff J. Blue sclerotics, fragile bones and deafness. Arch Ophthalmol 1934; 12:60–71.

163. Seedorff KS. Osteogenesis Imperfecta: A Study of Clinical Features and Heredity Based on 55 Danish Families Comprising 180 Affected Persons, Thesis, Copenhagen. Munksgaard Press, 1949:1–229, cited in Konigsmark and Gorlin.

164. Kosoy J, Maddox HE. Surgical findings in van der Hoeve's syndrome. Arch Otolaryngol 1971; 93:115–122.

165. Boulet SL, Rasmussen SA, Honein MA. A population-based study of craniosynostosis in metropolitan Atlanta, 1989–2003. Am J Med Genet A 2008; 146A(8):984–991.

166. Agochukwu NB, Solomon BD, Muenke M. Hearing loss in syndromic craniosynostoses: otologic manifestations and clinical findings. Int J Pediatr Otorhinolaryngol Dec 2014; 78(12):2037–47.

167. Tessier P. The definitive plastic surgical treatment of the severe facial deformities of craniofacial dysostosis. Crouzon's and Apert's diseases. Plast Reconstr Surg 1971; 48:419–442.

168. Franceschetti A, Klein D. Mandibulofacial dysostosis. New hereditary syndrome. Acta Ophthalmol 1949; 27:143–224.

169. Stovin JJ, Lyon JA, Clemmens RL. Mandibulofacial dysostosis. Radiology 1960; 74:225–231.

170. Hutchinson JC, Caldarelli DD, Valvassori GE et al. The otologic manifestations of mandibulofacial dysostosis. Trans Sect Otolaryngol Am Acad Ophthalmol Otolaryngol 1977; 84:520–528.

171. McKusick VA, Claiborne R, eds. Medical Genetics. New York, NY: HP Publishing, 1973:63–78.

172. Igarashi M, Filippone MV, Alford BR. Temporal bone findings in Pierre Robin syndrome. Laryngoscope 1976; 86:1679–1687.

173. Dozier TS, Duncan IM, Klein AJ, Lambert PR, Key LL, Jr. Otologic manifestations of malignant osteopetrosis. Otol Neurotol Jul 2005; 26(4):762–766.

174. Johnston CC, Lavy N, Lord T, Vellios F, Merritt AD, Deiss WP, Jr. Osteopetrosis. A clinical genetic, metabolic and morphologic study of the dominantly inherited benign form. Medicine 1968; 47:149–167.

175. Myers EN, Stool S. The temporal bone in osteopetrosis. Arch Otolaryngol 1969; 89:460–469.

176. Wong ML, Balkany TJ, Reaves J, Jafek BW. Head and neck manifestations of malignant osteopetrosis. Otolaryngology 1978; 86:585–594.

177. Wildervanck LS, Hoeksema PE, Penning L. Radiological examination of the inner ear of deaf mutes. Acta Otolaryngol 1966; 61:445–453.

178. Everberg G. Wildervanck's syndrome: Klippel-Feil's syndrome associated with deafness and retardation of the eyeball. Br J Radiol 1962; 36:562–567.

179. Sataloff RT, Spiegel JR, Hawkshaw MJ, Epstein JM, Jackson L. Cornelia de Lange syndrome. Arch Otolaryngol Head Neck Surg 1990; 116:1044–1046.

180. Marchisio P, Selicorni A, Bianchini S, et al. Audiological findings, genotype and clinical severity score in Cornelia de Lange syndrome. Int J Pediatr Otorhinolaryngol Jul 2014; 78(7):1045–1048.

181. Bergeron M, Chang K, Ishman SL. Cornelia de lange manifestations in otolaryngology: A systematic review and meta-analysis. Laryngoscope Apr 2020; 130(4):E122–E133.

182. Monday LA, Lemieux B. Etude audiovestibulaire dans 1'ataxie de Friedreich. J Otolaryngol 1978; 7:415–423.

183. Aggerbeck LP, McMahon JP, Scano AM. Hypobetalipoproteinemia: clinical and biochemical description of new kindred with Friedreich ataxia. Neurology 1974; 24:1051–1063.

184. Latham AD, Munro TA. Familial myoclonus epilepsy associated with deaf mutism in a family showing other psychobiological abnormalities. Ann Engen 1938; 8:166–175.

185. Globus JH, Strauss L. Progressive degenerative subcortical encephalopathy (Schilder's disease). Arch Psychiatry 1928; 20:1190–1228.

186. Lichtenstein BW, Rosenbluth PR. Schilder's disease with melanoderma. J Neuropathol Exp Neurol 1959; 15:229–231.

187. Anderson PE. Radiology of Pendred's syndrome. Adv Otorhinolaryngol 1974; 21:9–18.

188. Lindsay J. Profound childhood deafness: inner ear pathology. Ann Otol Rhinol Laryngol 1973; 5(suppl.):1–21.

189. Selkae DJ. Familial hyperprolinemia and mental retardation. Neurology 1969; 19:494–502.

190. McKusick V. Heritable Disorders of Connective Tissue. 3rd ed. St. Louis: Mosby, 1966:150.

191. Kang ES, Byers RD, Gerald PS. Homocystinuria: response to pyridoxine. Neurology 1970; 20:503–507.

192. Zeigler SM, Sloan B, Jones JA. Pathophysiology and pathogenesis of Marfan syndrome. Adv Exp Med Biol 2021; 1348:185–206.

193. Hamberis AO, Mehta CH, Valente TA, Dornhoffer JR, Nguyen SA, Meyer TA. The pattern and progression of hearing loss in Marfan syndrome: a study of children and young adults. Int J Pediatr Otorhinolaryngol Nov 2020; 138:110207.

194. Wolfberg J, Chintalapati K, Tomatsu S, Nagao K. Hearing loss in mucopolysaccharidoses: current knowledge and future directions. Diagnostics Aug 4 2020; 10(8):554.

195. Leroy JG, Crocker AC. Clinical definition of Hunter-Hurler phenotypes. A review of 50 patients. Am J Dis Child 1966; 112:518–530.

196. Robbins MM, Stevens HF, Linker A. Morquio's disease: an abnormality of mucopolysaccharide metabolism. J Pediatr 1963; 62:881–889.

197. Van Noorden GK, Zellweger H, Parseti IV. Ocular findings in Morquio-Ullrich's disease. Arch Ophthalmol 1960; 64:585–591.

198. Kolodny EH, Brady RO, Volk BW. Demonstration of an alteration of ganglioside metabolism in Tay-Sachs disease. Biochem Biophys Res Commun 1969; 37:526–531.

199. Steinberg G. Erblinche Augenkrankheiten und Ohrenleiden. V Ohr Nas Kehlkopfheik 1937; 42:320–345.

200. Keleman G. Tay-Sachs-Krankeit und Gehororgan. Z Laryngol Rhinol Otol 1965; 44:728–738.

201. Danish JM, Tillson JK, Levitan M. Multiple anomalies in congenitally deaf children. Eugen Quart 1963; 10:12–21.

202. O'Reilly S, Weber PM, Pollycove M et al. Detection of carrier of Wilson's disease. Neurology 1970; 20:1133–1138.

203. Gorlin RJ, Pindborg JJ. Symptoms of the Head and Neck. New York, NY: McGraw-Hill, 1964:41–46.

204. Jervell A, Lange-Nielsen F. Congenital deaf-mutism functional heart disease with prolongation of the QT interval and sudden death. Am Heart J 1957; 54:59–68.

205. Fraser GR, Froggatt P, James TN. Congenital deafness associated with electrocardiographic abnormalities, fainting attacks, and sudden death: a recessive syndrome. Q J Med 1964; 33:361–385.

206. Levine SA, Woodworth CR. Congenital deaf-mutism, prolonged QT interval, syncopal attacks and sudden death. N Engl J Med 1958; 259:412–417.

207. Nelson MD, Bennett DM, Lehman ME, Okonji AI. Dizziness, falls, and hearing loss in adults living with sickle cell disease. Am J Audiol Dec 5 2022; 31(4):1178–1190.

208. Todd GB, Serjeant FR, Larson MR. Sensorineural hearing loss in Jamaicans with SS disease. Acta Otolaryngol 1973; 76:268–272.

209. Kapoor E, Strum D, Shim T, Kim S, Sabetrasekh P, Monfared A. Characterization of sensorineural hearing loss in adult patients with sickle cell disease: a systematic review and meta-analysis. Otol Neurotol Jan 2021; 42(1):30–37.

210. Morgenstein KM, Manace ED. Temporal bone histopathology in sickle cell disease. Laryngoscope 1969; 79:2172–2180.

211. Urban GE. Reversible sensorineural hearing loss associated with sickle cell crisis. Laryngoscope 1973; 83:633–638.

212. Scotet V, L'Hostis C, Férec C. The changing epidemiology of cystic fibrosis: incidence, survival and impact of the CFTR gene discovery. Genes May 26 2020; 11(6):589.

213. Stanford GE, Dave K, Simmonds NJ. Pulmonary exacerbations in adults with cystic fibrosis: a grown-up issue in a changing cystic fibrosis landscape. Chest Jan 2021; 159(1):93–102.

214. Zettner EM, Gleser MA. Progressive hearing loss among patients with cystic fibrosis and parenteral aminoglycoside treatment. Otolaryngol Head Neck Surg Nov 2018; 159(5):887–894.

215. Kreicher KL, Schopper HK, Naik AN, Hatch JL, Meyer TA. Hearing loss in children with primary ciliary dyskinesia. Int J Pediatr Otorhinolaryngol Jan 2018; 104:161–165.

216. Sethi BR. Kartagener's syndrome and its otological manifestations. J Laryngol Otol 1975; 89:183–188.

217. Kartagener M. Zur Pathogenese der bronkiektasien, bronkiektasien bei Situs viscerum inversus. Beitr Klin Tuberk 1933; 83:489–501.

218. Anderson H, Filipsson R, Fluur E, Koch B, Lindsten J, Wedenberg E. Hearing impairment in Turner's syndrome. Acta Otolaryngol 1969; 247(suppl.):1–26.

219. Hamberis AO, Mehta CH, Dornhoffer JR, Meyer TA. Characteristics and progression of hearing loss in children with turner's syndrome. Laryngoscope Jun 2020; 130(6):1540–1546.

220. Anderson H, Lindsten J, Wedenberg E. Hearing deficits in males with sex chromosome anomalies. Acta Otolaryngol 1971; 72:55–58.

221. van Trier DC, van Nierop J, Draaisma JMT, et al. External ear anomalies and hearing impairment in Noonan syndrome. Int J Pediatr Otorhinolaryngol Jun 2015; 79(6):874–878.

222. Nightengale E, Yoon P, Wolter-Warmerdam K, Daniels D, Hickey F. Understanding hearing and hearing loss in children with Down syndrome. Am J Audiol Sep 18 2017; 26(3):301–308.

223. Glovsky L. Audiological assessment of a mongoloid population. Train Sch Bull 1966; 63:27–36.

224. Fulton RT, Lloyd LL. Hearing impairment in a population of children with Down's syndrome. Am J Ment Defic 1968; 73:298–302.

225. Balkany TJ, Mischke RE, Downs MP, Jafek BW. Ossicular abnormalities in Down's syndrome. Otolaryngol Head Neck Surg 1979; 87(3):372–384.

226. Sataloff J, Pastore PN, Bloom E. Sex-linked hereditary deafness. Am J Hum Genet 1955; 7:201–203.

227. Bernstein JM. Occurrence of episodic vertigo and hearing loss in families. Ann Otol Rhinol Laryngol 1965; 74:1011–1021.

228. Jorgensen MB, Kristensen HK. Frequency of histological otosclerosis. Ann Otol Rhinol Laryngol 1967; 76:83–88.

229. Linthicum FH, House HP, Althaus SR. The effect of sodium fluoride on otosclerotic activity as determined by strontium. Ann Otol Rhinol Laryngol 1972; 4:609–615.

# 16

# Hearing loss in children

ROBERT THAYER SATALOFF, MARY J. HAWKSHAW, AND PAMELA C. ROEHM

Childhood hearing loss is common and may hinder the normal development of speech and language. Even a mild hearing loss can produce measurable psychosocial problems for a child. Healthcare professionals can reduce the incidence and impact of handicapping hearing impairment through prevention and early detection. Doing so requires familiarity with the causes of hearing loss and astute attention to the signs of hearing impairment. Children are susceptible to nearly all the conditions discussed with regard to adults elsewhere in this book. This chapter is intended to emphasize some of the more common and important considerations in the pediatric population.

Hearing loss in children is of special importance because it often goes unrecognized for long periods of time and can create serious problems. Many children are compelled to repeat grades in school because of poor scholastic achievement, often the result of unsuspected and remediable hearing loss. Equally important is the social cost of truancy and other forms of antisocial behavior that is prevalent among children with undiagnosed hearing loss. The severe repercussions that hearing loss has on an individual's personality, both in childhood and in later life, require that the problem of hearing impairment

be recognized as being of high medical importance. Because the solution or amelioration of the problems depends largely on the early detection of hearing loss in children, the major responsibility rests with the general practitioner and the pediatrician.

The extent of the problem is recognized nationally from the data in many school studies. Most of these show that between 2.8% and 4% of school children have "significant hearing losses." These reports emphasize further that well over 80% of the hearing losses in these children are curable with adequate medical attention. Although the great benefit to be derived from routine testing in a school hearing screening program is apparent, facilities for testing preschool children with symptoms suggesting hearing loss also would be extremely valuable. In children below the age of 6, mild or even moderate hearing loss may be missed easily. 54% of the cases reported by the Chicago audiological screening clinics were found to have a loss of ≥ 35 dB for the speech frequencies, of which the parents were unaware.

A distinction should be made between the child with a hearing impairment and a child who is deaf. Deafness, at any age, is characterized as hearing that is nonfunctional for ordinary purposes. Even with a hearing aid, a deaf individual

DOI: 10.1201/b23379-16

has no real serviceable hearing. This problem is far different from that of the child whose hearing is impaired but useful (serviceable). A few schools are available for deaf students, providing a beneficial environment—socially and culturally—by specializing in deaf education. In addition to these institutions, deaf children are mainstreamed into public schools with the assistance of teacher's aides and assistive devices. This chapter discusses principally the hard-of-hearing child and stresses the need for correct diagnosis of hearing loss and deafness as early in infancy as possible as well as the importance of early intervention to help the child develop proper speech and communication skills.

## CLASSIFICATION OF HEARING LOSS

Hearing loss is classified as conductive (external or middle ear), sensorineural (inner ear or auditory nerve), mixed (sensorineural and conductive), or central (brain). It may be classified further as congenital (present at birth) or acquired (occurring after birth). Both congenital and acquired hearing loss may be conductive and/or sensorineural. Hereditary hearing loss may be congenital or acquired.

## COMMON CAUSES OF PEDIATRIC HEARING LOSS

### HEREDITARY CAUSES OF HEARING LOSS

Hereditary hearing loss may be part of a variety of syndromes, or it may occur without associated anomalies. Although dominant, recessive, and X-linked inheritance patterns have been implicated, most hereditary hearing loss is recessive. In recessive syndromes, while both parents must carry the trait, neither may necessarily have the syndrome. Consequently, special attention must be paid to recognizing the hereditary nature of these conditions. Genetic counseling can help parents determine the probability of their having

other affected children and ease the minds of those parents for whom the defect was a spontaneous mutation rather than a heritable disease. There are high-risk registries in the country to help track the incidence and epidemiology, manage, and prevent hereditary hearing loss. In addition, blood tests are available to identify many causes of genetic hearing impairment. Unfortunately, they are fairly expensive and often are not covered by insurance.

An extensive review of syndromes associated with hearing loss is presented in Chapter 15. In children, it is important to recognize that serious associated health problems such as renal disease (Alport syndrome) and cardiac anomalies leading to sudden death (Jervell and Lange-Nielsen syndrome) may have hearing loss as their only presenting sign. Therefore, every child with hearing loss requires a complete systemic evaluation. It is important to remember that hereditary hearing loss need not be present at birth. For example, in otosclerosis and von Recklinghausen disease, hearing loss may not appear until the teen or adult years. Developmental malformations of the inner, middle, or outer ears also may present with various degrees of hearing loss and deafness.

## PRENATAL CAUSES OF HEARING LOSS

Exposure to a variety of environmental factors during pregnancy, especially during the first or second trimester, can result in congenital hearing impairment. Usually, this kind of hearing loss is bilateral, sensorineural, and sometimes profound. Although some afflicted children may be helped with hearing aids, they often have severely handicapped communication abilities.

Rh incompatibility is among the more serious causes of congenital deafness. This type of hearing loss is usually the result of neural damage caused by hyperbilirubinemia secondary to erythroblastosis fetalis. Hearing loss due to Rh incompatibility is less common now because of current prenatal care dictating the Rh typing of mothers prior to delivery and the advent of RhoGAM® (Kedrion Biopharma Inc., Melville, NY) treatment by injection for the expectant mother.

Contracting rubella during the first trimester of pregnancy is another cause of congenital anomalies, including deafness. The rubella vaccine should be given to children routinely and to adolescents and adult women if serologic tests show them to be susceptible to the disease, provided that they are not pregnant and do not become pregnant until at least 3 months after immunization. Lack of serologic testing, however, should not be a deterrent to rubella immunization. Pregnant mothers should be counseled to recognize and avoid people with the disease. Although only initial studies have been performed, treatment of pregnant women who have contracted rubella with immune globulin may protect against congenital rubella syndrome in their children.

Other maternal infections, particularly viral infections, and syphilis, also may result in congenital hearing loss.

Ototoxicity from a wide variety of drugs and from exposure to radiation during the first trimester of pregnancy also may result in a child with hearing loss. Exposure to aminoglycoside antibiotics and other known ototoxic agents should be avoided. Pregnant women should be counseled not to take any medication or undergo any elective procedure, such as surgery requiring anesthesia, without consulting their obstetrician. When exposure to such ototoxic agents has occurred, infants should be screened for hearing loss.

## POSTNATAL CAUSES OF HEARING LOSS

Hypoxia, neonatal jaundice, and birth trauma may be causally related to hearing loss in the neonate. Premature birth and low birth weight also can be associated with hearing loss. When these events occur, there must be a high suspicion for hearing loss, and hearing screening and medical evaluation should be considered early. While congenital and hereditary forms of hearing loss may be among the more severe types, the more common causes of hearing loss in children are acquired.

### Outer ear causes of postnatal hearing loss

Acquired conductive hearing loss involving the outer ear occurs for many reasons. Cerumen impaction is undoubtedly the most common. As long as there is even a pinhole in the impacted wax, hearing is virtually unaffected, but when the external auditory canal is occluded completely by cerumen, substantial hearing loss results. Frequently, this happens during attempts to clean a child's ears with a cotton-tipped swab; however, manually cleaning the external ear canals is usually unnecessary. Ears ordinarily clean themselves and can be cared for externally with a washcloth. The old admonition to "put nothing smaller than your elbow in your ear" is a good one that will help prevent direct ear trauma. Small objects such as hairpins can cause considerable damage.

An extensive variety of foreign bodies (cotton, plastic toys, corn, peas, erasers, etc.) has been found in the ears of children; thus, children should be trained early not to put anything in their ears. When such a mishap occurs, an otologist should remove the foreign objects. Care must be taken to assess hearing, if possible, before removing the object and to manipulate the object deftly. Trying to remove a foreign body without proper equipment can cause middle or inner ear damage as a result of eardrum perforation or, more rarely, trauma to the ossicles. Attempts to wash out some organic (e.g., small vegetables) foreign bodies result in their swelling, greatly increasing the difficulty of removing them.

"Swimmer's ear," or otitis externa, can cause the ear canal to fill with debris and to swell, causing pain and conductive hearing loss. Scratching the ear canal skin with a cotton swab can aggravate or even initiate the condition. Just shaking water out of one's ears and letting them self-dry is generally adequate. Some physicians advocate a few drops of alcohol in the ears after swimming. However, this practice is usually not necessary in most children, and it may dry and "chap" the ear canal skin, possibly causing increased susceptibility to infection. The author (R.T.S.) recommends the gentle use of a hair blow-dryer on the lowest heat setting to dry the ear canal when "water in the ear" occurs.

Other causes of external-ear obstruction include growths of various types and trauma. Trauma also can result in perforation of the eardrum. Such perforations usually heal spontaneously. When they do not, closure of the perforation is desirable not only to improve hearing if there is hearing loss but also to prevent repeated middle-ear infections.

## Middle ear causes of postnatal hearing loss

Eustachian tube dysfunction often underlies middle ear disease in children. Suspicion should be high in children with large adenoids, allergies, cleft palate, and frequent ear infections. Serous otitis media, acute and chronic, is the most common cause of hearing loss in children. It results from negative middle ear pressure with respect to the barometric pressure external to the eardrum, and that causes collection of fluid in the middle ear space. This is correctable medically, with the use of antibiotics and decongestants, or surgically, with the insertion of pressure equalization tubes and/or eustachian tube dilation, allowing hearing to be restored. Additionally, any child with a cold or with eustachian tube dysfunction should be restricted from flying or exposure to other barotraumas.

Acute suppurative (infected fluid) otitis media causes hearing loss and needs aggressive treatment with antibiotics. Occasionally, a myringotomy is necessary. Chronic suppurative otitis media frequently requires surgical intervention to restore normal hearing. In many instances, the disease can be prevented by proper management of an antecedent acute otitis media or by keeping water out of an ear with a perforated eardrum. However, in some cases, it may herald more serious middle-ear disease such as cholesteatoma. Early diagnosis and management prevent more serious inner ear problems or other complications.

Forceful nose blowing during an upper respiratory infection may predispose the child to otitis media by forcing infecting organisms through the eustachian tube into the middle ear. While this is controversial, in the authors' judgment, forceful nose blowing should be avoided. Sniffing is harder to live with, but it is safer.

## Inner ear causes of postnatal hearing loss

Inner ear, or sensorineural, hearing loss (commonly called "nerve deafness") is generally irreversible, but not always. Both bilateral and unilateral sensorineural losses may affect a child's speech and language development. Acquired causes of sensorineural hearing loss include infection, ototoxic drugs, noise exposure, head trauma, tumors, autoimmune disease, and many others discussed elsewhere in this book.

Mumps is a classic cause of unilateral severe hearing loss, but a number of other viruses may be responsible as well. Because more serious infections such as meningitis and encephalitis often produce hearing loss, children who recover from these diseases should have their hearing tested. If hearing loss develops, it is usually bilateral and may be severe. It is important to diagnose congenital and acquired syphilis that have caused sensorineural hearing loss because they are treatable. Extension of a middle ear infection may result in inner ear damage.

Commonly used drugs may be ototoxic and cause inner ear damage. Antibiotics such as neomycin, kanamycin, vancomycin, and gentamycin are particularly damaging to the acoustic nerve and must be used with caution, especially in the presence of renal dysfunction. Streptomycin, used to treat tuberculosis, is also ototoxic. Serologic antibiotic levels should be monitored in many cases while children are being treated with these antibiotics, and drug dosing must be adjusted accordingly. Serial audiograms including high-frequency testing are also indicated when possible. Various diuretics, such as furosemide administered intravenously, produce hearing loss. Furosemide's toxicity is related to peak blood level; therefore, rapid intravenous infusion should be avoided. It is important to be aware of the many other medications that can cause hearing loss.

Lead is an environmental toxin that affects hearing. Children living in high-risk homes, that is, those predating World War II, should be screened for high lead levels.

Acoustic trauma can produce sensorineural hearing loss. Most commonly, children suffer this type of hearing loss from firecrackers and cap gun explosions. Such blast injuries also may produce eardrum and middle ear damage. Parents should recognize the hazards of these and other toys before they decide whether to buy them. Prolonged exposure to loud noise, such as music through ear inserts, can damage hearing.

When it is impossible to avoid noise, ear protectors should be worn.

Direct trauma may damage the outer, middle, or inner ear including but not limited to ossicular discontinuity, oval or round window perforation, hematoma formation, swelling, and cochlear hair cell damage. Residual scarring can interfere with the function and appearance of the ear and its structures; it can be quite difficult to treat satisfactorily. Children should never be "boxed" in the ear, and if a child's ear is injured enough to swell, the child should be evaluated by a physician. A blow to the ear also can produce a loud blast-like noise and pressure that can rupture the ossicles or cause a sensorineural hearing loss. A firm kiss on the ear can produce the same damage.

General head trauma can produce hearing loss. If a blow to the head is not severe enough to produce unconsciousness, it rarely produces hearing loss unless the ear was struck directly. However, fractures of the temporal bone often cause hearing loss. Automobile accidents account for most severe pediatric head injuries, although the prevalence of such injuries has decreased substantially because of seat belts and child car seats.

## INFANT HEARING IMPAIRMENT

A child may be born with a hearing deficit or acquire it in infancy before he/she develops speech. In either case, the symptoms are similar because the hearing loss occurred before speech development. The defect may be conductive, as in congenital fixation of the stapes footplate, ossicular defects, or aplasia of the outer or the middle ear. The hearing loss also may be sensorineural, as in hereditary nerve or hair cell dysfunction or in hearing loss resulting from Rh incompatibility, maternal rubella in the first trimester of pregnancy, anoxia, viral infections, or other causes. Congenital hearing losses are more commonly bilateral than unilateral. The impairment may run the gamut from very slight impairment to total loss of hearing in both ears.

Conductive hearing loss, especially if bilateral, may retard speech development somewhat and cause inattention; however, the child usually develops essentially normal speech patterns because he/she understands and can respond to loud speech. A child with moderate or severe sensorineural hearing loss usually shows not only a poor hearing response but also even more prominently, he/she may have absented or impaired speech. Sensorineural losses involving only the higher frequencies generally cause fewer symptoms and may go unnoticed until they are detected in a school hearing screening program.

When a parent brings a child to the physician and complains that the child is 3 years old and still cannot speak or seems to be "backward," disinterested, and inattentive, the first question that should arise in the mind of the physician is "Can this child hear?" One of the earliest clues to the presence of a hearing loss is delayed or defective speech. Temper tantrums in a speechless child, poor schoolwork, and many emotional disturbances may be caused by hearing impairment.

## HEARING AND SPEECH

To understand the problems associated with hearing impairment in children, one should be aware of the intimate relationship between hearing and speech development. Throughout infancy, a child listens to speech, learns to associate sounds with meaningful information, and subsequently mimics what is heard. By the age of 3, a normal-hearing child has developed most of his/her speech patterns. However, a child with no useful hearing will form little or no intelligible speech spontaneously because he/she cannot imitate what is never heard. If he/she passes silently through the early years ideally suited for language development, the individual will be handicapped in developing normal speech, education, and important social and emotional qualities. If he/she had a partial hearing loss accompanied by distortion, a defective speech pattern is likely to develop.

When a child is acquiring speech, he/she learns to pronounce vowels and consonants, combining them into meaningful sounds. In our audible frequency range, the vowels (a, e, i, o, and u) are low-frequency tones, whereas consonants (e.g., s, f, t, and g) are high tones. If a child has a high-frequency hearing loss, the vowels will be heard but the consonants will be inaudible or seem to be indistinct or distorted.

The child who has difficulty in correctly pronouncing certain sibilant sounds, particularly "s," was in the past likely to be described as "tongue-tied." Most of these children are in reality not tongue-tied but cannot pronounce high-frequency sibilants due to a hearing loss in that frequency range. To a child with such a high-frequency hearing loss, an "s" may sound like a "t," and in learning to pronounce words, he/she naturally will repeat only what is heard. If he/she does not hear accurately, the speech produced also will be inaccurate.

## DIAGNOSING HEARING LOSS EARLY

When a parent indicates that a child is inattentive and possibly hard-of-hearing, it is vital that the presence or the absence of hearing impairment be determined accurately and, in the event of a hearing loss, that its cause be determined. The question often is asked: "How old must a child be before his/her hearing can be tested?" Today, infants can be screened for hearing loss as young as 1–2 days old. Parents should never be told that a child is too young to have his/her hearing tested. The earlier a hearing loss is detected, and treatment is begun, the better.

Many states have adopted a newborn hearing screening (NHS) program designed to identify newborns with congenital hearing losses among the general population and to test infants who have at-risk conditions for hearing loss. NHS programs' primary goal is the early identification and treatment of congenital hearing loss. Although each state has adopted its own NHS program, many follow a sample protocol as follows. Otoacoustic emission (OAE) tests are performed on every newborn prior to hospital discharge. OAEs are inexpensive and a quick screening test of inner ear function. A newborn either passes or is referred for further assessment. If he/she is referred, a repeat OAE is performed 1 day later. If the retest result is also abnormal, a consultation is made with a hearing professional for a brainstem evoked-response audiometry (BERA or ABR).

Infants with a high risk of hearing loss are screened with a separate protocol. Indicators of a high risk of hearing loss are low birth weight, premature birth, *in utero* infections, family history of pediatric hearing loss, craniofacial anomalies, hyperbilirubinemia, neonatal use of ototoxic medications, low Apgar score, use of mechanical ventilation, or presence of a syndrome known to be associated with hearing loss. These infants have their hearing tested prior to discharge via a brainstem evoked-response test and OAEs, instead of just an OAE screening. If the newborn fails these tests, a consultation is made with an otolaryngologist. NHS programs are increasing the frequency of early identification of congenital hearing loss; however, the physician still needs to be attentive to the symptoms of acquired hearing loss in the pediatric population.

## HISTORY OF AUDITORY BEHAVIOR

Obtaining an accurate quantitative assessment of an infant's or a young child's hearing is frequently a very difficult task. In the case of younger children, it is often not possible to perform reliable air conduction tests, let alone bone conduction tests, due to uncooperative behavior. The principal responsibilities of the physician are (a) to be on the alert for the possible presence of hearing loss and (b) when findings are suspicious, to determine whether more definitive studies are warranted. Many methods are available to determine whether hearing loss is present. It is important to obtain an adequate history of the child's behavior from the parents. For example, a child who never answers or does not come when he/she is called but does react when the face of the caller is visible may have hearing loss. It is important in such cases to ask the parents whether they call the child by voice alone or whether, in addition, they stamp their foot or bang the table. The child who cannot be awakened at night by being spoken to in a loud voice should be evaluated for hearing loss, especially if his/her speech development is delayed or imperfect. Because similar negative responses often are obtained in the case of emotionally disturbed children or in children with retrocochlear lesions, careful differentiation is essential both through hearing tests and through other consultations. Certain auditory behavior patterns are prominent during an infant's development, and these should be explored to determine whether hearing loss is a likely etiology.

During the first 6 months, a baby should respond to his/her mother's voice before seeing her; he/she should be affected by sounds such as being startled, awakened, or amused. He/she even should be able to localize the mother's voice and should start to imitate certain simple sounds. Before the age of 1 year, the average child can be expected to obey simple commands and to understand several words, especially familiar names. By the age of 2, the child should start to speak simple words like "all gone" and "bye-bye." From then on, the child's vocabulary and understanding should continue to increase and become more comprehensive.

A careful history of auditory responses can lead the physician to a judgment of whether a parent's concern about her baby's hearing is justified.

## RESPONSE TO NOISEMAKERS

The reaction of a child less than 5 years of age to handclapping from behind, stamping the feet, or striking pans together does not always prove whether or not the child can hear. A response may be due to feeling vibration from the noisemakers; an absent response could be due to a variety of psychological or physiological reasons in the presence of normal hearing. If a child has some useful hearing and a vibrating tuning fork of 512 Hz is placed surreptitiously near one of his/her ears, he/she may either turn in the direction of the sound or otherwise indicate that the sound is heard. Handbells also may be used behind the child's back to see whether he/she turns around consistently when they are sounded. A positive response by the child in carefully conducted noisemaking tests generally is reliable, but in such tests, a negative response does not always indicate hearing loss. Noisemakers of different frequencies should be used to determine whether the response is better in the higher or the lower frequency range. True responses to the noisemakers must be carefully distinguished from random movement. Children up to 3 months of age respond more consistently to percussion than to voice sounds. Older children respond more readily to voice sounds and may respond better to moderately loud than to very loud voices and sounds. The examiner should remain carefully out of the child's line of sight to avoid visual reactions being mistaken for auditory responses. Reactions to look for are an eye-blink reflex, startle response, initiation of sucking or cessation of sucking movements, a pinna reflex, turning of the head, or other obvious signs. Responses to noisemakers usually cease after just a few observations. Not only do these gross hearing tests help determine whether there is a hearing loss, but they also warn of neurologic defects. A word of caution in the interpretation of these gross hearing tests: Noisemakers are only used as a screening tool and do not indicate the degree of hearing loss, nor can they identify a unilateral hearing loss as normal hearing in one ear only will provide a response.

## HEARING AND BEHAVIOR

Children with high-frequency hearing loss present a complex and often deceptive picture. Sometimes they seem to hear and to understand well, particularly when they are looking at the speaker or paying strict attention, but at other times, they seem to be inattentive and intellectually challenged, especially under some conditions for which the reason often is not apparent to a layperson. Most of the adverse effects of early hearing loss on the child's personality have their origin in the distorted communication caused by the inability to discriminate between high-frequency sounds.

From this nucleus, development of abnormal behavior and the maladjustment of the child to his/her immediate social environment are common. Most children with substantial hearing loss present behavior problems before the cause of their difficulty is recognized and before they are treated properly. It is the responsibility of the physician to be alert for hearing impairment. It is also important for the physician to be aware of the considerable variability in the effects of severe hearing loss, depending on whether its onset was before or after the age of 3 (when speech patterns in a child become reasonably well established), as well as other factors.

## ABNORMAL AUDITORY BEHAVIOR IN A NORMAL-HEARING CHILD

Whenever a physician suspects a hearing loss, he/she should seek more definitive and quantitative evaluations. Further hearing tests are in order when a child's speech defect involves the enunciation of sibilants, particularly the letter "s." Alternate testing often takes not only considerable time and patience but also special training and equipment. It should be done by an audiologist equipped and trained to perform such studies.

The hard-of-hearing child, the mentally delayed child, and the emotionally disturbed child often develop symptoms so similar that they obscure the diagnosis. Yet, it is essential to distinguish between these very different conditions in order to institute proper therapy and to offer a prognosis. Aphasia is very frequently confused with the sequelae of profound hearing loss. Damage to the brain may cause inability to comprehend speech, resulting in a receptive (verbal) aphasia, even though the ears and hearing are intact.

Studies have shown that there is not, as is accepted generally, a high incidence of hearing loss in the mentally delayed population. Initial tests may indicate a hearing loss, but when tests are repeated by a specially trained audiologist, they may reveal more hearing than the first tests suggested.

The autistic child is confused often with the hard-of-hearing child because he/she may not use speech and has limited attention to sound. Such a child, and children with other types of disorders that may be confused with hearing loss, must have an accurate diagnosis if each is to receive therapy appropriate to his/her condition. In such cases, referrals to other healthcare professionals can be valuable in determining a diagnosis.

In other instances, poor auditory behavior can be a symptom of an underlying central auditory processing disorder (CAPD). CAPDs can be present in the pediatric population alone or can co-occur with diagnoses of attention deficit disorder or attention deficit hyperactivity disorder. CAPDs generally manifest during elementary school-aged children when their listening demands and workloads increase dramatically. Children with CAPDs can have difficulty separating speech signals from noise, determining temporal cues, coding auditory inputs within the auditory cortex, and processing binaural stimuli. Typically, they have difficulty even concentrating on a written text in the presence of background noise because of the inability to filter out unwanted noise. It is important that the physician who suspects a CAPD in the presence or absence of a hearing loss refers the child to an audiologist and/or other professionals such as a neuropsychologist familiar with CAPD testing for a complete diagnostic work-up.

## HEARING TESTING BY THE AUDIOLOGIST

It is comparatively simple for the audiologist to test the hearing of older children because they are usually cooperative and give accurate responses to auditory signals. The situation is quite different with infants and young children who have little or no speech, especially if they have developed some antisocial patterns. The audiologist must perform a battery of tests, and the otologist considers their results in conjunction with the history, particularly the developmental history, and the physical examination. Just as with the use of noisemakers, caution must be exercised in interpreting test results performed with loudspeakers, as they are not ear-specific and will not reveal a unilateral hearing loss. There are several other hearing tests that can be performed to ensure that the child's responses to auditory signals reflect reliably the level of the child's hearing. Such tests include behavioral and nonbehavioral methods of testing hearing levels through calibrated test equipment. Impedance audiometry and evoked-response audiometry are especially helpful.

## BEHAVIORAL AUDIOLOGIC TESTS

### Speech reception tests

Speech tests generally require that the child have some language ability in order to give a response to the test material. In younger children, testing the ability of the child to hear speech rather than pure tones is useful in obtaining thresholds of sound awareness. The child is left in a quiet room and spoken to either through earphones, if he/she will accept them, or through loudspeakers. The tester may be in an adjoining room where he/she can control the loudness of the presentation level using calibrated equipment and can watch the responses of the child through an observation window. The child may respond to voice input by placing his/her hand to the earphone, ceasing play activities, or turning to the speaker during free-field testing. It is important to recall that a lack of a response does not necessarily mean that the child does not hear. Children aged ~2 generally can perform speech reception testing by repeating numbers, body parts, favorite words, or pointing to body parts or pictures.

## Behavioral observation audiometry

Behavioral observation audiometry (BOA) is a method of obtaining consistent responses to stimuli (tones and/or speech) for infants or mentally young patients. With BOA, a team approach generally is employed. The assistant remains in a quiet room with the patient, while the tester is located in a separate room with a viewing window. Speech and/or tones are presented through earphones, if tolerated, or loudspeakers. Calibrated noisemakers also can be used to generate stimuli. Both the assistant and the tester are responsible for observing responses to presented stimuli. Responses consist of quieting behavior, eye-blink reflex, startle response, change in sucking behavior or respiration rate, eye movement, or vocalizations. Normative data have been developed based on the infant's developmental age, as true thresholds of hearing cannot be obtained using this method.

## Visual reinforced audiometry

For children who have control and support of their head movements, visual reinforced audiometry (VRA) can be used as a testing method. VRA reinforces a child's response to a sound by presenting a positive visual reinforcement object timed with stimulus presentation. The child is conditioned to orient to a toy contained in a lighted box when a sound is presented. If the child looks when an auditory stimulus was not presented, the toy will not be visible. Localization ability is controlled in most infants aged 5–6 months. As with BOA, earphones are worn, if tolerated, or stimuli are presented through loudspeakers. Results influenced the child's cooperation and interest; therefore, as many auditory thresholds are gathered during a session as possible, and several sessions may be necessary to obtain a complete audiological picture.

## Conditioned play audiometry

In this method of testing, the child is conditioned to respond to the presence of speech or tones by placing a ring on a peg, dropping an object in a box, or other play activities. All the conditioned responses are coordinated with the presence of a stimulus, and a response without a stimulus is not rewarded. Any sort of game can be employed in conditioned play audiometry, as long as it maintains the child's attention without detracting from the task at hand (listening). This form of testing requires that the child be emotionally, physically, and intellectually able to cooperate; therefore, it is most effective with children aged 3–7 years. By the time a young child is in school, he/she usually can begin to respond to audiological testing similar to the way an adult responds by raising a hand or pressing a button in response to stimuli. However, the mental capacity and attention span for each child, regardless of chronological age, must be assessed in order to select the most appropriate method of testing.

## NONBEHAVIORAL AUDIOLOGIC TESTS

Impedance audiometry and evoked-response audiometry are discussed in Chapters 7 and 8, respectively. These tests are used commonly in assessment of hearing levels and are standard for evaluating hearing in children. Impedance audiometry usually is performed at the same time as a behavioral hearing test. The principles and procedures involved in testing children and adults are similar for impedance measurements.

## Brainstem evoked-response audiometry

BERA or ABR generally is performed after behavioral tests indicate a possible hearing loss or as a standard procedure for infants at high risk for hearing loss. The method of testing children with evoked-response equipment is similar to testing in adults. The best results are obtained when the child is sleeping or motionless, and testing can be performed during an infant's naptime. If a child is restless (often seen with children aged l–6) and cannot remain still for the duration of the test (up to 1 hour) a sedated evoked response may be requested. General anesthesia can be used.

## Otoacoustic emissions

Another method of screening can be used to nonbehaviorally test auditory responses. OAEs are present in all normal-hearing ears and in some ears with mild hearing losses. The accuracy and prevalence of OAEs generate an ideal method of screening for moderate-to-profound hearing losses. To record OAEs, the child is placed in a quiet room with a probe in the ear. No participation is required for this test; therefore, the child can be asleep. Soft clicks are presented to each ear individually, and the response levels are recorded for a range of frequencies from 750 to 5000 Hz. The presence of a response indicates the absence of a moderate-to-profound hearing loss. The duration of the test is 2–4 minutes per ear. OAEs are used routinely in NHS programs prior to the discharge of the infant from the hospital.

## Psychogalvanic skin resistance test

Many forms of auditory testing require the cooperation of the child giving subjective responses. Psychogalvanic skin resistance (PGSR) testing is rarely used anymore, having been replaced by BERA and other tests. Nevertheless, it is effective and may occasionally be appropriate. It is similar in principle to lie detector tests. In PGSR testing, active participation and cooperation of the child are not essential, except that they must accept earphones and remain reasonably quiet. The services of at least two people experienced with children are required; one works directly with the child and tries to keep the examination from becoming an unpleasant experience, and the other examiner operates the equipment. The test can be useful in some children and infants. Its reliability in proper hands has been established, but it is not definitive in all children. It must be viewed as a supplementary test to be correlated with other findings rather than as a single test providing all of the information desired. The testers must be not only experienced with children but also aware of the electronic and the psychological pitfalls inherent in this technique.

In brief, the child is taught to accept wearing a set of earphones, two small electrodes on his/her fingers, and another pair on the leg. He/she is then conditioned carefully so that each time sound is introduced through the headphones, it is followed a second later by a mild electrical shock to the calf of the leg. The shock must be almost imperceptible to the child and should not cause any obvious discomfort. The shock produces a change in sympathetic nerve activity, causing increased skin perspiration and reduced skin potential. The electrical effect is conducted from the finger electrodes to a recording device. When the child has been conditioned adequately, the shock is stopped except for reinforcement purposes, and the change in skin resistance continues in response to sound alone. In this manner, by reducing the intensity of the sound in the ear until at one level the skin resistance is affected and at a slightly weaker level it is not affected, it is possible to obtain a complete audiogram on most children.

## SCHOOL TESTING PROGRAMS

School hearing testing programs have major importance in the early detection of hearing loss in children of school age. Audiometry as used in these school tests is much more sensitive and exact in detecting early hearing defects than any office voice test. Therefore, physicians should be the first to understand the valuable preventative possibilities of these routine hearing tests. The detection of early hearing changes often makes it possible to take corrective action and to prevent further deterioration in hearing and behavior.

The pediatrician or the family doctor can render valuable service by suspecting hearing losses in school children who are brought to them because the children have been inattentive, or do poorly at school, or have had repeated ear infections. They should obtain the results of school hearing tests and should consider formal testing by an audiologist.

It is advisable to perform an audiogram on all such children, but even in the absence of an audiometer, a physician can obtain a wealth of information by means of a careful history and simple tests with a 512-Hz tuning fork and spoken words, such as speaking softly into each ear and asking the child to repeat words or phrases that a normal child should be able to hear. If a child hears and repeats softly spoken phrases properly, hearing may be within normal limits. However, it must always be borne in mind that many times children hear and yet do not respond. If it is assumed that the response is reliable and the child fails to hear a soft voice, the physician then should use a 512-Hz tuning fork to help determine whether the impairment is conductive or sensorineural. Such tests are not adequate substitutes for a formal audiogram. If the pediatrician or the general practitioner is unable to find the cause of a hearing loss or to suggest proper treatment, it is his/her obligation to refer the child to an otologist or a hearing clinic that can provide the required services.

## TREATMENT OF PEDIATRIC HEARING LOSS

Most patients visit a physician for relief of pain or discomfort or to allay their fears of cancer, deformity, or other serious disease. In contrast, a hearing loss is painless and rarely recognized as a direct threat to life or health. However, the social and the vocational consequences of impaired hearing are the driving forces that impel the adult patient to go to the physician. In the case of a child, the initiative almost never comes from the child but usually from a teacher or the parents. When the thought occurs to them that the child may have a hearing loss, they may realize the serious social and economic implications of hearing loss and seek a physician's counsel.

It is true that physicians cannot actually cure hearing loss in some cases. Certainly, they are incapable of restoring hearing in many cases of sensorineural hearing loss, but, as discussed elsewhere in this book, even sensorineural hearing loss can be improved in some patients such as those with autoimmune inner ear disease, syphilis, Lyme disease, hypothyroidism, sickle cell disease, and other etiologies. In any case, the physician can tell the patient or his/her parents whether medicine or surgery will help and, if not, the physician should mitigate greatly the social and the emotional consequences of hearing loss through rehabilitative measures.

Physicians and counselling can help to prevent unnecessary hearing loss by exercising care in the use of ototoxic drugs, particularly gentamicin, neomycin, and kanamycin. These drugs should be avoided especially in cases of urinary retention and kidney malfunction and should not be used if there are effective alternatives that are not ototoxic.

Families with a high prevalence of hearing loss should be guided in their marriage plans and possibly seek genetic counseling. Pregnant women should be cautioned against vaccination and exposure to certain diseases, particularly rubella, and animal feces (especially feline, which carries toxoplasma), during the early months of pregnancy. Anoxia in the newborn should be avoided meticulously by good obstetric and pediatric management, and high fevers and convulsions in infants should receive prompt and intensive treatment.

## CONDUCTIVE HEARING LOSS

Conductive hearing loss is the most treatable type of hearing loss, and generally, the loss can be cured completely or improved considerably. The following procedures may be indicated: cerumen debridement, removal of foreign bodies from the ear canal, adenoidectomy; myringotomy and tubes; eustachian tube inflation or dilation; treatment of otitis media, sinusitis, and/or allergies; and tympanoplasty or stapes surgery.

In treating infections of the middle ears, the physician should keep in mind the importance of appropriate antibiotic therapy, as well as the surgical principle of incision and drainage in those cases in which there is localized pus, such as in an attack of acute otitis media with a bulging eardrum.

Frequently, expert handling of such cases will prevent residual conductive hearing loss. Similar emphasis should be placed on a careful adenoidectomy, when it is indicated. Just because a child has had a tonsillectomy and adenoidectomy, it does not follow necessarily that regrowth of adenoids is not be the cause of persistent ear symptoms and conductive hearing loss. It is essential that the adenoids be removed properly. There may be adenoid tissue left in vital areas behind the eustachian tube orifices, marked regrowth, or even extensive scar tissue with damage to the eustachian tubes from adenoidectomies.

Whenever mastoidectomy is considered, hearing status must be given high priority. The type of operation performed should not only clear the infection but also preserve as much hearing as possible. It is possible also to close most perforated eardrums by tympanoplasty (with or without mastoidectomy) and thus improve some conductive hearing losses.

The physician can help prevent the important complications of hearing loss by forthrightly explaining the problems to the parents and assuming the role of guide and adviser in their efforts to compensate and adjust to the child's hearing impairment.

## SENSORINEURAL HEARING LOSS

In sensorineural hearing loss, the pathologic process is more likely to be irreversible. As yet, there is no available therapy that can restore the function of damaged sensorineural elements in the ear except when the loss is associated with specific causes such as those discussed above. Nevertheless, a great deal can be done to help children with handicapping hearing loss of this type, and in such cases, the physician must assume great responsibility. It is essential to explain to the parents why medical or surgical treatment is ineffective presently and why all efforts should be directed toward rehabilitation rather than toward a nonexistent cure that exposes the child to needless medical and surgical treatments. Nevertheless, prior to giving such advice, it is essential that the physician be absolutely certain he/she has not missed the diagnosis of a treatable or correctable cause of hearing loss. In profoundly deaf children, it is also important to consider potential candidacy for cochlear implantation.

The primary interest of the physician is not in how much hearing is lost. He/she is interested in how much hearing is left and what can be done to help the child use his/her residual hearing most effectively. We have found it unwise to tell a parent that his/her child has lost a certain percentage of hearing. It is far more helpful to say that the child has lost some hearing but that a certain quantity of hearing remains that can either be corrected medically, surgically, or enhanced by a hearing aid and special auditory training

procedures. The atmosphere that the physician creates should be positive rather than negative. The standard audiogram chart records hearing loss in terms of decibels, which can be perceived in a negative manner. The true purpose of hearing tests is to determine how much hearing is present.

## AURAL REHABILITATION

All children with hearing loss severe enough to interfere with their ordinary communication should receive, in addition to medical treatment, some form of auditory rehabilitation if their auditory deficit cannot be corrected. Usually a 30- or 35-dB hearing loss in the speech frequencies in the better-hearing ear or a marked high-frequency loss is considered to be sufficiently handicapping to interfere with communication. Such children must be taught to listen actively and pay strict attention to all sounds. They must be instructed carefully in how to get the most out of their residual hearing. The early application of a hearing aid and training in its use often will demonstrate to hesitant parents the realistic value of this approach and stimulate their wholehearted support and cooperation.

## HEARING AIDS

The hearing aid usually should be a behind-the-ear (BTE) or in-the-ear (ITE) instrument with an individually molded earpiece placed in the ear, or ears, that will give the child the most benefit. This may be in the ear that has worse or better hearing, depending on the degrees and the types of hearing loss present. Bone conduction hearing aids have specific uses and are suitable primarily for use in the presence of atresia of the ear canals or for chronically draining ears. They can either be worn with a headband or implanted surgically. When a diagnosis of hearing loss is established in an infant or a young child and the hearing loss is sensorineural, amplification generally will be necessary.

The least possible delay should be permitted in making maximum use of the residual hearing. There is convincing evidence that even young infants benefit from auditory amplification.

Exposure to the rhythm of music and the background nuances of speech are important for the infant and young child with a marked hearing loss. When an aid is fitted on the child, the parent should be encouraged to report the child's reactions and progress with amplification. In order to obtain optimal use of the aid, the parent should be alert constantly for any changes in the operation of the aid (the need for a new battery or adjustment, for example). Children usually are fitted with a BTE style of hearing aid for a number of reasons. Children's external ears and ear canals change shape rapidly over time, making the use of a custom ITE hearing aid very costly because of the need to remake the aid frequently. Earmolds that are connected to the BTE hearing aids can be made at much lower costs to the parents. It also is easier for the parent to control and care for the larger BTE and to confirm at a glance that the aid is being used Additional information about hearing aids is presented in Chapter 18, along with a discussion of cochlear implants.

## SPEECH READING AND AUDITORY TRAINING

In conductive hearing losses, adequate compensation can be secured, for the most part, by amplification. However, in sensorineural losses, amplification does not solve the problem of distortion, and the use of speech reading, and auditory training should be added to amplification as a component of aural rehabilitation.

In speech reading training, the basic goal is the strengthening of the powers of visual observation. This includes the coordination of lipreading with the interpretation of facial expressions and an intuitive grasp of the conversational trend.

The child's responses to speech tests will determine the type of auditory training that he/she will need. In many cases, the child will need auditory training before he/she is fitted with an individual hearing aid. This training may be necessary due to poor listening habits. In any case, the object of such training is to teach him/her that sounds have meaning and that sounds should be differentiated and identified. The specific goal is the development of discrimination of the sounds of speech.

## A TEAM OF SPECIALISTS

More than in many other conditions, the hard-of-hearing child requires the integrated attention of a team of specialists. One person cannot diagnose, treat, rehabilitate, and guide the parents and child in their efforts to overcome the communicative handicap imposed by hearing loss. It is the responsibility of the pediatrician (or sometimes the otologist) to act as the coordinator of the team, which frequently includes an otologist, an audiologist, a speech-language pathologist, a psychologist, and possibly a psychiatrist, as well as social workers and others.

In brief, the physician who suspects the presence of hearing loss in a child should first refer the child for quantitative hearing tests and an accurate diagnosis of the cause of the hearing loss. He/she must then determine whether the hearing loss is curable and what measures are necessary to remedy it as soon as possible. If the loss is irreversible and hearing aid(s) would assist the child, selection of a hearing aid and training the patient and parents in the use of amplification by an audiologist should be advised. Speech therapy should be provided by a speech-language pathologist who is familiar with the problems associated with hearing loss and understands the characteristics of amplified sound. If there is a psychological problem, a trained psychologist or psychiatrist should be asked for an evaluation.

The physician must always be available to guide and to support the parents and the child during the trying months following a hearing loss diagnosis. He/she can and should make every effort to relieve the parents of any guilt that they may feel regarding the birth of their hard-of-hearing child. Instead, the physician can guide their emotional involvement into constructive channels by encouraging them to start auditory training or sign language early and to raise the child in the healthiest environment possible, making the best use of all available methods of communication and effectively utilizing the child's residual hearing. The emotional stability of the child and his/her parents, and not merely the hearing problem, must receive farsighted attention. Referrals to parent and child support groups serve to assist the family in relating to others who have gone through a similar experience.

## SUMMARY

Hearing loss can result from hereditary or non-hereditary disorders as well as prenatal or post-natal exposure to a variety of diseases, toxins, or trauma. Hearing loss, particularly early in life, can have a profound, detrimental effect on a child's psychological and social development. The hearing professional who understands the development of normal auditory behavior is equipped best to detect children whose auditory behavior is pathologic and to screen such children for hearing loss. Recognizing conditions that predispose children to hearing loss encourages early recognition of high-risk groups, early detection of hearing deficits, and early aural rehabilitation. Attention to these factors can reduce both the incidence and impact of hearing loss in children.

# 17

# Diagnosing occupational hearing loss

ROBERT THAYER SATALOFF AND KATHERINE MULLEN

Occupational hearing loss is a specific disease due to repetitive injury with established symptoms and objective findings. The diagnosis of occupational hearing loss cannot be reached reliably solely on the basis of an audiogram showing high-frequency sensorineural loss and patients' histories that they worked in a noisy plant. Accurate diagnosis requires a careful and complete history, physical examination, and laboratory and audiologic studies. Numerous entities such as acoustic neuroma, labyrinthitis, ototoxicity, viral infections, acoustic trauma (explosion), head trauma, hereditary hearing loss, diabetes, presbycusis, and genetic causes must be ruled out, as they are responsible for similar hearing loss in millions of people who were never employed in noisy industries.

## DEVELOPMENT OF A NOISE STANDARD

Comprehensive understanding of the nature of occupational hearing loss has been hindered by the difficulties associated with scientific studies in an industrial setting. A brief review of the old literature and an in-depth discussion of the most comprehensive studies highlight the complexities of the problem and the clinical and scientific findings that form the basis for the guidelines set forth in this chapter.

In 1952, James H. Sterner, MD, conducted an opinion poll among a large number of individuals working with noise and hearing to investigate the maximum intensity level of industrial noise that they considered safe to hearing (**Figure 17.1**) (1). The wide range of estimates clearly demonstrated the lack of agreement among knowledgeable individuals and the futility of any attempt to establish meaningful guidelines by means of such polls.

In 1954, the Z24-X-2 Subcommittee of the American Standards Association (now American National Standards Institute [ANSI]) published its exploratory report on the relations of hearing loss to noise exposure (2). They concluded that on the basis of available data, they could not establish a "line" between safe and unsafe noise exposure. They presented questions that required answers before criteria could be formulated, such as: (a) What amount of hearing loss constitutes a sufficient handicap to be considered undesirable? (b) What percentage of workers should a standard be designed to protect? The report emphasized the need for considerably more research before "safe" intensity levels could be determined.

DOI: 10.1201/b23379-17

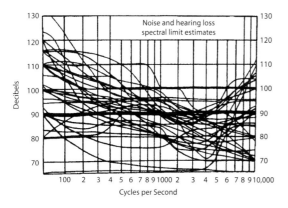

Figure 17.1 Noise and hearing loss spectral limit estimates.

Many authors between 1950 and 1971 proposed damage risk criteria, only some of which were based on stated protection goals. Articles are referenced in Table IX of the National Institute of Occupational Safety and Health's (NIOSH's) Criteria for Occupational Exposure to Noise (3). All these reports had limitations that precluded the adoption of any one of them as a basis for the establishment of standards. In 1973, Baughn (4) published an analysis of 6835 audiograms from employees in an automobile stamping plant, with employees divided into three groups on the basis of estimated intensity of noise exposure. Its validity as the basis for a national noise standard was seriously questioned by Ward and Glorig (5) and others because of shortcomings of non-steady-state noise exposures, vague estimates of noise dosage, auditory fatigue, and test room masking. Baughn's raw data were never made available to the Secretary of Labor's Advisory Committee for Noise Standard despite a formal request from that group.

A study by Burns and Robinson (6) avoided many of the deficiencies of previous studies but was based on a very small number of subjects exposed to continuous steady-state noise, particularly in the 82- to 92-dBA range. Workers were included who "change position from time to time using noisy hand tools for fettling, chipping, burnishing, or welding"—hardly continuous or steady state. Their report admitted to the inclusion of workers exposed to non-steady-state levels below 90 dBA. In fact, some workers were included whose noise exposure range varied by 15 dBA. The oft-quoted

Passchier-Vermeer report (7) was not based on an actual field investigation but was rather a review of published studies up to 1967. Some of these studies addressed the validity of measuring sound levels in dBA; none was really designed to be used as the basis for a noise standard.

As early as 1970, interested individuals from industry, labor, government, and scientific organizations discussed the concept of an Inter-Industry Noise Study. The project was started in 1974 for the stated purpose of gathering data on the effect of steady-state noise in the range of 82–92 dBA. While the results of such a study would obviously be of interest to those involved in noise regulation, the basic purpose of the study was scientific rather than regulatory. The detailed protocol has already been published (5) and will not be repeated here. Some of the important points are (a) clear definitions of the temporal and spectral characteristics of the noise; (b) noise exposures must fall between 82 and 92 dBA, with no subject exceeding a 5-dBA range (later modified to a 6-dBA range); (c) noise environment must be steady state throughout a full shift, with few, if any, sharp peaks of impact noise; (d) subjects, both experimental and control, must include men and women; (e) no prior job exposure to noise greater than 92 dBA for experimental subjects and 75 dBA for control subjects; (f) minimum of 3 years on present job; (g) all audiometric testing, noise measurement, equipment calibration, otological examinations, histories, and data handling to be done in a standardized manner, as detailed in the protocol; and (h) the original raw data to be made available to all serious investigators upon request at the conclusion of the study. Hearing levels were measured in 155 men and 193 women exposed to noise levels ranging from 82 to 92 dBA for at least 3 years, with a median duration of approximately 15 years; they were also measured in 96 men and 132 women with job exposure that did not exceed 75 dBA. Noise exposure was considered steady state in that it did not fluctuate more than ±3 dB from the midpoint as of the time of the first audiogram. As many subjects as possible were reexamined 1 year later and 2 years later.

Jobs involving some 250,000 employees were examined to find the 348 experimental subjects who met the criteria of the Inter-Industry Noise Study as of the time of entry. Within the range of 82–92 dBA, differences in noise intensity had no observable "effect" on hearing level. That is, the hearing levels of workers at the upper end of the noise intensity exposure were not observably different from the hearing levels of workers at the lower end of the noise exposure. Age was a more important factor than duration on the job in explaining differences in hearing level within any group. Comparisons between experimental and control subjects were made on an age-adjusted basis.

Differences between women exposed to 82–92 dBA and their controls were small and were not statistically significant. Differences between men exposed to 82–92 dBA and their controls were small and were not statistically significant at 500, 1000, and 2000 Hz. Levels in the noise-exposed group significantly exceeded those in the control group at 3000, 4000, and 6000 Hz by approximately 6–9 dB. At 8000 Hz, differences again became not significant.

There was no real evidence of a difference between noise-exposed workers and their controls with respect to the changes in hearing level during the course of their follow-up 1 and 2 years after initial audiograms. Changes were negligible for both groups.

It is important to note that the studies discussed, and the regulations promulgated to date concern themselves with exposure to continuous noise. Reports demonstrate that intermittent exposure to noise results in different effects on hearing (8). Although it may produce marked, high-frequency, sensorineural hearing loss, it does not have the same propensity to spread to the speech frequencies even after many years of exposure, as is seen with continuous noise exposure.

## AUDIOMETRIC FEATURES

The American College of Occupational Medicine Noise and Hearing Conservation Committee promulgated a position statement on the distinguishing features of occupational noise-induced hearing loss (NIHL) (9). This statement summarizes the currently accepted opinions of the medical community regarding diagnosis of occupational hearing loss. The American Occupational Medicine Association (AOMA) Committee defined occupational NIHL as a slowly developing hearing loss over a long time period (several years) as the result of exposure to continuous or intermittent loud noise. The committee stated that the diagnosis of NIHL is made clinically by a physician and should include a study of the noise exposure history. It also distinguished occupational hearing loss from occupational acoustic trauma, an immediate change in hearing resulting from a single exposure to a sudden burst of sound, such as an explosive blast. The committee recognized that the principal characteristics of occupational NIHL are as follows:

1. It is always sensorineural, affecting the hair cells in the inner ear.
2. It is almost always bilateral. Audiometric patterns are usually similar bilaterally.
3. It almost never produces a profound hearing loss. Usually, low-frequency limits are about 40 dB and high-frequency limits about 75 dB.
4. Once the exposure to noise is discontinued, there is no substantial further progression of hearing loss as a result of the noise exposure.
5. Previous NIHL does not make the ear more sensitive to future noise exposure. As the hearing threshold increases, the rate of loss decreases.
6. The earliest damage to the inner ears reflects a loss at 3000, 4000, and 6000 Hz. There is always far more loss at 3000, 4000, and 6000 Hz than at 500, 1000, and 2000 Hz. The greatest loss usually occurs at 4000 Hz. The higher and lower frequencies take longer to be affected than the 3000- to 6000-Hz range.
7. Given stable exposure conditions, losses at 3000, 4000, and 6000 Hz will usually reach a maximal level in about 10–15 years.
8. Continuous noise exposure over the years is more damaging than interrupted exposure to noise, which permits the ear to have a rest period.

On November 9, 2018, the American College of Occupational and Environmental Medicine (ACOEM) issued an evidenced-based statement regarding NIHL which can be viewed on updated the ACOEM website: https://acoem.org/Guidance-and-Position-Statements/Guidance-and-Position-Statements/Occupational-Noise-Induced-Hearing-Loss (10). In this statement, revisions to the criteria were suggested. The current language of the ACOEM criteria about NIHL is as follows:

- It is always sensorineural, primarily affecting the cochlear hair cells in the inner ear.
- It is typically bilateral since most noise exposures affect both ears symmetrically. Its first sign is a "notching" of the audiogram at the high frequencies of 3000, 4000, or 6000 Hz with recovery at 8000 Hz.
    - This notch typically develops at one of these frequencies and affects adjacent frequencies with continued noise exposure. This, together with the effects of aging, may reduce the prominence of the "notch." Therefore, in older individuals, the effects of noise may be difficult to distinguish from age-related hearing loss (presbycusis) without access to previous audiograms.
    - The exact location of the notch depends on multiple factors including the frequency of the damaging noise and size of the ear canal.
    - In early NIHL, average hearing thresholds at the lower frequencies of 500, 1000, and 2000 Hz are better than average thresholds at 3000, 4000, and 6000 Hz, and the hearing level at 8000 Hz is usually better than the deepest part of the notch. This notching is in contrast to presbycusis, which also produces high-frequency hearing loss but in a down-sloping pattern without recovery at 8000 Hz.
    - Although Occupational Safety and Health Act (OSHA) does not require audiometric testing at 8000 Hz, inclusion of this frequency is highly recommended to assist in the identification of the noise notch as well as age-related hearing loss.
- Noise exposure alone usually does not produce a loss greater than 75 dB in high frequencies and greater than 40 dB in lower frequencies. Nevertheless, individuals with non-NIHL, such as presbycusis, may have hearing threshold levels in excess of these values. Hearing loss due to continuous or intermittent noise exposure increases most rapidly during the first 10 to 15 years of exposure, and the rate of hearing loss then decelerates as the hearing threshold increases.

This is in contrast to age-related loss, which accelerates over time.

- Available evidence indicates that previously noise-exposed ears are not more sensitive to future noise exposure. There is insufficient evidence to conclude that hearing loss due to noise will progress once the noise exposure is discontinued. This is primarily based on a National Institute of Medicine report which concluded that, on the basis of available human and animal data, it was felt unlikely that such delayed effects occur. However, recent animal experiments indicate although there appears to be threshold recovery and no loss of cochlear cells following noise exposures to rodents, there is evidence of cochlear afferent nerve terminal damage and delayed degeneration of the cochlear nerve, thus suggesting that delayed effects could be seen in the future.
- Although the OSHA action level for noise exposure is 85 dB (8-hour time-weighted average), the evidence suggests that noise exposure from 80 to 85 dB may contribute to hearing loss in individuals who are unusually susceptible. The risk of NIHL increases with long-term noise exposures above 80 dB and increases significantly as exposures rise above 85 dB.
- Continuous noise exposure throughout the workday and over years is more damaging than interrupted exposure to noise, which permits the ear to have a rest period. At the present time, measures to estimate the health effects of such intermittent noise are controversial.
- Real-world attenuation provided by hearing protective devices may vary widely between individuals. The noise reduction rating of hearing protective devices used by a working population is expected to be less than the laboratory derived rating. Hearing protective devices should provide adequate attenuation to reduce noise exposure at the eardrum to less than 85-dB time-weighted average. In addition, technology is now available, which can provide an individualized attenuation rating for hearing protective devices and continuous monitoring of noise at the eardrum.
- The presence of a temporary threshold shift (TTS, i.e., the temporary loss of hearing, which largely disappears 16–48 hours after exposure to loud noise) with or without tinnitus is a risk indicator that permanent NIHL will likely

occur if hazardous noise exposure continues. Barring an ototraumatic incident, workers will always develop TTS before sustaining permanent threshold shift (PTS).

The ACOEM document also discusses additional considerations in the evaluation of workers with suspected NIHL, addressing several issues such as exposure to noise sources that affect the ear asymmetrically, the effect of additional impulse/impact noise on steady-state noise exposure, co-exposure to ototoxic agents, individual comorbidities, genetic predisposition and medical history that may be associated with hearing loss, non-occupational noise exposure, the impact of hearing loss and associated symptoms on worker communication and safety, early recognition of NIHL, age-correction, and emphasis on holistic and detailed evaluation of patients. The document also describes the role of an occupational and environmental medicine physician in diagnosing NIHL.

## SENSORINEURAL HEARING LOSS

Habitual exposure to occupational noise damages the hair cells in the cochlea, causing a sensory hearing loss. No damage to the outer or middle ear (conductive loss) can be caused by routine daily exposure to loud industrial noise. Ultimately, some of the nerve fibers supplying the damaged hair cells may also become damaged from many causes and result in a neural loss of hearing, as well.

## BILATERALITY OF OCCUPATIONAL HEARING LOSS

Both ears are equally sensitive to TTS and PTS hearing loss due to free-field occupational noise exposure, and, therefore, damage is equal or almost equal in both ears. If an employee working in a very noisy environment develops substantial one-sided nerve deafness, it is essential to find the cause and to rule out an acoustic neuroma, which commonly presents as unilateral sensorineural deafness. In weapons and range fire, the ear nearest the stock (left ear in a right-handed shooter) sustains damage before and to a somewhat greater degree than the other ear; however, a loss will generally be present to some degree bilaterally.

## THE 4000-Hz AUDIOMETRIC DIP

NIHL has been shown to be sensorineural in nature and usually bilateral; it also contains a characteristic frequency response known as the 4000-Hz dip. **Figure 17.2** shows a composite audiogram of the classic progress of many cases of occupational hearing loss. This pattern is actually more common in hearing loss caused by gunfire, but exposure to continuous noise, such as in weaving mills and some metal plants, also produces this pattern in which the earliest damage occurs between 3000 and 6000 Hz. Some noise sources, such as papermaking machines, can damage the 2000-Hz frequency somewhat before the higher frequencies, while noise exposures such as chipping and jackhammers characteristically damage the higher frequencies severely before affecting the lower ones. However, in general, the frequencies below 3000 Hz are almost never damaged by occupational noise without earlier damage to the higher frequencies.

It has been known for many years that prolonged exposure to high-intensity noise results in sensorineural hearing loss that is greatest between 3000 and 6000 Hz. In such cases, the classic audiogram shows a 4000-Hz dip in which hearing is better at 2000 and 8000 Hz (**Figure 17.3**). Unfortunately, the fact that noise produces this 4000-Hz dip has led some physicians to assume that any comparable dip is produced by noise. This error can lead to misdiagnosis and can result in undesirable medical and legal consequences.

Although there are numerous hypotheses that attempt to explain the 4000-Hz dip in NIHL (11–14), its pathogenesis remains uncertain. However, it is known that in most cases this loss initially affects hearing between 4000 and 6000 Hz and then spreads to other frequencies (15, 16). Frequencies higher than those usually measured clinically may be tested on special audiometers and are helpful in diagnosing NIHL in selected cases (17). This hearing loss may result from steady-state or interrupted noise, although the intensities required to produce comparable hearing losses differ (18), and controversy exists as to the nature of the actual cochlear damage (18–21). Other types of acoustic trauma, such as that from blast injuries, may result in other audiometric patterns or in a 4000-Hz dip, but they will not be considered in this discussion.

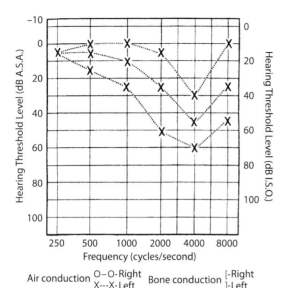

Figure 17.2 Series of audiometric curves showing a "classic" progressive loss that may be found in employees with excessive noise exposure. *Abbreviations*: ASA, American Standards Association; ISO, International Standards Organization.

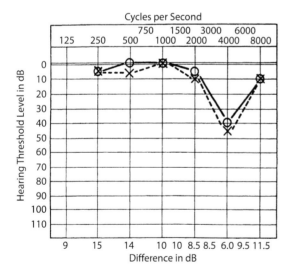

Figure 17.3 Typical 4000-Hz dip. In this audiogram and in all other audiograms in this chapter, bone conduction equals air conduction.

## DISCRIMINATION SCORES

In almost all cases of occupational hearing loss where the high frequencies are affected (even severely), the discrimination scores are good (over 85%) in a quiet room. If patients have much lower discrimination scores, another cause in addition to occupational hearing loss should be suspected.

## GRADUAL HEARING LOSS WITH EARLY ONSET

In addition to having the characteristics of a bilateral sensorineural hearing loss with a 4000-Hz dip, occupational hearing loss begins early with noise exposure and progresses gradually. Sudden deafness is not caused by noise that patients are exposed to regularly at their job: there are, of course, incidents of unilateral sudden deafness due to acoustic trauma from an explosion or similar circumstance. Other causes must be sought in sudden deafness in one or both ears regardless of occupational noise exposure.

Occupational hearing loss characteristically develops in the first few years of exposure and may worsen over the next 8–10 years of continued exposure, but the damage does not continue to progress rapidly or substantially with additional exposure beyond 10–15 years. Rarely will an employee working in consistent noise have good hearing for 4 or 5 years and then develop progressive hearing loss from occupational causes. Employees who retire after age 60 and develop additional hearing loss without continued noise exposure generally should not attribute this to their past jobs (22). The same pertains to employees who wear hearing protectors effectively and either develop hearing loss or have additional hearing loss.

## ASYMPTOTIC HEARING LOSS

Another characteristic of occupational hearing loss is that specific noisy jobs produce a maximum degree of hearing loss. This has been called asymptotic loss. For example, employees using jackhammers develop severe high-frequency, but minimal low-frequency, hearing losses. Employees working for years in about 92 dBA generally do not have over 20-dB losses in the low frequencies, and once they reach a certain degree of high-frequency hearing loss, little additional loss occurs. Many employees exposed to weaving looms experience a maximum of about a 40-dB loss in the speech frequencies, but they rarely have greater losses. If an employee shows a loss much greater than is typical for similar exposure, the otologist should suspect other causes.

## LIMITATIONS OF THE AUDIOGRAM

An audiogram showing a 4000-Hz dip is not, by itself, sufficient evidence to make a diagnosis of NIHL. In order to do so, one must have at least a history of sufficient exposure to noise of adequate intensity to account for the hearing loss. In the absence of this history, or with a history and findings suggestive of another origin, a thorough investigation must be done to establish the true cause of the hearing loss. It must be understood that it is not always possible to ascribe a hearing loss to a noise or to completely rule out other causes. If, however, the patient's noise exposure has been sufficient, and if investigation fails to reveal other causes of hearing loss, a diagnosis of NIHL can be made with reasonable certainty in the presence of supportive audiometric findings.

## OTHER CAUSES OF THE 4000-Hz DIP

### Viral infections

It is well known that viral upper-respiratory infections may be associated with hearing loss, tinnitus, and a sensation of fullness in the ears. This fullness is frequently due to inner ear involvement rather than middle ear dysfunction. Viral cochleitis may also produce either temporary or permanent sensorineural hearing losses, which can have a variety of audiometric patterns, including a 4000-Hz dip (**Figure 17.4**) (23). In addition to viral respiratory infections as causes of sensorineural hearing loss, rubella, measles, mumps, cytomegalic inclusion disease, herpes, and other viruses have been implicated (**Figure 17.5**).

### Skull trauma

Severe head trauma that results in fracture of the cochlea produces profound or total deafness. However, lesser injuries to the inner ear may produce a concussion-type injury, which may be manifested audiometrically as a 4000-Hz dip. Human temporal bone pathology in such cases is similar to that seen in NIHL (24). Similar findings also can be produced by experimental temporal-bone injury (14).

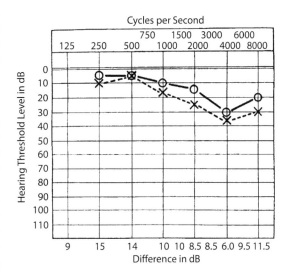

Figure 17.4 4000-Hz dip caused by viral cochleitis in a patient with no history of noise exposure.

## Hereditary (genetic) hearing loss

Hereditary sensorineural hearing loss results commonly in an audiometric pattern similar to that of occupational hearing loss (25–27). This may be particularly difficult to diagnose since hereditary deafness need not have appeared in a family member previously; in fact, many cases of hereditary hearing loss follow an autosomal-recessive inheritance pattern. There have been new developments in identification of genes associated with hereditary hearing loss, making it possible currently to identify specifically some forms of genetic hearing loss.

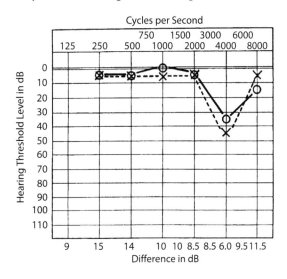

Figure 17.5 4000-Hz dip caused by a herpes infection in a patient without noise exposure.

## Ototoxicity

The most commonly used ototoxic drugs at present are aminoglycoside antibiotics, diuretics, chemotherapeutic agents, and aspirin (in high doses; see **Table 10.2**). When toxic effects are seen, high-frequency sensorineural hearing loss is most common and profound deafness may result, although a 4000-Hz dip pattern also may be seen (**Figure 17.6**) (21). Unlike damage caused by the other ototoxic drugs listed above, aspirin-induced hearing loss usually is only temporary, recovering after cessation of the medication.

## Acoustic neuroma

Eighth-nerve tumors may produce any audiometric pattern, from that of normal hearing to profound deafness, and the 4000-Hz dip is not a rare manifestation of this lesion (**Figures 17.7** and **17.8**) (28). In these lesions, low speech discrimination scores and pathological tone decay need not be present and cannot be relied on to rule out retrocochlear pathology. Nevertheless, asymmetry of hearing loss should arouse suspicion even when a history of noise exposure exists. There are several cases in which patients were exposed to loud noises producing hearing losses that recovered in one ear but not in the other because of underlying acoustic neuromas (M.D. Graham, personal communication).

## Sudden hearing loss

Each year, clinicians see numerous cases of sudden sensorineural hearing loss of unknown origin. Although the hearing loss is usually unilateral,

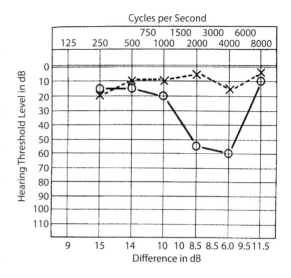

Figure 17.7 4000-Hz dip caused by right 3-cm acoustic neuroma.

it may be bilateral and show a 4000-Hz dip. This audiometric pattern may also be seen in patients with sudden hearing loss due to inner ear-membrane breaks (29, 30) and barotrauma (31, 32).

## Multiple sclerosis

Multiple sclerosis also can produce sensorineural hearing loss that may show almost any pattern and may fluctuate from severe deafness to normal threshold levels. An example demonstrating a variable 4000-Hz dip is shown in **Figure 17.9**.

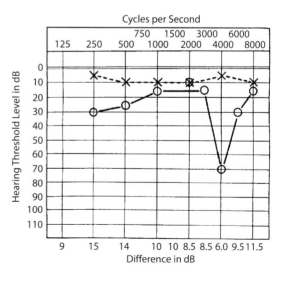

Figure 17.8 4000-Hz dip caused by 1-cm right acoustic neuroma.

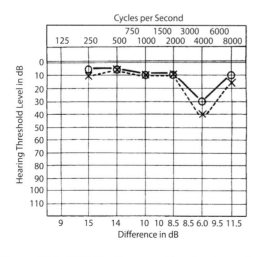

Figure 17.6 4000-Hz dip caused by streptomycin.

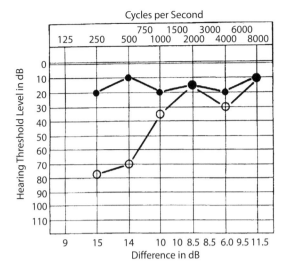

**Figure 17.9** Fluctuating sensorineural hearing in a patient with multiple sclerosis that includes a 4000-Hz dip. The lower (worse) test was obtained 3 months before the upper (better) test.

## Other causes

A variety of other causes may produce audiograms similar to those seen in NIHL. Such conditions include bacterial infections such as meningitis, a variety of systemic toxins (33), and neonatal hypoxia and jaundice. **Figure 17.10** illustrates one such sensorineural hearing loss that resulted from kernicterus due to Rh incompatibility.

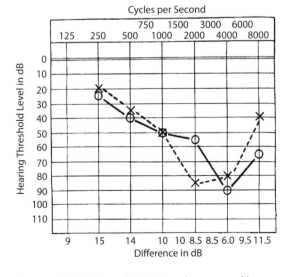

**Figure 17.10** Bilateral 4000-Hz dips caused by kernicterus due to Rh incompatibility.

## NOISE EXPOSURE HISTORY

It is important to recall that sound of a given frequency spectrum and intensity requires a certain amount of time to produce hearing loss in most subjects. While the necessary exposure varies from person to person, a diagnosis of NIHL requires a history of sufficient noise exposure. Guidelines for estimating how much noise is necessary to cause hearing loss in most people have been established by the scientific community and the federal government and are reviewed in this chapter. However, a reasonable assessment of patients' occupational noise exposure cannot be obtained solely from their histories, especially if compensation is a factor.

Patients who have worked for many years on weaving looms, papermaking machines, boilers, sheet metal riveters, jackhammers, chippers, and the like nearly always have some degree of occupational hearing loss. However, many other patients have marked hearing losses that could not possibly have been caused by their minimal exposures to noise. Almost all patients working in industry can claim that they have been exposed to a great deal of noise. It is essential, especially in compensation cases, to get more accurate information by obtaining, if possible, a written work history and time-weighted average of noise exposure from the employer. If a physician does not have firsthand knowledge of the noise exposure in a patient's job, definitive diagnosis should be delayed until such information is made available.

Some publications (5, 8) have suggested that exposures below 90 dBA can produce handicapping hearing losses in the speech frequencies. A critical review of the most quoted historical publications (34, 35) reveals serious shortcomings in study design that cast doubt on the conclusions drawn from these studies. However, new guidance outlined by the most recent ACOEM committee opinion suggests that occupational noise exposure to levels of 80–85 dB may contribute to hearing loss in some individuals (10). OSHA guidelines conservatively protect hearing and mandate initiation of a hearing conservation program and use of hearing protection when workers are exposed to noise levels at or above 85 dBA over 8 hours. The exact level at which exposure to occupational noise produces hearing loss has not been definitively reported in the literature. Even the authors of the Inter-Industry Noise Exposure studies, which are thought to be the best-conducted and monitored research projects relating hearing loss and noise exposure, emphasize the need for additional valid and reliable research. It can then be suggested that when a patient presents with hearing loss and occupational noise exposure between 85 and 90 dBA, a specific cause for their hearing loss should be ruled out before the diagnosis of occupational hearing loss is given. The term biological hypersensitivity to noise is often misused and requires clarification. Many physicians and attorneys have attributed patients' substantial sensorineural hearing loss to hypersensitivity to noise, even though the exposure was 85 dBA or less. There is no basis for such an opinion. Prolonged exposure to this type of noise level will not cause handicapping hearing loss in the speech frequencies. Biological hypersensitivity to noise does not mean that individuals exposed to mild levels below 90 dBA can sustain substantial hearing losses, but rather that in a group of employees habitually exposed to very loud noise (over 95 dBA) without hearing protectors, a few will have little or no hearing loss (so-called hard ears), most will have a fair amount of loss, and a few will sustain substantially greater losses because they are hypersensitive.

Many years of otologic studies and clinical experience have demonstrated certain symptoms and findings that are characteristic of occupational hearing loss. For instance, we know that employees do not suffer total or very severe sensorineural deafness in the speech frequencies even if they work for years in the loudest industrial noise areas. Several explanations have been proposed for this observation, for example: "the nerve-deafened ear acts as a hearing protector" and "what you don't hear doesn't hurt you." Even when noise exposure is very high and undoubtedly a contributing cause, all patients with severely handicapping losses in the speech frequencies should be studied carefully to find the underlying etiology.

Otologic history should include use, duration, effectiveness of hearing protection, type of noise exposure (including continuous or intermittent), dosage of exposure (daily hours and years), and presence of recreational noise exposure such as target practice, trap shooting, hunting, snowmobile use, motorcycling, and chain saw or power-tool use. Recreational exposure may contribute to NIHL. Employees should be advised to use hearing protectors during recreational exposure to loud noise. Infrequent exposures and intermittent exposures are far less hazardous than continuous daily exposures. It seems that if the ear has sufficient rest periods, damage to the speech frequencies is minimized.

## HISTOPATHOLOGY OF NOISE-INDUCED HEARING LOSS

Histologic studies of human inner ears damaged by noise reveal diffuse degeneration of hair cells and nerves in the second quadrant of the basal turn of the cochlea—the area sensitive to 3000- to 6000-Hz sounds (**Figures 17.11–17.13**) (21). Similar findings have been demonstrated in cochlear hair cells and first-order neurons in experimental animals exposed to loud noises, as discussed below. Further experimental studies in rodents have shown noise-induced injury to the stria vascularis, as well (36, 37), but there is some question as to the applicability of this finding to clinical medicine.

Comprehensive discussion of the histopathology of NIHL is beyond the scope of this book. The subject is controversial, and many questions remain unanswered. However, certain observations are of particular clinical interest and worthwhile reviewing, particularly those of Professor H. Spoendlin of Innsbruck, Austria (37).

The psychophysical effects of sound stimulation at various intensities include the following:

1. Adaptation is an immediate and rapidly reversible threshold shift proportional to the sound intensity at the frequency of stimulation.
2. TTS is pathological, metabolically induced fatigue. Its development and recovery are proportional to the logarithm of exposure time. It reverses slowly over a period of hours.
3. PTS, such as occupational hearing loss, develops by exposure to excessive noise for sufficiently long period of time.

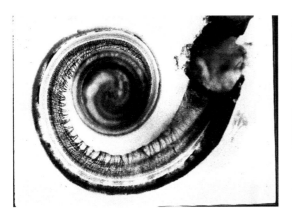

Figure 17.11 Normal cochlea from a 17-year-old woman with largely intact hair cells and neurons.

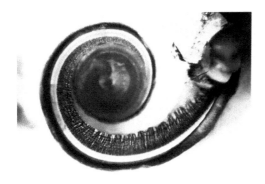

Figure 17.12 Cochlea showing hair cell and nerve loss that worsens progressively as it approached the basal end of the cochlea from a 77-year-old man.

The extended exposure time results in the destruction and eventual loss of the cells of the organ of Corti. Two mechanisms appear to be involved in this process:

1. In high-intensity noise exposure, there may be direct mechanical destruction.
2. In exposure to moderately intense noise, there is a metabolic decompensation with subsequent degeneration of sensory elements.

If a cochlea is examined shortly after even short-term exposure to extremely intense noise, it will show entire absence of the organ of Corti in the epicenter of the injured area. Moving laterally from the epicenter, the hair cells are swollen and severely distorted with cytoplasmic organelle displacement. More laterally, the cells reveal bending of sensory hairs. Further from the epicenter, but still in the area of damage, one finds only slight distortion of the outer hair cells. In addition to sensory damage, dislocation of the tympanic lamina cells, disruption of the heads of the pillar cells, holes in the basilar membrane, and other findings may be found.

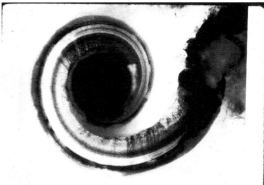

Figure 17.13 Cochlea from the left ear of an avid hunter showing severe loss of hair cells and nerves in the second quadrant of the basal turn, corresponding to 3000-/6000-Hz detection region.

After exposure to moderately intense acoustic stimuli, the nuclei of outer hair cells become extremely swollen. Swelling is also seen in the terminal unmyelinated portion of the afferent nerve fibers to the inner hair cells. This pathological condition of afferent nerve fibers is also seen in hypoxia. In both instances, it appears to result from metabolic derangement. Degeneration of mitochondria and alteration of the synaptic vesicles may be observed in the efferent nerve endings of the outer hair cells after long exposure (38).

TTS appears to cause only an increase in number and size of lysosomes, primarily in the outer hair cells, a finding probably also related to increased metabolic activity.

The localization of damage depends on the type of noise exposure. Exposure to white noise, multifrequency noise encountered under most industrial circumstances, usually produces damage in the upper basal turn of the cochlea, the 3000- to 6000-Hz frequency range in humans. Narrowband noise causes damage in different areas depending on the frequency of the noise; the extent of the damage increases with increasing intensity of the center frequency. These observations are true for continuous noise, impulse noise results in much more variability in the site of damage. The rise time of the impulse appears to be an important factor in the amount of hearing damage. Histologically, square-noise impulses appear to produce less damage than impulses with a gradual rising time of 25 milliseconds (37). The practical implications of this finding remain unclear.

The histological progression of cochlear injury over time is also of interest. Some of the mechanically or metabolically induced structural changes are reversible, whereas others progress to degeneration. Metabolically induced changes such as swollen nuclei in the outer hair cells and swollen nerve endings usually reverse, although scattered degeneration occurs. Severe distortion of cells often leads to degeneration and membrane ruptures, which may result in the disappearance of the organ of Corti in the area of injury. In places where the organ of Corti is completely destroyed, the cochlear neurons undergo slow, progressive retrograde degeneration over months. Eventually, about 90% of the cochlear neurons associated with the injured area disappear, including their spiral ganglion cells of origin. This retrograde neural degeneration usually is not observed when only outer hair cells are missing (39). No significant neural degeneration has been noted in adjacent areas. Thus, although histopathological changes progress even after acoustic stimulation has stopped, significant degeneration occurs only in regions where substantial hair cell destruction (hence, substantial hearing loss) has already occurred. Consequently, progressive histological changes do not imply progressive clinical hearing deterioration.

Histologically, maximal damage to the cochlea secondary to noise exposure is never total. Even under laboratory circumstances, there are always some sensory elements preserved in the cochlea. Moreover, for each exposure intensity, "saturation damage" occurs after a certain time. The time interval is short for high-intensity noise exposure and long for low-intensity noise exposure. Additional exposure to noise of the same intensity does not produce additional observable damage beyond this "saturation damage" limit. This histological finding corresponds to asymptotic hearing loss. Moreover, even under laboratory conditions, there is a great variability of cochlear damage produced by controlled noise exposure, especially following stimulation by moderately intense noise or impulse noise. These are the conditions encountered most commonly in an industrial environment. This histological and experimental evaluation corresponds to the biological variability (hard ears and soft ears) observed in industrial populations.

## OCCUPATIONAL NOISE EXPOSURE DURING PREGNANCY

During approximately the last two decades, questions have been raised about whether significant noise exposure during pregnancy has any adverse effect upon the fetus or pregnancy outcome. While definitive answers have not been established, a growing body of literature suggests that there may be an effect. Nurminen suggested the possibility that noise-induced stress in the mother might cause reproductive disturbances (40). It has been noted that high noise levels and shift work (especially rotating schedules that interfere with circadian rhythm) may have negative effects on both weight and length of gestation and that there have been suggestions that noise exposure and shift work correlated with menstrual disturbance and infertility. However, although Nurminen suggested that it would be prudent to consider high noise levels and shift work as reproductive risks, no evidence was presented to confirm or refute the hypothesis.

An effect of occupational noise on birth weight and gestational length was supported by evidence from the fetal noise exposure study (FENIX), a prospective cohort study of mother–child pairs in Sweden who were followed over a 16-year period. FENIX demonstrated that infants of mothers who worked full-time and were exposed to noise levels of either 75–85 dBA or >85 dBA had an increased risk of small-for-gestational age (odds ratios of 1.09:1 and 1.44:1, respectively) when compared to infants of mothers who worked full-time with low occupational noise exposure (< 75 dBA) (41). Infants of mothers who worked full-time and were exposed to either 75–85 dBA or > 85 dBA also had an increased risk for low birth weight indicated by odds ratios of 1.11:1 and 1.36:1, respectively (41). Preterm birth was found only among infants exposed to noise levels of 75–85 dBA in mothers who worked full-time (41). The increased risk for low birth weight and small-for-gestational size was attributed to the occupational noise itself, given that mothers who worked part-time or had high absenteeism from work did not show any increased risk for these birth outcomes.

Comorbidities of pregnancy such as pregnancy-related hypertensive disorders (gestational hypertension, preeclampsia, and eclampsia) can have a negative impact on birth outcomes. A prospective cohort study from Sweden indicated that mothers exposed to noise levels of 80–85 dBA during pregnancy had an increased risk of gestational hypertension and preeclampsia (42). This association was found to be even stronger in women who worked full-time and were first-time mothers. However, a meta-analysis revealed that occupational· noise exposure had no effect on the incidence of gestational hypertension, but it did show that exposure to occupational noise increased the risk of preeclampsia (43).

Lalande et al. (44) examined the hearing of 131 children whose mothers had worked while pregnant with that child, in noise ranging from 65 to 95 dB over 8-hour periods. They found a threefold increase in the risk of children having high-frequency hearing loss when their mothers had been exposed to noise in the range of 85–95 dBA and a significant increase in the risk of hearing loss at 4000 Hz when maternal exposures had involved a "strong component" of low-frequency noise. Evidence from the FENIX study supported the association between infants whose mothers had been exposed to noise ranging from 75 to 85 dBA and sensorineural hearing loss in the child (45). The association between hearing dysfunction and occupational noise exposure was strongest in the study when subgroup analysis was restricted to mothers who worked full-time and had a low absenteeism rate.

Research regarding fetal malformations or congenital abnormalities and occupational noise exposure is scarce and remains an important area for further investigation. A review reported that no studies found an association between occupational noise exposure and perinatal mortality, although two studies have demonstrated a link between occupational noise and congenital abnormalities (46). Shi et. al (47) found an association between occupational noise exposure and polydactyly, and Gong et al. (48) found an association between congenital heart disease and occupational noise exposure. This research expands the knowledge regarding the impact of noise on fetuses in foundational work done by Murato et al., who looked at the effects of noise and cadmium in mice (49). They found (not surprisingly) that cadmium was teratogenic, and there was no synergistic effect between cadmium and noise. In the groups exposed to continuous noise for 6 hours, total percentages of malformed fetuses were significantly higher than those in the control group, but there were no significant increases in total percentages of fetal malformations in the combined treatment groups in comparison with the groups, given the same dose of cadmium alone. The authors speculated that the magnitude of the teratogenicity due to noise might be so much weaker than that of cadmium that the effects were masked statistically. However, one must also consider the possibility that there was no effect.

While these papers certainly raise interesting questions, data to definitively support the association between occupational noise on fetuses and pregnancy outcomes are still scarce. Further study will be necessary to determine with certainty whether there is any fetal or maternal risk associated with occupational noise exposure.

## COFACTORS ASSOCIATED WITH OCCUPATIONAL HEARING LOSS

### NON-OCCUPATIONAL NOISE EXPOSURE

Habitual exposure to loud rock-and-roll and amplified music can produce hearing damage between 2000 and 8000 Hz. Occasional exposure, however, can be annoying to unaccustomed listeners but does not cause significant hearing damage in most cases. Sataloff et al. found potentially damaging noise levels at audience locations at a concert by the band Metallica™ (50). Peak levels reached 140 dBA, and audiodosimetry measurements revealed loudness equivalent levels between 95 and 111 dBA. Further, a single-blinded, randomized control trial found that music festival attendees who were exposed to sound pressure levels (SPLs) of 100 dBA and did not use ear plugs had a relative risk of a TTS of 5.5 when compared to attendees who used ear plugs during the festival (51). Derebery et. al (52) found TTSs of 10 dBA or greater in one-third of teenagers who attended a single rock concert. While single events are unlikely to cause measurable permanent hearing damage, such events repeated over time have the potential to cause PTSs.

In another venue often attended by the public, Sataloff et al. looked at noise levels in two movie theaters (53). They found maximum SPLs of approximately 97 dBA, but exposures over time were safe. Household noises such as vacuum cleaners, fans, and air conditioners generally do not damage hearing even though they may be disturbing. Despite some parental arguments to the contrary, it also appears that prolonged telephone use does not impair hearing. Mendes and Barrionuevo

(54) examined the hearing of 50 female telephone operators between 35 and 50 years of age who had been using earphones at work for 6-hour shifts for at least 10 years. They compared these subjects with an age-matched control group of 291 women who had not been exposed to earphone noise and whose telephone use was typical of that practiced by the general public. The control group also had not been exposed to noise levels in excess of 85 dB. The authors found that even telephone operators using earphones had no greater risk of hearing loss than the control group (54).

Exposure to ultrasonic noise, such as in certain commercial cleaners, does not affect hearing in the usually recorded frequencies (up to 8000 Hz). Community noises such as trolley cars, airplanes, noises from industrial plants, and sirens also ordinarily do not cause measurable hearing damage. A study recording noise exposure on the London underground over 13 years revealed that passengers were consistently exposed to SPLs above 80 dBA and that passengers were occasionally exposed to sound levels above 100 dBA (55). While this represents intermittent noise exposure at or above 80 dBA, more research is needed to address whether this poses a risk to hearing loss.

Although childcare facilities are boisterous environments charmed with loud exclamations of joy and dismay, they are often not considered capable of inducing hearing dysfunction in caretakers and children alike. However, Lissåker et al. listed child caretakers as the second most common worker exposed to 80–85 dBA in the FENIX study (42). Part of the noisy milieu stems from toys, and Yaremchuk et al. addressed the hazard that toys can have on child caretakers and children in a particularly interesting paper. (56). Guidelines for noise production of toys have been updated from the Voluntary Product Standards, PS 72-76, the Toy Safety Act of 1969 to the U.S. Consumer Product Safety Commission, American Society for Testing and Materials (ASTM) F963–17, and *Standard Consumer Safety Specification for Toy Safety*. Yaremchuk and her coauthors evaluated 25 toys purchased at a national toy store chain and measured SPLs at distances approximating ear level (2.5 cm) and a child's arm length (25 cm) from the surface of the toy. They found peak sound levels ranging from 81 to 126 dBA at 2.5 cm, and from 80 to 115 dBA at 25 cm. Some of their findings are summarized in **Tables 17.1–17.3**. They found that

at ear level, seven of the 25 toys tested exceeded 115 dBA, which OSHA recommends workers spend less than one-fourth of their day in proximity of even while wearing hearing protection. Six toys exceeded the 115 dBA at the "arm's length" distance of 25 cm. Yaremchuk et al. concluded that these toys posed significant noise hazards and advocated for regulations to measure SPLs at ear level, as well as at 25 cm. Despite the update to the legislation governing toy noise production, the recommendations from Yaremchuk et al. were not included and guidelines from ASTM International specify that toys should be tested 50 ± 1cm from the microphone. We continue to advocate for a change in the testing standards for the safety of children and child caretakers alike.

Table 17.1 Preliminary measure peak dBA of three trials with portable sound level meter (SLM) in double-wall sound booth

| Toys | dBA 2.5 cm | dBA 25 cm |
|---|---|---|
| Bike horn #1 | 120 | 108 |
| Bike horn #2 | 122 | 110 |
| Headset portable radio (Auto volume limiter) | 81 | NA |
| Guitar | 106 | 92 |
| Boom box music | 112 | 106 |
| Laser gun | 114 | 96 |
| Army gun | 113 | 110 |
| Whistle | 114 | 106 |
| Sonic shooter | 117 | 101 |
| X-ray phaser | 108 | 88 |
| Gatling gun | 110 | 104 |
| Toy drill | 106 | 91 |
| Telephone | 95 | 89 |
| Flute | 126 | 102 |
| Pop gun | 92 | 90 |
| Bicycle horn | 120 | 90 |
| Camcorder | 94 | NA |
| Keyboard #1 | 103 | 101 |
| Siren/Radio | 110 | 96 |
| Tape player #1 | 100 | 90 |
| Tape player #2 | 114 | 101 |
| Keyboard #2 | 104 | 86 |
| Beeper/Pager | 122 | 93 |
| Cassette recorder | 126 | 115 |
| Sound effects keyboard | 98 | 80 |

Table 17.2 Leq measures and spectral analysis of the 10 toys studied in detail

| Toys | Leq (dBA) at 2.5 cm | Leq (dBA) at 25 cm | Frequency spectrum (Hz) |
|---|---|---|---|
| Flute | 127 | 118 | 1000–1200 |
| Bicycle horn | 126 | 111 | 1000–3000 |
| Gatling gun | 119 | 116 | 800–4000 |
| Pop gun | 122 | 116 | 300–5000 |
| Army gun | 119 | 116 | 500–3000 |
| Telephone | 117 | 115 | 1500–2000 |
| Sonic shooter | 119 | 115 | |
| Cassette player (Feedback) | 119 | 116 | 700 |
| Machine laser gun | 117 | 116 | 700–8000 |
| Guitar | 117 | 115 | 500–5000 |

In our automobile-dependent society, motor vehicle accidents and airbag deployment are common. All of us with busy otology practices encounter claims in which hearing loss, tinnitus, and/or dizziness have allegedly been caused by an airbag deployment. Various literature summarized this subject (57, 58). In the report by Yaremchuk and Dobie (57), the authors noted that there had been an estimated 2.1 million airbag deployments in the preceding 10 years. Although the possibility of airbag-induced hearing impairment had been dismissed initially, later experience indicated that such hearing injury is possible. Airbags are deployed using either gas inflation, an explosive device, or hybrid devices. They deploy at speeds of approximately 200 miles per hour over 25–50 milliseconds. Hence, they produce impulse noise (a high-amplitude, short-duration pressure wave). This noise is comparable to a single rifle shot and is generally in the range of 160–170 dB SPL. Just as with a single rifle shot, most people exposed to airbag deployment do not sustain hearing damage. However, such an event is capable of causing otologic symptoms in some people under specific circumstances. For example, in drivers whose heads were turned to the side when the front airbag deployed and whose ears were struck directly by the inflating airbag, otologic injury is common. Similar contact may occur from a side airbag, but the position of side airbags usually precludes such an occurrence and usually places the driver's or passenger's ear more than 1 ft from the airbag deployed. Interestingly, although it seems counterintuitive, a closed vehicle actually helps protect against hearing injury from airbag deployment by preserving protective effects from low-frequency components that are lost through open windows. Most airbag noise is low frequency. People who sustain cochlear injury from acoustic trauma such as airbag deployment ordinarily recognize the injury promptly (at the scene or within approximately a day) unless there is some other major, related injury that distracts them. Readers who encounter this complex problem are encouraged to consult the articles by Yaremchuk and Dobie (57) and by McKinley and Nixon (58), as well as the classic literature cited in those publications, and more recent studies.

Table 17.3 Leq measurements, peak dBA, and peak latencies for the pop gun

| | 2.5 cm | 25 cm |
|---|---|---|
| Sample rate | 25 fs | 25 fs |
| Leq | 122.045 dBA | 115.833 dBA |
| L90 | 122.265 dBA | 115.902 dBA |
| L10 | 115.109 dBA | 115.09 dBA |
| A duration | 38.0711 ms | 3.56916 ms |
| A peak[a] | 123.217 dBA | 124.222 dBA |
| B duration | 96.1777 ms | 21.415 ms |
| B peak[b] | 123.105 dBA | 123.709 dBA |

[a] "A peak" is the first major amplitude peak of the sound and "A duration" is its latency.
[b] "B peak" is the second major peak and "B duration" is its latency.

## ASPIRIN

Limited research exists that investigates the interaction of aspirin and noise exposure on hearing loss. A study by Carson et al. (59) explored the interaction of different aspirin doses and presence of noise on the hearing of rats. Permanent hearing losses and hair cell damage were noted in all animals exposed to the noise condition; however, a greater amount of hair cell loss was observed in the animals with the highest dose of aspirin. Although some animal studies, like the one discussed above, have shown a relationship between NIHL and aspirin, its interaction on human hair cells and hearing loss is unknown at this time.

## SMOKING

Research studies have implicated smoking as a cofactor that may affect the degree and risk of occupational hearing loss. Past experiments investigating the correlation of smoking and high-frequency NIHL illustrate a higher risk of hearing loss (60–64). Several cross-sectional studies have shown that smoking is a risk factor for NIHL (60, 65–68). One study revealed that current smokers had an increased rate of hearing loss by a ratio of 1.39:1 with an increase in the trend based on the number of packs smoked per day (60). A meta-analysis found that current smokers had a pooled odds ratio of 2.05:1 for the risk of developing occupational NIHL, and it was noted that increased risk of occupational NIHL increased with increasing reported pack-years of cigarettes up until 15 years in a non-linear association (69). It has also been suggested that passive cigarette smoke exposure is a risk factor for hearing loss. A study found hearing loss at high and low frequencies and 4000 Hz in metal workers passively exposed to cigarette smoke (65). However, the results of these investigations have been inconsistent regarding the exact role smoking plays in occupational hearing loss, in some part due to poor controls of noise exposure levels in participants. Studies have suggested that smoking, by itself, does not increase the risk of occupational hearing loss; however, when coupled with elevated blood pressure and other cardiovascular risk factors, those workers have a higher risk of hearing loss (70, 71). One longitudinal investigation found that smoking was not an independent risk factor for occupational hearing loss, which highlights the need for research describing the underlying pathologic mechanism of smoking on occupational hearing loss (72).

## INDUSTRIAL SOLVENTS

Another group of cofactors has been the topic of experimental research in both humans and animals. Industrial solvents such as toluene, styrene, xylene, trichloroethylene, and carbon disulfide, by themselves or in mixtures, have been implicated in affecting the inner ear both with and without the presence of noise. The ototoxicity of solvents was supported by a meta-analysis that found that hearing loss among workers exposed to both noise and solvents was approximately three times more likely when compared to workers who were exposed to noise only or solvents only (73). The study also found that hearing loss in workers exposed to noise and solvents was almost twice as likely when compared to workers who were exposed to solvents alone (73). The rest of this discussion will focus on the current state of the literature of two commonly used solvents: toluene and styrene.

A review of audiograms and electronystagmography (ENG) results for workers in a paint and varnish plant revealed that 42% of those exposed to industrial solvents had high-frequency hearing losses as compared to 5% in the age-matched control group; 47.5% of that same group demonstrated abnormal ENGs vs. 5% in the control group (74). However, a study by Schäper et al. (75) did not find an association between toluene exposure level or duration and occupational noise exposure on hearing loss in a modern printing shop with exposure to toluene below 50 parts per million (ppm). These results differ from previous reports of the effect of toluene and noise on occupational hearing loss (76, 77), but the current study adds value because the authors measured individual worker exposure to toluene and noise. The study does not serve to refute the potential effect of toluene exposure on hearing loss but rather to suggest a level of exposure at which no significant hearing loss is found.

In investigating the effects of styrene and styrene plus noise exposure, Sliwinska-Kowalska et al. (78) found that exposure to the styrene increased the risk of hearing loss in humans; in addition, the styrene plus noise-exposed group had two to three times higher odds of developing hearing loss. The ototoxicity of styrene and noise was supported by an animal model study by Chen and Henderson (79), in which rats exposed to styrene and noise had greater threshold shifts, outer hair cell loss, and apoptosis of Deiters' cells than rats exposed to noise or styrene alone. However, rats in this study were exposed to noise levels and styrene doses higher than those found in industrial settings. Despite this, the study demonstrates that noise and styrene are ototoxic, and further research is needed to understand the exact ototoxic role of styrene.

## NON-ORGANIC HEARING LOSS

Due to the compensation and legal factors involved in occupational hearing loss, there are much larger numbers of individuals who present with non-organic hearing loss in supposed noise-induced loss cases. The diagnosing physician needs to be aware of possible non-organic components including functional hearing loss, functional overlay, and malingering.

Functional or psychogenic hearing loss results from the influence of psychological or emotional factors resulting in an inability to hear when the peripheral mechanism may be essentially normal. Patients with extreme anxiety or emotional conflicts may outwardly manifest their mental disturbances by converting them into hearing loss or other conversion disorders. Conversion disorders are an involuntary response, escaping from the extreme emotions that cannot be faced voluntarily. Functional hearing loss can also be noted in addition to actual organic, peripheral hearing loss. When this is evident, it is noted as functional overlay. Careful history taking and accurate audiometry will assist in the diagnosis of these non-organic components.

Unlike functional hearing loss, malingering is the intentional misrepresentation of one's hearing, usually for monetary or emotional gain. Individuals have been known to misrepresent their hearing for financial gain, to avoid work environments such as military deployment, to evade responsibility, or for purposes of gaining attention. Functional overlay can also exist in malingering hearing losses. Most malingerers are revealed by their inconsistent test results. In cases of unilateral malingering, the shadow curve that should be present due to interaural attenuation is often absent. For other cases, the pure-tone average is not consistent with the speech reception threshold. To try to find the malingerer's true thresholds, a number of techniques are useful in audiology. An ascending method of test presentation decreases their ability to estimate loudness; this is also reduced if smaller 1- to 2-dB steps are used instead of the traditional 5-dB steps. Physiological measures such as otoacoustic emissions and auditory brainstem response (ABR) also can be helpful in determining normal hearing, as can other special tests.

## CASE REPORTS

Chiefly because of OSHA requirements and greater emphasis on workers' compensation for occupational hearing loss, hundreds of thousands of employees will ultimately be referred to otologists for consultations. Otologists must provide expert advice on matters such as employing people with possible safety and communication problems, managing numerous otologic problems, and determining whether hearing loss is due to occupational noise or some other cause. The general characteristics of occupational hearing loss described can help guide physicians to a reasonably accurate diagnosis. In order to illustrate some of the numerous problems that have arisen in managing claims for occupational hearing loss, it may be helpful to review a series of actual cases that have come to workers' compensation court for adjudication. The histories are abstracted, and the findings of plaintiff's and defense's experts are abbreviated, but included in each case are important features that illustrate both justified and unjustified contentions.

In all these cases, the physical aspects of the otologic examination revealed no abnormalities unless specifically stated in the case report. Appropriate complete physical examination, blood studies, and other examinations were performed with no abnormalities found unless specifically stated in the report.

### CASE REPORT 1

A 63-year-old pipefitter, employed by a shipbuilding company for 40 years, had 10 years' exposure to chippers and ship "scraping" noise. Hearing loss developed gradually over many years, most pronounced after chipping exposure. He denied tinnitus, vertigo, and gunfire exposure. Audiometry (**Figure 17.14**) showed bilateral sensorineural hearing loss with fairly good residual hearing at 10,000 and 12,000 Hz, discrimination between 80 and 88%, and good speech reception. These findings are characteristic of occupational hearing loss due to prolonged exposure to intense noise such as chipping, and the history is consistent with the diagnosis. If presbycusis and hereditary deafness were factors, the highest frequencies would be more seriously involved and the discrimination score might be worse.

HEARING RECORD

JOSEPH SATALOFF, M.D.
ROBERT THAYER SATALOFF, M.D.
1721 PINE STREET    PHILADELPHIA, PA 19103

Name _____    Age _____

### Air conduction

| | | | Right | | | | | | | | Left | | | | | | |
|---|---|---|---|---|---|---|---|---|---|---|---|---|---|---|---|---|---|
| Date | Exam | Left mask | 250 | 500 | 1000 | 2000 | 4000 | 8000 | Right mask | 250 | 500 | 1000 | 2000 | 4000 | 8000 | AUO |
| | | | 35 | 40 | 45 | 50 | 70 | 60 | | 40 | 40 | 40 | 55 | 65 | 60 | |
| | | | | | | | | | | | | | | | | |
| | | | | | | | | | | | | | | | | |
| | | | | | | | | | | | | | | | | |
| | | | | | | | | | | | | | | | | |
| | | | | | | | | | | | | | | | | |
| | | | | | | | | | | | | | | | | |

### Bone conduction

| | | | Right | | | | | | | Left | | | | | |
|---|---|---|---|---|---|---|---|---|---|---|---|---|---|---|---|
| Date | Exam | Left mask | 250 | 500 | 1000 | 2000 | 4000 | | Right mask | 250 | 500 | 1000 | 2000 | 4000 | AUO |
| | | | 30 | 40 | 40 | 50 | 65 | | | 35 | 35 | 35 | 50 | 65 | |
| | | | | | | | | | | | | | | | |
| | | | | | | | | | | | | | | | |
| | | | | | | | | | | | | | | | |
| | | | | | | | | | | | | | | | |

### Speech reception / Discrimination

| Date | Right | Left mask | Left | Right mask | Free Field | Mic | | Date | % Score | Test level | List | Left mask | % Score | Test level | List | Right mask | Exam |
|---|---|---|---|---|---|---|---|---|---|---|---|---|---|---|---|---|---|
| | | | | | | | | | 82 | 60 | | | 88 | 60 | | | |
| | | | | | | | | | | | | | | | | | |
| | | | | | | | | | | | | | | | | | |

Discrimination    Right          Left

### High frequency thresholds

| | Right | | | | | | Left | | | | | |
|---|---|---|---|---|---|---|---|---|---|---|---|---|
| Date | 4000 | 8000 | 10000 | 12000 | 14000 | Left mask | Right mask | 4000 | 8000 | 10000 | 12000 | 14000 |
| | | 60 | 40 | 40 | | | | | 60 | 45 | 45 | |
| | | | | | | | | | | | | |

| Right | | Weber | | Left | | Hearing aid | | |
|---|---|---|---|---|---|---|---|---|
| Binne | Schwabach | | | Binne | Schwabach | Date | Make | Model |
| | | | | | | Receiver | Gain | Exam |
| | | | | | | Ear | Discrim | Counc |

Remarks

**Figure 17.14** Sensorineural hearing loss due to occupational noise exposure. Note the hearing recovery at 8000–12,000 Hz.

## CASE REPORT 2

A 67-year-old railroad brakeman had worked for 35 years and retired 2 years ago. About 7 years prior to this otologic examination, he had been examined for hearing loss by an otologist, who concluded, on the basis of the patient's history of working with excessive noise and vibration, that the patient had "sensorineural hearing loss due to prolonged exposure to noise and vibration." Only two audiograms were available (**Figure 17.15**), one taken in 1974 about 5 years prior to retirement and one in 1982,

3 years after retirement. Note the rather late onset of hearing loss and the progressive nature of the condition even over the past 4 or 5 years. This employee had been working in the same noise environment for many years, yet he did not notice the hearing loss until a few years prior to retirement. These factors help indicate that the diagnosis is presbycusis rather than occupational hearing loss. This is further substantiated by the fact that measurements revealed that this patient's exposure did not exceed 87 dBA, and he had not been exposed to the especially loud noises occasionally found in railroad employment.

HEARING RECORD

JOSEPH SATALOFF, M.D.
ROBERT THAYER SATALOFF, M.D.
1721 PINE STREET    PHILADELPHIA, PA 19103

Name _____    Age _____

### Air conduction

| | | | Right | | | | | | Left | | | | | | |
|------|------|-----------|-----|-----|------|------|------|------|------------|-----|-----|------|------|------|------|-----|
| Date | Exam | Left mask | 250 | 500 | 1000 | 2000 | 4000 | 8000 | Right mask | 250 | 500 | 1000 | 2000 | 4000 | 8000 | AUO |
| 1974 | | | 20 | 25 | 40 | 45 | 50 | 50 | | 15 | 25 | 45 | 45 | 50 | 55 | |
| 1982 | | | 30 | 30 | 45 | 60 | 65 | 70 | | 25 | 25 | 50 | 55 | 65 | 65 | |
| | | | | | | | | | | | | | | | | |
| | | | | | | | | | | | | | | | | |
| | | | | | | | | | | | | | | | | |
| | | | | | | | | | | | | | | | | |
| | | | | | | | | | | | | | | | | |
| | | | | | | | | | | | | | | | | |

### Bone conduction

| | | | Right | | | | | | Left | | | | | | |
|------|------|-----------|-----|-----|------|------|------|------------|-----|-----|------|------|------|-----|
| Date | Exam | Left mask | 250 | 500 | 1000 | 2000 | 4000 | Right mask | 250 | 500 | 1000 | 2000 | 4000 | AUO |
| 1974 | | | 20 | 20 | 35 | 50 | 45 | | 10 | 25 | 40 | 45 | 55 | |
| 1982 | | | 25 | 25 | 45 | 60 | 70 | | 25 | 30 | 45 | 55 | 70 | |
| | | | | | | | | | | | | | | |
| | | | | | | | | | | | | | | |
| | | | | | | | | | | | | | | |
| | | | | | | | | | | | | | | |

### Speech reception

| Date | Right | Left mask | Left | Right mask | Free field | Mic |
|------|-------|-----------|------|------------|------------|-----|
| | | | | | | |
| | | | | | | |
| | | | | | | |

### Discrimination

| | Right | | | | Left | | | | |
|------|---------|------------|------|-----------|---------|------------|------|-----------|------|
| Date | % Score | Test level | List | Left mask | % Score | Test level | List | Right mask | Exam |
| | | | | | | | | | |
| | | | | | | | | | |
| | | | | | | | | | |

### High frequency thresholds

| | Right | | | | | | Left | | | | |
|------|------|------|-------|-------|-------|-----------|------------|------|------|-------|-------|-------|
| Date | 4000 | 8000 | 10000 | 12000 | 14000 | Left mask | Right mask | 4000 | 8000 | 10000 | 12000 | 14000 |
| | | | | | | | | | | | | |
| | | | | | | | | | | | | |
| | | | | | | | | | | | | |

| Right | | Weber | Left | | Hearing aid | | |
|-------|-----------|-------|-------|-----------|----------|--------|-------|
| Binne | Schwabach | | Binne | Schwabach | Date | Make | Model |
| | | | | | Receiver | Gain | Exam |
| | | | | | Ear | Discrim | Counc |

Remarks _____

Figure 17.15 Hearing tests 5 years before and 2 years after retirement after 35 years as a railroad brake-man (with consistent noise exposure). Late onset of hearing loss, absence of 4000-Hz dip, exposure to only 87 dBA, and progression of loss suggest presbycusis or some other etiology, not occupational hearing loss.

# CASE REPORT 3

A 65-year-old railroad machinist worked around diesel engines for 25 years. He said he had been exposed to roaring diesel train engines for many years and that his hearing loss started many years ago and gradually got worse. He had occasional vertigo but no tinnitus. He denied any family history of hearing loss and was in good health. The audiologic studies showed a flat mixed hearing loss in both ears of about 60 dB, slightly worse in the higher frequencies. The bone conduction threshold was reduced but slightly better than the air conduction in the lower frequencies.

The otologist who first evaluated this patient diagnosed nerve deafness due to occupational exposure to diesel engines.

A later examination by another otologist showed the same audiologic findings but noted excellent bone conduction when a 500-Hz tuning fork was applied to the upper teeth. Discrimination was excellent. The diagnosis was otosclerosis with sensorineural as well as conductive hearing loss. In many older patients, bone conduction tests on the mastoid are not necessarily good indications of actual sensorineural function. Occupational noise did not cause this patient's hearing loss.

## CASE REPORT 4

A 36-year-old man began work in a paper mill in 1976. His occupation often involved exposure to noise levels in excess of 95 dBA throughout the workday. He also had a history of exposure to firearms, discharging a shotgun approximately 200–300 times annually. He is left-handed. In addition, he listened to loud music daily. Serial audiograms revealed development between 1976 and 1984 of an obvious dip at 4000 and 6000 Hz. Despite continued exposure to the same occupational and extracurricular noise sources, there is no evidence of significant deterioration after approximately his first 8 years on the job (**Figure 17.16**). This is typical of occupational hearing loss.

## CASE REPORT 5

A 45-year-old man gave a complex history of having been evaluated by four otologists. The patient claimed that he had been hit in September 1981 on the right side of his face by a landloader. He was not dazed or unconscious, and there was no bleeding or visible trauma, but he could not hear with his right ear immediately after the incident and had been

unable to hear since. He denied any hearing loss prior to the accident and also denied any familial hearing loss. In April 1982, an otologist performed a stapedectomy and the patient's hearing subjectively improved. He developed recurrent vertigo postoperatively. However, audiograms performed shortly after the surgery showed no evidence of hearing improvement compared with preoperative thresholds. The otologist stated that surgery was for otosclerosis and that, in his opinion, the otosclerosis had no relation to the accident. Another otologist who examined the patient because of his persistent vertigo agreed that the vertigo was postoperative, and that the diagnosis was otosclerosis, not related to the accident. The patient underwent unsuccessful right revised stapes surgery in an attempt to resolve his vertigo and restore his hearing. At the request of the plaintiff's attorney, another otologist examined this patient in March 1983. Remarks from his report are as follows:

> It is apparent from reviewing the records that the patient had a dormant otosclerosis which has been activated and aggravated by the head injury suffered [in 1981]. It is my opinion that without this trauma the otosclerosis would have remained dormant for many years.

NAME:

| | RIGHT EAR AIR CONDUCTION | | | | | | | LEFT EAR AIR CONDUCTION | | | | | | |
|-------|------|------|------|------|------|------|------|------|------|------|------|------|------|------|
| DATE | 500 | 1000 | 2000 | 3000 | 4000 | 6000 | 8000 | 500 | 1000 | 2000 | 3000 | 4000 | 6000 | 8000 |
| 10/76 | 5 | 5 | 5 | 10 | 20 | 40 | | 5 | 5 | 10 | 10 | 25 | 25 | |
| 8/81 | 5 | 0 | 5 | 10 | 50 | 35 | | 5 | 0 | 0 | 30 | 65 | 75 | |
| 8/82 | 5 | 10 | 5 | 20 | 50 | 30 | 30 | 5 | 5 | 5 | 20 | 55 | 35 | 25 |
| 8/83 | 5 | 0 | 5 | 30 | 55 | 35 | 40 | 10 | 10 | 10 | 20 | 35 | 30 | 20 |
| 7/84 | 0 | 0 | 0 | 20 | 40 | 65 | 30 | 5 | 5 | 10 | 10 | 50 | 30 | 20 |
| 1/85 | 0 | 5 | 0 | 35 | 60 | 65 | 25 | 0 | 0 | 10 | 25 | 50 | 25 | 10 |
| 1/86 | 0 | 0 | 0 | 25 | 70 | 50 | 25 | 0 | 5 | 0 | 20 | 50 | 15 | 10 |
| 2/87 | 5 | 0 | 0 | 20 | 70 | 80 | 25 | 0 | 5 | 5 | 25 | 50 | 20 | 10 |
| 8/87 | 5 | 0 | 0 | 25 | 65 | 65 | 20 | 5 | 0 | 0 | 15 | 40 | 30 | 20 |
| 9/88 | 0 | 0 | 0 | 25 | 65 | 60 | 20 | 0 | 0 | 0 | 25 | 35 | 25 | 20 |
| 9/89 | 5 | 5 | 5 | 30 | 70 | 70 | 30 | 5 | 5 | 5 | 30 | 35 | 20 | 15 |
| 11/90 | 0 | 0 | 0 | 25 | 65 | 65 | 30 | 0 | 0 | 0 | 25 | 40 | 20 | 10 |
| 5/91 | 5 | 0 | 0 | 25 | 65 | 60 | 25 | 0 | 0 | 0 | 25 | 40 | 20 | 10 |

Figure 17.16 Occupational hearing loss that does not progress substantially after approximately the first 10 years of exposure to noise.

In April 1984, another otologic evaluation was performed and the audiologic findings revealed conductive hearing loss with no sensorineural involvement on the right side, excellent bone conduction and discrimination, and a good chance of improving this patient's hearing and clearing up his other symptoms. The difference of interpretation of the etiology of this otosclerotic process is an important issue for otologists. There is no question that all otologists have seen otosclerosis progress to this degree and in this manner without being aggravated by trauma. The contention that trauma could produce this sudden aggravation of otosclerosis has not been substantiated by any valid and reliable otologic study. An otologist may form an opinion that this could have happened, but in order for such an opinion to carry weight or be defensible, it is important that it be creditably based on scientific studies and accepted by the medical community.

## CASE REPORT 6

A 65-year-old diabetic man worked in a noisy cannery for over 40 years, using hearing protectors only in the last 10 years. His ears had drained intermittently over a 40-year period, most severely in the left ear for the last 7 years. Otologic examination revealed a large left perforation, with scarring and thickening of the residual tympanic membrane. Audiometry of the left ear revealed better bone conduction than air conduction. Bone conduction was excellent by Weber's test. Audiometry of the right ear revealed sensorineural hearing loss. Discrimination scores were good bilaterally. Serial audiograms from 1975 to 1981 showed progressive deterioration of hearing in the left ear. One otologist diagnosed right-sided occupational sensorineural hearing loss and left-sided mixed hearing loss due to occupational exposure with superimposed infection. Another otologist, basing his opinion on the most recent (1981) audiogram, claimed the entire hearing loss was due to occupational noise exposure. At the deposition, it became evident that the deterioration of hearing in the left ear between 1975 and 1981 was not a result of cannery noise because the worker had worn hearing protection and had not been exposed to loud noise in that time period. Good discrimination scores helped indicate that a large portion of the hearing loss present before 1978 was attributed

to occupational noise exposure, although superimposed chronic otitis, tympanosclerosis, and presbycusis were contributory. It was determined that the actual amount of noise exposure that warranted compensation should be determined by the 1975 audiogram.

## CASE REPORT 7

A 57-year-old dye caster and screw conveyor operator worked in a machine shop for many years. In 1979, while working around a screw conveyor, he was subjected to an extremely loud sound for about 30 seconds. He had no discomfort, but his wife noted marked hearing loss that evening. His physician diagnosed "vascular accident resulting from intense noise exposure" and prescribed medication.

The consulting otologist noted disparity in hearing tests taken before and after the incident and expressed the following opinion: "The cause-and-effect relationship between the loud noise exposure and sudden hearing loss is real, particularly in view of the fact that he has had normal hearing previously." He advised studies to rule out the possibility of other "disease processes."

The employee put in a claim for occupational hearing loss compensation because of deafness produced by loud noise, particularly in his left ear. Studies revealed the presence of a left acoustic neuroma that was confirmed operatively. Details of this case are reported in Chapter 9. It is important to note that all studies, including a computed tomography (CT) scan, had missed this small tumor. It was diagnosed only because of the otologist's insistence that the patient undergo a myelogram or air-contrast CT scan. Currently, MRI would be used. An estimated 11% of acoustic neuromas can present as "sudden deafness" (80).

## CASE REPORT 8

A 50-year-old employee had worked since 1969 in a plant making tires. His annual audiograms showed normal hearing until 1973, when annual testing of his hearing was discontinued. He gave a vague history of a "press explosion" in 1975 with some ringing in his right ear, but he did not complain of hearing loss. The explosion was not confirmed either at the plant or in any medical records.

In 1976, he had fullness in his right ear that was diagnosed by his otologist as "eustachian tube blockage due to a temporomandibular joint problem." In 1976, he developed hearing loss and tinnitus in his right ear, causing the otologist to rule out an acoustic neuroma based on normal calorics, tomograms, and posterior fossa myelograms. In 1979, a myringotomy was done for right-ear blockage. In 1981, he had two vertigo attacks and his otologist diagnosed Ménière's disease. The employee retired in 1981 because of physical disabilities. In 1983, he applied for workers' compensation for hearing loss after being examined by his otologist and audiologist. His otologist's report included the following:

> The patient shows a bilateral sensorineural hearing loss, which appears to be worse on the right side. The Weber test lateralized to the left ear as would be expected with this audiometric configuration. Speech discrimination is reduced in both ears. Based on the long-time history of noise exposure in his occupation, it is very likely that a significant amount of the current hearing loss is probably related to noise.

The otologist representing the defense during litigation demonstrated clearly that:

1. The employee actually was not exposed to noise exceeding 88 dBA during his work and generally worked at much lower levels, chiefly in the loading department.
2. He worked for at least 4 years at the same job before developing any hearing loss.
3. The hearing loss started and became severe in his right ear long before the left ear became involved.
4. The hearing loss continued to get worse even after he retired in 1981.

The real cause for his hearing loss was probably related to his generalized arteriosclerosis, hypertension, peripheral vascular disease, and long-standing diabetes. In February 1981, he had transient cerebral ischemia attacks, arterial insufficiency of the left leg with occlusion of the left femoral artery, and stenosis of the common iliac artery, treated surgically. The employee's otologist and audiologist were apparently unaware of the patient's diabetes and peripheral vascular problems and surgery. Their impression of his job-related noise exposure, which they obtained from his history, was inaccurate. They were not aware that his actual noise exposure was not capable of producing his hearing loss. There is no question that this hearing loss was neither caused nor aggravated by the worker's job.

## SUMMARY

A diagnosis of occupational hearing loss must be based on specific criteria. Otologists rendering medical diagnoses or legal opinions for patients alleging occupational hearing loss must be careful to base their opinions on facts. The potential medical, legal, and economic consequences of lesser diligence are likely to be serious.

## REFERENCES

1. Fleming AJ, D'Alonzo CA, Zapp, JA. Modern Occupational Medicine. Philadelphia, PA: Lea & Febiger, 1954.
2. Exploratory Subcommittee Z24-X-2, American Standards Association. The relations of hearing loss to noise exposure, 1954.
3. National Institute for Occupational Safety and Health (NIOSH). Criteria document: Recommendation for an occupational exposure standard for noise, 1972.
4. Baughn WL. Relation between Daily Noise Exposure and Hearing Loss Based On the Evaluation of 6,835 Industrial Noise Exposure Cases. Aerospace Medical Research Lab., Wright Patterson AFB, Ohio. AMRL-TR-73-53, June 1973.
5. Ward WD, Glorig A. Protocol of inter-industry noise study. J Occup Med 1975, 17:760–770.
6. Burns W, Robinson DS. Hearing and Noise in Industry. London: Her Majesty's Stationery Office, 1970.
7. Passchier-Vermeer W. Hearing Loss due to Steady State Broadband Noise. Report

No. 55, Institute for Public Health, Eng., Leiden, The Netherlands, 1968.

8. Sataloff J, Sataloff RT, Yerg A, Menduke H, Gore RP. Intermittent exposure to noise: effects on hearing. Ann Otol Rhinol Laryngol 1983; 92(6):623–628.

9. Orgler GK, Brownson PJ, Brubaker WW, Crane DJ, Glorig A, Hatfield TR, Hanson R, Holthouser MG, Ligo RN, Markham T, Mote WR, Sataloff J, Yerg RA. American Occupational Medicine Association Noise and Hearing Conservation Committee Guidelines for the Conduct of an Occupational Hearing Conservation Program. J Occup Med 1987; 29:981–982.

10. Mirza R, Kirchner DB, Dobie RA, Crawford J, ACOEM Task Force on Occupational Hearing Loss. Occupational noise-induced hearing loss. J Occup and Environ Med. 2018; 60(9):498–501.

11. Schuknecht HF, Tonndorf J. Acoustic trauma of the cochlea from ear surgery. Laryngoscope 1960; 70:479–505.

12. Lawrence M. Current concepts of the mechanism of occupational hearing loss. Am Ind Hyg Assoc J 1964; 25:269–273.

13. Kellerhals B. Pathogenesis of inner ear lesions in acute acoustic trauma. Acta Otolaryngol 1972; 73:249–253.

14. Schuknecht HG. Pathology of the Ear. Cambridge, MA: Harvard University Press, 1974: 295–297, 300–308.

15. Gallo R, Glorig A. Permanent threshold shift changes produced by noise exposure and aging. Am Ind Hyg Assoc J 1964; 25:237–245.

16. Schneider EJ, Mutchler JE, Hoyle HR, Ode EH, Holder BB. The progression of hearing loss from industrial noise exposure. Am Ind Hyg Assoc J 1970; 31:368–376.

17. Sataloff J, Vassallo L, Menduke H. Occupational hearing loss and high frequency thresholds. Arch Environ Health 1967; 14:832–836.

18. Sataloff J, Vassallo L, Menduke H. Hearing loss from exposure to interrupted noise. Arch Environ Health 1969; 17:972–981.

19. Salmivalli A. Acoustic trauma in regular Army personnel: clinical audiologic study. Acta Otolaryngol 1967; (Suppl. 22):1–85.

20. Ward WD, Fleer RE, Glorig A. Characteristics of hearing losses produced by gunfire and steady noise. J Audiol Res 1961; 1:325–356.

21. Johnsson L-G, Hawkins JE Jr. Degeneration patterns in human ears exposed to noise. Ann Otol Rhinol Laryngol 1976; 85:725–739.

22. Gates GA, Cooper JC Jr, Kannel WB, Miller NJ. Hearing in the elderly: the Framingham cohort, 1983–1985. Part I. Basic audiometric test results. Ear Hear 1990; 11(4):247–256.

23. Sataloff J, Vassallo L. Head colds and viral cochleitis. Arch Otolaryngol 1968; 19:56–59.

24. Igarashi M, Schuknecht HF, Myers E. Cochlear pathology in humans with stimulation deafness. J Laryngol Otol 1964; 78:115–123.

25. Anderson H, Wedenberg E. Genetic aspects of hearing impairment in children. Acta Otolaryngol 1970; 69:77–88.

26. Fisch L. The etiology of congenital deafness and audiometric patterns. J Laryngol Otol 1955; 69:479–493.

27. Huizing EH, van Bolhuis AH, Odenthal DW. Studies on progressive hereditary perceptive deafness in a family of 335 members. Acta Otolaryngol 1966; 61:35–41, 161–167.

28. Graham MD. Acoustic tumors: selected histories and patient reviews. In: House WF, Lutje CM, eds. Acoustic Tumors. Baltimore, MD: University Park Press, 1979, 192–193.

29. Facer GW, Farell KH, Cody DTR. Spontaneous perilymph fistula. Mayo Clin Proc 1973; 48:203–206.

30. Simmons FB. Theory of membrane breaks in sudden hearing loss. Arch Otolaryngol 1968; 88:67–74.

31. Soss SL. Sensorineural hearing loss with diving. Arch Otolaryngol 1971; 93:501–504.

32. Freeman P., Edwards C. Inner ear barotrauma. Arch Otolaryngol 1972; 95:556–563.

33. van Dishoeck HAE. Akustisches Trauma. In: Berendes J, Link R, Zollner F, eds. Hals-Nasen-Ohren-Heilkunde. Band III. Stuttgart: Georg Thieme, 1966; 1764–1799.

34. Yerg RA, Sataloff J, Glorig A, Menduke H. Inter-industry noise study. J Occup Med 1978; 20:351–358.

35. Cartwright LB, Thompson RW. The effects of broadband noise on the cardiovascular system in normal resting adults. Am Ind Hyg Assoc J 1978; 653–658.

36. Johnsson L-G, Hawkins JE Jr. Strial atrophy in clinical and experimental deafness. Laryngoscope 1972; 82:1105–1125.

37. Spoendlin H. Histopathology of nerve deafness. J Otolaryngol 1985; 14(5):282–286.

38. Spoendlin H, Brun JP. Relation of structural damage to exposure time and intensity in acoustic trauma. Acta Otolaryngol 1973; 75:220–226.

39. Spoendlin H. Primary structural changes in the organ of Corti after acoustic over-stimulation. Acta Otolaryngol 1971; 71:166–176.

40. Nurminen T. Female noise exposure, shift work, and reproduction. J Occup Environ Med 1995; 37(8):945–950.

41. Selander J, Rylander L, Albin M, Rosenhall U, Lewné M, Gustavsson P. Full-time exposure to occupational noise during pregnancy was associated with reduced birth weight in a nationwide cohort study of Swedish women. Sci Total Environ 2019; 651:1137–1143.

42. Lissåker CT, Gustavsson P, Albin M, Ljungman P, Bodin T, Sjöström M, Selander J. Occupational exposure to noise in relation to pregnancy-related hypertensive disorders and diabetes. Scand J Work Environ Health 2021;47(1):33.

43. Wang Z, Qian R, Xiang W, Sun L, Xu M, Zhang B, Yang L, Zhu S, Zeng L, Yang W. Association between noise exposure during pregnancy and pregnancy complications: A meta-analysis. Front Psychol 2022; 13:1026996.

44. Lalande NM, Hetu R, Lambert J. Is occupational noise exposure during pregnancy a risk factor of damage to the auditory system of the fetus? Am J Ind Med 1986; 10(4):427–435.

45. Selander J, Albin M, Rosenhall U, Rylander L, Lewné M, Gustavsson P. Maternal occupational exposure to noise during pregnancy and hearing dysfunction in children: a nationwide prospective cohort study in Sweden. Environ Health Perspect 2016; 124(6):855–860.

46. Vincens N, Persson Waye K. Occupational and environmental noise exposure during pregnancy and rare health outcomes of offspring: a scoping review focusing on congenital anomalies and perinatal mortality. Rev Environ Health 2023; 38(3):423–438.

47. Shi J, Lv ZT, Lei Y, Kang H. Maternal occupational exposure to chemicals in the textile factory during pregnancy is associated with a higher risk of polydactyly in the offspring. J Matern Fetal Neonatal Med 2020; 33(23):3935–3941.

48. Gong W, Liang Q, Zheng D, Zhong R, Wen Y, Wang X. Congenital heart defects of fetus after maternal exposure to organic and inorganic environmental factors: a cohort study. Oncotarget. 2017;8(59):100717.

49. Murato M, Takigawa H, Sakamoto H. Teratogenic effects of noise and cadmium in mice: does noise have teratogenic potential? J Toxicol Environ Health 1993; 339(2):237–245.

50. Sataloff RT, Hickey K, Robb J. Rock concert audience noise exposure: a preliminary study. J Occup Hear Loss 1998; 1(2):97–99.

51. Ramakers GG, Kraaijenga VJ, Cattani G, van Zanten GA, Grolman W. Effectiveness of earplugs in preventing recreational noise–induced hearing loss: a randomized clinical trial. JAMA Otolaryngol Head Neck Surg 2016; 142(6):551–558.

52. Derebery MJ, Vermiglio A, Berliner KI, Potthoff M, Holguin K. Facing the music: pre-and postconcert assessment of hearing in teenagers. Otol Neurotol 2012; 33(7):1136–1141.

53. Sataloff RT, Rau G, Preston L. Noise exposure in movie theaters. J Occup Hear Loss 1998; 1(4):281–282.

54. Mendes RC, Barrionuevo CE. Risk of occupational hearing loss in telephone operators. J Occup Hear Loss 1998; 1(3):179–184.

55. Singh T, Biggs T, Crossley E, Faoury M, Mahmood A, Salamat A, Patterson T, Jayakody N, Dando A, Sipaul F, Marinakis K. Noise exposure on the London Underground, an observational study over a decade. The Laryngoscope 2020; 130(12):2891–2895.

56. Yaremchuk KL, Dickson L, Burk K. Noise level analysis of commercially available toys. J Occup Hear Loss 1998; 2(4):163–170.

57. Yaremchuk KL, Dobie R. The otologic effects of airbag deployment. J Occup Hear Loss 1999; 2(2–3):67–74.

58. McKinley RL, Nixon CW. Human auditory response to an air bag inflation noise: has it been 30 years. J Acoust Soc Am 1998; 104(3), Pt2:1769.

59. Carson SS, Prazma J, Pulver SH, Anderson T. Combined effects of aspirin and noise in causing permanent hearing loss. Arch Otolaryngol Head Neck Surg 1989; 115:1070–1075.

60. Barone JA, Peters JM, Garabrant DH, Bernstein L, Krebsbach R. Smoking as a risk factor in noise-induced hearing loss. J Occup Med 1989; 29(9):741–746.

61. Thomas GB, Williams CE, Hoger NG. Some non-auditory correlates of the hearing threshold levels of an aviation noise exposed population. Aviat Space Environ Med 1981; 9:531–536.

62. Chung DY, Wilson GN, Gannon RP, Hamernik RP, Henderson D, Salvi R. Individual susceptibility to noise. In: Hamernik RP, Henderson D, Salvi R, eds. New Perspectives in Noise-Induced Hearing Loss. New York: Raven Press, 1982, 511–519.

63. Drettner B, Hedstrand H, Klockhoff I, Svedberg A. Cardiovascular risk factors and hearing loss. Acta Otolaryngol 1975; 79:366–371.

64. Siegelaub AB, Friedman GD, Adour K, Seltzer CC. Hearing loss in adults: relation to age, sex, exposure to loud noise, and smoking. Arch Environ Health 1974; 29:107–109.

65. Mohammadi S, Mahdi Mazhari M, Houshang Mehrparvar A, Attarchi MS. Cigarette smoking and occupational noise-induced hearing loss. Eur J Public Health 2010; 20 (4): 452–455.

66. Pouryaghoub G, Mehrdad R, Mohammadi S. Interaction of smoking and occupational noise exposure on hearing loss: a cross-sectional study. BMC Public Health 2007; 7(1): 1–5.

67. Ferrite S, Santana VS, Marshall SW. Interaction between noise and cigarette smoking for the outcome of hearing loss among women: a population-based study. Am J Ind Med 2013; 56 (1): 1213–20.

68. Mizoue T, Miyamoto T, Shimizu T. Combined effect of smoking and occupational exposure to noise on hearing loss in steel factory workers. Occup Environ Med 2003; 60 (1): 56–59.

69. Li X, Rong X, Wang Z, Lin A. Association between smoking and noise-induced hearing loss: A meta-analysis of observational studies. Int J Environ Res Public Health 2020; 17(4):1201.

70. Cocchiarella LA, Sharp DS, Persky VW. Hearing threshold shifts, white-cell count and smoking status in working men. Occup Med 1995; 45:179–185.

71. Starck J, Toppila E, Pyykko I. Smoking as a risk factor in sensory neural hearing loss among workers exposed to occupational noise. Acta Otolaryngol 1999; 119:302–305.

72. Khaldari F, Khanjani N, Bahrampour A, Ravandi MR, Mianroodi AA. The relation between hearing loss and smoking among workers exposed to noise, using linear mixed models. Iran J Otorhinolaryngol 2020; 32(108):11.

73. Nakhooda F, Govender SM, Sartorius B. The effects of combined exposure of solvents and noise on auditory function–A systematic review and meta-analysis. S Afr J Commun Disord 2019; 66(1):1–1.

74. Sulkowski WJ, Kowalska S, Matyja W, Guzek W, Wesolowski W, Szymczak W, Kostrzewski P. Effects of occupational exposure to a mixture of solvents on the inner ear: a field study. Int J Occup Med Environ Health 2002; 15:247–256.

75. Schäper M, Seeber A, Van Thriel C. The effects of toluene plus noise on hearing thresholds: an evaluation based on repeated measurements in the German printing industry. Int J Occup Med Environ Health 2008; 21(3):191–200.

76. Morata TC, Fiorini AC, Fischer FM, Colacioppo S, Wallingford KM, Krieg EF, Dunn DE, Gozzoli L, Padrão MA, Cesar CL.

Toluene-induced hearing loss among rotogravure printing workers. Scand J Work Environ Health 1997; 23(4):289–298.

77. Chang SJ, Chen CJ, Lien CH, Sung FC. Hearing loss in workers exposed to toluene and noise. Environ Health Perspect 2006; 114(8):1283–1286.

78. Sliwinska-Kowalska M, Zamyslowska-Szmytke E, Szymczak W, Kotylo P, Fiszer M, Wesolowski W, Pawlaczyk-Lusczynska M.

Ototoxic effects of occupational exposure to styrene and co-exposure to styrene and noise. J Occup Environ Med 2003; 45:15–24.

79. Chen GD, Henderson D. Cochlear injuries induced by the combined exposure to noise and styrene. Hearing Research 2009; 254(1–2):25–33.

80. Sataloff RT, Davies B, Myers DL. Acoustic neuromas presenting as sudden deafness. Am J Otol 1985; 6(4):349–352.

# 18

# Hearing loss: Handicap and rehabilitation

ROBERT THAYER SATALOFF

The most obvious effect of hearing loss is its impact on auditory communication; however, the damaging effect of hearing loss on an individual's ability to function effectively in social and business life is far more critical. In some people, hearing loss can undermine natural optimism and confidence in one's ability to interact successfully with other people. If hearing loss is not addressed through medical treatment and/or rehabilitation, it can lead to insecurity, social withdrawal, paranoia, and impaired function in professional settings.

## EFFECT ON THE PERSONALITY

The impact of hearing loss varies by degree of loss, personality of the individual, and the individual's activity level. Interestingly, hearing loss can manifest as a great disability in people with comparatively mild hearing loss (e.g., otosclerosis or Ménière's disease), whereas some individuals with profound hearing losses may have severe disruption of communication without seriously affecting personality. The degree of impact depends on an individual's character—including mental, spiritual, societal, and economic resources—and other factors that determine one's reaction to hearing loss and the level of handicap it generates.

The effects of hearing loss cannot be restricted to physiology alone, as the mechanics of the ear cannot be divorced from the social aspects of hearing. Hearing is a phenomenon that utilizes peripheral pathways from the ears to the central pathways of the brain to form a complete understanding of acoustic signals; however, hearing is also our method of socialization. In any discussion of hearing, communication, deafness, and handicap, it is necessary to think of the person as a whole and not merely as a mechanism of hearing. For this reason, hearing loss concerns the otologist and the general practitioner, the pediatrician, the psychologist, the psychiatrist, and many others, including members of the legal profession.

## THE RELATIONSHIP BETWEEN HEARING AND SPEECH

To understand the basis for personality changes and communication handicaps that hearing loss may produce, it is necessary to recall the relationship between hearing and speech. It is known that the ear is sensitive to a certain frequency range and that speech falls within that range. Speech can be divided into two types of sounds: vowels and consonants. Roughly speaking, vowels fall into the frequencies <1500 Hz and consonants >1500 Hz. Vowels are relatively powerful sounds, whereas consonants are weak and sometimes dropped within everyday speech or not pronounced clearly. Vowels give power to speech; that is, they signify that someone is speaking, but they give very little

DOI: 10.1201/b23379-18

information about what the speaker is saying. To give specific meaning to words, consonants are interspersed among the vowels. Thus, it can be said that vowels alert the listener to the presence of speech, and consonants help the listener to understand or discriminate what the speaker is saying.

For example, the hard-of-hearing individual (B), whose audiogram is shown in **Figure 18.1**, would have difficulty hearing speech unless it was raised in volume. The difficulty lies in the low frequencies, causing the individual to have trouble hearing vowels and soft voices. However, if a voice were raised in volume, it would be heard and understood clearly. This illustrates a principal problem of loudness or amplification.

The person (A), whose hearing impairment is portrayed in **Figure 18.1**, has a high-frequency loss with almost normal hearing in the low frequencies. In applying this hearing loss to speech inputs, person (A) would hear vowels almost normally but would have difficulty in hearing and discriminating consonants. If a speaker raised his/her voice volume, the missing consonants would be emphasized only slightly and the loudness of the vowels may increase to a disturbing degree. The individual's primary problem is not *hearing* but *distinguishing*

what is heard. The vowels are heard and he/she is aware of someone speaking, but the patient cannot distinguish some of the consonants and misses the meaning of the conversation. This type of person would want the speaker to enunciate more clearly, pronouncing the consonants more distinctively rather than speaking louder. Hearing loss of this type, with its accompanying handicaps, is caused commonly by presbycusis, hereditary hearing loss, and certain types of congenital deafness.

## High-frequency hearing loss and distortion

High-frequency sensorineural hearing loss often causes deterioration of a person's ability to understand speech. In addition, music, certain voices, and especially amplified sound may sound hollow, tinny, and muffled. The hard-of-hearing person affected in this manner may first ask his/her companion to speak louder, but in spite of the louder speech, he/she may understand even less. Loudness may actually reduce discrimination in such individuals with high-frequency hearing loss due to distortion of the signal. Distortion occurs most frequently in people with high-frequency losses

JOSEPH SATALOFF, M.D.
ROBERT THAYER SATALOFF, M.D.
1721 PINE STREET    PHILADELPHIA, PA 19103

NAME _____

| DATE | AIR CONDUCTION | | | | | | | AIR CONDUCTION | | | | | |
|---|---|---|---|---|---|---|---|---|---|---|---|---|---|
| | 250 | 500 | 1000 | 2000 | 4000 | 8000 | | 250 | 500 | 1000 | 2000 | 4000 | 8000 |
| (A) | 15 | 20 | 40 | 60 | 45 | NR | | | | | | | |
| (B) | 50 | 50 | 40 | 30 | 30 | 35 | | | | | | | |

| RIGHT EAR BONE CONDUCTION | | | | | | LEFT EAR BONE CONDUCTION | | | | | |
|---|---|---|---|---|---|---|---|---|---|---|---|
| | | | | | | | | | | | |
| | | | | | | | | | | | |

SPEECH RECEPTION: Right _____ Left _____          DISCRIMINATION: Right _____ Left _____

(Each ear is tested separately with pure tones for air conduction and bone conduction, if necessary. The tones increase in pitch in octave steps from 250 to 8000 Hz. Normal hearing in each frequency lies between 0 and 25 decibels. The larger the number above 25 decibels in each frequency the greater the hearing loss. When the two ears differ greatly in threshold, one ear is masked with noise to test the other ear. Speech reception is the patient's threshold for everyday speech, rather than pure tones. A speech reception threshold of over 30 decibels is handicapping in many situations. The discrimination score indicates the ability to understand selected test words at a comfortable level above the speech reception threshold.)

Figure 18.1 Patients A and B have an average pure-tone loss of 40 dB, but their clinical hearing is substantially different.

because overall loudness also amplifies the low-frequency sounds, such as vowels, which they can hear at a normal level. Speaking in a louder voice creates overpowering vowels with relatively weaker consonants and does not improve the clarity of speech. It is easy to understand that people who have a high-frequency loss could easily become frustrated and confused in trying to follow a conversation.

## Dynamic aspects of hearing-loss handicap

Although compensation for occupational hearing loss demands the establishment of standardized values for hearing loss, from a medical and social aspect, a hearing loss is a personal issue to each individual and cannot be measured on a universal scale. Furthermore, just as hearing loss usually varies over time for an individual, the handicapping effects are also dynamic. They are changing even as this book is being written. With the development of new media for sound communication, an individual's hearing comes to assume even greater importance. For example, a hearing loss today is much more handicapping than it was before television, radio, and telephones began to play such major roles in education, leisure, and the business world. Today, the inability to understand on a telephone is indeed a handicap for the majority of people. The loss of just high-frequency sounds, to a professional or an amateur musician, or even to a high-fidelity fan, is also a handicap. The hearing loss of tomorrow probably will have a different handicapping effect from the hearing loss of today.

## REACTIONS TO HEARING LOSS

The manner in which people react to hearing loss varies considerably. Some may try to minimize or hide their impairment by making strenuous listening efforts, filling in missing information by guessing, and carefully concealing frustration by acting particularly pleasant and affable. His/her effort to "save face" may lead to numerous embarrassing situations through incorrect guessing. Toward evening, the person may be worn out from the efforts to hide his/her hearing handicap. Maintaining this façade often becomes fatiguing and can lead to nervousness, irritability, and instability.

More commonly, some people react to hearing loss by withdrawing and losing interest in their environment, particularly with impairments that have slow and insidious onsets. The personality change is reflected in an avoidance of social contacts and in a preoccupation with the individual's own misfortunes. These individuals may dismiss friends and make excuses to avoid social contacts that might cause the handicap to become more apparent to friends and to themselves.

## PSYCHOSOCIAL IMPACT OF HEARING LOSS

### Economic and family aspects

Hearing loss can affect an individual economically if the impairment affects job performance directly or if a decrease in social activity negatively affects one's professional effectiveness. For example, withdrawing from societal interactions during meetings may negatively affect an individual's ability to perform at work. The handicapped person may realize that he/she cannot perform the duties of the job and, rather than tolerate criticism regarding his/her alertness and proper interest in business, he/she may resign and step down to a position of less worthy potential. In another scenario, he/she may be passed over for a promotion or asked to resign due to lack of participation and apparent lack of interest in employment.

When a salesperson becomes hard-of-hearing, business often suffers and ambitions frequently are suppressed or surrendered if the individual does not proactively seek assistance. On the contrary, a hearing impairment may be regarded as advantageous instead of a handicap to a chipper or a riveter while at work. The hearing loss may make the noise from work appear to be not as loud as it is to fellow workers with normal hearing. Because there is little or no verbal communication in most jobs that produce intense noise, a hearing loss will not be apparent by an inability to understand verbal directions. However, when the hard-of-hearing person returns to a family after work, the situation assumes a completely different perspective. The individual may have trouble understanding what is said by children or a spouse. Conversation becomes more difficult when in the presence of background noise, such as running water or a television or if attention is focused elsewhere. This kind of situation frequently leads at first to mild disputes and later to serious family tension.

Marital strain is often a serious social consequence of an unaided hearing loss. The hearing spouse may accuse the individual with a hearing loss of inattention. The accusation is then denied with the hearing-impaired spouse claiming that the other mumbles. Over time, the frustration and strain of listening with a hearing loss cause the person to become inattentive, weakening the marital bond. The same difficulties noted at home are evident at meetings, visits with friends, and at religious activities. A person with hearing loss often withdraws from the places where he/she feels pilloried by the handicap. This includes social activities such as the movies, theater, or concerts. Little by little, family life and social interactions can be undermined by an untreated hearing loss.

## The plight of the elderly hearing impaired

Hearing loss in older persons, whether from causes associated with aging or owing to other sensorineural etiologies, is often quite severe. More severe to profound losses usually create a larger change in personality and lifestyle due to the challenges that listening now presents. Elderly individuals with hearing loss also find listening in the presence of multiple speakers or background noise especially difficult, as our ability to detect signals in noise diminishes with age. All too often, the unfortunate elderly person begins to believe that the inability to hear and understand a conversation is due to a deterioration of the brain. Family, friends, and stereotypes of the elderly population may reinforce this belief. People may ignore the hearing-impaired person in group conversations and assume that he/she does not know what is going on. Stereotypes of aging, such as physical and mental slowing, further undermine the elderly person's weakened self-confidence and hasten his/her withdrawal from society. The isolation caused by hearing loss can further delay elderly individuals from seeking medical attention to address their hearing handicap.

## Effect of profound hearing losses

In general, people with profound hearing losses are somewhat easier to help than borderline cases, as the former are under greater compulsion to admit that they have a handicap. People with borderline losses are more likely to hide their handicap and deny it, even to themselves. They conceal their hearing loss just as they try to conceal hearing aids if they can be induced, or are able, to use them. For people with mild losses, a hearing aid often becomes part of the handicap due to the stigma it contains. In contrast, people with severe losses perceive their major handicap as the communication difficulty that results from their hearing loss, in addition to some economic and social conflicts. Often individuals with profound hearing loss cannot hear warning signals such as fire alarms or telephone rings, unless they use an assistive device. They may be unable to maintain their jobs if listening for sounds or reliance on verbal communication is an integral part of their duties. Another challenging handicap for people with severe hearing losses is the inability to localize sound. This difficulty is particularly prominent when the hearing loss exists unilaterally or in the case of an asymmetrical hearing loss because two fairly symmetrical hearing ears are necessary to be able to localize the source and direction of sound.

Another interesting aspect of profound hearing loss is the change in the individual's clarity of speech over time. Speech deteriorates as he/she is unable to self-regulate tone, volume, and sound production due to the degree of hearing loss. Primary characteristics of speech become slurred S consonants in speech and a rigid and somewhat monotonous vocal quality. To counteract the inability to hear one's own voice, the individual may raise vocal volume, often to the point of shouting. After a while, he/she may find this unsatisfactory and lose interest in monitoring his/her speech, not realizing the deterioration that is occurring. Without the ability to monitor one's voice, the individual is unable to control vocal volume, modulation, and pronunciation accuracy. With the loss of this important monitoring system in people with profound hearing loss, various speech and voice changes usually occur.

## Effect on social contacts

Unlike other handicapped individuals, the hard-of-hearing have no outward signs of disability, and strangers can sometimes confuse imperfect hearing with imperfect intelligence. This misconception and similar attitudes can create a strained relationship between a speaker and a listener. The hard-of-hearing person may miss the depth of conversations, usually enriched by side remarks and innuendoes which are often unheard. This lack of a social connection eventually makes the person feel shut off from the normal-hearing world, making him/her prey to discouragement and hopelessness. Until a person loses some hearing, he/she hardly can realize how important it is to hear the small background sounds. These sounds help us feel alive and their absence makes life seem to be rather dull. Imagine missing the sounds of rustling leaves, footsteps, keys in doors, motors running, and the thousands of other little sounds that make human beings feel that they "belong."

## AURAL REHABILITATION

Hearing loss may be medically or surgically treatable, but for more permanent hearing losses, like most sensorineural hearing loss, a cure does not exist. However, a great deal can be done to help the individual compensate for hearing handicap and lead as normal a life as possible, minimizing effects on personality as well as social and economic status. This is all done through a method emphasized during World War II and described as "aural rehabilitation." Thousands of servicemen with hearing impairments were rehabilitated successfully through the large hearing centers established by the Army, the Navy, and the Veterans Administration. Although few such centers are available to civilians, many private otologists, audiologists, university centers, and hearing aid centers can provide rehabilitation measures for persons with handicapping hearing losses that cannot be corrected medically or surgically.

Almost everyone with a handicapping hearing loss can be helped by effective aural rehabilitation. The principal objective of such a program is to help the individual overcome hearing handicap through multiple components. The program includes the following:

1. *Giving the individual a clear understanding of the hearing problem* and explain why he/she has trouble hearing or understanding speech. This requires the otologist or audiologist to demonstrate to the patient how the hearing mechanism works and where the patient's pathology lies. The patient also should be given a clear understanding of the difference between hearing trouble and trouble in understanding what is heard. It also should be explained why he/she has more difficulty understanding speech in the presence of background noise or when several people are speaking simultaneously. The problems that might easily lead the patient to develop frustrations and personality changes should be explained clearly so that these problems can be met forthrightly and intelligently. The goal of aural rehabilitation is to prevent or mitigate psychosocial changes that may result from hearing loss.

2. *Psychological adjustment for each patient,* which involves giving the patient more penetrating insight into the personality problems that are already in evidence or likely to develop as a result of hearing loss. The individual also must be treated in relation to his/her job, family, friends, and way of life. Therapy does not use a generalized technique but must be designed specifically to meet the needs of the hearing-impaired individual. Frequently, it is advisable to carry out this part of the program not only with the patient but also with the patient's spouse or family because it is impossible to separate a person's individual problems from the problems of his/her family. At this point in the program, the patient must accept his/her hearing impairment as a permanent situation and not wait for a medical or surgical cure. Above all, confidence and self-assurance must be instilled in the patient. The patient must be encouraged to associate with friends and not become isolated because of difficulties in communication. It must be impressed on him/her that effectively using the hearing that remains allows him/her to achieve ambitions and carry on as usual with only minor modifications. The assistance of a psychologist specializing in hearing impairment can be invaluable at this stage.

3. *The fitting of a hearing aid, when it is indicated.* This is a vital part of the program, but before a patient can be expected to accept a hearing aid, he/she must be realistically prepared for it. Many people are reluctant to use hearing aids, and many who have purchased hearing aids never use them or use them ineffectively. Before a hearing aid is recommended, it is necessary to determine whether

the patient will be helped by it enough to justify purchasing one. This is particularly important in a sensorineural impairment in which the problem is more one of discrimination than of amplification. Older hearing aids did very little to improve a person's ability to understand but improved abilities to hear by making sounds louder. Recent hearing aid technology targets sensorineural losses with poorer discrimination, greatly improving the amount of benefit these individuals can receive from a hearing aid.

One of the most important things that a hearing aid does for people with hearing loss is it permits the individual to hear sounds with greater ease, removing the severe strain of listening. Although the individual may not be able to understand more with an aid than without one, he/she nevertheless receive great benefit from the device because it relieves tension, fatigue, and some of the complications of a hearing impairment. It also calls other people's attention to the hearing loss and encourages them to speak more clearly.

The patient who seeks early medical attention for hearing loss is wise in many respects. If the condition can be benefited by medical or surgical means, the patient often has a better chance of being helped if a diagnosis is established early in the condition. If a hearing aid is necessary and the patient acquires it quickly, he/she will experience a less drastic adjustment period while wearing the hearing aid. An adjustment period is necessary because the individual will hear sounds that have not been heard for a long time when wearing the hearing aids, such as the refrigerator hum, barking dogs, and shoes clicking on the floor. These sounds can be distracting at first, but the brain will adapt to a noisy environment if given an appropriate adjustment period.

Thousands of hearing aids, bought and then given a too brief or half-hearted trial, can be relegated to a bureau drawer. Overlong postponement in acquiring the aid is sometimes a factor in disuse. In addition, a patient's misguided expectations can lead to a diminished trial period. The patient often expects to hear normally with a hearing aid, when the condition of his/her residual hearing makes such a result impossible. Both the physician and the audiologist should make it clear to the patient that a hearing aid cannot be a perfect substitute for a normal ear, especially in the case of sensorineural hearing loss. Other common causes of disappointment with a hearing aid are an incompetent hearing aid salesperson and the patient's preoccupation with an "invisible" or inconspicuous aid, when a hearing aid that will be most effective in improving the ability to understand conversation should be purchased.

4. *Auditory training to teach the patient how to most effectively use residual hearing with and without a hearing aid.* If the patient can be helped with a hearing aid, he/she should also be made to realize that merely wearing the aid will not solve all his/her hearing and psychosocial problems. The patient needs to learn to use the hearing aid with maximum efficiency in situations such as person-to-person conversation, listening to people in groups and at meetings, and on the telephone. Above all, the patient must recognize the limitations of an aid and when to reduce its use in situations in which it would be a detriment.

Use of gestural cues and environmental cues can be beneficial to both the non-hearing aid user and the hearing aid user. The patient can be taught to use hearing more effectively by looking purposefully at the speaker's face and to develop an intuitive grasp of conversational trends so that he/she can fill in the gaps better than the average person.

5. *Speech reading—a broader concept of lip reading.* This is particularly important in patients who have profound hearing losses. It teaches the patient to obtain information from the speaker's face that cannot be obtained by sound communication. Patients can be taught to read the emotional tone of the conversation. They can also discern if a question or a statement was spoken based on facial expressions. Individuals with hearing loss can learn to use consonant information read from the speaker's lips to fill in missing pieces not heard by the patient. All people do a large amount of speech reading naturally, and a person can develop this faculty extremely well through excellent training, although some individuals have a greater aptitude for speech reading than others.

By cooperating with a carefully planned and competently presented rehabilitation program, almost all people with handicapping hearing loss can be aided not only to hear better but also, more importantly, they can be helped to overcome the many personal problems and psychosocial difficulties that may result from a hearing impairment.

One factor that often complicates helping hearing-impaired persons is the long delay in obtaining medical attention. It is difficult to get some people with hearing loss to admit that they have a hearing problem and it is even more difficult to convince them that they should consult a physician about it. This is one of the reasons that physicians often do not see patients until their hearing impairment has had years to create marked social and communicative problems, both for the patient and for family and friends.

In older people, this delay usually is the result of pride and denial (they think, "This could not happen to me!"). When hearing handicaps are neglected in children, it is more often due to a lack of adult recognition of the problem. The delay in diagnosis is more regrettable for children as many of the conditions that cause hearing loss in the pediatric population are treatable if they are detected early enough and other conditions can be prevented from progressing further. Too often, the symptom of inattentiveness is attributed to a child who fails to respond when spoken to, overlooking the possibility of a hearing loss.

The emphasis in this chapter on rehabilitative measures short of a medical or surgical intervention reflects the fact that a total cure—especially in adults—is not possible in many cases of hearing loss. The often dramatically successful middle-ear surgery is limited mainly to the treatment of otosclerosis who have a reasonably good spread between air- and bone conduction levels (air–bone gap). For such a surgery to have a chance of success, the patient must have a cochlea in at least fair working order and have a functioning auditory nerve. Unfortunately, these requirements are not met by a majority of hard-of-hearing patients. Yet, for those for whom medical surgery is not an option, rehabilitation often can do a great deal in helping them cope.

The physician can play an important part in helping patients overcome their psychological hurdles after a hearing aid, speech reading, and similar measures have been provided. The patient may still need help in adjusting socially, economically, and emotionally to the continuing handicap. One of our patients wrote a book for the hard-of-hearing public on living with a hearing handicap. He theorized that "above the ears there is a brain," an organ of often inadequately explored possibilities that can be used to solve many problems if properly used. He points out that people who do not use their brain for all it is worth really suffer from a handicap far more severe than a mere hearing impairment, leading him to a series of case histories of men, women, and children who have lived successfully with their hearing losses. Sometimes, these individuals have had the help of understanding parents and marriage partners, but, in other cases, they had success in the face of misunderstanding and discouragement. Sometimes, we prescribe this book for our patients (1).

The informed physician, working in close collaboration with an audiologist, is the ideal person to share his/her knowledge of the causes of hearing handicaps with patients to help them overcome the many hurdles that loom so much larger in the patient's mind than the hearing loss itself.

## HEARING AIDS

A hearing aid is a portable personal amplifying system used to compensate for a loss of hearing. Almost all hearing-impaired patients are candidates for a hearing aid, although some will receive greater benefits from their aid than others. Any patient who is motivated to use a hearing aid deserves a thorough evaluation and a trial with an appropriate instrument.

Patients with conductive hearing losses generally are the best candidates for hearing aids because they do not have a distortion problem and just need amplification. Many of these patients may also qualify for corrective surgery. However, all such patients should be advised that a hearing aid might be an effective, if somewhat bothersome, alternative to surgery. Because surgery for conductive hearing loss has been so satisfactory, most people wearing hearing aids are those who have nonmedically treatable losses, such as sensorineural hearing loss, or in whom corrective surgery has failed.

Patients with sensorineural hearing loss not only have difficulty perceiving loudness but also have trouble discriminating speech because of distortion present in their auditory system. Distorted voices become more difficult to understand when they are in the presence of background noise. A sophisticated hearing aid can help compensate for these difficulties by improving loudness perception and boosting the signal-to-noise ratio in noisy environments.

Modern technology allows for specific modifications of hearing aids, which can make a suitable hearing aid useful to almost any patient with hearing loss in the speech frequencies. For example, the frequencies of greatest loss can be emphasized selectively, while others are left unamplified. This is particularly helpful for patients who can hear low frequencies (vowels) but have substantial hearing loss for higher frequencies (consonants). Patients with recruitment may benefit from hearing aids with limited output to protect them from uncomfortably loud sounds. In addition, wearing a hearing aid alerts other people to the patient's hearing loss and frequently prompts them to speak more clearly.

## HEARING AID EVALUATION

Any patient with a hearing loss should have a thorough otologic and audiologic examinations before purchasing a hearing aid. Hearing loss may be merely a symptom of a more serious underlying disease. After being medically cleared, the patient should undergo a formal "hearing-aid evaluation."

It is necessary to know the patient's usable residual hearing for pure tones and speech, ability to hear speech in a noisy environment, and tolerance for loudness. With this information, the audiologist can choose the most audiometrically appropriate hearing aid. The final decision of the purchased hearing aid is based on the above audiometric considerations and the patient's lifestyle, activity level, preference, and income.

The ultimate criteria for a successful fitting are user acceptability and satisfaction. A hearing aid is traditionally given a trial period of 30–45 days, depending on individual state regulatory guidelines to determine successfulness of the fitting. A comprehensive follow-up education program should be arranged to help the user obtain maximum communication with amplification. Such a program might include auditory training (or retraining) and speech-reading lessons. If the patient's speech has deteriorated as a result of the hearing loss, speech-retraining therapy also is recommended.

## HEARING AID COMPONENTS

The basic parts of a hearing aid include a *microphone*, an *amplifier* circuit, a *receiver*, and a *power supply*. A *microphone* transduces acoustic energy into electrical energy, activated by sound waves impinging on the microphone diaphragm. The electrical energy is then fed into an *amplifier* circuit, which increases and adjusts the power of the electrical signal. The amplified signal activates the *receiver*, which changes the signal back into amplified acoustical energy to be delivered to the ear canal with increased intensity. The *power supply* of a hearing aid is usually a zinc-air battery cell.

## Earmolds

Earmolds provide a connection for the delivery of the sound to the ear from an amplifier source. Unless it is specifically designed as an "open" mold, the tight-fitting seal it provides is important in preventing acoustic leakage, known as feedback, between the microphone and the receiver. When a patient complains that his hearing aid is not working because it whistles, the earmold is usually not sealing properly or has not been inserted correctly. When a person complains that the aid is not amplifying well or not working at all, it may be because the canal portion is occluded with cerumen, the battery is dead, or for other mechanical reasons.

The earmold may be made of hard material such as Lucite or of soft materials with various trade names. Nonallergenic materials are also available for individuals with sensitive skin. The acoustic properties of the earmold and the length and the inside diameter of the connecting tube play an important part in the final acoustical characteristics of the amplified sounds that reach the ear. An improperly designed mold can produce discomfort and reduce markedly the acoustical response of the most carefully selected and adjusted hearing aid.

## Special considerations for abnormal ear anatomy and earmolds

Surgically altered external auditory canals and/ or auricles may pose special challenges when ear molds are required. Normal anatomy can be quite variable; however, anatomy is even more unpredictable in patients with congenital anomalies or those who have undergone ear surgery. An exhaustive review of possible anatomic distortions is beyond the scope of this discussion, but familiarity with basic principles should be helpful for anyone trying to create earmolds in patients with anatomic abnormalities.

Congenital abnormalities of the auricle vary from total absence to minimal disfigurement; birth defects of the external auditory canal range from total absence to mild narrowing. The ear canal may be not only narrow but also short in distance from the meatus toward the eardrum. In such cases, there may be a bridge of tissue at any point along the ear canal, walling off the eardrum; absence of the medial portion of the ear canal and eardrum, so the ear canal ends as a shallow pouch; or the eardrum may be laterally placed (uncommon except following surgery). In patients with atresia (absence of the ear canal), a bone conduction aid or implantable hearing aid is required unless an ear canal is created surgically. Reconstructive surgery is possible in virtually all cases, nearly always without injury to the facial nerve (which often is also abnormal). The amount of hearing loss present depends on the abnormality as well as on inner ear function.

During surgical reconstruction for congenital atresia, the surgeon faces several limitations, which help explain the challenges these patients pose when they require earmolds. First, the surgeon must be concerned about both function and cosmetics. Often there are two surgeons involved in caring for congenital atresia, particularly if it involves both the auricle and the ear canal. One creates an external ear, attempting to make it appear as normal as possible. The ear is often made of rib cartilage with a thin layer of skin over it. Even slight irritation from an earmold may cause erosion, infection, and loss of an entire reconstructed auricle. From a functional standpoint, the surgeon (often a different member of the surgical team) is interested in creating an ear canal, making an eardrum, and possibly creating or reconstructing ossicles. This processes is usually staged. The functional surgeon wants to make an ear canal that is as large as possible because they always re-stenose and end up smaller than they were when they left the operating room. The position of the ear canal

is dictated by the position of the middle ear, which often is misplaced anteriorly and inferiorly and does not coincide with the cosmetically desirable ear canal position. The cosmetic and functional otological surgeons create compromises that permit acceptable appearance and function.

An earmold can be used postoperatively as a surgical packing and/or as an assistive device used with a hearing aid. One of the authors (R.T.S.) often uses an earmold postoperatively as a stent to help maintain a large ear canal; this technique has not been reported previously. Often, the earmold is created in the operating room. The ear block is cut down so that it is as small as possible and then placed against the grafted tympanic membrane. A mold is shaped to the contours of the entire surgical defect. A thin coating of antibiotic drops or ointment is placed in the ear prior to application of earmold material, as the procedure is "clean" rather than completely sterile. When the mold is sent for processing, it is important to specify that it should not be shortened. This mold is intended to go all the way to the eardrum to help maintain ear canal size. Additionally, a large bore in the earmold will enable passage of some air and low-frequency sound into the ear canal. We make a second mold immediately in the operating room and leave it in the ear to function as surgical packing and stenting. We use a medium-viscosity silicone impression material to make this mold. This will prevent the material from distorting or stretching the ear canal after surgery, without generating too much pressure from the application syringe. It is removed 1 week following surgery, and the permanent mold with the large bore is placed in the ear. It can be removed for cleaning once or twice daily, coated lightly with antibiotic ointment and reinserted. This technique usually results in final ear canal anatomy that is not only adequate in size but also of a shape that will hold an earmold. However, this technique is not used widely, yet.

Earmolds for surgical ears can also have retention problems due to the nature of reconstructive surgery. Most ear canals that have been created surgically are fairly straight, and they may be somewhat flared at the meatus. This can sometimes create problems with mold retention. If they cannot be overcome by mold design, surgery is sometimes necessary to narrow the lateral aspect with the meatus slightly to create a small ridge to help hold the earmold or to widen the medial aspect of the ear canal, also creating an anatomic indention that will stabilize the mold. If the meatus is soft and "floppy" after surgery, and if there is plenty of soft tissue between the skin and cartilage or bone, a hard, acrylic material may be the most suitable for an earmold, although a softer material can certainly be used. However, if the postsurgical anatomy presents a hard, inflexible meatus with thick skin adherent to bone, a softer, silicon material may be preferable, providing a better seal and greater comfort. In addition, softer material also may work better when the anterior wall of the external auditory canal has been removed during surgery, and the remaining anterior canal wall communicates with the region of the temporomandibular joint. In such cases, there is more ear canal motion than normal during chewing and talking; soft mold materials tend to work better than acrylic molds for excessive motion.

Chronic ear surgery in adults or children also may result in anatomic abnormalities. Simple mastoidectomy or "intact canal wall" mastoidectomy ordinarily leaves the ear canal undisturbed. However, both modified radical mastoidectomy and radical mastoidectomy involve removing the ear canal and creating a cavity. The difference between the two classifications is determined primarily by which structures are left in the patient. In a radical mastoidectomy, the eardrum, malleus, and incus are removed, and only the stapes (with or without its superstructure) is preserved. If a portion of the eardrum or additional ossicles can be saved, then the procedure becomes a modified radical mastoidectomy. In either case, the posterior wall of the external auditory canal should be removed to the level of the vertical portion of the facial nerve, and the inferior wall of the ear canal should be widened and beveled toward the mastoid tip. Because it is usually necessary to clean mastoid cavities, the meatus is also widened markedly (meatoplasty). It is often possible to place a mold and begin using a hearing aid within 8–12 weeks following the time of surgery, but healing will cause alterations in size and shape for 6–12 months. So, it may be necessary to remake earmolds periodically and patients should be warned of this potential inconvenience. Making molds for patients with mastoid cavities is not usually a major problem. Additional ear block material may be required, but there is usually enough irregularity in the shape of the canal, meatus, and cavity to assure that there are curves and indentations that will help stabilize a mold.

Many patients who have mastoid cavities suffer repeated ear infections because of infections medial to the earmold. Although this problem may be solved by venting when it is appropriate, the repeated infections are usually not the fault of the earmold (assuming that there is no allergic reaction to the mold material). Rather often, they are related to pockets of residual disease or moisture from the upper respiratory tract and middle ear that has not been sealed off from the rest of the mastoid cavity (a "tubal ear"). In the vast majority of cases, if hearing aid use is necessary in patients who are plagued with repeated otitis, the problem can be solved by revision surgery.

## TYPES OF AIDS

There are four types of wearable hearing aids: the body aid, the eyeglass aid, the behind-the-ear (BTE) aid, and the in-the-ear (ITE) aid.

### The body aid

Owing modern micro-technology, the body aid is now rarely dispensed. It is a large, high-powered instrument worn on the body and connected to the earmold. Body aids offer wide ranges of amplification and usually are used by patients who have severe hearing impairments. The microphone, amplifier, and battery are located in the case, which is worn on the body or carried in a pocket. The receiver is connected to the amplifier by a long wire and is attached directly to the earmold. This separation of receiver and microphone helps eliminate acoustical feedback in high-amplification instruments. Body aids can be fit to losses of 40- to 110-dB HL.

### The eyeglass aid

Another classic aid that is rarely dispensed is the eyeglass aid. The amplifying unit is housed in the arm of the eyeglasses and connects to the earmold by a short length of tubing. Eyeglass hearing aids are appropriate for hearing losses of up to >70-dB HL. With special modifications, they can be used for even greater losses. Their use is limited due to poor cosmetics of the device and because of better technology available currently.

## The behind-the-ear aid

BTE hearing aids currently dominate the market for fitting of severe to profound losses, an application previously reserved for body aids and eyeglass aids. All of the necessary components of the amplifying system, including the battery, are held in a single case worn BTE. The amplified sound is then fed to the ear via a plastic hook attached to the tubing of an earmold. This design provides adequate separation of microphone and receiver to reduce acoustical feedback, which is common in severe hearing losses. These aids can be used for losses in the 25- to 110-dB HL range, making them the most flexible instruments available on the market.

## The in-the-ear aid

ITE instruments are the most widely dispensed hearing aids in North America today. Micro-digital technological developments allow for the entire hearing aid system to be housed inside the earmold shell. The aids can be used for losses in the 25- to 80-dB HL range. There are several different styles of ITE instruments available for dispensing: full shell, half shell, canal, and completely-in-the-canal (CIC), listed, respectively, from largest to smallest shell size. One drawback to the smaller ITE sizes is that they cannot provide as much amplification as the larger shells, making them inappropriate for more severe of hearing loss.

## PERFORMANCE CHARACTERISTICS

All hearing aids have certain performance characteristics that must be taken into account when matching a patient to the best possible aid. The five most commonly considered characteristics are acoustic gain, acoustic output, basic frequency response, frequency range, and distortion. *Acoustic gain* is the decibel difference between the incoming signal reaching the hearing aid microphone and the amplified signal reaching the ear. *Acoustic output*, also called *saturation sound pressure level* (SSPL), is the highest sound pressure level an aid is capable of producing. This parameter is important in assuring that the aid will not produce uncomfortably loud sounds, especially for patients with sensorineural hearing loss and recruitment and that it will amplify the sound adequately for the

patient. The *basic frequency response* is the curve found most commonly on the manufacturer's specification sheets. It describes the relative gain achieved at each frequency. Many conventional hearing instruments have external tone controls that can amplify or suppress certain frequencies, according to the needs of the user. For example, a hearing loss may involve only the frequencies of ≥2000 Hz. By appropriate selection or by manipulation of the tone controls, the hearing aid can be adjusted so that it will not amplify frequencies <2000 Hz. The *frequency range* is a calculated measure of the high- and low-frequency limits of usable amplification for an individual instrument. This is also important to determine if an aid is adequate for a user's hearing loss. *Distortion* of the acoustic signal is measured electronically and the output of the hearing aid must meet specifications established by the American National Standards Institute (ANSI).

## HEARING AID CIRCUITRY

### Analog hearing aids

Analog hearing aids were the first type of hearing aids available to consumers. They were best suited for amplification of signals in a generally quiet environment. Conventional instruments were adjusted manually (with a screwdriver) through a variety of potentiometers. External output and gain tone potentiometers extended the applicability of the hearing aid to a wider range and patterns of hearing loss. Once these controls were adjusted properly, the wearer should not change them.

### Analog–digital hybrids

The next technology to become available in the hearing aid industry was analog–digital hybrid, also known as programmable hearing aids. These hearing aids allow for digital, computerized control of analog circuits and offer far more precision in the fitting process than is available in conventional analog hearing aids. Initial programming was more involved and time consuming, which may increase the price of the fitting. The improved sound quality, frequency shaping capabilities, and enhanced output controls make the analog–digital hybrid a more flexible option for hearing aid users.

## Digital hearing aids

The most current state of the art in hearing aid circuitry is the digital hearing aid, the most dynamic and flexible instrument available to consumers. A digital instrument takes an acoustic input, changes it into binary data, performs any amplification and special modifications, and then transduces it back to an acoustic form to be delivered to the patient's ear. As the signal is in a binary form, an unlimited number of enhancements can be performed by a digital hearing aid. For example, digital hearing aids are designed to amplify a broader set of inputs—keeping soft sounds soft and audible, medium sounds are comfortably amplified, and loud inputs are perceived as loud but not uncomfortable. These instruments provide for an expanded dynamic range to sounds, especially useful for patients with recruitment. Digital instruments clearly offer the best sound quality and the most flexibility in fitting.

## CONTROLS

Digital technological advances have made signal processing capabilities far superior to those designs of the past. In particular, the features listed below have improved the quality of sound to make it seem natural and far more pleasing to the listener.

## Proprietary speech-enhancing algorithms

With the digitalization of amplification, each manufacturer has developed a mathematical formula to improve speech sounds prior to the amplification stage. Utilizing the splitting of the speech band into smaller elements, these areas are controlled to package sound for better understanding and enjoyment.

## Automatic gain control

Automatic gain control (AGC) circuits maintain the overall intensity of the output and prevent it from reaching an individual's uncomfortable listening level, effectively keeping sound within a maximum comfort range. The level at which this circuit is activated can be preset by an audiologist or a hearing-aid dispenser. The AGC is especially useful for those individuals with sensorineural hearing loss who do not tolerate loud sounds well. Digital technology now allows this control to occur inside specific frequency sections providing a superior means of adjustment than in the past.

## Noise suppression features

Noise suppression circuits and dual microphone technology function to reduce unwanted background noise by either improving the signal-to-noise ratio using noise suppression or using noise cancellation. This technology allows for improved speech understanding by modifying the speech areas. These features can be particularly useful in noisy environments such as a crowded restaurant or party. Noise suppression features should be considered especially for patients who are actively presented with speech-in-noise difficulties.

## Feedback reduction

Feedback is an acoustical output from a hearing aid, often characterized as a "whistle" or a "squeal." Feedback often occurs at high frequencies with a loose-fitting earmold or in the presence of an occluded ear canal. Feedback reduction circuits eliminate acoustic feedback caused by large peaks in the frequency response of hearing aids. These nonlinear peaks can cause harmonic and intermodulation distortion, generating user dissatisfaction with the instrument. There are other ways of reducing acoustic feedback, but they involve compromising overall acoustic gain. Some methods of feedback reduction are low-pass notch filters (hard rejects), which filter the peaks in the frequency response, frequency shifting circuits, and phase cancellation. These methods of feedback reduction generally increase user satisfaction with the instrument by reducing feedback during everyday activities such as chewing and smiling. Feedback reduction features are only available in digital and programmable instruments.

## Volume

Most hearing aids have a volume control by which the user can vary the intensity of the signal reaching the ear. In some aids, the volume control also acts as an on–off switch. In the newer circuitry, the hearing aid may not have a volume control because the circuit modifies its output based on the loudness of the input, automatically adjusting the volume of the hearing aid. The digital circuits, depending on the size of the shell, have the option of adding a manual volume control or activating the control allowing for some wearer control over the function.

## Switches and buttons

Some hearing aids have a separate switch for turning the aid on and off. Also incorporated into this switch may be a telephone (T) position for using the telephone. The telephone receiver is placed over the magnetic field of the hearing aid with the switch in this position. The hearing aid is then set to receive only the magnetic signal of the telephone. After completion of the call, the switch is returned to the microphone (M) position to receive acoustical signals again. Some instruments have an MT position that allows the user to receive both magnetic and acoustical signals through the hearing aid at the same time. The telephone position also can be used with various assistive listening devices that use a magnetic field to transmit signals.

Recent technology has developed memory or program buttons on digital and programmable hearing aids. Multiple-memory hearing aids allow the user to scroll through preprogrammed settings in the hearing aid based on the person's listening environment. An audiologist can load acoustical programs, such as a quiet, noise/party, telephone, or music program, which modifies the output of the hearing aid. In one memory setting, the hearing aid may provide a generous low-frequency response; in another, the hearing aid changes directional characteristics to suppress background signals. Switching between memory positions allows the user to optimize hearing aid function in different listening environments.

## THE HEARING AID USER

Any patient with abnormal hearing may be a candidate for amplification. In general, when the thresholds in the speech frequencies are ≥25 dB, a hearing aid could be helpful, even if only one ear is involved. When both ears are involved and have usable residual hearing, binaural amplification is often recommended. Binaural amplification has been shown to be advantageous for three reasons—binaural summation, elimination of the head shadow, and binaural squelch. Binaural summation is the perception of a sound as louder (~3 dB) when it is presented binaurally vs. monaurally (2, 3). When an individual is aided monaurally and speech is presented to an unaided ear, a head shadow effect is created where high-frequency speech signals are attenuated up to 16 dB because they cannot travel around objects as well as low-frequency sounds due to short wavelengths (4). Binaural hearing aids eliminate the head shadow effect by abolishing the need for sound to travel around the head to be detected. The third advantage to a binaural hearing aid fitting is called binaural squelch, which is the reduction in perceived noise or reverberation by the auditory system when the two ears are symmetrically stimulated, thus enhancing speech detection in noise (5, 6). All three of these well-researched advantages should be presented to patients when discussing monaural vs. binaural hearing aid fittings.

Not all patients are receptive to using a hearing aid, as a stigma is often attached to hearing loss. It is not uncommon for a patient to refuse an aid or become upset over the recommendation. A few moments of calm, sensitive counseling may be invaluable. Associations of hearing aids with "getting old," mental incompetence, and physical unattractiveness (especially in teenage patients) can be dispelled by a sensitive physician or audiologist.

## Hearing aids in children

Studies have demonstrated that even a mild hearing loss in infancy and early childhood can have an effect on learning and development. A child with a hearing loss that cannot be corrected medically or surgically should be fitted with a hearing aid as soon as the hearing loss is diagnosed. This may be even as early as the age of ≥6 months. With the advent of newborn hearing screenings, more children with hearing loss are identified at an earlier age, decreasing the impact the hearing loss might have had on their language and development. A properly fitted hearing aid is usually well tolerated by the child because of the benefit he/she receives from it. In general, children should be fitted with binaural amplification in order to maximize auditory input for speech–language development and to provide sound localization capabilities.

## NONCANDIDACY FOR A HEARING AID

There are a few circumstances under which fitting a proper hearing aid may be difficult or impossible. In certain ears, the use of an earmold may be medically contraindicated. This precludes the use of the majority of hearing aids, except those with open canal earmolds or bone conduction receivers. Some ears, particularly in cochlear hearing loss, are extremely sensitive to loud sounds despite the fact that they have substantially reduced hearing thresholds. Such a narrow *dynamic range* may make a hearing aid more bothersome than helpful. A similar situation is seen in ears with severely reduced discrimination ability. A hearing aid, in the latter scenario, would only be useful for sound awareness.

On August 25, 1977, the Food and Drug Administration established rules regulating professional and labeling requirements and conditions for the sale of hearing aids. In accordance with this regulation, the hearing aid dispenser or audiologist should advise a prospective user to consult a licensed physician (preferably an ear specialist) if any of the following conditions exist:

1. Visible congenital or traumatic deformity of the ear;
2. History of active drainage from the ear within the previous 90 days;
3. History of sudden or rapidly progressing hearing loss within the previous 90 days;
4. Acute or chronic dizziness;
5. Unilateral hearing loss of sudden or recent onset within the previous 90 days;
6. Audiometric air–bone gap ≥15 dB at 500, 1000, and 2000 Hz;
7. Visible evidence of significant cerumen accumulation or a foreign body in the ear canal;
8. Pain or discomfort in the ear.

The law "permits a fully informed adult to sign a waiver statement declining the medical evaluation for religious or personal beliefs." The dispenser or audiologist shall not sell a hearing aid until he/she receives a signed waiver or statement from a licensed physician indicating that the patient's "hearing loss has been medically evaluated and the patient may be considered a candidate for a hearing aid." This FDA law also requires a 30-day trial period during which the aid(s) can be returned.

## SPECIAL HEARING AID SYSTEMS

### CROS systems

When a patient has one ear that is not suitable for amplification, sound can be routed from the unaidable side to the better hearing side. This is especially helpful when trying to hear a conversation from the unaidable side. However, it does not restore the ability to localize the direction of the sound source.

*CROS* is an acronym for contralateral routing of signals. The microphone is placed on the unaidable side, and the amplifier and receiver are located on the better hearing ear. The amplified sound is carried across the head via a wire, through a pair of eyeglasses, or by a radio signal and fed to the better ear by a tube to an open earmold. This arrangement is most useful in cases of unilateral hearing loss with up to a mild loss on the better hearing ear. A variety of modifications of the CROS principle have extended its applicability.

### BICROS systems

Bilateral contralateral routing of signals (BICROS) is used for patients with an asymmetric bilateral hearing loss. Microphones are placed on both sides of the head, and the amplifier is placed on the more aidable ear. The amplified sound is fed only to the aidable ear via tubing and an occluding earmold. In cases where the aidable ear has a high-frequency hearing loss, a similar arrangement with an open earmold or an open BICROS is more appropriate. The BICROS can be thought of as a microphone on the unaidable ear and a hearing aid on the aidable side that also receives information from the contralateral side of the head.

### Transcranial CROS

A *transcranial CROS* is similar to the CROS system, except that the signal is delivered to the better hearing ear by vibrating the bones of the skull. A deeply fit CIC hearing aid is manufactured and placed in the unaidable ear. The sound output of the CIC then travels to the better hearing ear via bone conduction. A transcranial CROS is indicated generally for individuals who have normal bone-conduction thresholds in their better hearing ear.

## IROS system

In patients with mild hearing losses or in whom hearing is normal in the lower frequencies with a precipitous drop off in the higher frequencies, the ipsilateral routing of signals (IROS) system is used. This employs an open earmold to allow the normally heard low-frequency signals to enter the ear naturally and vent off unwanted amplified frequencies. The hearing aid is then set to provide enhanced high-frequency emphasis.

## High-frequency hearing aids

Several companies are now producing an alternative to IROS hearing aids for users with precipitous, sloping hearing losses. Instead of using an open earmold, these hearing instruments are designed with special tubing that is inserted into the ear canal, leaving the canal more open than a large IROS vent. The specially designed tubing allows for more low-frequency information to pass into the ear canal naturally where the patient's hearing is normal. The hearing aid is either manually or computer programmed to provide amplification in the high frequencies where the patient's hearing loss is located. In order to measure the response of this special hearing aid, the audiologist or dispenser must use the new ANSI average called the SPA or "Special Purpose Average" to determine the gain and SSPL output. These new high-frequency emphasis aids show promise of providing benefit to those who have previously not been able to wear amplification.

## Bone conduction hearing aids

Bone conduction hearing aids are useful for patients with atresia or stenosis of the ear canal, microtia of the pinna, or those with chronic drainage. They are a nonsurgical alternative to deliver sound to an affected ear with a conductive hearing loss. A bone conduction vibrator attached to a headband is placed on the mastoid bone. The vibrator is connected to a body-worn processor that transmits the acoustic signal and transfers it to a mechanical one. Although the bone conduction hearing aid is a nonsurgical method of delivering sound to an ear, its output is limited by the presence of distortion at high intensity levels and the inability to provide large amounts of amplification.

# IMPLANTABLE DEVICES

## Bone-anchored hearing aids

An improvement on bone conduction hearing aids is the *bone-anchored hearing aid*, BAHA™ (Entific Medical Systems Inc., Sweden). Similar devices are available from other companies. Similar to the bone conduction instruments, it is useful for patients with conductive hearing losses that are unaidable due to ear malformations or chronic drainage. The BAHA utilizes an external bone-conduction processor that is attached to a titanium screw implanted in the temporal bone. Because the skull is directly stimulated, more amplification can be delivered to the better hearing ear without as much distortion. Besides being used for conductive losses, the BAHA has been approved by the FDA for patients with unilateral sensorineural hearing loss to be applied as an alternative to a CROS hearing aid. Currently, the device is recommended for patients with bone conduction thresholds in the speech frequencies no worse than 25-dB HL (with no speech frequency worse than 40-dB HL) and air conduction thresholds not better than 40-dB HL. Its principle disadvantage is the presence of the bone anchor that protrudes permanently though the skin.

## Middle ear implants

A *middle ear implant*, known as the Vibrant® Soundbridge®, is used to treat mild-to-severe sensorineural hearing losses. It involves a vibrating ossicular prosthesis device implanted through the mastoid bone in a surgical procedure under local or general anesthesia. The prosthesis is then controlled by a magnetically attached external processing device, similar to a BTE hearing aid. The processor transmits the amplified signal to the prosthesis and is adjusted based on the individual's hearing loss.

## Cochlear implant

A cochlear implant is analogous in many ways to a hearing aid. It is used in very carefully selected patients with severe profound bilateral sensorineural hearing loss, too severe to be aided effectively with hearing aids. A cochlear implant involves surgical placement of electrode bundles directly into the cochlea. The electrodes are controlled by a processor worn on the outside of the head, either BTE or on the body, which sends electrical impulses along the bundles to the acoustic nerve. The cochlear implant initially began with only a single-electrode array device. This design has been supplanted by multichannel devices, which provide a more complex signal and generally better speech discrimination than the original single channel system. Cochlear implants produce true sound; however, the outcome (hearing ability) with an implant varies by patient. Some individuals are very successful with cochlear implants, even being able to use the telephone with their implant; other patients are limited to having only sound awareness. Patients who undergo cochlear implant surgery require intense rehabilitation in order to learn how to use the device optimally. Cochlear implants are currently approved for use in adults and children. As technology improves, the criteria change. Candidates no longer have to be profoundly deaf. Patients with moderate hearing loss and even with unilateral hearing loss may benefit from a cochlear implant.

## Brainstem implants

Auditory brainstem implants (ABIs) are useful for patients who have undergone removal of acoustic tumors for neurofibromatosis type 2 (NF2). The surgery for acoustic tumor removal in NF2 patients typically ablates hearing bilaterally. The ABI provides sound awareness for those patients by implanting electrodes in the brainstem. This implantation is typically done during the surgery to remove the acoustic tumors. The electrodes bypass the severed acoustic nerves and transmit sound directly to the auditory brainstem nuclei. Through extensive auditory retraining therapy, the implant recipients learn to associate the new acoustical information to assist in detection of environmental sounds and some speech information.

## ASSISTIVE DEVICES

There are many inexpensive convenience items available to hearing-handicapped persons. If a patient's hearing aid is not equipped with a telephone switch, the patient may benefit from a volume control inset placed on his/her telephone or an amplified telephone. A battery-operated, pocket-sized telephone amplifier is also available for travel. For patients with profound hearing losses, an auxiliary receiver may be installed in home and office telephones. This allows the patient's secretary or spouse to hear the incoming message and repeat it so that the patient can lip-read and respond directly into the telephone. Specialized aids are available for patients with particular occupational needs, such as transistorized switchboard amplifier for telephone operators.

Telecommunications device for the deaf (TDD) or teletypewriter (TTY) devices are telephone devices for the deaf or profoundly hearing-impaired person. TDDs and TTYs use a typewriterlike keypad with a printout or LED display. They can communicate with one another with text messages or can be used to communicate with a hearing person by using a relay system. Most states have a telephone relay service through which the typed message is transmitted to an operator who then reads the message to the hearing contact and types the replies back to the hearing-impaired individual. Telephones (TT) also are available.

Detecting routine auditory signals such as the telephone or doorbell is a special problem for the hearing-impaired. The telephone company can provide a variety of bells and buzzers, either frequency adjustable or amplified, which may help solve the problem. Auxiliary devices such as flashing lights also are available. Waking devices that vibrate can replace an alarm clock. Lights, vibrators, and specialized sound signals can be connected to sound-sensing devices. These may be placed, for example, in a baby's room so that they can be activated by the sound of a cry.

Personal amplification systems are available for listening to television or at a social event. These systems typically include an amplifying headset and direct audio input from a remote microphone. They allow the speaker to talk directly into the microphone and effectively cut back on the background noise. The reduction in background noise improves the signal-to-noise ratio, thus improving comprehension.

Many other convenience devices are available as well. Earphones and loudspeakers for radio and television listening are useful and relatively inexpensive. An induction coil device or telephone switch in the hearing aid can be used with the radio or television to selectively amplify the desired signal without amplifying the surrounding noise. Even electronic stethoscopes are available for the hearing-impaired physician and nurse. It is worthwhile for all professionals in the health-care delivery system to be familiar with the complexities of both the problems and the solutions of hearing loss. Only in this way can we provide optimum care and maximize the quality of life of the many afflicted members of our society.

## ACKNOWLEDGMENT

The authors are grateful to Tracy M. Virag, Caren J. Sokolow, and John Luckhurst for their contributions to the chapter on this topic in the previous edition.

## REFERENCES

1. Van Itallie PH. How to live with a hearing handicap. New York, NY: Paul S. Erikson, 1963.

2. Hirsh I. The influence of interaural phase on interaural summation and inhibition. J Acoust Soc Am 1948; 20:544–557.

3. Licklider J. The influence of interaural phase relations upon the masking of speech by white noise. J Acoust Soc Am 1948; 20:150–159.

4. Feston J, Plomp R. Speech reception threshold in noise with one or two hearing aids. J Acoust Soc Am 1986; 79:465–471.

5. Byrne D. Binaural hearing aid fitting: research findings and clinical application. In: Libby E, ed. Binaural Hearing and Amplification. Chicago, IL: Zenetron, Inc., 1980.

6. Ross M. Binaural versus monaural hearing aid amplification for hearing-impaired individuals. In: Libby E, ed. Binaural Hearing and Amplification. Chicago, IL: Zenetron, Inc., 1980.

# 19

# Hearing protection devices

DANIEL EICHORN, BRIAN McGOVERN, AND ROBERT THAYER SATALOFF

## INTRODUCTION

There are three main means of preventing noise-induced hearing loss in the work environment: engineered controls, administrative controls, and personal protective equipment (PPE). The most effective means of preventing noise-induced hearing loss is to remove the worker from hazardous noise. Employers must try to reduce noise levels in industrial work environments when it is not possible to move the employee. High-intensity noise sources may need to be treated by covering surfaces with acoustically absorbent materials. Administrative controls encompass rotating jobs and shifts so that employees have reduced exposure to noisy equipment and job sites. However, that may not be feasible as companies and crews may not have the sufficient workers, capital, or resources to support a rotation. If engineered and administrative controls are insufficient, Occupational Safety and Health Act (OSHA) requires employers to provide employees with hearing protection devices (HPDs). Hearing protectors should provide immediate, effective protection against occupational hearing loss without substantially compromising safe, effective communication.

An effective HPD serves as a barrier between the noise and the hair cells of the cochlear, where noise-induced damage to hearing occurs. A wide variety of HPDs are available, including ear inserts, earmuffs, and canal caps. Ear inserts or earplugs provide an acoustical seal in the outermost portion of the ear canal. Earmuffs are worn over the external ear and provide an acoustical seal against the head. Canal caps provide an acoustical seal at the entrance of the external ear canal.

## PROTECTOR TYPES

### EAR CANALS

Ear canals differ widely in size, shape, and position among individuals and between ears of the same individual. Ear canal asymmetry can contribute to challenges in obtaining a proper fit in both ears. Earplugs should be chosen that are adaptable to a wide variety of ear canal configurations in order to prevent a mismatch between the canal size and size of the HPD.

DOI: 10.1201/b23379-19

Ear canals vary in cross-section from ~3 to 14 mm, with a large majority falling in the range of 5–11 mm. Most ear canals are elliptically shaped, with a bend to direct sound toward the front of the head.

HPDs generally are classified according to the manner in which they are worn. The three best-known types are ear inserts, canal caps, and earmuffs.

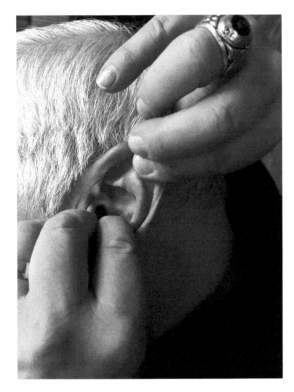

Figure 19.1 Recommended method for inserting earplugs.

## INSERTS

Ear inserts or earplugs fit directly inside the ear canal. Earplugs can be subcategorized into formable, premolded, and custom-molded. The space for an insert earplug is small. The entrance of the ear canal can be opened and straightened by pulling the external ear directly from the head upward and backward with the opposite hand (**Figure 19.1**). For comfort and plug retention, the ear canal must return approximately to its normal configuration once the protector is seated.

A properly fit earplug depends on a seal along the entire circumference of the ear canal walls. Ear inserts are supplied in three general configurations (**Figure 19.2**).

Earplugs can be made from a variety of materials. Cotton is the least effective protector, providing little attenuation, and it is not recommended. Custom-made HPDs generally are made from a thermoplastic or silicone material. Use of these materials allows earplugs to be made to fit the exact size and shape of the user's ear canal. Custom earplugs are able to provide a significant amount of attenuation. These earmolds tend to fit the most comfortably, making them the most likely to be worn as intended. Custom earmolds are reusable. However, the material does deteriorate after long-term usage.

Formable ear inserts are made from soft, compressible foam. These earplugs come in one to three sizes. The material is compressed or gently rolled to insert into the ear canal. Once inserted, these earplugs expand to fill the ear canal and should be held in place while the foam decompresses to form an airtight seal. Once the foam seals the ear canal completely, formable earplugs provide a high attenuation value. Foam plugs tend to be difficult to insert properly into the ear. Annual employee education should instruct users to proper use of the earplugs. These earplugs may be washed and reused but do need replacement often.[1,2] Some individuals, especially women and young children, may have difficulty rolling conventional foam plugs small enough to fit a small ear canal. Some manufacturers do offer a small-size expandable foam earplug.[2,3]

Premolded earplugs are available in specific sizes and shapes, although are generally manufactured as "one-size-fits-most" for small, medium, or large ear canals. It is important to be aware that a person may need a different size earplug for each ear due to canal asymmetry.[2] They are commonly made from plastic, rubber, or silicone. The most common premolded earplug styles are the single flange and triple flange. Insertion technique is slightly different for premolded earplugs and is achieved through a gentle rocking motion of the plug until the canal is sealed. Premolded earplugs are washable and reusable but do deteriorate and should be replaced periodically. They are convenient to carry, and in dusty or dirty environments, the tips do not require manipulation, rolling, or handling.[1,2]

All earplugs have the advantage of being small and lightweight. In warm environments, ear inserts tend to be the most comfortable HPD. It is easy to combine earplugs with other safety equipment, such as hard hats and safety goggles.

Earplugs require specific fitting instructions. Improperly seated earplugs will not provide the intended attenuation. Occasionally, ear inserts come loose. Excessive jaw movement may unseat earplugs.

Often, earplugs are soiled. A custom-made earmold will need proper cleaning. Foam inserts are disposable and are thrown away after use. It may be difficult to monitor earplug use as some inserts sit deeply inside the worker's ear canal.

Some people are more prone to cerumen impaction than others. Earwax naturally migrates from inside the ear canal to the outside. Earplugs that temporarily occlude the ears rarely cause significant problems with wax impaction. If the ear becomes filled with earwax, it should be removed by a doctor.

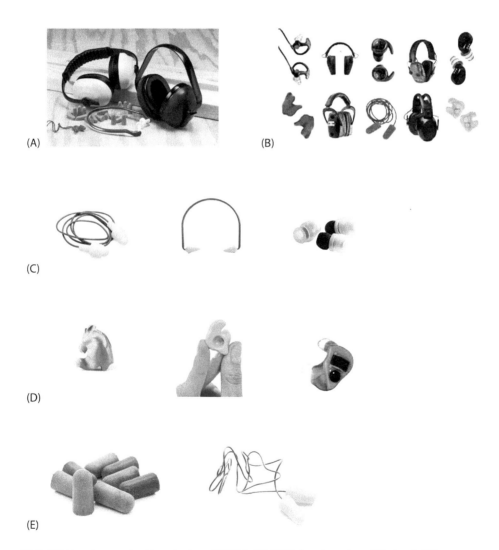

(A)

(B)

(C)

(D)

(E)

Figure 19.2 (A) Hearing protection devices (HPDs), (B) HPD for shooting, (C) sized, (D) custom molded, and (E) moldable.

## CANAL CAPS

Protectors that cannot be strictly classified as earplugs or earmuffs are more broadly described as concha-seated protectors. Canal caps fall into this category. Canal caps are usually conical in shape and resemble earplugs on a flexible plastic or metal band. The device may be worn over the head, behind the neck, or under the chin. The earplug tip of a canal cap may be made of formable or premolded material. Newer models have adjustable headbands to match the shape of a user's head and ear positions more effectively.[1,2]

Although sizing is not a problem, good insertion instruction is essential with this type of HPD. Concha-seated HPDs are inserted similar to earplugs. The outer ear is pulled up and back, and the tip of the cap is inserted into ear, pushing it into place. Insertion is most reliably achieved by placing one earplug at a time. Canal caps are reusable, and the caps do need to be replaced periodically. However, they should be cleaned.

Sound attenuation with canal caps is achieved by sealing the external opening of the ear canal (**Figure 19.3A–C**). Canal caps are ideal for employees who are constantly removing and replacing their HPDs as they can be easily left to hang around the head or neck and replaced when hazardous noise restarts. They are not designed for continuous, long-term use.

Canal caps do not fit deeply into the ear canal; they only close the ear opening. Therefore, they do not provide as much attenuation as earmuffs or earplugs. These HPDs provide maximum protection at frequencies >1000 Hz. The attenuation <1000 Hz is considerably less by ~15–20 dB.

## EARMUFFS

Earmuffs are designed to be worn over the ears to reduce the level of noise reaching the inner ear (**Figure 19.4A–D**). The effectiveness of earmuffs depends on a hermetic seal between the ear cushion and the outer ear. The ear cups are made of plastic, padded with acoustic foam, and joined by an adjustable headband. The headband can be worn over the top of the head, to the rear of the head, or under the chin. With proper hardware, earmuffs can be attached to hardhats. Sponge wedges are available to fill any openings between the earmuffs and safety glasses. Proper headband tension needs to be present to ensure a tight seal over the outer ears.

Most earmuffs have similar designs. Seal materials lining the ear cups that are placed against the skin should be made of a nontoxic material. Fit, comfort, and general performance of comparable models do not vary widely.

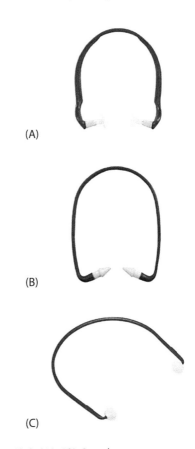

(A)

(B)

(C)

Figure 19.3 (A)–(C) Canal caps.

If maximum protection is required, the protector ear cups must be formed of a rigid, dense, imperforate material. The size of the enclosed volume within the muff shell is directly related to the low-frequency attenuation. Ear seals should have a small circumference so that the acoustic seal takes place over the smallest possible irregularities in head contour. This minimizes air leaks caused by jaw and neck movements.

The ear cup is filled with an open-cell material to absorb high-frequency resonant noises.

The material placed inside the cup should not contact the external ear. Contact may cause discomfort or soiling of the lining. Perspiration may cause the ear cup cushion material to become stiff or shrink. Fluid-filled cushions have the additional problem of leakage. Most earmuffs are equipped with easily replaceable seals to provide adequate protection.

Maintenance of the earmuffs is essential for maximum protection. The plastic or foam cushions can be cleaned with warm, soapy water. The inside of each earmuff should not get wet. When not in use, earmuffs should be placed in open air to allow moisture to evaporate.

Earmuffs have the advantage of having one size fit most users. Adjustable arms connected to the ear cups let the user adjust to a comfortable fit. The attenuation provided from earmuffs tends to be consistent among wearers. Employers can easily monitor earmuff use because of their size and visibility. Ear infection is not a contraindication to use.

Less protection is expected when earmuffs are worn over hair or glasses. Obstructions should be minimized; otherwise, the expected attenuation will not be provided. Earmuff use is difficult in warm environments and in close quarters. Warm environments make earmuff use uncomfortable. Perspiration tends to stick to the ear cup lining, and, as a result, they can feel hot and heavy in some conditions. Head maneuvering while wearing earmuffs in close quarters is restricted. Headband suspension forces can become reduced with usage. Reduced tension means that the ear cups are not being held to the ears tightly enough to ensure maximal attenuation.

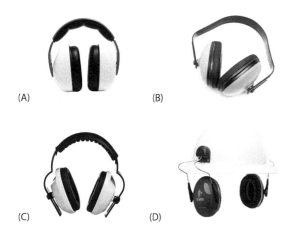

(A)　　　　　(B)

(C)　　　　　(D)

Figure 19.4 (A)–(D) Muffs.

# COMBINING EARPLUGS AND EARMUFFS

Both earplugs and earmuffs should be worn if the worker's time-weighted noise exposure exceeds 100 dBA (**Figure 19.5**). However, using double protection does not provide double attenuation. Use of earplugs and earmuffs provides an additional 5 dB of protection. The employee wearing both earmuffs with a noise reduction rating (NRR) of 25 and earplugs with the NRR of 30 would be provided with ~35 dB of total attenuation. The National Institute for Occupational Safety and Health (NIOSH) cautions that even double protection may be insufficient if time-weighted average exposures exceed 105 dBA.

## PROTECTOR PERFORMANCE CHARACTERISTICS, LIMITATIONS, AND CONCERNS

The protection afforded by a hearing protector depends on its design and on several physiological and physical characteristics of the wearer.[4] While wearing a HPD, sound energy can reach the inner ears by four different pathways: bone conduction, HPD vibration, leaks through the HPD, and leaks around the HPD (**Figure 19.5**).

At sufficiently high noise levels, noise will reach the inner ear through regular air conduction travel, as well as through bone conduction. The practical limits set by the bone and tissue conduction thresholds and the vibration of the protector vary considerably with the design of the protector and with the wearer's anatomy. For example, external ear canal and meatus anatomical characteristics that influence these limits are the shape of the ear canal opening, the length of the cartilaginous and bony portions of the canal, and the total length and diameter.[5] Approximate limits for plugs and muffs are shown in **Figure 19.6**.[6,7]

There are several important limitations and concerns that should be addressed if hearing protectors are to provide optimum noise reduction. Limitations primarily involve sound quality while a HPD is in place, limits of attenuation, and potential for impeding communication. Sound quality and potential for impeding communication will be discussed under 'Concerns', as these often have a subjective component unique to each user. Acoustical leaks through and around the protectors are central to limiting attenuation and must be minimized. A well-fit, imperforate HPD will provide a higher NRR than a porous HPD (**Figures 19.7** and **19.8**).

The following rules should be followed to minimize loss of attenuation due to acoustical leaks:

1. HPDs should be made of imperforate materials. If it is possible for air to pass freely through the material, noise will be able to pass as well.
2. The HPD should make a good seal in the ear canal or over the external ear. Reduction of a sound is dependent on preventing leakage.
3. Hearing protectors should be comfortable to wear. Uncomfortable devices are not used consistently.
4. Earmuffs should not be worn over long hair, poorly fit eyeglasses, or other obstacles.

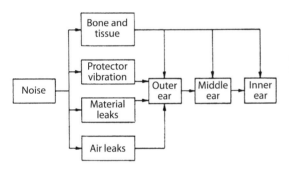

Figure 19.5 Noise pathways to the inner ear.

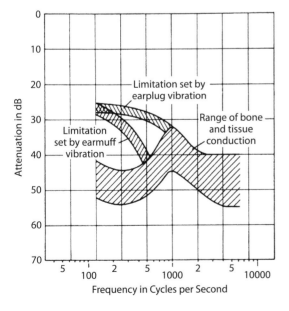

Figure 19.6 Practical protection limits for plugs and muffs.

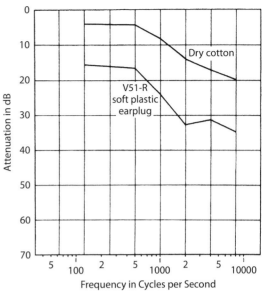

Figure 19.7 Mean attenuation characteristics of a well-fitted, imperforate earplug and an earplug made of dry cotton.

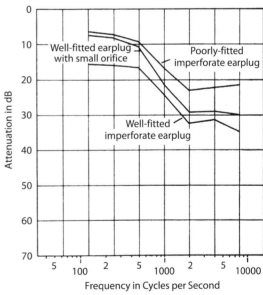

Figure 19.8 Mean attenuation characteristics of an earplug.

Hearing protector device use is not without concerns from employees and employers. Frequently cited reasons for workers to not wear their HPDs include discomfort, interference in hearing speech and warning signals, sound quality while using a HPD, and the belief that hearing loss is going to occur, regardless of HPD use. HPDs have been shown to reduce spatial perception in different ways based on the type of hearing protection. Earmuffs have a larger effect on localization while inserts have a larger effect on speech awareness.[8] Special care must be taken to ensure that the HPD is fit to the user. A comfortable device that provides appropriate attenuation (neither less nor more) has the best chance of being used.

The comfort of the HPD must be considered within the context of the wearer's external ear anatomy, manual dexterity and physical movements, and demands. Anatomical issues such as external ear canal length, shape, diameter, canal volume, and canal contour are important for the comfort of the HPD but also maintain relevance for achieving the necessary noise attenuation.[5] In 2003, the NIOSH conducted a survey evaluating physical factors and HPD comfort. Pressure exerted by HPD against the ear canal was one factor studied. Foam plug HPDs were found to exert the same pressure on any diameter of the external canal; however, premolded HPDs were found to be more favorable for larger diameter external auditory canal meatuses compared to smaller diameter ones. HPD placement was studied in a 2018 paper exploring noise attenuation levels and comfort of earplugs. Premolded earplugs in this study were found to require the least amount of repositioning and be the easiest to use. Foam plugs were found to be the most difficult to place, and training on placement was only partially effective.[5,9]

Another important aspect of HPD use and a concern that can increase resistance to HPD use is the occlusion effect. This describes an amplification of lower frequency sounds that occurs when a HPD or other insertion device is in the ear canal. Examples include a perceived difference in one's own voice or an easier time listening to his/her own body sounds such as heartbeat, breathing, or peristalsis. While this may not impede attenuation the same way an improperly fitting HPD may, it may contribute substantially to HPD comfort and thus its use.

In addition to physical comfort, a concern of equal, if not more, merit in some cases for workers is psychological discomfort resulting from impaired communication. Specifically, concerns exist regarding sound recognition/detection, sound localization, speech intelligibility, and listening effort. This is important because it can compromise situational awareness around potentially hazardous work conditions. A study by Smalt et al. in 2019 found that signal-detection performance was significantly degraded in quiet settings with passive HPDs. However, active HPDs showed variability in the degree of signal degradation based on the gain setting chosen in their internal software.[10] These results are not necessarily surprising as one of the goals of an ideal HPD is adequate noise attenuation. Sound localization has been studied more comprehensively, but results have been somewhat conflicting. Several studies have shown HPD use significantly degrades sound localization performance, namely in terms of identifying a quadrant in space where a sound is presented. On the other hand, a systematic review and meta-analysis of the effectiveness of HPDs done in 2019 showed that wearing HPDs neither improved or worsened sound localization.[11] Differences in the results of these studies are likely due to differences in study methodology as the systematic review had included studies that tested both passive and active HPDs which may have different mechanisms of attenuation.

As mentioned earlier, compromised situational awareness can augment hazardous work conditions. One way to measure this has been by measuring cognitive load, or listening effort, through visual reaction time during a dual task. Speech intelligibility and listening effort are closely related in that poorer speech intelligibility requires increased listening effort and as a result can produce cognitive fatigue.[10,11] This cognitive fatigue is manifested through added working memory demands. HPDs can increase the listening effort of the participant which subsequently can increase cognitive fatigue, especially in very noisy environments. Cognitive fatigue is also increased from degraded sound localization, but this may be alleviated with practice and training. However, the realization of how acclimation to given HPD may be difficult may be a deterrent to use. Despite these speech and communication concerns with HPD use, it is unclear what role the increased cognitive fatigue has on job performance.[10–13] Theoretical impacts are decreased productivity, increased workplace accidents and injuries, or less consistent use of HPDs.

It is important to acknowledge that a given HPD concern for one user may not be the same for another. For example, not all groups experience the same magnitude or quality or sound localization degradation or speech intelligibility issues. Workers with hearing loss often state that use of a HPD adds to existing hearing loss. This can be partially alleviated with active or level-dependent HPDs and worsened with conventional (passive) hearing protectors. Noise-induced hearing loss affects higher frequencies, between 3000 and 6000 Hz. Many consonant sounds are heard in at ~3000 Hz. A hearing loss in the high frequencies may cause speech discrimination problems. The attenuation curves provided for HPDs show that most of the attenuation is obtained in the higher frequencies. Active noise reduction HPDs can provide substantial benefits for hearing-impaired users.[14] In fact, in laboratory-setting experiments, users with moderate-to-severe hearing impairment experienced the largest benefit in speech recognition performance based on word recognition scores. Conversely, these same participants showed large decrements in speech recognition using conventional (passive) hearing protection compared to unprotected listening. It is unclear how this translates into a noisy work environment, but certain devices may add to the existing discrimination problems and the audibility of warning signals in selected cases. Individuals with hearing impairment should be given additional considerations and hearing protectors should be individualized accordingly.

Wearing hearing protectors in very noisy areas makes it easier for normal hearing employees to understand conversations, instructions, and signals. Workers wearing protectors do not need to raise their voices as much as employees with no protection in the same noisy environment. This has implications for speech intelligibility depending on the level of noise in an area or for jobs with a high mental workload such as control room operators and computer-based work in process or manufacturing industries. HPDs may reduce speech intelligibility at background noise levels between 60 and 70 dBA but improve speech intelligibility at background noise levels approximately between 80 and 90 dBA. In industrial work environments where the signal-to-noise level is usually negative, HPDs can substantially improve verbal communication while also preventing noise-induced hearing loss. However, for employees exposed to more favorable signal-to-noise ratios or medium noise levels with or without a high mental workload, the HPD with the minimum NRR while maintaining acceptable communication comfort should be worn to avoid overprotection.[15–17]

Education programs should stress that noise-induced hearing loss is avoidable. Ear protection can protect employees from future noise-induced hearing loss. Discomfort can be avoided with properly fit HPDs.

These concerns help illustrate that protector comfort is often the first aspect considered by wearers, and noise attenuation is second. This may be counterintuitive to the purpose of wearing a HPD, but the most effective HPD is the one worn consistently. The next section will discuss other types of HPDs and any concerns relevant to their use.

| F(Hz) | Correction |
|---|---|
| 25 | − 44.7 |
| 32 | − 39.4 |
| 40 | − 34.6 |
| 50 | − 30.2 |
| 63 | − 26.2 |
| 80 | − 22.5 |
| 100 | − 19.1 |
| 125 | − 16.1 |
| 160 | − 13.4 |
| 200 | − 10.9 |
| 250 | − 8.6 |
| 315 | − 6.6 |
| 400 | − 4.8 |
| 500 | − 3.2 |
| 630 | − 1.9 |
| 800 | − 0.8 |
| 1,000 | 0.0 |
| 1,250 | + 0.6 |
| 1,600 | + 1.0 |
| 2,000 | + 1.2 |
| 2,500 | + 1.3 |
| 3,150 | + 1.2 |
| 4,000 | + 1.0 |
| 5,000 | + 0.5 |
| 6,300 | − 0.1 |
| 8,000 | − 1.1 |
| 10,000 | − 2.5 |
| 12,500 | − 4.3 |
| 16,000 | − 6.6 |
| 20,000 | − 9.3 |

Figure 19.9 A-frequency weighting adjustments.[18]

## OTHER HEARING PROTECTION DEVICES

## MUSICIAN'S EARPLUGS

Musicians can sustain occupational hearing loss (see Chapter 32), although usually to a lesser extent than typical industrial workers. Whenever possible, high-risk performance environments should be altered. Alterations include distancing the musician from the sound source, using acoustic baffles, repositioning some instrumentalists, and other measures. When environmental modifications are not enough or not feasible, a HPD should be used. Musicians generally use earplugs more commonly than earmuffs. Normal earplugs tend to have a high-frequency emphasis because these frequencies are damaged first by noise. The high-frequency emphasis compromises the musician's perception of sound quality. Musicians' earplugs differ from standard foam earplugs in that musicians' earplugs are custom molded with a passive filter to attenuate with a flatter frequency response than standard ear protectors. This gives sound a truer quality. Adding an acoustic filter to earmolds enables uniform attenuation across the frequency range. A slightly different filter can be used to roll-off high-frequency information slightly. Another method of adjusting earplugs is the addition of a tuned vent. Tuned vents let low frequencies pass and high frequencies become attenuated. Musicians' earplugs may not be appropriate for hearing protection in high-level industrial noise.

The largest barrier for this population is long-term adoption of HPDs. Survey responses of musicians showed that although 71% had tried to use hearing protection in the past, only 8% consistently wore hearing protection.[19,20] The reasons given for lack of use included not feeling as if their hearing was at risk, expense, issues with comfort and sound perception, and the occlusion effect, which is a particular concern for vocalists and instrumentalists using mouth pieces. The occlusion effect is a phenomenon whereby self-generated sounds (usually speech, chewing, swallowing, breathing, etc.) are perceived as louder when the ears are covered. This can apply to musicians generating sound from their body with a hearing protector in place, as opposed to musicians generating sound from outside their body such as pianists or string players.[19–21]

Vocalists have reported distortions of timbre and dynamics, which can be a substantial disadvantage in a highly competitive professional environment. Instrumentalists in ensemble settings have cited inability to assess the sound of their own instrument, difficulty hearing others, and subsequent problems of balance and intonation. Brass players appear to have the lowest rate of HPD use, specifically trumpet players. This is thought to be due to the loudness of the trumpet.[21] The occlusion effect and sound perception issues tend to be reduced with the use of custom musicians' plugs, although they are incompletely eliminated. This appears to be the primary reason for the low rate of adoption. Another important reason for the low rate of HPD adoption among musicians is limited awareness of HPDs and their importance. Survey responses regarding this issue have shown as few as 3% of musicians have thought of using a hearing protector.[22]

However, despite these barriers to consistent HPD use among musicians, there are musicians who choose to wear HPDs. Musicians with existing hearing loss tend to have a high rate of HPD use. This is important because it suggests that increased awareness and education on the benefits of HPDs could result in improved long-term use, as musicians appear more likely to use them after some degree of noticeable hearing impairment.

Understanding the effect of hearing protection use on musical performance and musician experience is critical to achieving consistent use. Several performance factors such as dynamic range of intensities (differentiating loud and quiet sounds), pitch matching, and timbre recognition may be amenable to improvement through acclimatization. Studies have shown that performance scores in these measures improve with trial number and familiarity.[23–25] Providing time to practice with and acclimate to a new HPD may be a way to improve HPD use among musicians. Such time to practice may need to be only a few short sessions before improvement is noticed.[21] In terms of musician experience, HPDs are felt by musicians to impact coloration (muffled and dull sound) more than comfort, dynamics, or articulation, and foam earplugs are more uncomfortable than musician ear plugs.[21]

Advances in adoption of hearing protector device use among musicians is needed. Emphasis should be placed on increasing awareness regarding the risks of noise exposure especially in a musical context, providing opportunities for acclimatization to HPD use, instituting safety policies to increase adoption rates, and developing technological advances to musician earplugs. Further research should focus on performance measures of HPDs within different musical contexts (solo, group, large ensemble, various genres, and others) and between different instruments.[26]

## IN-EAR MONITORS

In-ear monitors are HPDs with high-fidelity speaker systems built inside. In-ear monitors are used instead of conventional floor monitors. The earpiece itself acts as a HPD by reducing unwanted noise enabling the user to monitor himself/herself and the instruments at lower sound intensity levels, while providing balanced amplification across frequencies of sound. This custom signal-to-noise ratio may provide some hearing protection if used responsibly but may not be sufficient for very loud music such as produced by some heavy metal bands or industrial hearing protection.

They were developed originally for musicians and performers to be able to hear themselves on stage. They have provided two benefits: the performer does not need to rely on traditional stage monitor speakers and potentially can minimize noise-induced hearing loss.

In-ear monitors can be worn as a straight-wired, over-the-ear hook, or in-ear with a memory foam tip. One common feature among all brands of in-ear monitors is that they produce a balanced sound profile. This is in contrast to many consumer-brand earbuds that emphasize lower frequency (bass) sounds. Comfort, ease of use, and lightweight materials are emphasized in the design of professional in-ear monitors to promote long durations of use.

Performers often can set the levels that they prefer while performing which can allow for more sustained use. The output levels of in-ear monitors are substantially lower than floor monitors; however, care should be taken when setting levels because they still can produce a dangerous level of sound, especially over longer exposure times.[27]

## COMMUNICATION HEADSETS

Communication headsets are used primarily for broadcast, studio, film, and television applications as well as for professional sports such as American football, baseball, and racing. The headsets allow for increased communication, while providing sound attenuation through the use of dual headsets with a microphone. The headphone transducers feature extended frequency responses. The result is clear and audible speech.

Noise cancellation principles (active noise control) are a key design feature for these HPDs. In general, for successful noise cancellation to occur, a microphone collects the targeted ambient sounds and sends them to a small amplifier. The amplifier generates sound waves that are exactly out of phase with the desired sounds. This process of destructive interference can improve the signal-to-noise ratio. In communication headsets, a noise-canceling microphone picks up ambient noise through one or two apertures: one at the user's ear and in some models, one also located in the mouthpiece microphone.[28] This arrangement allows a portion of the low-frequency noise to be canceled and preserve speech.[29,30]

These electronic communication systems may improve speech clarity when used in high-level noise environments as they are typically more effective at cancelling low-frequency background noise. The improved perceptions of the speaker's own voice allow better voice modulation. Also, some distortion that often accompanies loud speech and shouting can be avoided. The listener can adjust the electronic gain control to obtain a level of undistorted speech that will provide the best reception. An exception may be found in very high levels, above ~130 dB overall, where speech perception is not always improved by the use of earplugs under communication headsets.

In noise fields >120 dB with reference to 0.0002 µbar overall, noise may be attenuated at the microphone by noise shields encasing the sensing element. Efficient noise-attenuating shields tightly held around the mouth may be used with microphone systems to transmit intelligible communication in wide-band noise levels exceeding 140 dB. Communication headsets can be a reliable HPD for many occupations, including control room operators and industrial or factory workers who rely on clear, verbal communication for safety.

## ELECTRONIC EAR PROTECTION

Electronic hearing protection can be divided into two categories: devices to improve short-range communications in noisy environments and devices to provide entertainment during work or play. These devices are also known as noise canceling earmuffs and active earmuffs. However, the technology used in electronic ear protection devices is not synonymous with noise cancellation. Various compression and filter techniques are used to improve communication in noise. In this context, compression refers to digital technology that converts physical sound waves into digital code. This digital code can be converted into an entirely different sound depending on the programming of the digital circuit. This process compresses sounds over a certain dB sound pressure level (SPL) to eliminate dangerous noise peaks in a user's environment.[31,32] Users can adjust the frequency range that is transmitted and the filtration level of high- and low-frequency noise. FM radio earmuffs are included in the electronic hearing protection category. These hearing protectors have an FM radio receiver built into the headphones. Other devices (such as a CD player) can be connected to these headphones.

## HEARING PROTECTION, HEARING LOSS, AND HEARING AIDS

## USE OF HEARING AIDS IN NOISE

A problem frequently faced by the hearing conservationist is the employee who uses a hearing aid, works in noise, and is required to use hearing protection. Amplification also has the potential to make otherwise safe noise levels dangerous. Hearing aids are personal amplifiers that compensate for a deficit in hearing. Sounds reaching the hearing aid microphone are amplified. Use of hearing aids may make warning signals easier to hear. However, use of hearing aids in noisy industrial setting is not recommended in most situations. Moderate-intensity sounds will be amplified

by the hearing aid. This has the potential to make typically safe noise environments for normal hearing potentially dangerous for workers using hearing aids. Modern hearing aids have maximum power output (MPO) limitations and compression strategies to limit dangerous sound levels, but these controls are designed for relatively short exposure periods. Furthermore, hearing aids that are set for a conductive or mixed hearing loss can have MPOs set well above the 80-dBA range. A conductive hearing loss also can protect a worker's inner ear from damaging noise levels, but special care should be taken by the worker's otologist and audiologist to ensure safe time-weighted noise levels are maintained.[33]

Workers with hearing loss may have difficulty hearing warning signals at baseline, and a conventional passive noise-reduction HPD may exacerbate this problem, thus posing a safety hazard to themselves and others. However, active noise-reduction HPDs may provide substantial benefits for speech perception as users can adjust the gain to achieve a favorable, yet safe, signal-to-noise ratio.[14]

The hearing-impaired worker and employer should be aware of the hearing aid being used. If workers are unable to perform their job because of the severity of their hearing loss, a transfer to a less noisy area is recommended. Efforts should be made to assist the employee before a transfer occurs.

## OTHER PRECAUTIONS

Earmolds worn with the hearing aid fail to provide adequate noise attenuation. Also, hearing aids advertised as having automatic noise suppression are not adequate for use in industrial noise. The circuit cannot work fast enough to reduce intense, transient noise. It is important to be aware of this, as many modern hearing aids are advertised as being able to suppress noise above a predetermined upper limit. If in doubt, hearing aid documentation and manual should be inspected, or the manufacturer should be contacted.

## NOISE REDUCTION RATING

Code of Federal Regulations, Title 40, Section 211, states that manufacturers are required to show the NRR on the label of HPDs. The NRR is a simplified method of describing the amount of hearing protection a device provides. There are three standards for estimating the amount of attenuation provided. None of the methods specify minimum performance qualities or approve of a single type of HPD.

The most common method of characterizing sound attenuation (American National Standards Institute [ANSI] Z24.22) is the real ear attenuation at threshold (REAT) method. Described in 2005, this method finds the difference between the minimum levels of sounds that can be detected while ears are occluded and unoccluded.[34-36] The change in hearing between the two conditions is called a threshold shift. This standard was revised with ANSI S3.19 and again with ANSI S12.6. The original standard data used pure-tone stimuli in an anechoic chamber. The revisions are based on 1/3 band octave noise presented at random incidence in a nondirectional sound field. The REAT method is intended primarily for continuous usage conditions to provide estimates of performance in the given field.[37,38] A problem with the NRR system is to ensure that the descriptor value does not sacrifice the estimated attenuation for simplicity. These methods often underestimate laboratory-derived methods for sound attenuation. The methods tend to give high weighting to the low-frequency noise, whereas high-frequency performance is not given the same consideration. Other methods have been developed to get around the shortcomings of the NRR.

Another problem with the NRR system is that the values obtained are derived from controlled conditions in a laboratory setting. According to research, 98% of workers are predicted to achieve the protection level set by the NRR; however, in practice fewer than 5% may actually reach this.[39,40] One proposed metric to help resolve these differences is the personal attenuation rating (PAR) measured in dBA. This is defined as the SPL incident upon the ear due to the application of a hearing protector. The PAR is a measure of the attenuation achieved by an HPD fit at the level of the individual. A device called the field attenuation estimation system (FAES) is critical to performing ecologically valid experiments that are comparable to experiments used to determine the NRR. The PAR is used currently in many countries as an adjunct to the NRR.[41-42]

The intention of the NRR was to calculate the exposure under the hearing protector by subtracting the NRR from the C-weighted unprotected noise level. However, noise levels are measured using the A-weighted scale. An additional 7 dB should be subtracted from the labeled NRR when working with the A-weighted noise levels to estimate the A-weighted noise level under the protector.

## AMOUNT OF PROTECTION PROVIDED IN PRACTICE

A comparison of the noise analysis of a particular noise exposure and the levels specified by the chosen hearing conservation criterion should be used to determine the amount of bands noise reduction required. The hearing conservation criteria are often expressed in octave bands. The amount of noise reduction required can be determined by subtracting the SPLs specified by the criteria from the exposure levels measured in corresponding octave bands. Hearing protection should provide attenuation within each of these bands to meet the noise reduction requirements. Mandatory methods for estimating the adequacy of hearing protector attenuation are specified in Appendix B of the OSHA Hearing Conservation Amendment (see Chapter 37).

Hearing conservation criteria based on the A-frequency weighting may be used following the NIOSH method described subsequently:

*Step 1*: Take sound level measurements in octave bands at the point of exposure.
*Step 2*: Subtract from the octave-band levels (in decibels) obtained in Step 1 the center frequency adjustment values for the A-frequency weighting shown in **Figure 19.9**.
*Step 3*: Subtract the A-weighted octave bands calculated in Step 2 from the attenuation values provided by the protector for each corresponding octave band to obtain the A-weighted octave-band levels reaching the ear while wearing the hearing protector.
*Step 4*: Calculate the equivalent A-weighted noise level reaching the ear while wearing the hearing protector by adding the octave-band levels as shown in **Figure 19.10**. An alternative method for adding decibels is as follows:

| Sum ($L_R$) of dB Levels $L_1$ and $L_2$ | | |
|---|---|---|
| Numerical Difference Between Levels $L_1$ or $L_2$ | $L_3$: Amount to be Added to the Higher of $L_1$ or $L_2$ | |
| 0.0 to 0.1 | 3.0 | Step 1: Determine the difference between the two levels to be added ($L_1$ and $L_2$). |
| 0.2 to 0.3 | 2.9 | |
| 0.4 to 0.5 | 2.8 | |
| 0.6 to 0.7 | 2.7 | |
| 0.8 to 0.9 | 2.6 | |
| 1.0 to 1.2 | 2.5 | Step 2: Find the number ($L_3$) corresponding to this difference in the table. |
| 1.3 to 1.4 | 2.4 | |
| 1.5 to 1.6 | 2.3 | |
| 1.7 to 1.9 | 2.2 | |
| 2.0 to 2.1 | 2.1 | |
| 2.2 to 2.4 | 2.0 | Step 3: Add the number ($L_3$) to the highest of $L_1$ and $L_2$ to obtain the resultant level ($L_R = L_1 + L_2$). |
| 2.5 to 2.7 | 1.9 | |
| 2.8 to 3.0 | 1.8 | |
| 3.1 to 3.3 | 1.7 | |
| 3.4 to 3.6 | 1.6 | |
| 3.7 to 4.0 | 1.5 | |
| 4.1 to 4.3 | 1.4 | |
| 4.4 to 4.7 | 1.3 | |
| 4.8 to 5.1 | 1.2 | |
| 5.2 to 5.6 | 1.1 | |
| 5.7 to 6.1 | 1.0 | |
| 6.2 to 6.6 | 0.9 | |
| 6.7 to 7.2 | 0.8 | |
| 7.3 to 7.9 | 0.7 | |
| 8.0 to 8.6 | 0.6 | |
| 8.7 to 9.6 | 0.5 | |
| 9.7 to 10.7 | 0.4 | |
| 10.8 to 12.2 | 0.3 | |
| 12.3 to 14.5 | 0.2 | |
| 14.6 to 19.3 | 0.1 | |
| 19.4 to ∞ | 0.0 | |

Figure 19.10 Table for combining decibel levels of noise with random frequency characteristics.

Equivalent dBA =

$$10\log_{10}\left( \text{antilog}_{10}\frac{L_{125}}{10} + \text{antilog}\,\frac{L_{250}}{10} + \cdots + \text{antilog}\,\frac{L_{8000}}{10}\right)$$

where $L_{125}$ is the SPL of the A-weighted octave band centered at 125 Hz, $L_{250}$ is the A-weighted octave-band level at 250 Hz, etc.

*Example*: The first and second columns in **Figure 19.11** contain octave band SPL data measured in a textile mill weaving room. The third column shows the same octave-band data, but with an A-frequency weighting (using **Figure 19.9**). The mean and mean − 1 standard deviation (SD) attenuation values for a good earmuff HPD (**Figure 19.11**) are listed under 1 and 2 of the fourth column heading. By definition, 50% of the persons

wearing this hearing protector can be expected to have less than the mean attenuation values, and ~14% can be expected to have less than the mean − 1 SD. Octave-band levels reaching the ear canal while wearing the HPD are listed for mean and mean − 1 SD attenuation values under the last column heading. The octave-band exposure levels listed in each of the last two columns may be added (using **Figure 19.10**) to determine the decibel exposure levels while wearing hearing protectors. In this example, the exposure level for those receiving the mean attenuation values from the protector would be 66 dBA, and for those receiving mean − 1 SD values, the exposure level would be 71 dBA. Either exposure level while wearing hearing protectors is obviously well < 90 dBA.

| Octave Band Center Frequency in Hz | Weaving Room Spectra in dB | | Weaving Room Spectrum with A-Weighting in dB | Muff-Type Protector Attenuation in dB | | Resultant Exposure to Inner Ear in dB | |
|---|---|---|---|---|---|---|---|
| | | | | (1) | (2) | (1) | (2) |
| 125 . . . . . . . . . . 90 | (less 16 =) | 74 | 16 | 9 | 58 | 65 |
| 250 . . . . . . . . . . 92 | (less 9 =) | 83 | 21 | 15 | 62 | 68 |
| 500 . . . . . . . . . . 94 | (less 3 =) | 91 | 31 | 23 | 60 | 68 |
| 1,000 . . . . . . . . . . 95 | (less 0 =) | 95 | 42 | 30 | 53 | 65 |
| 2,000 . . . . . . . . . . 97 | (plus 1 =) | 98 | 43 | 32 | 55 | 66 |
| 4,000 . . . . . . . . . . 95 | (plus 1 =) | 96 | 45 | 35 | 51 | 61 |
| 8,000 . . . . . . . . . . 91 | (less 1 =) | 90 | 34 | 22 | 56 | 68 |
| Overall . . . . . . . . . . 103 dB | | 102 dB(A) | | | 66 | 75 dB(A) |

Figure 19.11 Protection provided by ear protectors worn in a weaving room noise environment.

Two factors must be considered when selecting hearing protectors to meet the noise reduction requirements. First, the HPD attenuation values determined in the laboratory are not always an accurate representation of the noise reduction capability of the protector. Second, the protection provided by hearing protectors varies considerably among wearers and among the ways the protectors are worn. There are also significant differences in performance among some protectors of the same model. Standard deviations of 3–7 dB are commonly found in subjective measurements of protector attenuation at any test frequency. Therefore, attenuation values may have a range of ± 14 dB for 95% confidence limits. The variability in the amounts of protection provided must be considered along with the mean attenuation values when selecting a hearing protector for a particular application.

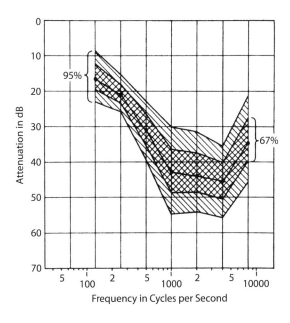

Figure 19.12 Mean attenuation characteristics of a good muff-type protector plotted with one and two standard deviation shaded areas (67% and 95% confidence levels). Attenuation values determined according to the ANSI specifications using pure-tone threshold shift technique. *Abbreviation*: ANSI, American National Standards Institute.

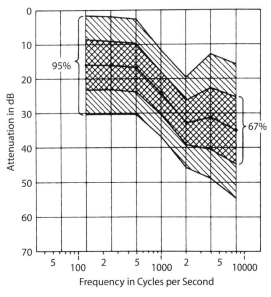

Figure 19.13 Mean attenuation characteristics plotted with one and two standard deviation shaded areas for a well-fitted imperforate earplug. Attenuation values determined according to the ANSI specifications using pure-tone threshold shift technique. *Abbreviation*: ANSI, American National Standards Institute.

Confidence limits of 100% of employees protected all the time are desirable. However, the spread of attenuation values is so great that very high-level confidence limits are not plausible. A practical choice is the mean attenuation – 1 SD, which would provide confidence limits ~86% level. This confidence limit would be very similar to the limits set by most of the present rules and regulations concerning noise exposure levels, which also have been limited by practical considerations.

In common practice, a much more simple method is used and provides fairly comparable results. To estimate the effective noise reduction, subtract 7 dB from the supplied NRR and divide that number by 2. For example, if an ear protector is reported to have a NRR of 27 dB, subtract 7 dB, then divide that value by 2, leaving 10 dB. So, the expected attenuation in the field would be 10 dB. If the environment exposed the person to noise levels of 95–99 dB, this would be an appropriate ear protector.

Additional methods of determining NRRs are presented in Appendix B of the OSHA Noise Amendment. An update to OSHA's Field Operations Manual on January 27, 1984, described administrative guidelines that only required protective measures in most situations. Citations will only be issued if engineering controls are feasible and either the "employee exposure levels are so high that the hearing protectors alone may not reliably reduce noise levels" or "the costs of controls are less than the cost of an effective hearing conservation program."

The point at which hearing protectors can reliably reduce a noise level is 100 dBA. Above this level, hearing protector NRR must be derated by 50% and must reduce exposures below 90 dB.

When calculating hearing protection effectiveness for comparison to engineering controls (50% derating), the 7-dB adjustment must be used along with the 50% derating. Therefore, to be effective for levels of 106 dBA, the NRR published by the manufacturers must be at least 39 dB, that is, (39 − 7)/2 = 16 dB. This will result in an exposure level of 90 dBA (106 − 16 = 90).

It is possible for a particular hearing protector with a published NRR to have four different NRRs used by OSHA. A protector with an NRR of 30, as noted under OSHA Appendix 2, maintains the 30 NRR of noise if measured on the C scale (dBC) and only 23 if measured on the A scale (dBA). For comparison to engineering controls, the NRR is 15 dBC and 11.5 dBA.

Because the effective protection provided by a given set of hearing protectors can only be approximated in most field applications, a hearing monitoring program is essential for all persons wearing hearing protectors. Fortunately, a very large majority of noise exposures are at relatively low levels, and the proper use of good HPDs can provide adequate attenuation for a large majority of persons exposed to these noises (**Figures 19.12** and **19.13**).

In summary, the use of a good ear protector can provide sufficient attenuation in the majority of work environments where engineering controls cannot be used successfully. For the few workers exposed to noise levels in excess of 115 dBA over long periods of time, special care should be taken to ensure that the best HPDs are used properly, and hearing thresholds are monitored regularly. For higher exposure levels over extended time periods, it may be necessary to use a combination of ear inserts and earmuffs and/or to limit the time of exposure (**Figure 19.14**). Hearing protectors will provide adequate protection for only a small percentage of wearers when worn in levels >125 dBA for 8 hours/day.

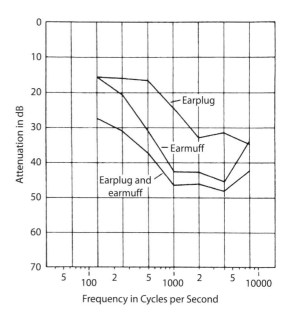

Figure 19.14 Mean attenuation characteristics of a muff and an earplug worn separately and together.

## NOISE REDUCTION AND COMMUNICATION

Workers should be able to communicate with each other and to hear warning signals in many different high-noise environments while wearing HPDs. The effect of noise on communication depends on the spectrum of the noise. Communication difficulties tend to occur when the noise has high-level components in the speech frequency range, 400–3000 Hz. A review of speech interference studies shows that conversational speech begins to be difficult when the speaker and listener are separated by ~2 ft in noise levels of 85 dBA.[43,44] Many noisy areas exist in work environments, and the additional attenuation of hearing protection often makes communication difficult. However, some studies indicate that the use of HPDs in noisy environment may improve speech perception.[10,11]

## COMMUNICATION WHILE WEARING PROTECTORS

Wearing HPDs obviously interferes with speech communication in quiet environments. Wearing a conventional set of earplugs or earmuffs in noise levels >90 dB in octave bands (or 97 dBA for at spectra) may improve speech intelligibility for normal hearing ears.[44,45] The improvement in speech perception occurs because speech-to-noise ratios are kept nearly constant. Additionally, the protected ear does not distort from overdrive caused by the high speech and noise levels. The efficiency in abnormal ears has not been demonstrated as conclusively.

The concept of an occluded ear hearing better in noise is difficult for the worker to accept. To gain acceptance, the HPD should be tried in a quiet environment. Workers tend to be attracted to hearing protectors advertised as providing a *filter*, allowing the low frequencies in the speech range to pass but blocks the noise. Some of these filter-type devices do provide better communication scores in quiet environments, and they may be a good choice for use in areas where there are intermittent exposures to moderately high noises. However, in steady-state noise levels greater than ~90 dB in octave bands, the conventional ear inserts or earmuffs provide communication scores that are at least as good as filter type (**Figures 19.15** and **19.16**) and provide better overall protection.[45,46]

## CHECKING HEARING PROTECTION ATTENUATION

When an employee is fitted with hearing protection, how can the technician determine that the HPD is reducing noise and to what degree? Frequent audiometric testing can show whether any change in hearing thresholds have occurred and if they can be attributed to noise exposure. Some companies conduct a hearing test after plugs have been fitted and compare these test results against those obtained without the earplugs in place. This *fit-test* gives the technician an idea of the attenuation provided by the HPD.

There are many ways to conduct a fit-test, from simple to complicated. A preliminary method of determining whether the HPD is working properly is to perform a Rinne tuning-fork test. Workers should notice a temporary conductive hearing loss while wearing their HPDs. With the HPD in place, a vibrating fork is placed on the mastoid and then moved to the entrance of the ear canal. If the protector is properly sized and fitted, the subject will indicate that the sound was louder at the mastoid than at the ear canal. An additional method to check adequate fit as well as the noise level around a worker is the NIOSH Sound Level Meter App.[3]

A more complicated and also more objective technique involves the PAR. This is the person-specific noise attenuation rating obtained while wearing a given hearing protector. The PAR can be determined by a number of ways; however, perhaps the most objective method is from the field microphones in workers' real ears (F-MIRE) method. The F-MIRE setup includes a single, dual-element microphone attached to thin flexible tubing. One tubing and microphone runs through or around an earplug and measures SPLs in the ear canal, while the other measures a wearer's external sound field. A sound is played for a duration of 10 seconds and measured by both microphones simultaneously. This produces an exact number, and it produces much less variability than a NRR calculated from a laboratory setting. One source of variability stems from problems with the tubing. For example, the tubing can leak sound around or through its walls if not properly positioned or sealed.[47–49]

NIOSH has developed a commercially available fit-test called the HPD Well-Fit™. The HPD Well-Fit™ has solved limitations of previous fit-testing programs that rendered them impractical

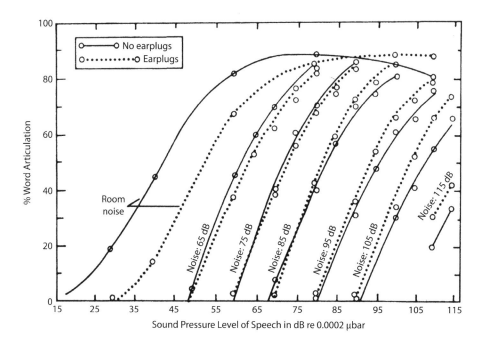

**Figure 19.15** The relationship between articulation and speech level with noise level as the parameter.

for use in the workplace. These limitations had included expensive and bulky equipment mixed with long testing times. Now, a reliable fit-test such as the HPD Well-Fit™ only takes as long as 4–7 minutes to complete as opposed to tests that lasted 30 minutes or more. The test produces a PAR for each employee, and the speed of the test facilitates re-training, re-fitting, and re-testing in a reasonable amount of time.[50,51]

## CHARACTERISTICS OF SUCCESSFUL EAR PROTECTOR USERS

There is a significant difference in the age, level of education, and years of noise exposure between workers identified as successful hearing protector users and those identified as unsuccessful users,

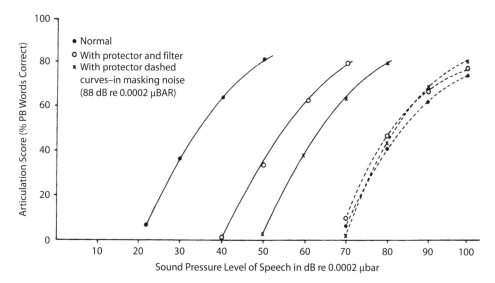

**Figure 19.16** Average articulation curves with and without protector in quiet and with thermal masking noise.[45]

according to Lt. Col. Kenneth Aspinall, Brooke Army Medical Center, Fort Sam Houston, TX.

Aspinall discussed the results of a questionnaire he administered to workers to determine which personality traits and attitudes are associated with the successful use of hearing protectors. Successful users were well informed about the dangers of noise exposure and the use of hearing protectors, concerned about their overall health, and have a higher incidence of hearing loss. They tended to be motivated to wear HPDs, without reminder from supervisors. These workers perceived their supervisors as being highly interested in their compliance with the hearing protection plan.

Aspinall said the old adage *the older you are, the wiser you get* seems to apply to the use of hearing protectors. The average age of the 200 workers he identified as successful hearing protection users was 39 years, with an average education level of 12.7 years, and average noise exposure of 14.1 years. This is consistent with a more recent study that has examined attitudes toward noise among young people. These studies have shown that there tend to be fewer concerns regarding noise and its negative effects and that there are more barriers to protective action.[52]

The study found that successful users wore their HPDs during unannounced inspections, were rated successful users by their supervisors, and rated themselves as successful users. Unsuccessful HPD users were not observed wearing hearing protectors, were rated poorly by their supervisors, and rated themselves as unsuccessful users.

Some employees express concern over the possibility of the use of hearing protection causing ear infections. Regular wearing of HPDs does not normally increase the likelihood of contracting ear infections. Some users may develop irritation from earplug use. Nondisposable earplugs should be washed before reuse. Earmuff cushions should be wiped periodically.

## DOCUMENTS

The OSHA Noise Standard, 29 CFR 1910.95 and Regulation 7 of the Environmental Regulations for Workplace (1993) standard states that employees exposed to 8 hours of ≥85 dB should be provided with HPDs from their employers at no charge.

To encourage the employees to wear the hearing protectors, employers should provide a variety of hearing protection options as there are several personal factors that influence consistent use (as discussed above). The employers need to ensure that the HPDs are worn properly. Educating employees of how to use and care for their HPD is recommended.

## EMPLOYEE EDUCATION

The Amendment to the Noise Standard is very specific concerning the need for employee education and the steps necessary to secure that education. Employers are required to institute training programs for employees exposed to noise levels at ≥85 dB for an 8-hour time-weighted average. Training must be completed individually or in groups annually. The hearing conservation program should be updated to educate about current HPDs and work processes. Each training session should address the effects of noise on hearing. Education programs should discuss the purpose of HPDs, their advantages and disadvantages, attenuation of different types of devices, and instructions on fitting, care, and use of HPDs. Additionally, the purpose and importance of audiometric monitoring should be explained.

If audiometric testing indicates the presence of a standard threshold shift (STS), the Amendment delineates follow-up procedures. Employees should be notified in writing within 21 days of the presence of STS. Employers must ensure HPD use, re-fit and re-instruct regarding HPD use, refer for an audiological and otological examination, and informed of medical evaluation results in the event of a threshold shift.

If further audiometric testing on employees exposed to noise levels <8-hour time-weighted average of 90 dBA indicates that STS is not persistent, the employee should be informed. The employee may also discontinue required use of HPDs.

Employee education is also important from the perspective of improved compliance with HPDs and achieving acclimatization with a novel HPD. Sound localization performance can be affected negatively by HPD use and is often most pronounced in the early stages of use. A study in 2015 demonstrated that with proper training, improvements in sound localization accuracy can be achieved.[10,53] Although training may be a mild deterrent to use of a HPD, the advantages of use likely outweigh the disadvantages.

## NEW EMPHASIS ON ENGINEERING CONTROLS

Revised in 2002, OSHA put forth a hearing conservation program that emphasized engineering and administrative controls for reducing occupational noise exposure over PPE. HPDs are the mainstay of this PPE category. Engineering controls were deemed to be the most effective at reducing workplace noise. New technologies, innovations, and applications are being developed each year. Each development can be classified as either a type of source treatment, pathway treatment, or receiver treatment.[54-56] Before implementation, they generally are put through the following feasibility tests:

1. Hearing protectors alone cannot reliably reduce the noise levels, especially when noise levels exceed 100 dBA.
2. Engineering and administrative controls would cost less than that required to run the hearing conservation program.
3. Engineering and administrative controls do not necessarily have to reduce noise to or below the exposure limit. Controls and hearing device protection use are required to reduce the levels.

Engineering controls may not be required if the employer can show that the ongoing hearing conservation program is protecting employees. Also, if the hearing conservation program is less costly than engineering controls, then those controls may not be required. If it would cost less to bring a plant in compliance with a hearing conservation program or if that program can be improved, engineering controls may not be required. However, if improvements to the program cannot be made and engineering controls are not available, the employer may be cited. The employer can be certain of a citation for a serious violation if hearing protection is required, but not used.

## REFERENCES

1. Hearing Protectors. National Institute on Deafness and Other Communication Disorders. 2020. NIH Pub. No. 20-DC-8122. Accessed July 18, 2023. https://www.nidcd.nih.gov/health/hearing-protectors.
2. Provide Hearing Protection. Centers for Disease Control and Prevention. 2013. Accessed July 18, 2023. https://www.cdc.gov/niosh/noise/prevent/ppe.html#:~:text=Know%20how%20much%20hearing%20protection,reduce%20noise%20by%2010%20dB.
3. Noise and Hearing Loss. National Institute for Occupational Safety and Health. 2023. Accessed August 19, 2023. https://www.cdc.gov/niosh/noise/about/noise.html#:~:text=Loud%20noise%20at%20work%20can,over%20an%20eight%2Dhour%20workday.
4. von Gierke HE, Warren DR. Protection of the Ear from Noise: Limiting Factors, Benox Report, University of Chicago, pp. 47–60 (Dec. 1, 1953).
5. Samelli AG, Gomes RF, Chammas TV, Silva BG, Moreira RR, Fiorini AC. The study of attenuation levels and the comfort of earplugs. Noise Health 2018; 20(94):112–119.
6. Nixon CW, von Gierke HE. Experiments on the bone-conduction threshold in a free sound field. J Acoust Soc Am 1959; 31:1121–1125.
7. Unpublished work by Paul L. Michael at The Pennsylvania State University.
8. Snapp HA, Millet B, Schaefer-Solle N, Rajguru SM, Ausili SA. The effects of hearing protection devices on spatial awareness in complex listening environments. PLOS ONE. 2023 Jan 12; 18(1):e0280240.
9. Toivonen M, Pääkkönen R, Savolainen S, Lehtomäki K. Noise attenuation and proper insertion of earplugs into ear canals. Ann Occup Hyg 2002; 46(6):527–530.

10. Smalt CJ, Calamia PT, Dumas AP, et al. The effect of hearing-protection devices on auditory situational awareness and listening effort. Ear Hear 2020; 41(1):82–94.

11. Kwak C, Han W. The effectiveness of hearing protection devices: a systematic review and meta-analysis. Int J Environ Res Public Health 2021 Nov 7; 18(21):11693.

12. Byrne DC, Palmer CV. Comparison of speech intelligibility measures for an electronic amplifying earmuff and an identical passive attenuation device. Audiol Res 2012; 2(1):e5.

13. Tufts JB, Frank T. Speech production in noise with and without hearing protection. J Acoust Soc Am 2003; 114(2):1069–1080.

14. Giguère C, Laroche C, Vaillancourt V. The interaction of hearing loss and level-dependent hearing protection on speech recognition in noise. Int J Audiol 2015; 54 Suppl 1:S9–S18.

15. Karami M, Aliabadi M, Golmohammadi R, Hamidi Nahrani M. The effect of hearing protection devices on speech intelligibility of Persian employees. BMC Res Notes 2020; 13(1):529. Published 2020 Nov 11.

16. Ljung R, Israelsson K, Hygge S. Speech intelligibility and recall of spoken material heard at different signal-to-noise ratios and the role played by working memory capacity. Appl. Cognit. Psychol 2013; 27:198–203.

17. Fernandes JC. Effects of hearing protector devices on speech intelligibility. Appl Acoust 2003; 64(6):581–590.

18. American National Standard Specification for Sound Level Meters, S1.4-1971, American National Standards Institute, New York, 1971.

19. Crawford K, Willenbring K, Nothwehr F, Fleckenstein S, Anthony TR. Evaluation of hearing protection device effectiveness for musicians. Int J Audiol 2023 Mar; 62(3):238–244.

20. Federman J, Ricketts T. Preferred and minimum acceptable listening levels for musicians while using floor and in-ear monitors. J Speech Lang Hear Res 2008 Feb; 51(1):147–159.

21. Boissinot E, Bogdanovitch S, Bocksteal A, Guastavino C. Effect of hearing protection use on pianists' performance and experience: comparing foam and musician earplugs. Front Psychol 2008; 13:886861.

22. Pouryaghoub, G, Mehrdad R, Pourhosein S. Noise-induced hearing loss among professional musicians. J Occup Health 2017; 59:33–37.

23. Kozowksi E, Zera J, Mlynski R. Effect of musician's earplugs on sound level and spectrum during musical performances. Int J Occup Saf Ergon 2011; 17:249–254.

24. Rawool V, Buñag R. Levels of music played by Caucasian and Filipino musicians with and without conventional and musicians' earplugs. J Am Acad Audiol 2019; 30:78–88.

25. Killion MC. Factors influencing use of hearing protection by trumpet players. Trends Amplif 2012; 16(3):173–178.

26. Bockstael A, De Bruyne L, Vinck B, Bottledooren D. Hearing protection in industry: companies' policy and workers' perception. Int J Ind Ergon 2013; 43:512–517.

27. Thomas C. What are in-ear monitors? All you need to know about this special category of earphones. Soundguys. May 5, 2023. Accessed August 18, 2023. https://www.soundguys.com/what-are-in-ear-monitors-90955/.

28. Bose. Bose Noise Cancelling Headphones 700. 2021. 14–59. Accessed August 19, 2023. https://www.bose.com/p/bose-noise-cancelling-headphones-700/NC700-HEADPHONEARN.html

29. Soper T. Behind-the-scenes with NFL sideline technology: Microsoft and Bose power team communication. Geekwire. October 6, 2017. Accessed August 18, 2023. https://www.geekwire.com/2017/behind-scenes-nfl-sideline-technology-microsoft-bose-power-team-communication/.

30. Seol HY, Kim SH, Kim GY, Jo M, Cho YS, Hong SH, Moon IJ. Influence of the noise-canceling technology on how we hear sounds. Healthcare 2022 Aug 2; 10(8):1449.

31. NRA Shooting Illustrated Staff. The science behind electronic hearing protection. NRA. February 7, 2021. Accessed August 18, 2023. https://www.shootingillustrated.com/content/the-science-behind-electronic-hearing-protection/.

32. Talcott KA, Casali JG, Keady JP, Killion MC. Azimuthal auditory localization of gunshots in a realistic field environment: effects of open-ear versus hearing protection-enhancement devices (HPEDs), military vehicle noise, and hearing impairment. Int J Audiol 2012; 51(Suppl 1):S20–S30.

33. Dolan TG, Maurer JF. Noise exposure associated with hearing aid use in industry. J Speech Hear Res 1996 Apr; 39(2):251–260.

34. Berger EH. Methods of measuring the attenuation of hearing protection devices. J Acoust Soc Am. 1986; 79(6):1655–1687.

35. Berger EH, Royster LH, Driscoll DP. The noise manual. American Industrial Hygiene Association: Falls Church, Virginia, Fifth Edition; 2003.

36. ISO 4869-1, Acoustics; Hearing Protectors, Part 1: Subjective Method for the Measurement of Sound Attenuation. International Organization for Standardization: Geneva, Switzerland; 1990.

37. Gauger D, Berger EH. A new hearing protector rating: the noise reduction statistic for use with a weighting (NRSA); a report prepared at the request of the U.S. EPA, reviewed and approved by ANSI S12/WG11, EAR0404/HP; U.S. EPA: Indianapolis, IN, USA, 2004.

38. Berger EH, Franks JR, Behar A, et al. Development of a new standard laboratory protocol for estimating the field attenuation of hearing protection devices. Part III. The validity of using subject-fit data. J Acoust Soc Am 1998; 103(2):665–672.

39. Murphy, WJ, Themann CL, Murata TK. Field-Testing NIOSH HPD Well-Fit: Off-Shore Oil Rig Inspectors in Louisiana and Texas; EPHB Report 360-11, DHHS-CDC-NIOSH; U.S. National Institute for Occupational Safety and Health (NIOSH): Washington, DC, USA, 2015.

40. Copelli F, Behar A, Ngoc Le T, Russo FA. Field Attenuation of Foam Earplugs. Saf Health Work 2021; 12(2):184–191.

41. Behar A, Wong W. Fit testing of hearing protectors. Can Acoust 2010;38(3):90–91

42. Canadian Standards Association Z94.2-14 Hearing protection devices - Performance, selection, care, and use. CSA. 2014.

43. Webster JC. Updating and interpreting the speech interference level (SIL). J Audio Eng Soc 1970; 18:114–188.

44. Pollack I, Pickett JM. Making of speech by noise at high sound levels. J Acoust Soc Am 1958; 30:127–130.

45. Kryter KD. Effects of hearing protective devices on the intelligibility of speech in noise. J Acoust Soc Am 1946; 18:413–417.

46. Michael PL. Hearing protectors—Their usefulness and limitations. Arch Environ Health 1965; 10:612–618.

47. Hager LD, Voix J. Individual field fit testing of hearing protectors – a Field-MIRE approach. In: Conference of the American Society of Safety Engineers (ASSE), Seattle. 2006.

48. Chiu C-C, Wan T-J. Individual fit testing of hearing-protection devices based on microphones in real ears among workers in industries with high-noise-level manufacturing. Int J Environ Res Public Health 2020; 17(9):3242.

49. Berger EH, Voix J, Hager LD. Methods of fit testing hearing protectors, with representative field test data. Hearing Loss: 9th International Congress on Noise as a Public Health Problem. 2008, Foxwoods, CT.

50. Murphy WJ, Stephenson MR, Byrne DC, Themann CL. NIOSH HPD Well-Fit™. Centers for Disease Control and Prevention: National Institute for Occupational Safety and Health. 2013. Accessed August 24, 2023. https://blogs.cdc.gov/niosh-science-blog/2013/05/31/well-fit/

51. Murphy WJ, Stephenson MR, Byrne DC, Witt B, Duran J. Effects of training on hearing protector attenuation. Noise Health 2011; 51(13):132–141.

52. Degeest S, Corthals P, Keppler H. Evolution of hearing in young adults: Effects of leisure noise exposure, attitudes, and beliefs

toward noise, hearing loss, and hearing protection devices. Noise Health 2022 Apr–Jun; 24(113):61–74.

53. Casali, JG, Robinette, MB. Effects of user training with electronically-modulated sound transmission hearing protectors and the open ear on horizontal localization ability. Int J Audiol 2015; 54(Suppl 1):S37–S45.

54. U.S. Department of Labor, Occupational Safety and Health Administration. OSHA Technical Manual (OTM) Section III: Chapter 5: Noise. July 6, 2022. Accessed August 19, 2023, https://www.osha.gov/otm/section-3-health-hazards/chapter-5#appendixf.

55. Bauer ER, Spencer ER, Smith AK, Hudak RL. Reducing noise-induced hearing loss in longwall coal mine workers: NIOSH's approach. National Institute for Occupational Safety and Health: Atlanta, Georgia; 2007.

56. Hearing Conservation. Occupational Safety and Health Administration. 2002 (revised). OSHA 3074. Accessed August 19, 2023. chrome-extension://efaidnbm nnnibpcajpcglclefindmkaj/https://www.osha.gov/sites/default/files/publications/osha3074.pdf

# 20

# Tinnitus

ROBERT THAYER SATALOFF AND CAMRYN MARSHALL

Tinnitus, or noise in the ear, is one of the most challenging problems in otology and medicine. It has been speculated that tinnitus may be the result of a continuous stream of otoacoustic discharges along the auditory nerve to the brain caused by abnormal irritation in the sensorineural pathway. Although no sound is reaching the ear, the spontaneous nerve discharge may cause the patient to experience a false sensation of sound. Although this theory sounds logical, there is as yet no scientific proof of its validity.

Tinnitus is a term used to describe perceived sounds that originate within the person rather than in the outside world. Although nearly everyone experiences mild tinnitus momentarily and intermittently, continuous tinnitus is abnormal, but not unusual. The National Center for Health Statistics reported that ~32% of all adults in the United States report having had tinnitus at some time.[1] Approximately 6.4% of people with tinnitus describe it as debilitating or severe. The prevalence of tinnitus increases with age up until ~70 years and declines thereafter.[2] This symptom is more common in people with otologic problems, although tinnitus also can occur in patients with normal hearing. Nodar reported that ~13% of school children with normal audiograms reported having tinnitus at least occasionally.[3] Sataloff et al. studied 267 normal elderly patients with no history of noise exposure or otologic disease and found 24% with tinnitus.[4] As expected, the incidence is higher among patients who consult an otologist for any reason. Fower questioned 2000 consecutive patients, 85% of whom reported tinnitus.[5] Heller and Bergman and Graham found that 75% of patients complaining of hearing loss reported tinnitus.[6,7] According to Glassgold and Altmann, ~80% of patients with otosclerosis have tinnitus, and House and Brackmann reported that 83% of 500 consecutive patients with acoustic neuromas had tinnitus.[8,9]

DOI: 10.1201/b23379-20

One of the surprising features of tinnitus is that not everybody has it. After all, the cochlea is exquisitely sensitive to sounds, and relatively loud sounds are being produced inside each human head such as the rushing of blood through the cranial arteries and the noises made by muscles in the head during chewing. The reason an individual rarely hears these body noises may be explained partially by the way that the temporal bone is situated in the skull and by the depth at which the cochlea is embedded in the temporal bone. The architecture and the acoustics of the head ordinarily prevent the transmission of these noises through the bones of the skull to the cochlea and thus to consciousness, even though the cochlea is built and situated in a way so that it can respond to very weak sounds normally transmitted by the air from outside the head. Only when there are certain changes in the vascular walls, perhaps caused by atherosclerosis, or in the temporal bone structure, does the ear pick up these internal noises. The patient may hear his/her own pulse because of a vascular disorder, and it may seem to be louder when the room is quiet or at night when trying to go to sleep. Pressing on various blood vessels in the neck occasionally stops this type of tinnitus.

Although it is usually just troublesome, tinnitus also may serve as an early sign of auditory injury. For example, high-pitched ringing or hissing may be the first indication of impending cochlear damage from ototoxic drugs, a clear signal that a drug should be stopped, or its dosage reduced whenever possible. Generally, the tinnitus disappears, and no measurable hearing loss results, though in some instances the noises may persist for months or even years.

Among the common drugs capable of producing tinnitus are aspirin and quinine in large doses, and especially diuretics, aminoglycoside antibiotics, and chemotherapy drugs. These drugs should be used with extreme caution, especially when kidney function is deficient as this can lead to decreased drug excretion and, therefore, elevated levels of the drug in the body, exacerbating the tinnitus.

Among the common misconceptions about tinnitus is that it is idiopathic and incurable. Neither of these assumptions is always correct. Awareness of conditions that cause tinnitus, however, has not been as helpful to tinnitus research as might be expected. Recognizing a causal relationship has not shed much light on the actual mechanisms by which internal sounds are created.

Tinnitus is a difficult problem for the physician and patient in all cases. Tinnitus may be either subjective (audible only to the patient) or objective (audible to the examiner, as well). Objective tinnitus is comparatively easy to detect and localize because it can be heard by the examiner using a stethoscope or other listening device. It may be caused by glomus tumors, arteriovenous malformations, palatal myoclonus, and other conditions. Subjective tinnitus is much more common; unfortunately, it cannot be confirmed with current methods of tinnitus detection.

While the etiology of tinnitus is often unknown, neuroscientists and otolaryngologists have begun to elucidate a possible mechanism for subjective tinnitus. It is thought to be an aberrancy in the central auditory circuits. In the case of hearing loss, the input (sound detection) is lower than what the central circuit expects, and therefore, there is a release of inhibition. In animal models, lower-than-expected input results in increased neural firing and neural synchrony within the brainstem dorsal and ventral cochlear nuclei, the midbrain, the thalamus, and the cortex.[10] Many other mechanisms have been suggested including by the author (R.T.S.) who has hypothesized that subjective tinnitus is often due to denervation hypersensitivity analogous to phantom pain. This phenomenon could occur anywhere in the auditory pathway where a synapse is exposed to ambient neurotransmitter due to death of the hair cell or nerve that should have joined with and protected the exposed synapse.

Consequently, it is usually difficult to document its presence and quantify its severity, although a few tests are available to help with this problem. Although the character of tinnitus is rarely diagnostic, certain qualities are suggestive of specific problems. A seashell-like tinnitus is often associated with endolymphatic hydrops, swelling of the inner ear membranes associated with Ménière's syndrome, syphilitic labyrinthitis, trauma, and other conditions. Unilateral ringing tinnitus may be caused by trauma, but it is also suggestive of acoustic neuroma. Pulsatile tinnitus (PT) raises suspicion for underlying cardiovascular disease or vascular abnormalities, increased intracranial pressure, or neoplasm. Benign problems are more common than tumors.

A focused, detailed history and physical examination (with comprehensive testing) are the primary tools for diagnosis of tinnitus and allow a healthcare professional to differentiate benign tinnitus etiologies from dangerous causes such as arteriovenous malformations or glomus jugulare and to determine potential treatment options. Chronicity, location, and laterality, associated hearing changes, can impact on the patient's well-being and provide helpful guidance for evaluation and management. When evaluating the history of a tinnitus (ear noise) problem, the following questions should be asked:

**Yes/No**

___ ___   1.  Are your noises localized?

    ___ Right ear             ___ Head

    ___ Left ear              ___ Cannot localize

    ___ Both ears           ___ If both, which ear is worse? Right/Left/Neither

___ ___   2.  How long have you had ear noises? (Indicate which ear, and for how long)

Right/Left/Both

How long have they been bothersome?

    ___ Days

    ___ Weeks

    ___ Months

    ___ Years

Right/Left/Both

___ ___   3.  Was there a particular incident (head cold or other URI, explosion, etc.) that seems to have started your noises?

If yes, please describe:

___ ___   4.  Has the noise changed since it first appeared?

If yes, please describe:

___ ___   5.  Is it constantly present, or does it fluctuate (good days/bad days)?

___ ___   6.  Is it episodic (comes and goes)?

If yes, during what percentage of the time is it usually present during waking hours?_____%

___ ___   7.  If it is episodic, are you completely free of noises between attacks?

___ ___   8.  Recently, have attacks occurred *more* frequently?

___ ___   9.  Recently, have attacks occurred *less* frequently?

___ ___  10.  Are the noises more apt to occur at a particular time of the day?

If yes, when? ___ Morning ___ Day time ___ Evening ___ Night ___ None

___ ___  11.  Is there any activity that brings on the noises or makes them worse?

If yes, describe:

___ ___  12.  Are the noises worse when you are under stress?

___ ___  13.  Are the noises worse when you are tired?

___ ___  14.  Are there any foods or substances to which you are exposed that aggravate the noises?

If yes, please check the following that apply:

    ___ Alcohol            ___ Coffee

    ___ Cigarettes         ___ Chocolate

    ___ Excessive salt     ___ Other, describe:

___ ___  15.  Are the noises worse during any season?

If yes, when: ___ Summer ___ Fall ___ Winter ___ Spring

___ ___  16.  Is there anything you can do to decrease the noises or make them go away?

If yes, describe:

___ ___  17.  Are there any activities or sounds that make the noises less disturbing?

If yes, describe:

**Yes/No**

___ ___ 18. Does the noise sound the same in both ears?

Please characterize the noise.

___ Ringing            ___ Heartbeat

___ Whistling        ___ Bells

___ Buzzing         ___ Hissing

___ Seashell-like (ocean roar) ___ Voices

___ ___ 19. What medications or treatments (medications, maskers, biofeedback, etc.) for the noises have you tried?

Please list:

___ ___ 20. Have any of them helped?

If Yes, please list:

___ ___ 21. To which of the following would you compare the loudness of your noise?

___ A soft whisper           ___ A diesel truck motor

___ An electric fan         ___ A jet taking off

___ ___ 22. Is the loudness fairly constant?

___ ___ 23. Does it vary *slightly* from day-to-day?

___ ___ 24. Does it vary *widely* from day-to-day?

___ ___ 25. Please rate the severity of the noises on a scale from 1 to 10. (Please check)

___ Mild (1, 2)             Aware of it when you think about it

___ Moderate (3–5)      Aware of it frequently, but able to ignore most of the time; occasionally interferes with falling asleep.

___ Severe (6–8)          Aware of it all the time, very disturbing; often interferes with activities, communication, etc.

___ Very severe (9, 10)    Aware of it all the time, interferes with daily activities, communication, and sleep; has changed your behavior.

___ ___ 26. Do you think your tinnitus interferes with your ability to hear?

___ ___ 27. Do you think other people should be able to hear the noises?

___ ___ 28. Do the noises sound as if they are coming from:

___ Inside your head ___ Outside your head

___ ___ 29. Are your head noises ever voices?

If yes, what do they say to you?

___ ___ 30. Do you have a feeling of fullness in your ears?

___ ___ 31. If yes, does it fluctuate with the noises?

___ ___ 32. Has anyone else in your family had tinnitus?

___ ___ 33. Do you have a hearing loss?

___ ___ 34. Do you have dizziness?

In some cases, the answers to these questions, combined with other information obtained through history taking, physical examination, and audiologic and other testing, permit the identification of a specific cause of tinnitus. For example, ringing tinnitus associated with fluctuating ear fullness and hearing loss during straining can be caused by a perilymph fistula. This is a fairly common injury following trauma. Seashell-like tinnitus associated with ear fullness and fluctuating hearing loss unassociated with straining or forceful nose blowing suggests endolymphatic hydrops. Tinnitus may be amenable to treatment in some cases. The tinnitus physical examination includes evaluation of the ears, eyes, musculoskeletal system, neurologic, vascular, and other systems. Audiologic examination should be performed promptly when tinnitus is diagnosed.

Information also can be obtained about the effect of tinnitus on the individual. Recently, instruments have been developed to measure tinnitus handicap. One of the best divides is a 25-question assessment divided into functional, emotional, and catastrophic response categories.[11,12] This Tinnitus Handicap Inventory (THI) is well-designed and psychometrically validated, but it still depends entirely upon voluntary, subjective responses.[13] Objective criteria for detecting exaggerated responses (malingering) have not been developed, yet. Similar handicap indices have also been proposed for dizziness and hearing loss.[14–16] In general, the American Academy of Otolaryngology-Head and Neck Surgery Foundation advises against the use of imaging studies in patients with nonpulsatile bilateral tinnitus, symmetric hearing loss, and an otherwise normal history and physical examination.[17] Magnetic resonance imaging (MRI) with and without contrast is performed in asymmetric, unilateral, nonpulsatile tinnitus to evaluate for vestibular schwannoma, vascular abnormalities such as ischemia, and other pathologies. Temporal bone CT without contrast (sometimes with) or CT angiography is recommended for the investigation of PT. Ultrasonography can be used to evaluate for extracranial carotid artery stenosis, followed by CT angiography or MRI/MRA.[17] However, this recommendation is not endorsed by all experts, and many neurologists advocate imagining in other tinnitus patients, as well.

## DIAGNOSTIC SIGNIFICANCE OF THE DESCRIPTION OF TINNITUS

Because tinnitus, like pain, is subjective, it can be described by the patient only by comparing it with some familiar noise. The patient may say it sounds like the hissing of steam, the ringing of bells, the roar of the ocean, a running motor, buzzing, or machine shop noises. Very often it is difficult for the patient to localize the noise in the ears; he/she may not be able to tell from which ear it is coming, or it may sound as though it were in the center of his/her head. Some people report that the noises are not in their ears at all but inside the head. Quite frequently, a patient will claim that the noise is in one ear and not in the other; yet, when by some surgical or medical intervention the noise is stopped in the symptomatic ear, the patient then notices the noise in the contralateral ear. This means that the patients can localize the tinnitus to

the ear in which it was louder but do not realize that it is present also in the opposite ear.

How the patient describes the tinnitus is sometimes of diagnostic significance, although the description alone cannot be depended upon for etiological judgments. For example, a low-pitched type of tinnitus is more common in otosclerosis and other forms of conductive hearing loss. Sounds like ringing and hissing are more common in sensorineural hearing loss. The ocean-roaring type of noise or a noise like a hollow seashell held to the ear is reported most often in patients with Ménière's syndrome.

Patients sometimes say that the ear noises are so loud that they are unable to hear what is going on around them. They claim also that if only the ear or head noises would stop, they would be able to hear better. Unfortunately, this is not usually the case. It is possible to measure how loud these noises actually are. These measurements show that tinnitus rarely is louder than a very soft whisper (5–10 dB above hearing threshold), and it is actually the concomitant hearing loss or a psychological disturbance, rather than the masking effect of the tinnitus, that prevents patients from hearing. This is known as the psychological model of tinnitus, initially proposed by Hallam, Rachman, and Hinchcliffe in 1984.[18] Although this model is largely theoretical, it is supported by the benefits that cognitive behavioral therapy (CBT) has in patients with tinnitus.

## PHYSICAL EXAMINATION AND TESTING

Patients with tinnitus deserve a comprehensive neurotologic assessment in order to determine whether there is any serious or underlying cause of the tinnitus. After a thorough history, a physical examination includes complete head and neck assessments, including an examination of the cranial nerves. Objective tinnitus, or tinnitus that can be perceived by the examining physician on cranial auscultation, or with a Toynbee tube, should be differentiated from subjective tinnitus, in which only the patient can hear the tinnitus. Previous otologic such as hearing loss, prior ear surgery, infections, pain, or drainage is relevant. Other neurotological testing of cerebellar and other functions should be performed, as indicated. In addition to a routine audiogram, testing commonly includes assessment of hearing at frequencies not tested routinely; brainstem evoked-response audiogram (BERA); balance tests such as electronystagmogram (ENG) and computerized dynamic posturography (CDP); otoacoustic emission (OAE) testing; imaging studies (MRI, computerized tomography [CT], single-photon emission computed tomography [SPECT], and positron emission tomography [PET]). Blood tests for diabetes, hypoglycemia, hyperlipoproteinemia, Lyme disease, syphilitic labyrinthitis, thyroid dysfunction, collagen vascular disease, autoimmune inner ear disease, and many other conditions also should be considered. A review of the patient's medication regimen is also required, as many medications are ototoxic, including aspirin, antibiotics (oral aminoglycosides), chemotherapeutic agents (cisplatin), ACE inhibitors, loop diuretics, proton pump inhibitors, benzodiazepines, and antimalarials (quinine and chloroquine).[19] Such comprehensive evaluation can identify a treatable cause of tinnitus in a substantial number of patients, although not a majority.

## AUDIOMETRY IN THE PRESENCE OF TINNITUS

Occasionally, when an audiogram is performed on a patient with marked tinnitus, he/she complains of inability to detect the tone produced by the audiometer because of the tinnitus. That is a real problem, and it can be handled best by modifying the technique of audiometry. Instead of sounding a tone on the audiometer for a second or less, it is best to present quickly interrupted or warbled tones so that the patient can distinguish the discontinuous audiometer tone from the constant tinnitus. In this way, the test will determine the threshold more accurately than by using the routine method of tone presentation.

If the tinnitus is unilateral, the character of a patient's tinnitus can be determined by asking him/her to match it with sounds applied to the good ear. This is done using tinnitus-matching audiometer circuitry. Both the frequency and intensity usually can be identified. This information is helpful for quantitative diagnostic and rehabilitation

purposes. The presence of residual tinnitus inhibition after masking also has useful therapeutic implications, as discussed subsequently.

## TINNITUS WITH A NORMAL AUDIOGRAM

It is standard procedure in otologic practice to perform an audiogram on every patient who complains of tinnitus. If the otoscopic findings are normal and the audiogram shows normal hearing from the lowest frequencies to 8000 Hz, and yet the patient complains of tinnitus, several causes should be considered: (1) hearing defects >8000 Hz or at "in-between" frequencies not tested during routine audiogram, (2) vascular and neurologic disorders, (3) functional causes, (4) retrocochlear disease such as an acoustic neuroma, and (5) temporomandibular joint (TMJ) abnormality.

## TINNITUS WITH HIDDEN HIGH-FREQUENCY HEARING LOSSES

Tinnitus and hearing loss are associated so frequently with each other that some physicians attribute tinnitus to a psychological disturbance if the audiogram shows normal hearing. Such a diagnosis is hardly justified. A psychological diagnosis should be made based on positive clinical findings rather than on normal audiogram results. Studies show that many patients who complain of ringing or hissing tinnitus may have perfectly normal hearing in the frequencies that routine audiometers test, that is, 250, 500, 1000, 2000, 3000, 4000, 6000, and 8000 Hz. However, when the hearing is tested at higher frequencies up to 20,000 Hz, it is not uncommon to find a hearing deficit in the ear in which the patient claims to have tinnitus. In addition, the standard audiogram shows thresholds only at a few fixed octave frequencies. The hearing damage may well be at a point intermediate between these routinely tested frequencies. For example, a 40-dB loss at 3500 Hz would not be seen on a standard audiogram because hearing is routinely measured at 2000 and 4000 Hz.

**Left Ear–Air Conduction**

| 250 | 500 | 1000 | 2000 | 4000 | 8000 | 10000 | 12000 | 14000 |
|-----|-----|------|------|------|------|-------|-------|-------|
| 5 | 5 | −5 | −10 | −10 | −5 | 15 | 10 | 5 |

**Right Ear–Air Conduction**

| 250 | 500 | 1000 | 2000 | 4000 | 8000 | 10000 | 12000 | 14000 |
|-----|-----|------|------|------|------|-------|-------|-------|
| 5 | 0 | −5 | −10 | 5 | 5 | 35 | 30 | 35 |

Figure 20.1 *History*: Audiogram of a 38-year-old woman with fullness in her right ear and high-pitched constant tinnitus for several months. No obvious cause. She had had eustachian tube inflations, allergic desensitization, bite correction, and nose treatments without help. *Otologic*: Normal. *Audiologic*: Normal hearing with high tone hearing loss > 8000 Hz. *Classification*: High-tone sensory hearing loss. *Diagnosis*: After further questioning, the patient subsequently associated the onset of tinnitus with a bad cold. Hearing loss and subsequent tinnitus are probably due to viral cochleitis.

Continuous frequency audiometry is a tremendous help in cases of this type. **Figures 20.1** and **20.2** relate cases of tinnitus that were diagnosed as functional because no hearing loss was found during routine audiometry. However, more detailed hearing tests revealed the presence of auditory damage which could well account for the patients' tinnitus.

## PULSATILE TINNITUS

PT should be differentiated from nonpulsatile symptoms, as the etiologies often differ. While nonpulsatile tinnitus is often idiopathic, the underlying etiology of PT can be identified in 70% of patients with a thorough history and physical examination.[18] PT is described by patients as a perception of rhythmic sound, often similar to a heartbeat, and is typically unilateral. Pulse-synchronous PT and pulse-asynchronous PT should be differentiated. Pulse-synchronous PT is likely due to abnormal blood flow in the vasculature of the head, neck, or ear. Pulse-asynchronous PT is usually from a mechanical etiology. A low pitch is usually venous, whereas a high pitch often is arterial. Full physical examination, audiological testing, and imaging are required in PT evaluation.

The causes of PT can either be structural, metabolic, vascular malformations, or aneurysms. Structural causes can be seen on MRI (usually paragangliomas or schwannomas). Tensor tympani, stapedius, or soft palate spasm, anemia, and hyperthyroidism are metabolic causes of PT. Hypervitaminosis B6 is a possible medicinal cause, although it may also be associated with nonpulsatile tinnitus. Arterial etiologies of PT include carotid artery stenosis, dissection, fibromuscular dysplasia, aneurysm, arteriovenous malformations, aberrant internal carotid artery, and arteriovenous fistula. PT due to a venous source usually is associated with turbulent sigmoid sinus, lateral sinus, or jugular bulb blood flow; or enlarged condylar veins, transverse sinus, sigmoid sinus, or internal jugular vein stenosis, or high riding jugular bulb, although many of these conditions can be asymptomatic. So, care must be exercised before ascribing causation to them for PT.[19]

## TINNITUS AND OTOSCLEROSIS

Tinnitus usually is low-pitched and described as buzzing or, occasionally, a roaring sound in patients with otosclerosis. Sometimes the patient may say he/she hears a pulsing noise timed to his/her heartbeat. In some patients with otosclerosis, the tinnitus is even more disturbing than the hearing loss. However, not all patients with otosclerosis have tinnitus, and some with very severe otosclerosis deafness deny ever having had tinnitus. In most instances, tinnitus will disappear or diminish during the course of many years of hearing impairment. Tinnitus is uncommon in older patients who have had long-standing otosclerosis.

In view of all that has been learned about the pathology of otosclerosis, it might be thought that it would be possible to eliminate tinnitus by correcting the fixation of the stapedial footplate. This is not necessarily so. Many patients who have had successful stapes surgery and a return to almost normal hearing have found that the tinnitus seems to persist, although it may not be as loud as it was prior to surgery. Yet in other patients, tinnitus seems to subside completely when hearing is restored surgically. Rarely, it even may worsen. It would appear, then, that there are other factors besides stapes fixation in the etiology of tinnitus associated with otosclerosis. Otosclerosis eventually produces sensorineural hearing loss in many cases, and tinnitus may be related to the same etiology.

## TINNITUS IN MÉNIÈRE'S DISEASE

One of the most disturbing and persistent types of tinnitus is associated with Ménière's disease. It generally is described as an ocean roar or a hollow seashell sound. In the early stages of Ménière's disease, tinnitus often persists all the time and becomes the most disturbing symptom of the disease. Many patients would even sacrifice their hearing to get rid of the tinnitus, but unfortunately, there is no guaranteed therapy, not even surgery, that will ensure the resolution of the tinnitus. Fortunately, tinnitus and inner ear involvement are restricted in most patients to one ear. However, when both ears are affected, the psychological impact on the patient may become a serious challenge to both the patient and the physician.

## TINNITUS AFTER HEAD TRAUMA OR EXPOSURE TO NOISE

Ringing tinnitus is experienced commonly after a blow to the external ear or close exposure to a sudden very loud noise such as the explosion of a firecracker or the firing of a gun. In most instances,

**Left Ear–Air Conduction**

| 250 | 500 | 1000 | 2000 | 4000 | 8000 | 10000 | 12000 | 14000 |
|-----|-----|------|------|------|------|-------|-------|-------|
| 0 | −5 | −5 | −5 | 0 | −10 | −5 | 0 | 5 |

**Right Ear–Air Conduction**

| 250 | 500 | 1000 | 2000 | 4000 | 8000 | 10000 | 12000 | 14000 |
|-----|-----|------|------|------|------|-------|-------|-------|
| −10 | −5 | −5 | −10 | −5 | 45 | 30 | 35 | 60 |

Figure 20.2 *History*: An 18-year old woman with ringing tinnitus 8 weeks after fall on right side of head, with unconsciousness. Skull was fractured, and she had vertigo and bleeding from right ear. For 6 weeks, she had light-headedness. A persistent ringing tinnitus is present. *Otologic*: Normal. *Audiologic*: Note the loss in the very high frequencies in the right ear. *Classification*: Sensorineural hearing loss. *Diagnosis*: Direct trauma to the inner ear.

the tinnitus is accompanied by high-frequency hearing loss. If the hearing loss is temporary, the tinnitus often subsides in a few hours or days. If permanent hearing loss has occurred from damage to the inner ear, ringing tinnitus may persist for many years or permanently.

The close relationship between head injury and tinnitus is clear in the classic cartoon that portrays an individual knocked out by a punch on the jaw or a blow on the head, complete with "seeing" stars and bells ringing in his ears. The bells portray the tinnitus that the patient hears after a severe blow. The noise probably is caused by a concussion of the cochlea. The damage seems to be reversible most of the time because the ringing gradually subsides in most patients.

## "ACOUSTIC NEURITIS," ACOUSTIC NEUROMA, AND MISCELLANEOUS CAUSES

For want of a more specific etiology, tinnitus often is attributed to neuritis (inflammation) of the acoustic nerve, especially if a high-tone deafness accompanies it. It is not known precisely whether the irritation or inflammation actually injures the nerve itself, but at least some of the damage probably occurs in the cochlea. Diseases such as hepatitis, influenza, and other viral diseases frequently result in high-pitched tinnitus, tentatively attributed to cochleitis or acoustic neuritis. Tinnitus may also be associated with presbycusis, impacted cerumen on the eardrum, and many other causes. It rarely is associated with infection of the middle ear.

Acoustic neuroma is a benign tumor of the cerebellopontine angle. It may cause tinnitus (often the first symptom) by damaging the acoustic nerve or auditory pathways in the brainstem by compression. Tinnitus may be caused by other cerebellopontine angle neoplasms, as well, including meningioma, cholesteatoma, and vascular malformation. Similar compression and nerve damage/irritation can be caused by the anterior–inferior cerebellar artery vascular loop if this blood vessel is in contact with the auditory nerve or its root-entry zone. Tumors within the brainstem are also capable of causing tinnitus. These serious conditions highlight the need for thorough evaluation in patients who complain of tinnitus; MRI should be considered especially in any patient with unilateral tinnitus.

## TEMPOROMANDIBULAR JOINT PROBLEMS

The pathophysiology of how dental malocclusion or TMJ disparity can cause tinnitus is not known, but there are some patients whose tinnitus has resolved with adequate TMJ treatment. The evidence conflicts with the assumption that all these cases are of emotional origin. Only a few patients with malocclusion ever complain of tinnitus, and even when malocclusion and tinnitus are present in the same patient, it does not follow necessarily that the dental abnormality causes the tinnitus. As dental correction is sometimes a formidable undertaking, one might consider a noninvasive treatment to indicate whether a complete corrective procedure would be likely to stop tinnitus. Such a procedure may consist of placing a plastic prosthesis (bite block) over the lower molars at night. If there is a noticeable improvement in tinnitus after a satisfactory trial period, then more permanent measures may be indicated. Indiscriminate or radical efforts to alleviate tinnitus by correcting malocclusion and subsequent TMJ symptomatology without a valid therapeutic test to establish the causal relationship should be avoided. Many otologists question the reality of any true relationship between dental malocclusion or TMJ dysfunction and tinnitus despite the frequency of association of TMJ problems with ear pain.

## FUNCTIONAL CAUSES

For all reasons enumerated, a diagnosis of functional or psychological tinnitus should be made with great caution. Nevertheless, in some patients with normal hearing and tinnitus, a tentative diagnosis of functional tinnitus may have to be considered. The patients should be differentiated into two categories. Malingering occurs when the patient does not perceive an abnormal noise and is aware of the fact, but claims to have tinnitus, usually for secondary gain (such as a lawsuit). True functional or "hysterical" tinnitus is psychiatric in etiology and disappears following effective psychotherapy. It is also extremely rare. Excessive functional response to existing tinnitus is the most common category of the three. Most such patients become so preoccupied with their tinnitus that they continue to talk about it to their friends and will consult numerous doctors and nonmedical persons for relief that is not forthcoming. Unfortunately, the otologist can do little to cure such patients of their tinnitus when the cause is not known. However, it may be possible to help the patient to adjust to the auditory disorder through psychological counseling, tinnitus maskers, habituators, and sometimes medications. Although it has not been proven, in the author's experience, patients with severe auditory processing disorders tend to be particularly disturbed by tinnitus which might be ignored by many patients. In these cases, neuropsychological testing and intervention may prove extremely valuable. It is helpful in such cases to bear in mind that tinnitus itself is really not very loud, but many patients overreact to their symptoms and allow their tinnitus to assume distressing proportions.

## PEDIATRIC TINNITUS

Tinnitus can start at any age. Even in adults, physicians should determine whether tinnitus was present during childhood. Tinnitus often goes undiagnosed especially in young children because they do not always realize that the sound that they hear is abnormal and should not be present. Of course, some children do complain about ear noise and seek medical care.

The presentation of tinnitus in pediatric patients is largely identical to the presentation in adults.[19] Tinnitus in children may cause long-lasting hearing and concentration impairment, particularly in children with a central auditory processing disorder. Prompt diagnosis is important.

Children often present with both tinnitus and hearing loss (conductive hearing loss more so than sensorineural hearing loss). Nonpulsatile tinnitus is usually due to disruption of the middle- and inner ear structures, and children may not require imaging if hearing loss is not present, although the decision about imaging is dependent on the clinical judgment of the otolaryngologist. Inner ear anomalies such as semicircular canal dysmorphism, enlarged vestibular aqueduct, and cochlear hypoplasia are seen commonly in children with tinnitus. Children with PT benefit from both CT and MRI imaging, with up to 70% etiology detection. MRI is the first-line imaging modality in evaluating a child with PT, although a CT scan is complimentary in the full evaluation of the nerves, middle and inner ear structures, and regional vessels.[20]

## MANAGING THE PATIENT WITH TINNITUS

Unless a correctable, structural, or metabolic cause is found, tinnitus is usually not curable. Most patients adjust well to their tinnitus, but some are extremely disturbed by it. An enormous number of medications have been used to treat tinnitus, most without success. Tinnitus maskers (devices similar to hearing aids) are recommended by some physicians, but their value is also limited for the vast majority of tinnitus sufferers. These devices introduce a noise into the ear that the patient can control. Some patients find this helpful, but most do not. External masking with a radio or fan is helpful to many people, especially at night if the tinnitus interferes with their ability to fall asleep. Many patients find tinnitus less disturbing if they wear a hearing aid. Consequently, in a patient with concomitant tinnitus and even mild hearing loss, it may be worthwhile to try amplification sooner than one ordinarily would in a patient not troubled by tinnitus.

Some patients become so obsessed with the noises in their ears that they become emotionally disturbed and are unable to sleep at night, reporting that the noise keeps them awake. This happens mainly in highly "anxious" individuals, but the problem requires much patience and understanding on the part of the physician. Reassurance and encouragement are very helpful, and symptomatic therapy for tinnitus, whatever is available, should be provided. One practical suggestion is for the patient to put an automatic timer on his/her radio and play it when going to sleep. After an hour or two, the automatic timer shuts off the radio, and by then the patient is fast asleep. Music from the radio may mask the patient's tinnitus by masking and distracting his/her attention from endogenous noises. A similar effect may be achieved with white noise generated either by a fan or another electronic device.

In managing a patient with tinnitus, it is advisable to have a forthright talk with the patient to explain the most likely cause of the tinnitus and that there is not yet a specific cure for it. It is nevertheless possible, in most instances, to mitigate the problem and alleviate the patient's excessive concern about the symptoms. If a hearing aid is indicated, its daily use usually makes the patient less aware of tinnitus by focusing attention on other matters. Everyday noises definitely help to mask tinnitus in most patients. However, when the patient takes off the hearing aid at night, the tinnitus may become more noticeable. Electronic tinnitus maskers and biofeedback techniques have been developed and proven helpful for some patients. Periods of tension and stress also tend to make tinnitus more troublesome. Most people with tinnitus who keep themselves occupied, especially at work, are less bothered by their noises.

CBT can be a particularly effective treatment for idiopathic tinnitus with well-established, moderate-to-high-quality-based evidence and allows patients to develop alternative coping strategies to improve their quality of life. Targeting secondary symptoms rather than the tinnitus tone itself with CBT, neurofeedback, and neuromodulation are superior to placebo.[16] Comorbid conditions with tinnitus, such as depression, anxiety, sleep disturbance, impaired cognition, and general disability, may be managed with pharmacotherapy. This may include nortriptyline and sertraline (depression and anxiety), tricyclic antidepressants (disability and other problems), and trazodone or melatonin (sleep disturbance).[16]

The use of tranquilizers, constructive suggestions, and specific cures for conditions such as otosclerosis and Ménière's disease are important therapeutic regimens in managing the patient with tinnitus. In many cases, the tinnitus subsides gradually or even suddenly for no obvious reason. Medical attention to related vascular abnormalities such as hypertension, Buerger's disease, and atherosclerosis is recommended. Hypnosis is helpful in some instances. Psychotherapy and encouragement may be of tremendous value.

There are also treatments that have been advocated for patients with tinnitus, but for which convincing evidence of efficacy may not be available. Nevertheless, they have been helpful anecdotally in some patients and may be considered in selected cases. These include benzodiazepines, anticonvulsants, Ginkgo biloba, Niacin, Lipoflavonoid, nicotinamide adenine dinucleotide (NAD), gabapentin, nitrous oxide, and transcranial magnetic or electrical stimulation. In addition, acupuncture, transcutaneous electrical nerve stimulation, bimodal (auditory and somatosensory) stimulation, hyperbaric oxygen, and microvascular decompression of the vestibulocochlear nerve have been studied, though evidence for their value in treating tinnitus is insufficient.[19]

## TINNITUS MASKERS, HABITUATORS, AND RETRAINING

There are various methods of temporary relief from tinnitus such as hypnosis and biofeedback. One method may prove quite effective for one patient and provide no relief for another. The use of a tinnitus masker may alleviate symptoms for some people. A masker is almost always considered but usually prescribed only after other methods have failed.

A tinnitus masker is a hearing aid-like instrument that produces a narrow band of noise centered around the pitch of the patient's tinnitus. These instruments are available as a masker alone or in a combination of hearing aid/masker.

Before a masker can be fitted, a tinnitus evaluation must be performed. The evaluation involves taking a detailed history of the individual's tinnitus, as well as matching the pitch and intensity of the tinnitus as closely as possible. It should be noted also whether the tinnitus is unilateral or bilateral. After the tinnitus is matched, the minimal masking level is determined. This is the level at which the masking noise is perceived above the patient's tinnitus.

Finally, the patient is assessed to determine whether residual inhibition is present. This is a temporary cessation or lessening of the tinnitus for a few seconds to several minutes following the presentation of a masking noise to the affected ear. The presence of residual inhibition suggests a good prognosis for the successful use of a masker.

A habituator is a device somewhat like a tinnitus masker. Habituators are used primarily to treat patients with hyperacusis (hypersensitivity to noise), but they may be helpful in some tinnitus patients, as well. A habituator supplies the ear with a constant, soft sound stimulus so that the ear is never in silence. Theoretically, this activates or "primes" inhibitory neurons and improves their ability to respond to and suppress external stimuli. In some cases, this approach also seems to help suppress tinnitus. Tinnitus retraining programs have proven useful and are becoming progressively more sophisticated.

Finally, the use of low-level laser therapy (LLLT) with red (630–700 nanometers) and infrared (800–1000 nanometers) light has been investigated preliminarily as a possible treatment for tinnitus. LLLT is thought to promote tissue regeneration, reduce inflammation, and relieve pain, and when focused on the cochlea and middle ear, it has been reported to relieve tinnitus. LLLT lasts anywhere from 6 to 15 minutes, and its therapeutic effect may last up to 15 days.[21]

## SURGERY

A few patients are truly distraught and disabled by tinnitus. In some patients, tinnitus persists even in a totally deaf ear. Such patients may be candidates for vestibulocochlear nerve section, an intracranial procedure in which the eighth cranial nerve is cut. However, this procedure is only successful in relieving tinnitus 50%–70% of the time, and as mentioned previously, evidence supporting this surgery continues to be limited. If it is reasonably certain that severe tinnitus in a non-hearing ear is coming from the ear rather than more centrally in the auditory pathway, eighth nerve section is reasonable. However, it usually is not possible to localize the tinnitus source in the auditory pathway with absolute certainty. If the tinnitus is believed to be associated with a vascular loop (malpositioned blood vessel) compressing this same nerve, microvascular decompression can be performed through the posterior fossa. This procedure may be helpful, but the tinnitus must be extremely disturbing in order to justify an operation of this magnitude. Patients should also be informed that tinnitus may worsen following any ear surgery, as can one's hearing.

Unilateral or bilateral cochlear implantation (CI) surgery for auditory rehabilitation often suppresses tinnitus. It is thought that CI restoration of acuity in the central auditory pathways and neuroplasticity affect the perception of tinnitus. Indications now include unilateral deafness. So, it is preferable to try CI before considering eighth cranial nerve section because CI can not only suppress tinnitus but also restore some hearing ability, unless CI is contraindicated for a medical reason. While most literature demonstrates the benefits of CI on tinnitus, tinnitus may conversely be a complication of this surgery.[22]

## CURRENT RESEARCH

Research into the causes of tinnitus poses unique problems. Paramount is the fact that tinnitus is a purely subjective phenomenon. Unlike hearing loss, which can be measured objectively, the only way to know that a patient hears noises is for the subject to report that fact. Naturally, experimental animals cannot make such a report even if researchers impart artificial tinnitus. For example, large quantities of aspirin predictably produce a temporary tinnitus. In addition, exposure to extremely loud noise, sufficient to cause a measurable temporary threshold shift, generally produces temporary tinnitus. If an experimental animal could report the tinnitus, various techniques could be used to try to make it go away.

In hearing research, animals frequently are trained and conditioned to perform accurate audiograms. Unfortunately, similar techniques are not suitable for tinnitus. Conditioning for hearing loss works because the animals are trained to respond to an intermittent signal such as the tone from an audiometer. As experimentally induced tinnitus is present constantly, a trained animal will adapt to it and cease to respond. Although some of these technical difficulties may be solved, at present research depends primarily on either histologic studies or the use of living humans. Histologic, pharmacologic, and biochemical studies directed toward understanding the hair cells of the inner ear, nerves, blood flow, and neurotransmitters are underway and have produced interesting information. So far, however, very little of it has had proven clinical value in the etiology and treatment of tinnitus.

Any healthcare clinician treating a severe tinnitus sufferer knows that finding volunteers for experimental treatments is easy. Some patients with tinnitus are miserable and anxious to try anything that may help. Investigators have used everything from garlic to electrical stimulation of the cochlea (first in the 19th century and more recently in the 1970s and 1980s), to masking, and to surgery. A long list of drugs has been tried without consistent success. These drugs range from benign medications such as vitamin A to ototoxic drugs used therapeutically for medical labyrinthectomy such as streptomycin and gentamycin.

The phenomenon of OAEs is also interesting for tinnitus researchers and clinicians. OAEs are acoustic energies that can be detected by inserting a miniature microphone directly into the external auditory meatus and measuring the response emitted back through the eardrum. It has been established that many people do have OAEs that they cannot hear (not tinnitus). Therefore, these emissions cannot be considered a dependable guide to the presence or absence of tinnitus in experimental animals. It should be noted that OAEs are only present and recordable in people with hearing levels of 35- to 40-dB HL or better. With worse hearing loss, detectable OAEs should not be expected.[23]

## FUTURE RESEARCH

To better understand tinnitus, additional research is needed. Certain facts, however, have become clear. First, the sounds that encompass tinnitus are produced by many different causes. Their mechanisms may be located anywhere within the auditory pathway from the eardrum to the cortex. Mechanical causes of tinnitus, such as earwax impacted against an eardrum and palatal myoclonus, may be understood, and treated. Other causes and mechanisms located in the cochlea or central nervous system are unclear. Future human and laboratory research is essential. Research projects using humans need to be carefully designed, with minimal risks and approval by the Federal Food and Drug Administration if they are performed in the United States. This research should attempt to systematically localize and categorize tinnitus sources and to interrupt the tinnitus through pharmacologic (preferably),

electrical, or surgical means. Laboratory research probably will not be fruitful or practical for the professional investigator until a useful animal model has been developed. Until that time, the greatest benefit probably will come from further study of the neuropharmacology that affects the ascending and descending auditory pathways. Tinnitus remains among the most challenging problems for hearing healthcare professionals, researchers, and, especially, patients.

## REFERENCES

1. National Center for Health Statistics. Hearing status and ear examination: Findings among adults. United States 1960–1962. Vital and Health Statistics, Series 11, No. 32. Washington, DC: U.S. Department of HEW, 1968.
2. Reed GF. An audiometric study of two hundred cases of subjected tinnitus. Arch Otol 1960; 71:94–104.
3. Nodar RH. Tinnitus aurium in school-age children: survey. J Aud Res 1972; 12:133–135.
4. Sataloff J, Sataloff RT, Luenenburg W. Tinnitus and vertigo in health senior citizens without a history of noise exposure. Am J Otol 1987; 8(2):87–89.
5. Fower EF. Tinnitus aurium: its significance in certain diseases of the ear. NY State J Med 1912; 12:702–704.
6. Heller MR, Bergman M. Tinnitus aurium in normally hearing persons. Ann Otol Rhinol Laryngol 1953; 62:73–83.
7. Graham JM. Tinnitus in children with hearing loss. CIBA Foundation Symposium 85, Tinnitus, London, UK, 1981:172–181.
8. Glassgold A, Altmann F. The effect of stapes surgery on tinnitus in otosclerosis. Laryngoscope 1966; 76:1624–1632.
9. House JW, Brackmann DE. Tinnitus: Surgical treatment. CIBA Foundation Symposium, Tinnitus, London, UK, 1981:204–212.
10. Haider HF, Bojić T, Ribeiro SF, Paço J, Hall DA, Szczepek AJ. Pathophysiology of subjective tinnitus: triggers and maintenance. Front Neurosci 2018; 12:866. Published 2018 Nov 27. doi:10.3389/fnins.2018.00866
11. Newman CW, Jacobson GP, Spitzer JB. Development of the Tinnitus Handicap

Inventory. Arch Otolaryngol Head Neck Surg 1996; 122:143–148.

12. Newman CW, Wharton JA, Jacobson GP. Retest stability of the Tinnitus Handicap Questionnaire. Ann Otol Rhinol Laryngol 1995; 104:718–723.

13. Newman CW, Sindridge SA, Jacobson GP. Psychometrically adequacy of the Tinnitus Handicap Inventory (THI) for evaluating treatment outcome. J Am Acad Aud 1998; 9:153–160.

14. Jacobson GP, Newman CW. The development of the Dizziness Handicap Inventory. Arch Otolaryngol Head Neck Surg 1990; 116:424–427.

15. Ventry I, Weinstein BE. The Hearing Handicap Inventory for the elderly: a new tool. Ear Hearing 1982; 3:128–134.

16. Newman CW, Weinstein BE, Jacobson GP, Hug GA. The Hearing Handicap Inventory for adults: psychometric adequacy and audiometric correlates. Ear Hear 1990; 11:176–180.

17. Dalrymple SN, Lewis SH, Philman S. Tinnitus: diagnosis and management. Am Fam Physician 2021; 103(11):663–671.

18. Hallam RS, Rachman S, Hinchcliffe R. Psychological aspects of tinnitus. Contributions to Med Psych 1984; 3:31–53.

19. Narsinh KH, Hui F, Saloner D, et al. Diagnostic approach to pulsatile tinnitus: a narrative review. JAMA Otolaryngol Head Neck Surg 2022; 148(5):476–483. doi:10.1001/jamaoto.2021.4470

20. Salman R, Chong I, Amans M, et al. Pediatric tinnitus: The role of neuroimaging. J Neuroimaging 2022; 32(3):400–411. doi:10.1111/jon.12986

21. Infrared Therapy Is the Most Effective Treatment for Tinnitus Among Those Tested: Study. Published July 8, 2023. Accessed July 13, 2023. https://www.theepochtimes.com/health/infrared-therapy-is-the-most-effective-treatment-for-tinnitus-among-those-tested-study_5371617.html?welcomeuser=1

22. Borges ALF, Duarte PLES, Almeida RBS, et al. Cochlear implant and tinnitus-a meta-analysis. Braz J Otorhinolaryngol 2021; 87(3):353–365. doi:10.1016/j.bjorl.2020.11.006

23. Graham MD, Sataloff RT, Kemink JL. Tinnitus in Ménière's disease: response to titration streptomycin therapy. J Laryngol Otol 1984; 98(12 suppl 9):281–286.

# 21

# Dizziness

ROBERT THAYER SATALOFF, HYE RHEE CHI, AND PAMELA C. ROEHM

In addition to deafness and tinnitus, vertigo is an important symptom associated with disorders of the ear. The ultimate relationship of the vestibular portion of the labyrinth to the cochlea makes it easy to understand the reason why many diseases and lesions, such as Ménière's disease, affect both hearing and balance. Some diseases, like mumps, classically affect only the cochlea. Certain toxins and viruses affect only the vestibular portion without affecting the hearing. Intense noise affects only the cochlea.

## VERTIGO

Vertigo, like deafness and tinnitus, is a subjective experience and is a symptom, not a disease. Its cause must be sought carefully in each case. The term "dizziness" or "vertigo" is used by patients to describe a variety of sensations, many of which are not related to the vestibular system. It is convenient to think of the balance system as a complex conglomerate of senses that each send the brain information about one's position in space. Components of the balance system include the vestibular labyrinth, the eyes, neck muscles, proprioceptive nerve endings, cerebellum, and other structures. The supranuclear oculomotor systems integrate information from various sites and are especially important for maintaining spatial orientation and permitting an individual to function during complex motion. The vestibular system and related structures are integral components of these systems. Within the inner ear, the cochlea performs audition, and the semicircular canals and other structures of the labyrinth perform vestibulation.

Vestibulation is the automation stabilization of the eyes relative to material space during normal patterns of movement, such as locomotion. It is a prerequisite for clear vision in these circumstances. The *vestibular system* includes structures responsible for several reflexes that are essential for normal balance function. These include the vestibuloocular reflex (VOR), vestibulospinal reflex (VSR) which includes the vestibulocolic reflex (VCR), and the

DOI: 10.1201/b23379-21

cervico-ocular reflex (COR). The vestibular system works in concert with the saccadic, pursuit, optokinetic, fixation reflex, and vergence systems. If all sources provide information in agreement, one has no equilibrium problem. However, if most of the sources tell the brain that the body is standing still, for example, but one component says that the body is turning left, the brain becomes confused, and we experience dizziness. It is the physician's responsibility to systematically analyze each component of the balance system to determine which component or components are providing incorrect information and whether correct information is being provided and analyzed in an aberrant fashion by the brain. Typically, labyrinthine dysfunction is associated with an abnormal sense of motion. It may be true spinning, a sensation of being on a ship or of falling, or simply a vague sense of imbalance when moving. In many cases, it is episodic. Fainting, light-headedness, body weakness, spots before the eyes, general light-headedness, tightness in the head, and loss of consciousness are generally not of vestibular origin. However, such descriptions are of only limited diagnostic help. Even some severe peripheral (vestibular or eighth nerve) lesions may produce only mild unsteadiness or no dizziness at all, such as seen in many patients with acoustic neuroma. Similarly, lesions outside the vestibular system may produce true rotary vertigo, as seen with trauma or microvascular occlusion in the brainstem, and with cervical vertigo.

Dizziness is a relatively uncommon problem in healthy individuals. In a study of 267 normal senior citizens, Sataloff et al. (1) found only a 5% incidence of dizziness in contrast to a 24% incidence of tinnitus. However, most of the population are not as healthy as the highly selected sample in this study. Initial physicians' visits involve a complaint of dizziness or imbalance in 5–10%, accounting for >11 million physician visits annually (2).

Dizziness is the most common reasons for a visit to a physician in patients >65 years of age, and this symptom may cause patients to fall. Approximately one-third to one-half of people aged ≥65 fall each year, and the consequences can be serious (3). Falls result in approximately 95% of 300,000 hip fractures per year, and this injury carries a 10% mortality rate.

Falls are the leading cause of death by injury in people > 75 years of age. Dizziness is also a common consequence of head injury. According to the Centers for Disease Control and Prevention (CDC) Surveillance Report, about 2.5 million Americans had traumatic brain injury-related emergency room (ER) visits annually (4). Unintentional fall accounted for causing 47.9% of the head injuries. A majority of the patients with serious head injuries complain of dizziness for up to 5 years following the injury, and many are disabled by this symptom (5). Dizziness may also persist for long periods of time following minor head injury (6).

Causes of dizziness are almost as numerous as causes of hearing loss, and some of them are medically serious (multiple sclerosis, acoustic neuroma, diabetes, cardiac arrhythmia, etc.). Consequently, any patient with an equilibrium complaint needs a thorough examination. For example, although dizziness may be caused by head trauma, the fact that it is reported for the first time following an injury is insufficient to establish causation without investigating other possible causes. While recording the history from a patient with equilibrium complaints, at least the following questions should be asked:

1. When did you first develop dizziness?
2. What is it like (light-headedness, blacking out, tendency to fall, objects spinning, you spinning, loss of balance, nausea, or vomiting)?
3. If you or your environment is spinning, is the direction of motion to the right or left?
4. Is your dizziness constant or episodic?
5. If episodic, how long do the attacks last?
6. How often do you have attacks?
7. Have they been more or less frequent recently?
8. Have they been more or less severe recently?
9. Under which circumstance did your dizziness first occur?
10. Exactly what were you doing at the time?
11. If you first noted dizziness after a head injury, how many hours, days, or weeks elapsed between the injury and your first imbalance symptoms?
12. Did you have any other symptoms at the same time, such as neck pain, shoulder pain, jaw pain, ear fullness, hearing loss, or ear noises?
13. Did you have a cold, the flu, or "cold sores" within the month or two prior to the onset of your dizziness?
14. Are you completely free of dizziness between attacks?
15. Do you get dizzy rolling over in bed?

16. If so, to the right, to the left, or both?
17. Do you get dizzy with position change?
18. If so, does your dizziness occur only in certain positions?
19. Do you get dizzy from bending, lifting, straining, or forceful nose blowing?
20. Do you have trouble walking in the dark?
21. Do you know of a cause for your dizziness?
22. Is there anything that will stop the dizziness or make it better?
23. Is there anything that will bring on an attack or make your dizziness worse (fatigue, exertion, hunger, certain foods, menstruation, etc.)?
24. Do you have any warning that an attack is about to start?
25. Once an attack has begun, does head movement make it worse?
26. Do you have significant problems with motion sickness?
27. Do you get headaches in relation to attacks of dizziness?
28. Do you get migraine headaches?
29. Are there other members of your family with migraine headaches?
30. Does your hearing change when you are dizzy?
31. Do you have fullness or stuffiness in your ears?
32. If yes, does it change when you have an attack of dizziness?
33. Have you had previous head injuries?
34. Have you ever injured your neck?
35. Do you have spine disease like arthritis (especially in the neck)?
36. Have you had any injuries to either ear?
37. Have you ever had surgery on either ear?
38. What drugs have been used to treat your dizziness?
39. Have they helped?
40. Do you have hearing loss or tinnitus?
41. Do you have any other medical problems (diabetes, high or low blood pressure, history of syphilis, other)?
42. Does your occupation involve head or neck strain?
43. Do you do any recreational activities that could injure your head and neck including (soccer, wrestling, and others)?
44. Is there any association between eating and your dizziness?
45. Have you ever received psychotherapy?
46. Do you have any family members with dizziness?
47. Are you pregnant?

It is important to pursue a systematic inquiry in all cases of disequilibrium not only because the condition is caused by serious problems in some cases but also because many patients with balance disorders can be helped. Many people believe incorrectly that sensorineural hearing loss, tinnitus, and dizziness are incurable, but many conditions that cause any or all of these may be treated successfully. It is especially important to separate peripheral causes (which are almost always treatable) from central causes such as brainstem contusion in which the prognosis is often worse.

## PHYSICAL EXAMINATION

In patients with dizziness, physical examination should include a complete assessment of the head and neck, hearing evaluation, evaluation of extraocular motion, and the presence of nystagmus (discussed subsequently) or papilledema in selected cases; testing for Hitselberger's sign (decreased sensation in the external auditory canal associated with pressure on the facial nerve from lesions such as acoustic neuromas) and Hennebert's sign (clinically, subjective dizziness caused by air pressure applied to the tympanic membrane during pneumotoscopy); and evaluation of the cranial nerves. These patients should also be tested for dysdiadochokinesis, dysmetria, and drift. Additional balance and gait testing should be performed, including at least Romberg and/or Tandem Romberg maneuvers. The patients should be evaluated for tremor, ticks, slurring of speech, and any other symptoms or signs of neurological dysfunction.

Every examination of the head and neck must include a careful search for spontaneous nystagmus, especially if vertigo is a complaint. A brief test can be done by first asking the patient to look straight ahead, holding his/her head straight, and then asking the patient to move his/her eyes from side to side. Normally, no nystagmus is present in an individual who is gazing straight ahead, but > 50% of people have a slight unsustained nystagmus when they are looking > 20–30 degrees to the right or the left. This is a normal reaction called end-point nystagmus and generally lasts only a few seconds. In pathological nystagmus of vestibular pathway origin, there is generally a slow and a fast component. The nystagmus is aggravated by looking in the direction of the fast component, and the nystagmus is named (to the right or the left), depending on the direction of the fast component. The nystagmus may be prolonged when it is pathological. In central nervous system disorders, it may persist for months. In acute attacks of Ménière's disease, it may last for several days or as long as the attack continues. In positional vertigo, the episode may be fleeting and last only as long as the head is held in a certain position. The nystagmus usually is weaker if the test position is repeated quickly. When marked nystagmus occurs spontaneously, and the patient does not complain of vertigo, it is suggestive of damage to the central nervous system or of congenital ocular nystagmus. Vertigo that accompanies spontaneous nystagmus also may suggest a central nervous system defect, but other conditions may produce the same symptoms, such as acute episodes of Ménière's disease, toxic labyrinthitis, and positional vertigo. Certain drugs, notably barbiturates and alcohol, also may produce nystagmus. Whenever pathological nystagmus is present, comprehensive otologic and neurological studies are indicated. Nystagmus can normally be induced by warm or cool irrigation. The caloric response causes nystagmus. Electronystagmography (ENG) or videonystagmography (VNG) will document the presence and direction of nystagmus, particularly if it is severe. VNG testing has the advantage of being able to record and analyze eye movements. The ability to observe and record eye movements in real time allows detailed monitoring of subtle findings that may not be as apparent.

However, the physician's eye is an order of magnitude more sensitive than the VNG machine in detecting fine nystagmus, and there is no substitute for good clinical examination. Clinical examination can be enhanced through Dix–Hallpike testing, a head impulse test (HIT or video HIT), head heave test (HHT), and many other maneuvers.

## BLOOD TESTS

A high percentage of the numerous conditions that cause hearing loss may also cause dizziness. Therefore, in many cases evaluation of a dizzy patient includes blood tests such as a complete blood count, fasting glucose or 5-hour glucose tolerance test (looking for hypoglycemia that provokes dizziness), cholesterol, triglycerides, FTA, Lyme titer, thyroid function tests, ANA, rheumatoid factor, sedimentation rate, and tests for autoimmune inner ear disease. Tests such as B12 and folate levels, screening blood tests for lead or other toxic substances, and viral screens also may be appropriate. Occasionally, dizziness also may be a presenting symptom of HIV/AIDS.

## VESTIBULAR TESTING

The balance system is extremely complicated, and ideal tests have not been developed. Research is currently underway to develop tests that will assess accurately the entire, composite functioning of the balance system and test each component in isolation. At present, the most commonly performed test is VNG for evaluation of inner ear functionality. Posturography is also used.

A brief review of vestibular physiology is helpful in understanding balance tests. The semicircular canals are arranged in three planes at right angles to each other ($x$, $y$, and $z$ axes) and work in pairs. The cupulae of the semicircular canals are stimulated by movement of endolymphatic fluid, and each canal causes the nystagmus in its own plane. That is, the horizontal canal produces horizontal nystagmus, the superior canal causes rotary nystagmus, and the posterior canal produces vertical nystagmus. Caloric testing stimulates primarily the horizontal semicircular canal and gives little or no information about function of the superior and posterior semicircular canals in most cases. The position of gaze and plane of the head are of great importance in vestibular testing, especially when the semicircular canals are stimulated by rotation rather than water irrigation. For rotary testing, it is useful to remember that ampullopetal flow (toward the cupulae) produces greater stimulation than ampullofugal flow (away from the cupulae) in the horizontal semicircular canal, but the opposite is true for the superior and posterior canals. Therefore, the response to rotation represents the combined effect of stimulating the sensory system of one semicircular canal while suppressing that of its counterpart on the other side of the body. Using rotational excitation and selective head position may be used to give information about the semicircular canals that is difficult or impossible to obtain from caloric stimulation. The clinical value of this additional information is controversial, and rotational testing is not common in the United States (although it is used more frequently in the UK).

## ELECTRONYSTAGMOGRAPHY

Electro-oculography is used to evaluate nonvestibular supranuclear oculomotor systems. These portions of the test battery include calibration, which assesses cerebellar function, gaze nystagmus, sinusoidal tracking, and optokinetic nystagmus. Vestibular tests include the detection and measurement of spontaneous nystagmus, Dix–Hallpike testing for positioning nystagmus, positional nystagmus testing, and caloric irrigations. Caloric irrigations usually are performed on one ear at a time, alternately using warm or cool stimuli. Simultaneous, bithermal stimulation and ice-cold stimulation are valuable in selected cases. The test may give useful information about peripheral and central abnormalities.

Caloric testing stimulates primarily the horizontal semicircular canal and gives little or no information about the function of the superior and posterior semicircular canals in most cases. The direction of gaze and plane of the head are of great importance in vestibular testing, especially when the semicircular canals are stimulated by rotation rather than thermal stimulus. For rotary testing, the response represents the combined effect of stimulating the sensory system of one semicircular canal while suppressing that of its counterpart on the other side of the body. Although this test does give some peripheral lateralizing information, it is especially informative about the integration of the vestibular signals in the brainstem (the central portion of the VOR). Rotational excitation and selective head position may be used to obtain information about the vertical semicircular canals which is difficult or impossible to deduce from caloric stimulation. Test interpretation relies on the knowledge that ampullofugal endolymphatic flow (away from the cupulae) produces nystagmus toward the opposite side in the horizontal

semicircular canal, whereas the opposite is true for the vertical canals. Rotational testing is not widely available in the United States. It allows measurement of eye movements with eyes opened or closed and permits quantification of the fast and slow phases, time of onset and duration, as well as other parameters. Although some centers use only horizontal leads, the use of both horizontal and vertical electrodes is preferable. ENG must be done under controlled conditions with proper preparation which includes avoidance of drugs (especially those active in the central nervous system). Even a small drug effect may cause alterations in the electronystagmographic tracing. The test is performed in several phases. These include calibration which assesses cerebellar function, gaze nystagmus, sinusoidal tracking, optokinetic nystagmus, spontaneous nystagmus, Dix–Hallpike testing, position testing, and caloric testing. The test may give useful information about peripheral and central abnormalities in the vestibular system. ENG/VNG measures the VOR whereas computerized dynamic posturography (CDP) measures not only the VOR but also VSR and other functions. Research suggests that CDP is also valuable in distinguishing organic from nonorganic dysequilibrium, an asset that is particularly valuable in some cases of alleged disability (7–11). Interpretation is complex. **Table 21.1** summarizes ENG/VNG findings and their meaning. ENG/VNG is especially helpful when a unilaterally reduced vestibular response is identified in conjunction with other signs of dysfunction in the same ear. In such cases, it provides strong support for a peripheral (eighth nerve or end organ) cause of balance dysfunction.

## VIDEONYSTAGMOGRAPHY

Although the older technique of measuring eye movements via changes in corneoretinal potential (ENG) is still in use, VNG has gained its popularity. In current practice, VNG is one of the essential components in recording eye movement and detecting spontaneous and induced nystagmus. Unlike ENG in which electrodes are used to gauge corneal–retinal potential changes, VNG utilizes a source of infrared light and binocular lenses combined with a video camera. It allows for visualization of multidirectional and torsional eye movement, and digital image processing measures eye movements accurately from the center of participant's pupils. This makes it possible to quantitatively measure the speed of the slow phase in different types of nystagmus, latency, saccade accuracy and velocity, and vestibular gain in ocular tracking and optokinetic nystagmus (12). Given the effectiveness in visualizing the direction of eye movement, VNG can be used for diagnosis of positional nystagmus such as benign paroxysmal positional vertigo (BPPV) (12). ENG is capable of similar information, but resolution is superior with VNG.

The use of VNG may be limited in patients with severe claustrophobia as the test requires patient to be placed in a dark and confined room while wearing tightly fitted goggles. This may induce anxiety and result in poor patient tolerance, making it challenging to complete the test. Additionally, VNG should be avoided in patients with significant palpebral ptosis, as ptosis can partially or completely obstruct the pupils, leading to inaccurate digital measurement of the eye movements. Other conditions such as degenerative retinopathies, diabetes, hypertensive retinopathies, and retinitis pigmentosa have the potential to affect the corneal–retinal potential, thereby altering the validity of the test results of ENG, but these conditions have little or no effect on VNG. Furthermore, the cost and availability of newer technology and equipment may pose challenges for patients in rural or medically underserved communities, limiting their access to VNG testing.

## DYNAMIC POSTUROGRAPHY

For approximately 50 years, platforms have been used to try to assess more complexly integrated functioning of the balance system. Static posture platforms with pressure were used to measure body sway while patients tried to maintain various challenging positions such as Romberg and Tandem Romberg maneuvers. Movement was measured with eyes closed and opened. The tests had many drawbacks including inability to separate proprioceptive function and to eliminate visual distortion. In 1972, Nasher (13) introduced a system

of dynamic posturography (DP) which has been developed into a test system which is now available commercially.

DP uses a computer-controlled moveable platform. In other words, both the platform and visual surround move, tracking the anterior–posterior sway of the patient. The visual surround and platform may operate together or independently. It is capable of creating visual distortion or totally eliminating visual cues. The platform can perform a variety of complex motions, and the patient's body sway is detected through pressure-sensitized strain gauges in each quadrant of the platform, which is believed to mimic the real-world scenario. In doing so, the test can isolate and quantify the use of perceptual information utilized for balance control. The typical sensory organization test (SOT) protocol requires patient to maintain balance during six test procedures and movement coordination through a variety of sudden platform movements. Balance strategies are assessed using visual, vestibular, and somatosensory integration with musculoskeletal movement coordination. As the result, DP provides a great deal of information about total balance function that cannot be obtained from tests such as ENG or VNG alone. DP provides a better window into patient's balance maintenance abilities during real-world situations.

## ROTARY CHAIR TESTING

Rotary chair testing helps identify whether dizziness is due to dysfunction in the inner ear or brain. Caloric testing (ENG/VNG) generally is considered the gold standard for identifying unilateral vestibular dysfunction. Rotary chair testing is the gold standard for detection of bilateral vestibular dysfunction. ENG/VNG is performed to evaluate most people with suspected labyrinthine dysfunction. Rotary chair testing is obtained when bilateral disease is suspected or when more sophisticated information is required. It evaluates the VOR and the central vestibular system. Rotational chair testing has no contraindications such as neck trauma, which is not the case with ENG/VNG. In rotary chair testing, rotation is computer controlled and extremely accurate. It is well-tolerated and even can be performed in children. Rotary chair testing has been used for decades, and there is extensive literature on the technique. In addition to bilateral semicircular canal paresis, common indications include equivocal or inconclusive ENG/VNG results, evaluation of vestibular compensation, ototoxicity management, and testing of special populations including children and handicapped individuals. Rotary chair testing assesses the integrity of VOR and suppression of that reflex. The tests are complementary. Unlike caloric testing, rotary chair testing stimulates both ears and vestibular organs simultaneously as the head rotates through a specific plane.

Caloric testing assesses the vestibular system at a frequency of only 0.003 Hz, but rotary chair testing assesses from 0.01 Hz through 0.64 Hz. Common rotary chair tests include sinusoidal harmonic acceleration (SHA), VOR suppression, and the velocity step test. Other subtests may include slow harmonic (sinusoidal) testing in darkness, high-velocity or high-frequency sinusoidal rotation, rotation with fixation on head-fixed targets to evaluate suppression, optokinetic after-nystagmus, tilted-axis rotation (OVAR), rotation with fixation on earth-fixed targets, and optokinetic testing. Rotary chair testing allows monitoring of the VOR over time, which is important because the phase abnormality and symmetry in VOR recover in some patients following vestibular injury.

## VESTIBULAR-EVOKED MYOGENIC POTENTIALS

Vestibular-evoked myogenic potential (VEMP) testing is based on the VCR between the saccule and the sternocleidomastoid muscle. The pathway is from the saccule to the inferior vestibular nerve to the lateral vestibular nucleus to the lateral vestibulo-spinal tract to cranial nerve XI to the sternocleidomastoid muscle. Cervical vestibular evoked myogenic potential (cVEMP) testing reflects the inferior vestibular nerve, and saccule reflects activity of the superior vestibular nerve and utricle. Amplitude asymmetry of 30%–47% or more is abnormal. VEMP may be abnormal in superior semicircular canal dehiscence, vestibular,

neuronitis, spinocerebellar, degeneration, multiple sclerosis, Ménière's syndrome, and other conditions. Responses may be augmented with Ménière's syndrome and absent or delayed with migraine. Clinically, the test is used most commonly for suspicion of superior semicircular canal dehiscence in which responses are evolved at 60–75 dB versus the 90–100 dB required in normal ears.

## IMAGING STUDIES

Brain and internal auditory canal imaging may be extremely valuable in documenting the nature and extent of physical abnormalities causing dizziness in selected cases and in establishing the organic basis of the equilibrium complaint. When CT, MRI, or MRA shows a definitive lesion within the vestibular pathway consistent with the individual's history, this information can be extremely helpful in developing appropriate plan of care. When these studies are negative, however, one cannot conclude that the dizziness is not organic in etiology. New dynamic imaging studies such as positron emission tomography (PET) and single-photon emission computed tomography (SPECT) may be helpful in some such cases, as may other techniques or brain mapping (including EEG) (14).

Vascular ultrasounds also may be extremely helpful in selected cases, especially in patients complaining of positional vertigo. For example, vertebral ultrasound can be performed with the neck in neutral, flexed, and extended and turned positions. The position that the patient associates with dizziness should always be tested. If positioning provokes symptoms that occur simultaneously with cessation of vertebral artery blood flow, and if the dizziness resolves when the position is changed and vertebral artery flow is restored, it is reasonable to diagnose vertebrobasilar insufficiency. In some cases, this problem can be resolved surgically, although noninvasive measures may be adequate.

In addition to cervical vascular compromise, dizziness can be caused by abnormalities in the cervical spine, especially in the first three cervical vertebrae. MRI of the cervical spine, spine X-ray, and/or cervical spine CT may be appropriate in selected patients.

Table 21.1 Interpretation of ENG

| Test | Finding | Description | Interpretation | Comments |
|---|---|---|---|---|
| Calibration | Ocular dysmetria (Calibration overshoot) | Greater than 50% of calibrations | Cerebellar of brainstem | *Caution*: Eyeblink artifact, alcohol intoxication |
| Gaze nystagmus | | Use 20° and/or 30° | | Test detects gaze nystagmus and paresis of ocular deviation |
| | Normal or end-point | Nystagmus at 40° or more, rarely at 30° | Normal | |
| | Vertical | | May be normal | Upward more common than downward. (See "Spontaneous Nystagmus") |
| | Vertical without associated horizontal gaze nystagmus | | Suggests midline or bilateral lesion in the upper pons or midbrain | Opiates and Demerol may cause vertical nystagmus |
| | Vertical upbeating | | Medulla, pons, or anterior vermis | May occur in metabolic derangements |
| | Vertical downbeating | | Usually caudal brainstem | May be enhanced by lateral gaze and may beat obliquely |
| | Rotary nystagmus | | CNS lesion | |
| | Bilateral, equal horizontal gaze nystagmus | Fast phase in direction of eye deviation. Intensity increased with increasing eye deviation (except congenital nystagmus) | Brainstem lesion or drug effect (especially barbiturates, diphenylhydantoin, and alcohol) | |
| | Bilateral, unequal horizontal gaze nystagmus | | Organic CNS pathology, probably *not* drug effect | |
| | Unilateral horizontal gaze nystagmus | | May be from intense spontaneous nystagmus (vestibular) | May elicit spontaneous nystagmus that has been suppressed. If there is spontaneous nystagmus in the same direction > 8° with eyes closed, then it is not a central sign |

*(Continued)*

Table 21.1 (Continued) Interpretation of ENG

| Test | Finding | Description | Interpretation | Comments |
|------|---------|-------------|----------------|----------|
| Periodic alternating nystagmus | | | CNS lesion, usually caudal brainstem | |
| Rebound nystagmus | | | CNS lesion, usually cerebellar | |
| Pendular nystagmus | | | Congenital or severe visual impairment | |
| Square wave jerks | | | If present with eyes opened, CNS lesion usually in cerebellar system | May be normal behind closed eyes, especially in anxious patient |
| Ocular myoclonus | | | CNS lesion, usually dentatorubral | Usually associated with chronic movements of the larynx and palate |
| Internuclear ophthal-moplegia | | | CNS lesion, usually medial longitudinal fasciculus | If unilateral, it is usually of vascular etiology; bilateral is associated with multiple sclerosis |
| Sinusoidal tracking | Saccadic pursuit | Saccadic eye jerks in the direction of stimulus movement, break up of smooth pursuit | Central oculomotor lesion usually involving the brainstem<br>May be caused by barbiturates | Enhanced gaze nystagmus may appear toward the extremes of the sinusoidal pattern<br>Usually associated with gaze nystagmus and bilateral gaze optokinetic diminution |
| Spontaneous nystagmus | | Recorded in vertical position with eyes closed and open | | |
| | Normal vertical | | May be normal | Occurs normally in ~8% with eyes closed, usually upbeating may be more intense than 10°/second |
| | Normal horizontal with eyes closed | | Normal | Occurs normally in 15%–30%, speed < 7° |
| | Normal horizontal eyes open | | "Normal" or functional | Only voluntary nystagmus |

(Continued)

Table 21.1 (Continued)

| Test | Finding | Description | Interpretation | Comments |
|------|---------|-------------|----------------|----------|
| | Vestibular | 1. "Jerks," with slow and fast phases<br>2. Primarily horizontal<br>3. Conjugate<br>4. Suppressed by visual fixation. Often enhanced by eye closure. Must be >7°/second | Usually is peripheral but may be central in the area of the vestibular nuclear complex | |
| | Congenital | 1. May be pendular or spikelike<br>2. May change with gaze or fixation distance<br>3. Eye closure direction or abolishes it<br>4. There is no oscillopsia<br>5. Convergence usually suppresses the nystagmus<br>6. Almost always horizontal | | On vertical gaze horizontal pendular component may disappear, but a vertical component rarely develops; makes vestibular and OKN very difficult to see |
| | Ocular or "fixation" noncongenital | May resemble congenital nystagmus | From chronic visual abuse, such as "miner's nystagmus" Pendular may also be caused by opiates | |
| | Central | Failure of fixation suppression; may be horizontal, vertical, or rotary | • Usually, brainstem or cerebellar | |
| | Convergence nystagmus | Jerk-type, course, disconjugate | • Usually, a dorsal midbrain lesion | |
| Optokinetic nystagmus (OKN) | | Slow phase in direction of movement, fast-phase refixation in opposite direction | • Normal | Larger stimulus pattern gives less variability; abnormalities must be present at both stimulus speeds; abnormality may be asymmetry (difference between the two directions) or bilateral diminution; vertical asymmetry is often more severe. Test should be done at two speeds |

(Continued)

Table 21.1 (Continued) Interpretation of ENG

| Test | Finding | Description | Interpretation | Comments |
|------|---------|-------------|----------------|----------|
| | Isolated or predominant vertical OKN abnormality | | • Indicates high midbrain lesion or upper pons, bilateral or midline; central oculomotor pathology<br>• Vertical OKN abnormality is rare from hemisphere lesions unless very diffuse | Slight OKN asymmetry may be normal (usually downbeating predominant)<br>Beware of eye blinks |
| | Horizontal OKN asymmetry | *Asymmetry*<br>1. Poorly formed—slow phase broken up by rapid jerks<br>2. Slow-phase speed asymmetry<br>This may be converted in some cases to poorly formed by increasing stimulus speed | | Greater than 8°/second nystagmus may appear to produce horizontal OKN asymmetry, as may strabismus, longstanding unilateral blindness, extraocular muscle paresis, and peripheral ocular pathology; horizontal OKN abnormality with normal gaze test usually indicates cerebral hemisphere lesion<br>Lateral lesions of pons and midbrain below the oculomotor nucleus cause OKN predominance away from the lesion. (Clinical usefulness is low.) In cerebral hemisphere lesions (generally temporal parietal or occipital), OKN abnormalities beat toward the side of the lesion |
| | Horizontal OKN abnormality with gaze nystagmus paresis | | • Usually indicates brainstem or cerebellar lesion | |

(Continued)

Table 21.1 (Continued)

| Test | Finding | Description | Interpretation | Comments |
|------|---------|-------------|----------------|----------|
| | Bilateral diminution | | • Bilateral or midline brainstem lesions or lack of cooperation | |
| Dix–Hallpike test | | No nystagmus or weak nystagmus with eyes closed | • Normal | Rapid movements from sitting to head-hanging and turned position for 30 seconds or duration of nystagmus up to $1\frac{1}{2}$ minutes<br>If longer, it is considered persistent; if positive, it is repeated to test fatigability; should be substantial decrease by third trial<br>Nystagmus is often rotary but measured on horizontal and vertical leads<br>Vertical is often greatest |
| | Classic response | *Classic response*<br>1. Latency of 0.5–8 seconds in most cases<br>2. Transient "paroxysmal" response, rapid crescendo in 2–10 seconds, then diminuendo<br>3. Dizziness often severe<br>4. Fatigability<br>*Additional characteristics:*<br>a. Hearing and calorics often normal<br>b. Usually, unilateral<br>c. Nystagmus usually downward pathologic ear | • Classic response is a peripheral sign, although some cerebellar lesions may produce a similar response | Much more common in patients > 55 years of age; posttraumatic dizziness, chronic middle ear infection, fistula, and idiopathic (benign) paroxysmal positional vertigo are associated with a classical response that may occasionally be seen following stapes surgery |

(Continued)

Table 21.1 (Continued) Interpretation of ENG

| Test | Finding | Description | Interpretation | Comments |
|------|---------|-------------|----------------|----------|
| | Nonclassical response | | • Nonlocalizing but is more likely to be central than is classical response | |
| Direction-changing nystagmus with eyes opened | | | • CNS pathology | |
| Position test | | Slow movement to various head positions (sitting, supine, head right, head left, right lateral, left lateral, head hanging) for 30 seconds each | | |
| | Positional nystagmus | Slow phase of < 7°/second, in position other than sitting eyes forward. Like spontaneous nystagmus (present head upright with eyes centered) but present in at least one other position or changing direction or intensity of a spontaneous nystagmus | • Idiopathic | |
| | Type IA | Nylen's classification (Aschan modification) I Persistent (at least 1 minute) (A) Type IA—direction changing (with different positions) | • Greater than 7°/second is pathologic but nonlocalizing, although IA tends toward central | Drugs may cause type IA, especially alcohol, barbiturates, and other sedatives, aspirin, and quinine |
| | Type IB | (B) Type IB—direction fixed | • IB tends toward peripheral | |
| | Type II | Transitory (gone within 1 minute) It is also known as "positioning" nystagmus | • Type II is usually a partially elicited "paroxysmal nystagmus" | |

Table 21.1  (Continued)

| Test | Finding | Description | Interpretation | Comments |
|---|---|---|---|---|
| Caloric test | | | | May be done with cold stimulus only or bithermal; bithermal widely practiced, with temperatures equally above and below body temperature (30° and 44°); maximum speed of slow component is measured |
| | Unilateral weakness | Compare right ear versus left ear Unilateral weakness is > 20% difference | • Peripheral sign involving primary vestibular fibers or end-organ. • Could include a vestibular nucleus lesion. | |
| | Directional preponderance | Compare right-beating versus left-beating responses Directional preponderance is > 30% difference | • Nonlocalizing | |
| | Bilateral weakness | *Bilateral weakness:* < 7°–10°/second | • Either bilateral peripheral pathology (such as ototoxicity) or central pathology involving the vestibuloocular arc reflex area. If central, optokinetic test is usually abnormal | Antihistamines, tranquilizers, and barbiturates may also decrease response |
| | Failure of fixation suppression | Test for suppression by visual fixation. Abnormal, if nystagmus with eyes open is equal to or greater than with eyes closed | • Unusually central lesion but may be caused by peripheral ocular pathology, contact lenses, or sedation (especially barbiturates) | |

*(Continued)*

Table 21.1 (Continued) Interpretation of ENG

| Test | Finding | Description | Interpretation | Comments |
|------|---------|-------------|----------------|----------|
| Simultaneous bilateral bithermal calorics | | Patient in 30° supine position, bilateral simultaneous 30° stimulation, then 44° stimulation 5 minutes later | | |
| | | Eye movement recorded for 30 seconds following irrigation. | | |
| | | Position if there are three beats of nystagmus in the most active 10-second period (correcting for pre-existing nystagmus) | | |
| | Type I | No nystagmus | • Type I—normal or symmetrically hyperactive or symmetrically hypoactive | |
| | Type II | Nystagmus in one direction with cold and opposite direction with warm | • Type II—usually hypoactive labyrinth; rarely hyperactive | |
| | Type III | Direction of nystagmus is constant | • Type III—usually vestibular abnormality but nonlocalizing | |
| | Type IV | Nystagmus with one temperature, but not the other | • Type IV—usually vestibular abnormality but nonlocalizing | |

*Abbreviation:* ENG, Electronystagmography.

## CT AND MRI STUDIES

In all patients with dizziness, imaging studies should be considered. In particular, MRI scan is an invaluable tool in detecting acoustic neuroma, other cerebellopontine angle tumors, multiple sclerosis, and advanced ischemia, as well as other conditions. Temporal bone CT may be helpful to detect not only middle ear disease but also cochleovestibular anomalies and, particularly, abnormalities in the cochlear aqueduct or vestibular aqueduct. High-resolution coronal temporal bone CT imaging also detect presence of superior semicircular canal dehiscence. Such anomalies have important diagnostic and therapeutic implications. If clinical presentation is concerning for vascular insufficiency, CT angiogram or MR angiogram may be performed to evaluate the patency of vasculature (15).

## EVOKED VESTIBULAR RESPONSE

Evoked vestibular response testing is analogous to brainstem auditory evoked testing. However, vestibular-evoked potentials are still not being used clinically. Current research indicates that this test is likely to be valuable in the near future, and clinical trials to assess its efficacy are already underway.

For selected patients, vestibular therapy exercises (short of a comprehensive, extended physical therapy program) can be extremely helpful. They usually are supervised by an otologist or audiologist. Such exercises have proven particularly effective for benign position paroxysmal vertigo (BPPV). Classically, such patients develop vertigo in the supine position when their heads are turned to one side, especially when their necks are extended so that the involved ear is below the horizontal. Usually, the onset of the vertigo and torsional nystagmus is delayed from 1 to 40 seconds. It usually disappears within 1 minute, but its intensity varies during the episode. Frequently, the vertigo is less intense if the patient assumes the position again immediately following resolution of symptoms. The etiology of BPPV usually is attributed to either cupulolithiasis (debris or otoconia from the utricle adherent to the cupula of the posterior semicircular canal, increasing gravity-induced sensitivity) or canalithiasis (debris or otoconia that are free floating in the endolymph of the posterior semicircular canal, causing endolymphatic fluid movements as they fall when the head is turned into the provoking position, thereby creating fluid movement that affects the cupula). The therapeutic approaches to BPPV involve either dislodging the debris embedded on the cupula and/or floating the debris out of the semicircular canal or habituating the response of the central nervous system to the positional vertigo. There are several different approaches, only a few of which will be summarized briefly here. Brandt–Daroff habituation exercises must be performed several times a day. The patient starts in the sitting position and is moved rapidly into the position that causes vertigo. The patient remains in that position until the vertigo stops, after which he/she sits up again. Sitting up frequently results in rebound vertigo. After remaining sitting for 30 seconds, the patient moves rapidly to the mirror image position on the opposite side for 30 seconds and then sits up. The sequence is repeated again until the vertigo diminishes. The exercises are repeated every 3 hours until the patient has two consecutive days without vertigo.

The Semont maneuver is based on a single treatment. The side of involvement is determined, and the patient is moved quickly into the position that causes dizziness, with the head turned into the plane of the posterior semicircular canal. This position is maintained for 2–3 minutes. The patient is then moved rapidly through the sitting position and then down into the opposite position, taking care to maintain alignment of the neck and head. If moving into the second position does not cause vertigo, the head is shaken abruptly a few times, theoretically to free the canal debris. This position is maintained for 5 minutes. The patient is then moved slowly to a seated position and must remain upright (including while asleep) for 48 hours. The provoking position must be avoided for a week.

The Epley maneuver is probably the most popular approach at present. It also theoretically moves the debris by placing the patient in the provoking position for 3–4 minutes. Then, the head is extended further and turned to the opposite position (the patient may be turned onto his/her side so that the head is turned toward the floor). This position is also held for 3–4 minutes. After sitting up slowly, the patient must remain upright for 48 hours and avoid the provoking position for at least 5–7 days. Epley has advocated using vibration over the mastoid during the procedure to help move the debris out of the region of the posterior semicircular canal. Most practitioners have achieved satisfactory results without the use of vibration.

Single treatment approaches like the Epley maneuver utilize Dix–Hallpike position. Habituation approaches generally do not depend on Dix–Hallpike positions. The Brandt–Daroff habituation exercises are summarized briefly. Methods advocated by Norre and DeWeerdt, and those of Norre and Becker, use specific movements to determine treatment positions and protocols that are individualized depending upon patients response (although the Dix–Hallpike positions may be included, as well, and are utilized routinely in the Brandt–Daroff method). The habituation exercises are similar in many ways to the Cawthorne–Cooksey exercises (and other protocols) that have proven useful for unilateral vestibular hypofunction.

For more specific information regarding these exercises and other approaches to vestibular rehabilitation, the interested reader is referred to the book *Vestibular Rehabilitation* by Susan Herdman which provides an excellent, practical, and well-referenced review of the topic.

## VIDEO HEAD IMPULSE TEST

As cited by Alhabib and Saliba, the HIT was described in 1988 by Curthoys and Halmagyi as a means of testing the VOR (16). This simple bedside test involves monitoring eye movements while the patient fixates on a stationary target and the head is rotated to the right or to the left. To minimize involvement of the oculomotor pathway, the patient's head is moved using small amplitude, high velocity, and high acceleration to study VOR of individual semicircular canals. In normal patients, the VOR effectively maintains the target image at the center of visual field by generating compensatory eye movement in an equal and opposite direction from the head movement, allowing the eye to appear stationary in space during multidirectional head movements. However, in patients with vestibular loss or hypofunction, the VOR fails to produce reflexive eye movement in the opposite direction of the head movement. Consequently, a quick catch-up saccade, either overt (visible) or covert (invisible), adjusts the eye back to the target after and during head movement, respectively (17). Since covert saccade begins during head movement, it cannot be detected by a naked eye.

In order to overcome the limitations of the bedside test in detecting covert saccades and providing a quantitative assessment of the vestibular–ocular reflex, the video HIT (vHIT) was developed. The vHIT uses a high-speed and high-resolution camera to measure head movements, VOR gain, latency, and peak velocity of saccades. VOR gain, calculated as the ratio of eye rotation to head movement, serves as an indicator of vestibular function. In individuals without vestibular abnormalities, VOR gain should equal 1. However, in cases of unilateral vestibular loss, the ipsilateral vestibular nerve fails to generate an equivalent neural response, resulting in disproportionate eye movement relative to the head velocity. As a result, VOR gain becomes significantly diminished, reflecting relative reduction in eye movement (18). Analysis of VOR asymmetry can aid in diagnosing vestibular hypofunction. If vHIT results are normal, caloric testing still may be necessary to exclude potential peripheral etiologies of vertigo (16).

## DYNAMIC IMAGING STUDIES

Although the value of new dynamic imaging studies such as PET and SPECT in patients with dizziness and tinnitus has not been fully clarified, it is important to be aware of these tests and their possible applications.

PET is a technique that permits imaging of the rates of biological processes, essentially allowing biochemical examination of the brains of patients *in vivo*. PET combines CT with a tracer kinetic assay method employing a radiolabeled biologically active compound (tracer) and a mathematical model describing the kinetics of the tracer as it is involved in a biological process. The tissue tracer concentration measurements needed by the model is provided by the PET scanner. A three-dimensional (3D) image of the anatomic distribution of the biological process is produced. The technique is feasible because four radio isotopes ($^{11}$C, $^{13}$N, $^{15}$O, and $^{18}$F) emit radiation that will pass through the body for external detection. Natural substrates can be labeled with these radio isotopes, preserving their biochemical integrity. Positrons are emitted from an unstable radio isotope, forming a stable new element of anatomic weight one less than the original isotope. The emitted positron eventually combines with an electron, forming positronium. Because a positron is essentially an anti-electron, the two annihilate each other, and their masses are converted to electromagnetic energy. This process emits two photons 180° apart, which can escape from the body and can be recorded by external detectors.

The value of PET in patients with dizziness and tinnitus has not been investigated as thoroughly as the value of other imaging modalities, including CT, MRI, and SPECT (discussed subsequently). However, as Jamison et al. (19) point out, PET adds another dimension to our understanding of the brain by demonstrating metabolic alterations. PET quantitates local tissue distribution of radio nucleotides that are distributed through the brain according to function. Commonly measured functions include local cerebral metabolism, cerebral blood flow, cerebral oxygen utilization, and cerebral blood volume. Langfitt et al. (20) compared CT, MRI, and PET in the study of brain trauma, which often results in dizziness and tinnitus. Although they studied only a small number of patients, they found that PET showed metabolic disturbances that extended beyond the structural abnormalities demonstrated by CT and MRI and missed by xenon-133 measurement of cerebral blood flow. Although much additional research is needed to determine the appropriate uses of PET and to interpret meaningfully the abnormalities observed, PET appears sensitive to dysfunctions that are not detected by more commonly available studies.

SPECT is also a form of emission tomography. It utilizes a technique that detects photons one at a time rather than in pairs like the photons detected with PET. SPECT also uses a radioactive tracer introduced intravenously. Because the photons are detected one at a time, in the presence of multiple photon emission, there is no simple spatial correlation. Therefore, the origin of photons in SPECT has to be traced using collimation, a process through which electromagnetic radiation is shaped into parallel beams. ECT provides images that are not nearly as sharp as transmission CT, and ECT images must be collected over a much longer period. Both static and dynamic SPECT studies may be performed. One particularly useful technique involves the use of technetium-99m HM-PAO (Tc-99m HM-PAO), a lipophilic chemical microsphere that crosses capillary walls freely. Within the brain, it is converted to a hydrophilic form that cannot leave the brain. Only a portion of the Tc-99m HM-PAO is converted, with the remainder diffusing back into the blood stream. The amount cleared by back diffusion depends on blood flow. As with PET, good studies on SPECT in dizziness and tinnitus are lacking. One study looked at the value of SPECT in assessing dizzy patients with suspected vascular etiology and found abnormalities in 15 of 18 patients. Significant alterations in cerebral blood flow were identified in the absence of any structural lesions identified by CT or MRI studies (21–23). Useful inferences can also be drawn from research on head injury. Abdel-Dayem et al. (24) compared Tc-99m HM-PAO SPECT with CT following acute head injury. SPECT has the following advantages: (1) It reflects profusion changes. (2) It was more sensitive than CT in demonstrating lesions. (3) It demonstrated lesions at an earlier stage than CT. (4) It was more helpful in separating lesions with favorable prognosis than those with unfavorable prognosis. Roper et al. (25) also compared Tc-99m HM-PAO SPECT with CT in 15 patients with acute closed head injury. They also found that SPECT can detect focal disturbances of cerebral blood flow that are not seen on CT. They observed that SPECT distinguished two types of contusions: those with decreased cerebral blood flow and those with cerebral blood flow equal to that of the surrounding brain. Bullock et al. (26) found SPECT useful in mapping blood–brain barrier defects (including delayed blood–brain barrier lesions) in 20 patients with acute cerebral contusions and four with acute subdural hematomas. Ducours et al. (27) found SPECT abnormalities on 9 out of 10 patients with normal transmission CT following craniofacial injury. Oder et al. (28) suggested that SPECT may help improve outcome prediction in patients with persistent vegetative state following severe head injury, and Morinaga et al. (29) used SPECT to demonstrate regional brain abnormalities in six patients with hyponatremia following head injury. The abnormalities observed on SPECT improved when the hyponatremia corrected.

Although extensive additional research and clinical experience are needed to clarify the roles of dynamic imaging studies, it appears likely that they may be useful to document abnormalities in patients with dizziness and/or tinnitus. The author (R.T.S.) has now had several patients in whom SPECT revealed the otherwise undetected organic basis for dizziness. A few cases involved posttraumatic dizziness, but others did not. For example, SPECT on a woman with episodic vertigo and normal ear function revealed a perfusion abnormality in the temporal lobe. Subsequent EEG confirmed an epileptic focus in this area, and her dizziness was controlled with antiseizure medication.

As Duffy observed, brain-imaging procedures, such as CT scan, PET, MR (nuclear magnetic resonance), and BEAM (brain electrical activity mapping), represent different windows upon brain and function. They provide separate but complimentary information (30).

## PERIPHERAL CAUSES

Vestibular disturbance may be suspected with a history of vertigo described as motion, particularly if associated with tinnitus, hearing loss, or fullness in the ear. However, even severe peripheral disease of the eighth cranial nerve or labyrinth may produce vague unsteadiness rather than vertigo, especially when caused by a slowly progressive condition such as acoustic neuroma, as mentioned earlier. Vascular loop compression (usually by the anterior inferior cerebellar artery) and internal auditory canal stenosis may cause the same symptoms. Similarly, central disorders such as brainstem vascular occlusion may produce true rotary vertigo typically associated with the ear. Therefore, clinical impressions must be substantiated by thorough evaluation and testing (31).

One of the most common causes of peripheral vertigo is BPPV. In BPPV, the vertigo attack often occurs briefly with movement of the head due to displacement of calcium-carbonate crystals, or otoconia, which can contact the cupula of the ampulla of a semicircular and cause an aberrant neuronal discharge that results in vertigo. The posterior semicircular canal is most often the source of the difficulty. Classically, there is a slight delay in onset, and if the maneuver is repeated immediately after the vertigo subsides, subsequent vertiginous responses are less severe. In general, BPPV is not associated with deafness or tinnitus.

Therapy for this condition is symptomatic. The initial step in managing BPPV is by performing repositioning maneuvers in an attempt to dislodge otoconia from the otolithic membrane. Therefore, repositioning maneuvers and vestibular exercises help more than prescribing medications for symptom control especially in patients with posterior canal involvement. When the condition is disabling, it may be cured surgically by dividing all or part of the vestibular nerve. In most cases, hearing can be preserved. If the problem can be localized with certainty to one posterior semicircular canal, an alternate surgical procedure called singular neurectomy may be considered.

Another type of vertigo associated with abnormality in the vestibule is Ménière's. The vertigo is classically of sudden onset, relatively brief in duration, and reoccurs in paroxysmal attacks. During the attack, it generally is accompanied by an ocean-roaring tinnitus, fullness in the ear, and fluctuating hearing loss. Occasionally, there may be some residual imbalance between attacks, but this does not happen often. Similar symptoms may accompany inner ear syphilis and certain cases of diabetes mellitus, hyperlipoproteinemia, or hypothyroidism. The symptoms are caused by endolymphatic hydrops that distends Reissner's membrane in the cochlea.

In some cases, vertigo and imbalance can be elicited by exposure to loud noises or alterations in pressure within the affected ear. These symptoms also can occur in superior semicircular canal dehiscence. Thus, they are most diagnostic for Ménière's syndrome.

This syndrome is characterized by the creation of a third window in the temporal bone connecting the superior semicircular canal with the middle cranial fossa. The presence of this osseous defect can give rise to episodes of vertigo and oscillopsia (32). Examples of such triggers include listening to loud music, attending concerts, encountering certain auditory frequencies, and performing actions like blowing the nose or straining. Patients affected by this syndrome may also experience symptoms of autophony, hyperacusis, pulsatile tinnitus, and hearing loss. For patients with severe, debilitating symptoms, surgical repair of the bony dehiscence can be considered as a potential treatment option.

Certain viruses such as herpes classically produce vertigo by involving the peripheral endorgan or nerve. The attack usually is of sudden onset associated with tinnitus and hearing loss, and it subsides spontaneously. In the absence of tinnitus and hearing loss, the virus is assumed to have attacked the nerve itself, and this condition is called vestibular neuritis. Certain toxins readily produce vertigo. Well-known vestibular toxins include aminoglycosides, platinum-based chemotherapies, organophosphates, heavy metals, and carbon monoxide poisoning.

Whenever a patient complains of vertigo and there is evidence of chronic otitis media, it is essential to determine whether there is presence of a cholesteatoma that is eroding into the semicircular canal and causing the vertigo. Vertigo can be present also with certain types of otosclerosis that involve the inner ear. In all such cases, the specific cause of the vertigo should be determined, and whenever possible, proper therapy based on the specific cause should be instituted. Perilymph fistula as a cause of vertigo is particularly amenable to surgical treatment, as are autoimmune inner ear disease, hypoglycemia, hypothyroidism, allergy, and other causes.

## NERVOUS SYSTEM INVOLVEMENT AND OTHER CAUSES

Vertigo involving the central nervous system is an urgent problem and must be ruled out in every case, especially in those cases in which it is associated with other symptoms outside the ear.

Certain symptoms strongly suggest that the cause of the vertigo must be sought in the central nervous system. If spontaneous nystagmus is present and persists, the physician should look for associated neurological signs such as falling and papilledema. This is especially true if the condition has persisted for a long time, and if the nystagmus is not horizontal and directional. If the rotary vertigo is associated with loss of consciousness, the physician should suspect also that the vertigo originates in the central nervous or cardiovascular system. The association of intense vertigo with localized headache makes it mandatory to rule out a central lesion.

Among the common central nervous system causes of vertigo are (a) vascular crisis, (b) tumors of the posterior fossa, (c) multiple sclerosis, (d) epilepsy, (e) encephalitis, and (f) concussion.

The vertigo in a vascular crisis is of sudden onset and generally is accompanied by nausea and vomiting as well as tinnitus and deafness. In many instances, there is involvement of other cranial nerves. In a special type of vascular crisis such as Wallenberg's syndrome, there is thrombosis of the posterior–inferior cerebellar artery or vertebral artery, resulting in sudden overwhelming vertigo, dysphagia, dysphonia, and Horner's syndrome, as well as other neurological findings. The episode often is so severe that death may supervene.

It is also possible to have a much more discrete vascular defect in the vestibular labyrinth without an involvement of the cochlea. This usually results in an acute onset of severe vertigo. Recovery is rather slow, and the vertigo may persist as postural imbalance. The nystagmus may subside, but unsteadiness and difficultly in walking may continue much longer.

A still milder form of vascular problem related to vertigo occurs in hypotension and vasomotor instability. These people have recurrent brief episodes of imbalance and instability, particularly after a sudden change of position such as suddenly arising from tying their shoelaces or turning quickly. Histamine sensitivity may play an important role in this type of vertigo, especially when migraine attacks also are present.

In multiple sclerosis, vertigo is commonly a symptom, but it is rarely severe enough to confuse the picture with other involvement of the vestibular pathways. In epilepsy, vertigo occasionally may be a premonitory sensation before an epileptic attack, but unconsciousness usually accompanies the attack and helps to distinguish the condition.

Epilepsy and migraine may also be associated with dizziness—so can many toxins (ingested, inhaled, and transdermal). A complaint of vertigo in postconcussion syndrome is extremely common. The vertigo usually is associated with movement of the head or the body, severe headache, and marked hypersensitivity to noise and vibration. The patients usually are jittery, tense, and very touchy.

Of special interest to the otologist is the vertigo that sometimes is associated with a lesion of the posterior cranial fossa and particularly with an acoustic neuroma. It is a standing rule in otology that when a patient complains of true vertigo, an acoustic neuroma must be ruled out. This is especially true when the vertigo is accompanied by a hearing loss or tinnitus in one ear. Vertigo is not always a symptom in all posterior fossa lesions, but when it occurs, a number of simple tests help to establish the possibility that a tumor is present.

Other occasional causes of vertigo are encephalitis, meningitis, direct head injuries, and toxic reactions to alcohol, tobacco, and other drugs such as streptomycin, as well as many other conditions.

Not all vertigo is of pathological origin. Regardless of vestibular disease, the number of hair cells in the vestibular system decreases with age (18). Aging also leads to degeneration of the vestibular ganglion and neuronal connections of the otolith organs and semicircular canals, contributing to overall vestibular hypofunction (33). In the central nervous system, there is gradual atrophy of neuronal mass in the brainstem, cerebellum, thalamus, and vestibular cerebral cortical circuits. When combined with musculoskeletal weakness and visual impairment, as well as diminished dexterity, patients become more susceptible to falls and experience increased morbidity and mortality.

This inevitably progressive decline in the vestibular system can have multifactorial causes, and the supportive (and preventative) care (including expert vestibular and fall-prevention therapy) is often the optimal management approach.

## CERVICAL VERTIGO

Cervical vertigo may be due to muscle spasm compromising neck motion or interfering with the perception of orientation of the neck, vertebral artery compression by osteophytes, or direct compression of the spinal cord. Interestingly, one-half of the proprioceptive receptors for the vestibular spinal tracts are located in the deep cervical musculature, with the rest being in the joint capsules of cervical vertebrae one to three (C1–C3). A majority of the proprioceptive information required for maintaining equilibrium comes from the muscle and joint capsule receptors. Whiplash and other spinal injury affect the output from these receptors, giving the brain a false impression of the neck's orientation in space. This information conflicts with information from elsewhere in the balance system, and the resulting confusion is cervical vertigo.

Basilar artery compression syndrome is another condition associated with head motion, particularly neck extension. It is due to compression of the basilar artery with resultant interference with blood flow to the brainstem. This diagnosis cannot be made with certainty without objective confirmation through arteriography or other tests.

Carotid sinus syndrome and psychic disturbances frequently produce vertigo that may be confused with vertigo of vestibular origin. Taking a careful history and testing the carotid sinus make it possible to distinguish these conditions.

## HEARING IMPAIRMENT AND DIZZINESS

To date, balance is known to be achieved from intricate integration of visual stimuli, somatosensation, and vestibular function. However, a recent study by Campos et al. suggests potential added impact of hearing in balance (34).

This recent suggestion is derived from the idea of close anatomic and physiologic relationship between hearing and vestibular organs sharing similar mechanoreceptors. Consequently, it is postulated that the decline in hearing may be associated with the functional loss of vestibular system (35). However, the extent of this association between hearing and balance and the assessment of balance enhancement obtainable through the utilization of sound amplification devices merit further comprehensive investigation.

## TREATMENT

Dizziness of central etiology will not be discussed in detail. In general, when dizziness is caused by cerebral, cerebellar, or brainstem contusion, it is associated with other neurologic problems and is difficult to treat. The outlook for dizziness caused by vestibular injury is better.

Many medications are helpful in controlling peripheral vertigo. Meclizine is among the most common. It causes drowsiness in many people, but it is often effective in controlling vertigo. Scopolamine, administered through a transdermal patch, is also effective in controlling dizziness of labyrinthine etiology.

However, its side effects limit its use in many patients who are bothered especially by mouth dryness and dilation of the pupils causing blurred vision. Diazepam is also effective in suppressing vertigo, but long-term use of this potentially habit-forming drug should be avoided when possible. Prochlorperazine also helps many patients, sometimes producing good clinical improvement with low doses of 5–10 mg once in the evening. In hydrops, diuretic therapy with hydrochlorothiazide decreases vertigo, stabilizes hearing, and decreases fullness and fluctuation in many patients.

Patients with positional vertigo present special problems. It is helpful to distinguish BPPV from cervical vertigo. BPPV occurs when the patient's head is turned in a certain position. Typically, vertigo is induced when the patient rolls to one side in bed. Typically, ENG shows a short delay before onset of nystagmus, and the severity of nystagmus decreases with repeat testing. BPPV is generally not helped by medications such as Meclizine and

Diazepam. Vestibular exercises which provoke vertigo and develop compensatory pathways and suppression are preferable (**Table 21.2**).

Cervical vertigo usually is accompanied by limitation of neck motion and tenderness. Turning the neck into certain positions causes dizziness, and symptoms can sometimes even be provoked by pressure over certain tender points in the neck or over the greater occipital nerve. Many treatments have been suggested for cervical vertigo. However, cervical manipulation and physical therapy generally produce the best results.

If dizziness is caused by a perilymph fistula, and if the patient seeks medical attention promptly, a short period of bed rest may be the first line of treatment. If the symptoms persist after 5 days of bed rest, or if they have been present for a long period of time before the diagnosis is made, surgical repair is warranted. This is accomplished with local anesthesia through the external auditory canal. The perilymph leak in the oval window or round window (or both) is repaired. Because of the hydrodynamics of the ear, the incidence of recurrent fistula formation is high, and the risks of permanent sensorineural hearing loss, tinnitus, and disequilibrium are substantial.

## PHYSICAL THERAPY

The value of physical therapy in patients with balance disorders increased over the past 15 years preceding the publication of the edition. It is useful in patients who have failed conventional treatment and in those who have persistent minor equilibrium problems after partially successful treatment. Often, physical therapy can be utilized in conjunction with medical and the treatment for symptom improvement. Due to the complexity of vestibular disorder, physical therapy for balance disorders is quite specialized. The physical therapy team must have considerable interest and expertise in balance disorders, special equipment for balance rehabilitation, and willingness to devote substantial energy and resources to balance rehabilitation. Most physical therapy departments do not have experience and expertise in this problem, and their results with patients having balance disorders are not encouraging. However, when a trained team is involved, it can be extremely beneficial in minimizing the risk of fall, improving gait and balance, and thus enhancing the patient's quality of life. Such therapy is useful not only in patients with vestibular disorders but also in patients with central disequilibrium, and it is often the only help we have to offer for that population.

## OCCUPATIONAL THERAPY

Both physical therapy and occupational therapy fall within rehabilitative sciences and share many similarities. However, each approach carries distinct methods when addressing patient's balance disorders. While physical therapy utilizes an exercise-based approach to alleviate vestibular evoked central and other balance dysfunctions, occupational therapy focuses on modifying daily activities and the external environment to reduce the physical and psychosocial impact of living with dizziness. This is achieved through careful analysis of the patient's daily routine, conducting screening to identify potential symptom triggers, and evaluating the risk of falls at home and/or in the workplace. The ultimate goal of occupational therapy is to facilitate appropriate changes in lifestyle or environment that optimize the patient's ability to resume daily activities.

When used appropriately, occupational therapy, in addition to physical therapy, can provide comprehensive care in improving individual's quality of life. Thus, understanding of the role of occupational therapy and appropriate referral are essential to providing patient care.

## SURGERY

Most vertigo is managed predominantly conservatively. If medical treatments for peripheral vertigo fail, several surgical approaches may be considered. For endolymphatic hydrops, endolymphatic sac decompression provides relief of dizziness in ~70% of people. Despite the 30% failure rate, it is appropriate in selected cases. Vestibular nerve section is a more definitive procedure. This may be performed by entering the posterior fossa through the mastoid or just behind the sigmoid sinus. The eighth nerve is divided, preserving cochlear fibers, and sectioning the vestibular division of the eighth nerve. The author's experience parallels that of other authors reporting success rates > 90% with this procedure. If there is no usable hearing, the entire eighth nerve can be divided. Interestingly, this procedure does not appear to improve the success rate substantially. Failures are probably due to

Table 21.2 Vestibular exercises (Cawthorne's exercises)

Aims of exercise

1. To loosen up the muscles of the neck and shoulders, to overcome the protective muscular spasm and tendency to move "in one piece."
2. To train movement of the eyes, independent of the head.
3. To practice balancing in everyday situations with special attention to developing the use of the eyes and the muscle senses.
4. To practice head movements that cause dizziness and thus gradually overcome the disability.
5. To become accustomed to moving about naturally in daylight and in the dark.
6. To encourage the restoration of self-confidence and easy spontaneous movement.

All exercises are started in exaggerated slow time and gradually progress to more rapid time. The rate of progression from the bed to sitting and then to standing exercises depends upon the dizziness in each individual case.

(A) Sitting position—without arm rests

    1. Eye exercises—at first slow, then quick.

        a. Up and down.
        b. Side to side.
        c. Repeat (a) and (b), focusing on finger at arm's length.

    2. Head exercises—head movements at first slow, then quick.
    3. Shrug shoulders and rotate, 20 times.
    4. Bend forward and pick up objects from the ground, 20 times.
    5. Rotate head and shoulders slowly, then fast, 20 times.
    6. Rotate head, shoulders, and trunk with eyes open, then closed, 20 times.

(B) Standing

    7. Repeat 1.
    8. Repeat 2.
    9. Repeat 5.
    10. Change from a sitting position to standing position, with eyes open, then shut.
    11. Throw ball from hand to hand (above eye level).
    12. Throw ball from hand to hand under knees.
    13. Change from sitting to standing and turn around in between.
    14. Repeat 6.

(C) Walking

    15. Walk across room with eyes open, then closed, 10 times.
    16. Walk up and down slope with eyes open, then closed, 10 times.
    17. Do any games involving stopping, or stretching and aiming, such as bowling, shuffleboard, etc.
    18. Stand on one foot with eyes open, then closed.
    19. Walk with one foot in front of the other with eyes open, then closed.

disequilibrium produced by a lesion more central in the vestibular pathway or located elsewhere in the vestibular system altogether (the other ear). Despite all efforts, it is not possible to identify such conditions in all patients prior to surgery.

Occasionally, it is impossible to determine which ear is responsible for dizziness, especially if there are signs of abnormality bilaterally. In such cases, bilateral medical labyrinthectomy is possible. This procedure takes advantage of the ototoxicity of streptomycin. Patients must be selected carefully (36), and the procedure must be carefully controlled. When bilateral labyrinthectomy is complete, patients generally adapt well so long as they have visual cues. However, they are not able to function in total darkness.

## VESTIBULAR IMPLANTS

Reduction or complete loss of bilateral vestibular function results in postural instability, an unsteady gait, disequilibrium, oscillopsia, and visual impairment. Surprisingly, the prevalence of bilateral vestibular hypofunction (BVH) is higher than previously recognized. According to the United States National Health Interview Survey conducted in 2008, 28 out of every 100,000 U.S. adults are affected by severe-to-profound BVH (37). Approximately 1.8 million adults worldwide were diagnosed with severe BVH (12). The absence of vestibular reflex imposes debilitating limitations in performing daily activities, requiring conscious effort to walk without falling, and resulting in a higher socioeconomic burden, including unemployment.

The vestibular implant is an exciting new advancement designed to restore the vestibular reflex in patients with BVH that is currently undergoing clinical trials (38). To date, vestibular implants have demonstrated surprising adaptation capabilities to artificial vestibular signals. The components of the vestibular implant are structured similarly to those in cochlear implants. It consists of an external motion sensor and processor anchored to the skull, which translates mechanical multidimensional motion into an electrical signal. Electrical pulses are delivered to the branches of the vestibular nerve using three stimulating electrodes, selected from a total of nine electrodes implanted in the three semicircular canals. An additional reference electrode is utilized. The generated signal is then transmitted to the brain via electrodes implanted in the vestibular organ. The encoding of the rotational velocity of the head movement in 3D space is achieved by modulating the pulse rates and amplitudes of the stimulation through the electrodes. The stimulation settings are adjusted as necessary to optimize the strength and selectivity of vestibular nerve branch stimulation during device activation and subsequent testing sessions. This adjustment is guided by the speed and direction of the perceived head motion and reflex head and eye movements. Although the vestibular implant is still in the development phase, the release of a functional product into the commercial market could provide life-altering improvement in the quality of life for many patients suffering from bilateral vestibular dysfunction.

## SPECIAL CONSIDERATIONS IN INDUSTRY

Tinnitus and especially vertigo present special problems in industry. They are both usually subjective complaints that may be difficult to document objectively. Tinnitus is common but rarely disabling. It may be quite disturbing to some individuals. However, only in rare cases is it severe enough to interfere with the ability to work or even to interfere very much with quality of life on a daily basis. There are exceptions, of course.

However, vertigo and other conditions of disequilibrium may be disabling, particularly for people working in hazardous jobs. A person who loses his/her balance even momentarily may be injured or injure others if the person is working around sharp surfaces, rotating equipment, driving a forklift, or working on ladders or scaffolding. There are many other examples of occupations that are not possible for people with disequilibrium disorders. The problem is even worse in conditions that typically cause intermittent severe disequilibrium, such as Ménière's syndrome. Our inability to test the balance system thoroughly makes it impossible to disprove a worker's contention that he has spells of dizziness. For example, if a worker is struck in the head while performing his job and claims that he has intermittent "dizzy spells" afterwards, even if he has a normal videonystagmogram, his assertion may be true. Even if malingering is suspected, in the absence of objective proof, if a physician contests the claim and declares him fit to return to work, both the physician and the industry may incur substantial liability if the worker suffers a period of disequilibrium and seriously injures himself or other workers. Considerable research is needed to develop more sophisticated techniques of assessing equilibrium despite recent advances (8–11, 13).

## CLASSIFICATION

Dizziness and especially vertigo can be very disabling symptoms and are often accompanied by nausea, vomiting, anxiety, headache, and other complaints. Symptoms may be constant, occur in episodic "attacks," frequently without warning, or may be constant with exacerbations. Some findings on clinical examination may be entirely objective, such as a severe spontaneous nystagmus, whereas others may be entirely feigned, for example, an alleged posttraumatic ataxia of gait. Many others fall between these extremes. Clinical and laboratory assessments are used to establish data that determine impairment and disability classification. Organizing the history, physical and laboratory findings help simplify and clarify this process. However, the processes of classifying impairment should be performed in accordance with the American Medical Association (AMA) Guides to the Evaluation of Permanent Impairment using the most current update as discussed in Chapter 43.

## SYMPTOMS ELICITED BY HISTORY

1. No complaint of dizziness/unsteadiness.
2. Mild dizziness, does not interfere substantially with daily activities.
3. Mild-to-moderate dizziness, interferes with some activities but they can be resumed.
4. Moderate dizziness, interferes with many activities, but important activities can usually be accomplished with effort and with lifestyle adjustments.
5. Severe dizziness, interferes with most activities. Unable to drive or ambulate without assistance.
6. Profound dizziness, bedridden, or wheelchair-dependent.

## SIGNS ON PHYSICAL EXAMINATION

1. None.
2. Mild unsteadiness with reduced visual or proprioceptive input.
3. Paroxysmal positioning nystagmus or moderate unsteadiness with reduced visual or proprioceptive input.
4. Staggering when walking with the eyes closed.
5. Inability to stand or walk without the assistance of another individual, even with eyes open.

## LABORATORY TEST RESULTS

Laboratory test results correlate well with, and indeed are the primary measure of, impairment of function, but they may not correlate well with disability. This is especially true if the brain and related structures are intact, and if the onset of the impairment occurred months or years prior to the evaluation.

Nevertheless, laboratory test results are usually helpful in determining whether there is a physical basis for the individual's complaints.

In correlating symptoms with laboratory tests, it is useful to rate the overall results of the tests as follows:

1. Normal.
2. Mildly impaired test results.
3. Moderately impaired test results.
4. Markedly impaired test results.
5. Complete loss of function on testing.
6. Consistency between history, examination, and test results that is not in keeping with organic etiology.
7. Inconsistency between history, examination, and test results that is not in keeping with organic etiology.

The outcome of the symptoms evaluation, the physical signs, and the laboratory test results should be correlated, with emphasis on the validated symptoms, that is, those confirmed by the history, physical findings, and the results of laboratory tests, as best representing the subject's true state of disability.

## CONSISTENCY

1. Consistency between history, symptoms, physical examination, and laboratory tests.
2. Inconsistency between history, symptoms, physical examination, and laboratory tests.

## CONCLUSION

Although dizziness is a common and vexing problem, it is not hopeless. The clinician should search diligently for the etiology in every patient with dysequilibrium. If we are enthusiastic about evaluating and treating dizzy patients and assume that we will be able to find a treatable cause (until proven otherwise), that assumption will prove right surprisingly often. In virtually all cases, patients feel better following comprehensive evaluation. Under the best of circumstances, a treatable etiology is found, and their dizziness is eliminated. Under the worst circumstances, at least they understand that "no stone has been left unturned" and that they have nothing serious or life-threatening that is responsible for their problem. Physical therapy, medications, and sometimes surgery can usually be used to at least improve each patient's ability to function, if not to eliminate symptoms altogether. Dizziness is a common problem that is challenging to both patients and physicians, and it is important for all of us to remember that every patient can be helped at least to some extent if we try hard enough.

# REFERENCES

1. Sataloff J, Sataloff RT, Lueneberg W. Tinnitus and vertigo in healthy senior citizens with a history of noise exposure. Am J Otol 1987; 8(2):87–89.

2. U.S. Department of Health and Human Services. Public Health Services. National Center for Health Statistics Series 13, No. 56, 1978.

3. Jenkins HA, Furman JM, Gulya AJ, Honrubia V, Linthicum FH, Mirko A. Dysequilibrium of aging. Otolaryngol Head Neck Surg 1989; 100:272–282.

4. Centers for Disease Control and Prevention, National Center for Injury Prevention and Control. Surveillance report of traumatic brain injury-related emergency department visits, hospitalizations, and deaths—United States, 2014. Atlanta (GA): Centers for Disease Control and Prevention; 2019.

5. Gibson WPR. Vertigo associated with trauma. In: Dix MR, Hood JD, eds. Vertigo. Chichester, New York: John Wiley & Sons, 1984.

6. Mandel S, Sataloff RT, Schapiro S. Minor Head Trauma: Assessment, Management and Rehabilitation. New York, NY: Springer-Verlag, 1993.

7. Goebel JA, Sataloff RT, Hanson JM, Nashner LM, Hirshout DS, Sokolow CC. Posturographic evidence of nonorganic sway patterns in normal subjects, patients and suspected malingers. Am Acad Otolaryngol Head Neck Surg 1997; 117(4):293–302.

8. Cevette MJ, Puetz B, Marion MS, Wertz MS, Wertz ML, Muenter MD. A physiologic performance on dynamic posturography. Otolaryngol Head Neck Surg 1995; 112:678–688.

9. Coogler CE. Using computerized dynamic posturography to accurately identify non-organic response patterns for posture control. Neurol Rep 1996; 20:12–21.

10. Hart CV, Rubin AG. Medico-legal aspects of neurotology. Otolaryngol Clin North Am 1996; 29(3):503–516.

11. Krempl GA, Dobie RA. Evaluation of posturography in the detection of malingering subjects. Am J Otol 1998; 19:619–627.

12. Ganança MM, Caovilla HH, Ganança FF. Electronystagmography versus videonystagmography. Braz J Otorhinolaryngol. 2010 May–Jun; 76(3):399–403. doi: 10.1590/S1808-86942010000300021. PMID: 20658023; PMCID: PMC9442181.

13. Nasher LN. A model describing vestibular detection of body sway motion. Acta Otolaryngol 1971; 72:429–436.

14. Herdman SJ. Vestibular Rehabilitation. Philadelphia, PA: F.A. Davis, 1994:1–377.

15. Fakhran S, Alhilali L, Branstetter BF 4th. Yield of CT angiography and contrast-enhanced MR imaging in patients with dizziness. AJNR Am J Neuroradiol. 2013 May; 34(5):1077–1081. doi: 10.3174/ajnr.A3325. Epub 2012 Oct 25. PMID: 23099499; PMCID: PMC7964658.

16. Alhabib SF, Saliba I. Video head impulse test: a review of the literature. Eur Arch Otorhinolaryngol. 2017 Mar; 274(3):1215–1222. doi: 10.1007/s00405-016-4157-4. Epub 2016 Jun 21. PMID: 27328962.

17. Janky KL, Patterson JN, Shepard NT, Thomas MLA, Honaker JA. Effects of device on video head impulse test (vHIT) gain. J Am Acad Audiol. 2017 Oct; 28(9):778–785. doi: 10.3766/jaaa.16138. PMID: 28972467; PMCID: PMC5749241.

18. Anson ER, Bigelow RT, Carey JP, Xue QL, Studenski S, Schubert MC, Agrawal Y. VOR gain is related to compensatory saccades in healthy older adults. Front Aging Neurosci. 2016 Jun 24; 8:150. doi: 10.3389/fnagi.2016.00150. PMID: 27445793; PMCID: PMC4919329.

19. Jamison D, Alavi A, Jolles P, Chawluk J, Reivich M. Positron emission tomography in the investigation of central nervous systems disorders. Radiol Clin North Am 1988; 26(5):1075–1088.

20. Langfitt TW, Obrist WD, Alavi A et al. Computerized tomography, magnetic resonance imaging, and positron emission tomography in the study of brain trauma. Preliminary Observations. J Neurosurg 1986; 64(5):760–767.

21. Boni F, Fattori B, Piragine F, Bianchi R. Use of SPECT in the diagnosis of vertigo syndromes of vascular nature. Acta Otorhinolaryngol Ital 1990; 10(6):539–548.

22. Laubert A, Luska G, Schober O, Hesch RD. Die digitale Subtraktionsangiographie (DSA) und die Jod-123-Amphetamin-Szintigraphie (IMP-SPECT) in der Diagnostik von akuten und chronischen Innenohrschwerhörigkeiten [Digital subtraction angiography and iodine 123 amphetamine scintigraphy (IMP-SPECT) in the diagnosis of acute and chronic inner ear hearing loss]. HNO 1987; 35(9):372–375.

23. Tuohimaa P, Aantaa E, Toukoniitty K, Makela P. Studies of vestibular cortical areas with short-living 1502 isotopes. ORL J Otorhinolaryngol Relat Spec 1987; 45(6):315–321.

24. Abdel-Dayem HM, Sadek SA, Kouris K et al. Changes in cerebral perfusion after acute head injury: comparison of CT with Tc-99m HM-PAO SPECT. Radiology 1987; 165(1):221–226 [published erratum appears in Radiology 1988; 167(2):582].

25. Roper SN, Mena I, King WA et al. An analysis of cerebral blood flow in acute closed-head injury using Tc-99m HM-PAO SPECT and computed tomography. J Nucl Med 1991; 32(9):1684–7.

26. Bullock R, Statham P, Patterson J, Wyper D, Hadley D, Teasdale E. The time course of vasogenic oedema after focal human head injury—evidence from SPECT mapping of blood brain barrier defects. Acta Neurochir Suppl 1990; 51:286–288.

27. Ducours JL, Role C, Guillet J, San Galli F, Caix P, Wynchank S. Cranio-facial trauma and cerebral SPECT studies using N-isopropyliodo-amphetamine (123I). Nucl Med Commun 1990; 11(5):361–367.

28. Oder W, Goldenberg G, Podreka I, Deecke L. HM-PAO-SPECT in persistent vegetative state after head injury: prognostic indicator of the likelihood of recovery? Intensive Care Med 1991; 17(3):149–153.

29. Morinaga K, Hayaski S, Matsumoto Y et al. CT and 123I-IMP SPECT findings of head injuries with hyponatremia. No To Shinkei 1991; 43(9):891–894.

30. Duffy FH, Burchfiel JD, Lombroso CT. Brain electrical mapping (BEAM): A method of extending the clinical utility of EEG and evoked potential data. Ann Neurol 1979; 5:309–321.

31. Sataloff RT, Hughes M, Small A. Vestibular "Masking": a diagnostic technique. Laryngoscope 1987; 7:885–886.

32. Palma Diaz M, Cisneros Lesser JC, Vega Alarcón A. Superior semicircular canal dehiscence syndrome - diagnosis and surgical management. Int Arch Otorhinolaryngol. 2017 Apr; 21(2):195–198. doi: 10.1055/s-0037-1599785. PMID: 28382131; PMCID: PMC5375705.

33. Arshad Q, Seemungal BM. Age-related vestibular loss: current understanding and future research directions. Front Neurol. 2016 Dec 19; 7:231. doi: 10.3389/fneur.2016.00231.PMID: 28066316; PMCID: PMC5165261. [published erratum appears in: Front Neurol. 2017 Aug 21;8:391].

34. Campos J, Ramkhalawansingh R, Pichora-Fuller MK. Hearing, self-motion perception, mobility, and aging. Hear Res 2018; 369(Nov), 42–55. doi:10.1016/j.heares.2018.03.025

35. Zarei H, Norasteh AA, Lieberman LJ, Ertel MW, Brian A. Balance control in individuals with hearing impairment: a systematic review and meta-analysis. Audiol Neurotol 2023; doi: 10.1159/000531428.

36. Graham MD, Sataloff RT, Kemink JL. Titration streptomycin therapy for bilateral Ménière's disease: a preliminary report. Otol Head Neck Surg 1984; 92(4):440–447.

37. Ward BK, Agrawal Y, Hoffman HJ, Carey JP, Della Santina CC. Prevalence and impact of bilateral vestibular hypofunction: results from the 2008 US National Health Interview Survey. JAMA Otolaryngol Head Neck Surg. 2013 Aug 1; 139(8):803–810. doi: 10.1001/jamaoto.2013.3913. PMID: 23949355; PMCID: PMC4839981.

38. Guyot JP, Perez Fornos A. Milestones in the development of a vestibular implant. Curr Opin Neurol. 2019 Feb; 32(1):145–153. doi: 10.1097/WCO.0000000000000639. PMID: 30566413; PMCID: PMC6343951.

# 22

# Facial paralysis

ROBERT THAYER SATALOFF, ARIANNE ABREU, AND MARY J. HAWKSHAW

The facial nerve courses with the auditory nerve and in a complex pattern through the ear and mastoid before distributing its fibers to the facial muscles. It also gives off several branches for functions other than facial motion. Because of the close anatomic and embryologic association of the facial nerve with the ear (1), physicians should be aware that facial nerve abnormalities may accompany other ear problems. Such abnormalities may include paralysis, hemifacial spasm, ear canal pain/numbness, hearing sensitivities, taste distortion, and dry mouth. Facial paralysis is the most common malady, and physicians concerned with ear problems should at least be acquainted with this condition.

## ANATOMY

The motor fibers of the facial nerve run from the facial nucleus in the brainstem, bending around the abducens nucleus, course from the brainstem across a short expanse of posterior fossa, enter the internal auditory canal in its anterior/superior compartment, become covered with bone in its labyrinthine segment as it leaves the internal auditory canal, course anteriorly, bend at the geniculate ganglion, course horizontally and vertically through the mastoid, exit through the stylomastoid foramen, and innervate muscles of facial expression. It also carries special sensory fibers for taste, preganglionic parasympathetic fibers to the lacrimal and submandibular glands, and sensory fibers to the skin of the posterior/superior aspect of the external auditory canal. Decreased sensation in this region is called a positive Hitselberger's sign and is common in the presence of lesions that cause pressure on the facial nerve, such as an acoustic neuroma. Several other branches within the temporal bone also can be tested, including, the greater superficial petrosal nerve which supplies preganglionic parasympathetic fibers to the lacrimal gland for tearing, the nerve to the stapedius muscle which helps regulate sound, and the chorda tympani nerve which supplies taste to the ipsilateral two-thirds of the tongue, and preganglionic parasympathetic fibers to the ipsilateral submandibular gland. Any portion of the nerve may be involved by disease or injury.

Facial paralysis is a relatively common affliction. The condition often involves one side of the face and can be abrupt or progressive in onset.

DOI: 10.1201/b23379-22

If the muscles cease working altogether, the condition is facial paralysis. If the muscles are merely weak, the condition is facial paresis. For the rest of this chapter, we will use the word "paralysis" to refer to complete paralysis or severe paresis. Facial paralysis can create cosmetic and functional deficits that may be extremely troublesome to patients. It results in drooping of the face, inability to close the eye (which exposes it to dryness and injury), and incompetence of the corner of the mouth (which may cause drooling of liquids and difficulty articulating some sounds). It also can cause facial spasm, hyperacusis (sound sensitivity), dysgeusia (altered taste), dry mouth, and eye dryness/excessive tearing due to both inability to close eye as well as decreased innervation to lacrimal gland.

One of the principle problems in management of facial paralysis is a widespread tendency within many sectors of the medical community to under-evaluate and misdiagnose the problem. In 1821, Sir Charles Bell studied the innervation of the facial musculature and named the motor nerve of the face the "facial nerve." Soon, all conditions of facial paralysis came to be known as "Bell's palsy." As time passed, the true cause of many cases of facial paralysis was discovered. Bell's palsy is now the name used to describe only those cases of facial paralysis in which the cause cannot be determined. Unfortunately, many physicians still diagnose "Bell's palsy" without going through the comprehensive evaluation necessary to diagnose and treat important causes of facial paralysis.

## EVALUATION

It is always important to take a through history when evaluating facial nerve paralysis. Both associated symptoms and the rate of onset help in forming a differential. The details of a comprehensive ear, nose, and throat examination, cranial nerve assessment, and audiometric testing will not be reviewed in this chapter, but these should be performed in the setting of facial paralysis. They are similar to those assessments performed in patients with hearing problems or suspected facial neuroma. However, it is important that when examining patients with facial paralysis,

the severity of their paralysis should be recorded using a standardized grading system. The House–Brackmann grading system is most widely used due to its ease of use. It is grading on a scale of 1–6. Grade I is normal. Grade VI is completely paralyzed. Grade II is almost normal. Grade V is almost completely paralyzed. The difficult distinctions come between Grade III and Grade IV. In Grade III facial paresis, the paralysis is obvious, but there is both forehead motion and eye closure. In Grade IV paresis, the patient can no longer obtain complete eye closure and the forehead is paralyzed. It is also useful to consider resting and dynamic motion of the face. The upper, middle, and lower division of the face should be evaluated individually, as well as involuntary movement. The House–Brackmann grading system does not account for segmental deficits in facial nerve paralysis or synkinesis (improper nerve innervation discussed later). There are a number of other, more detailed grading scales including the Facial Nerve Grading Scale 2.0 and Sunnybrook Grading Scale that offer zonal assessments. There is also an app-based facial nerve assessment called the eFACE that looks at static, dynamic, and synkinesis parameters. However, the House–Brackmann system is used most widely.

Specific work-up can be targeted depending on the patient's history and clues from the physical exam. Blood work for Lyme titers should be considered in the setting of a target rash on physical exam. Serologic testing for autoimmune diseases can be considered especially in middle-aged women and patients with facial paralysis alternating sides. Metabolic evaluation for diabetes and hypothyroidism and the many other conditions mentioned later in this chapter should also be performed. Radiological assessment is also similar and generally includes MRI with enhancement of the entire course of the facial nerve from the brainstem, through the temporal bone, and into the parotid gland and facial muscles especially in the setting of recurrent, ipsilateral, and progressive facial nerve paralysis when considering tumor as an etiology. Temporal bone CT is useful in identifying areas of bone destruction secondary to infection as well as possible temporal bone fracture in patients with a history of trauma. CT and MRI imaging of the brain helps especially when there are other neurological defects on exam and there is concern about possible stroke.

There are several other specific tests for the facial nerve, and facial nerve electrical testing warrants further discussion.

## FACIAL NERVE TESTING

Facial nerve testing is done routinely when a motor abnormality is observed (see the Case Report). However, tests may also be helpful in the absence of obvious motor abnormalities, especially if a pressure lesion is suspected, such as acoustic neuroma or vascular compression.

## CASE REPORT

A 32-year-old male who was injured at work. He was thrown against the wall striking the right side of his head. He was stunned for a few seconds and had short-term retrograde amnesia. He also had headache and minor memory deficits following the injury. One day after the accident, he noted complete right peripheral facial paralysis. Neurotologic examination was normal expect for facial paralysis and a positive Hitselberger's sign on the right. Audiogram revealed a small 4000-Hz dip on the right (**Figure 22.1**) with an even smaller dip on the left. CT and MRI were normal. Electroneuronography (ENoG) 3 months after injury still revealed 100% electrical degeneration on the right. The patient had declined facial nerve decompression. Partial recovery of voluntary facial motion occurred over the next several months.

Facial paralysis is common after penetrating trauma, fractures, or surgery. It is seen less frequently after minor head trauma and is felt to be due to edema within the facial nerve canal, particularly in the labyrinthine segment where the nerve leaves the internal auditory canal to enter the middle ear, because this is the most narrow segment. The slight 4000-Hz audiometric dip is typical following inner ear concussion.

## SIMPLE TOPOGNOSTIC TESTS

The validity and reliability of topognostic facial nerve testing have not been proven. Nevertheless, they often provide helpful information regarding the site of a facial nerve lesion. A modified Schirmer tear tests helps determine whether the lesion is proximately distal to the greater superfacial petrosal nerve and auricular ganglion. The stapedius reflex decay test establishes this relationship to the stapedius muscle. Testing of taste on the anterior two-thirds of the tongue, or testing salivary flow from the submandibular glands, locates the lesion in relation to the chorda tympani nerve. Peripheral branches of the facial nerve can be tested with a facial nerve stimulator. Although minimal nerve excitability testing is performed most commonly, maximal nerve excitability may provide more information. It usually requires 1 or 2 mA of current above the nerve threshold. Assessment of all of these tests is subjective.

**PATIENT:**

**RIGHT EAR AIR CONDUCTION**          **LEFT EAR AIR CONDUCTION**

| DATE | 250 | 500 | 1000 | 2000 | 4000 | 8000 | | 250 | 500 | 1000 | 2000 | 4000 | 8000 |
|------|-----|-----|------|------|------|------|--|-----|-----|------|------|------|------|
|      | 20  | 15  | 15   | 15   | 30   | 15   |  | 5   | 10  | 5    | 5    | 20   | 10   |
|      |     |     |      |      |      |      |  |     |     |      |      |      |      |
|      |     |     |      |      |      |      |  |     |     |      |      |      |      |

**SPEECH RECEPTION:**

R: 15 dB          L: 5 dB

Figure 22.1 Audiogram of Case Report.

## ELECTROMYOGRAPHY

Electromyography is a test complementary to ENoG. It looks at the function of the motor end plates in a muscle. It is performed by placing a needle into the facial muscles to measure resting potentials and recruitment with intentional movement. Standard facial electromyography records muscle action potentials produced by voluntary efforts to move muscles. The signal is monitored on an oscilloscope that measures voltage waves visually and acoustically. Neuromuscular function and degeneration can be detected by different patterns. These patterns include fibrillation which is a sign of a denervated muscle, polyphasic potentials which are signs that the nerve is recovering, and an absence of signal which suggests a non-functional neuromuscular complex.

## ELECTRONEURONOGRAPHY

ENoG is similar to electromyography except that it uses surface electrodes and evoked rather than volitional stimuli. A stimulating electrode is placed over the main trunk of the facial nerve at the stylomastoid foramen, and a recording electrode is placed over the muscle to be tested. This technique allows measurement of latency and conduction velocity, although latency has proven a more useful measure. Recording of threshold is possible. However, supramaximal stimuli are generally used. Several parameters can be measured and have proven useful clinically.

ENoG is a measure of the facial nerve action potential and is quantified in terms of amplitude as measured in millivolt. A comparison is made between the nerve response on the "poor" side vs. the "good" side, and a percent weakness is calculated for the "poor" side. This test is recommended most commonly for unilateral severe or complete facial nerve paralysis as it is performed as a ratio comparing the two sides of the face. It is also important to note that when nerves are damaged, there is a process of anterograde injury called Wallerian Degeneration in which nerve units degenerate distal to the site of injury. For this reason, testing usually should be performed several days after paralysis occurs to determine extent of injury once propagation of damage occurs.

The protocol for the test is as follows: The patient should first be instructed to relax as much as possible in order to minimize any muscle artifact from the response following electrode application. Electrode impedance is measured to ensure adequate recordings. The patient is then instructed to smile or contort his or her face to allow the tester to determine and set an appropriate sensitivity level for recording. An electrical current is then applied to the "good" side. Stimulator placement is critical, and often a small amount of pressure at the stimulation sites is required in order to obtain clear and reliable recordings. Stimulus intensity as measured in milliamperes is gradually increased until the maximum tolerance level of the patient is reached, and recordings become stable. Stimulation is then stopped, and maximum and minimum points are selected and plotted along the response curve. These values are subtracted from one another in order to obtain the amplitude of the response. The same protocol is then followed for the opposite or "poor" side. It is critical that maximum stimulation to this side of the face meet but not exceed that of the better side. This allows for a more exact comparison between the two responses. Once amplitude measures are obtained for both nerves, a percent weakness on the "poor" or involved side may be calculated as follows:

$$\frac{Poor\ side\ amplitude}{Good\ side\ amplitude} \times 100 = (x)$$

then $100 - (x) = $ percent weakness on poor side. A difference of $\geq 17\%$ between the two responses is considered significant. Decompression of the facial nerve is considered at more than 90% weakness. At that point, the injury is considered severe enough that odds of recovery are better with surgical intervention.

## CAUSES OF FACIAL PARALYSIS

There are many causes of both acute and chronic facial nerve paralysis. Although most cases of facial paralysis are idiopathic, there are many other diagnoses that must be ruled out prior to making that diagnosis of exclusion. This chapter will cover briefly only a few of those etiologies. Facial paralysis can be congenital. That is, some people are born with paralysis of one or both sides of the face. Congenital paralysis may result from various causes including genetic defects and anatomic malformations. However, acquired facial paralysis is much more common.

Infection and inflammation are well established causes of facial nerve paralysis. This is most commonly due to a viral process, particularly herpetic, and is often associated with a herpetic cold sore or "fever blister." Herpes zoster ("Shingles") may also be etiologic. The triad of facial paralysis, otalgia, and vesicles around the ear is known as Ramsay Hunt syndrome. This problem may also involve the hearing nerve which runs in close proximity to the facial nerve. Other viral etiologies include EBV, CMV, HIV and COVID-19. Bacterial infections of the ear (otitis media and malignant otitis externa) and brain (meningitis) can also cause facial paralysis, as do Lyme disease (from ticks) and syphilis. Facial paralysis has also been associated with toxic effects from exposure to heavy metals such as lead, and immunologic response following injections for tetanus, rabies, and polio. Metabolic conditions, including diabetes, hypothyroidism, and pregnancy, as well as autoimmune conditions such as sarcoidosis may also precipitate facial paralysis. In addition, vascular problems including stroke and vasculitis can cause paralysis. It is important to consider a stroke of the upper brain if facial paralysis spares the forehead.

Trauma is also an important cause of facial paralysis, particularly temporal bone fractures associated with motor vehicle accidents or falls. Due to the position of the otic capsule (inner ear) in the temporal bone, as well as the close anatomic association of the facial nerve and cochlear (hearing) nerve, patients with temporal bone fractures can have different types of hearing loss, as well. Facial lacerations and surgical trauma (facial paralysis is a potential complication of ear, brain, and parotid gland surgery) can also precipitate facial nerve paralysis.

Facial paralysis may also be the presenting sign of a tumor. The tumor may be benign or malignant. It may occur anywhere along the course of the facial nerve, which starts in the brainstem, courses circuitously through the ear encased in a tight, bony canal, exits the mastoid bone at the skull base, and spreads through the parotid gland and out along the face. Tumors of the facial nerve itself (facial neuromas and facial nerve hemangiomas) commonly present with facial paralysis. So do cancerous tumors of the skull base, middle ear, parotid gland, and upper neck.

Facial paralysis occurs rarely with acoustic neuromas, despite the fact that compression of the facial nerve by these tumors is common. Other growths of the temporal bone that may cause facial paralysis include cholesteatoma, glomus tumor, and neuromas of other nerves. Facial paralysis may also be caused by neoplasms outside the temporal bone. When a parotid neoplasm presents with facial paralysis, the lesion is almost always malignant.

A variety of other conditions may be associated with facial paralysis or paresis including hemifacial spasms which may be due to vascular loop compression of the facial nerve, Melkersson–Rosenthal syndrome (facial nerve paralysis, recurrent facial edema, and a fissured tongue), barotrauma, and, of course, Bell's palsy. However, because facial paralysis may be secondary to many serious conditions, physicians should not accept a cavalier diagnosis for "Bell's palsy" but should pursue a credible diagnosis based on systematic comprehensive evaluation. Tumors and many of the other conditions mentioned may be treated effectively, particularly if they are diagnosed early.

## TREATMENT

Treatment for facial paralysis is directed at the underlying diagnosis. In general, treatment also can be divided into acute and chronic, the former targeted at the underlying condition and the latter targeted at rehabilitating the face and protecting the eye. There is overlap between the two.

In the acute setting, the use of antiviral medications is controversial but strongly considered especially when herpetic or other viral causes of facial paralysis are suspected early in the course of disease. If a specific disease or tumor is identified, it is treated appropriately, and in many cases, facial nerve function can be restored. Regardless of the cause and chronicity, symptomatic treatment is important, particularly eye protection. The eye should be treated with artificial tears and/or a more long-lasting artificial lubricant. At night, the eye should be taped shut with tape running horizontally along the upper lid toward the side of the face. The tape should not cross the lash line. When it does, it may invert the lashes and scratch the cornea. These measures are taken to prevent exposure keratitis (damage to cornea) which is of particular concern when there is a poor Bell's phenomenon (the eyeball does not rotate up when the eye is closed) or when there is simultaneous fifth cranial nerve pathology resulting in decreased corneal sensation. In these cases, it is important to protect the eye aggressively and usually surgically. Surgical intervention can involve implantation of a gold or platinum weight, surgical tarsorrhaphy (attachment of upper and lower eyelids), and/or medial or lateral canthoplasty (eyelid reconstruction).

If no cause is found and the condition is truly Bell's palsy, various treatments are available. Treatment may involve observation, use of high-dose corticosteroids, or surgery. Antiviral medications often are preferred in conjunction with steroids. When treating with high-dose steroids, a proton pump inhibitor or similar medication should be used as prophylaxis for stomach ulcers.

In more acute settings of idiopathic facial nerve paralysis, surgery (facial nerve decompression) is the last resort. However, it should be considered if electrical excitability decreases by 90% or more; if facial paralysis is sudden, total, and associated with severe pain; and in selected other situations. In general, if recovery from facial paralysis begins within 3 weeks, recovery is excellent and total. If recovery does not start until after 3 months, it is usually imperfect. In these cases, the nerve usually develops some degree of synkinesis (inappropriate neuromuscular function). This is due to recovering nerve fibers sprouting along different tracts to muscles. This causes difficulty coordinating facial expression and results, for example, in a slight smiling of the lips when the person closes his/her eyes. "Crocodile tears" and "gustatory sweating" result similarly from misdirected nerve fibers that should have gone to salivary glands. In these cases, when the patient eats, tears fall from the eyes and the side of the face perspires.

When facial paralysis is noted in a more chronic setting (>12 months), it is unlikely that the nerve will recover fully. For that reason, it is important to consider other treatment modalities. Treatment at this stage is often focused on rehabilitating the face and depends on the specific deficits. There are both flaccid (no movement) and non-flaccid (spastic movement) paralysis in the chronic setting. Treatment is either focused on reinnervating a target muscle or reanimating the face. Reinnervation can be done by repairing a severed nerve, replacing the nerve with another nerve or by using synthetic nerve. Reanimation is considered when the

end muscles no longer have function and can be divided into static and dynamic options. Usually, it is focused on restoring the function of a target segment of the facial nerve. Static options have been discussed previously and involve eyelid weights, eyebrow lifts, and suspension of the mouth. Dynamic options include transferring a muscle to restore movement. When the problem is muscle spasticity or synkinesis, the muscle or nerve can be surgically cut to alleviate distress. There are also nonsurgical management options of chronic facial nerve paralysis including physical therapy as well as botulinum toxin injections for management of spastic muscles.

## PROGNOSIS

Prognosis is dependent on timing of facial nerve paralysis as well as severity at around the time of onset. Ultimately, treatment of the underlying cause may help alleviate symptoms of facial nerve paralysis depending on the cause. Patients with uncomplicated, idiopathic facial nerve paralysis often improve in the first 3 months. These patients usually can be managed on an outpatient basis with a specialist. The medical specialists most involved in caring for Bell's palsy are neurotologists, subspecialists of otolaryngology who deal with disorders of the ear and related structures including the facial nerve and the ear–brain interface.

Bell's palsy always recovers, at least partially, although recovery may take as long as a year. If the face remains paralyzed without recovery of facial function, the diagnosis of Bell's palsy is generally wrong, and the true etiology should be sought again. Because any disturbance of facial function is potentially so problematic and possibly quite serious, it is essential for any physician encountering this affliction to complete a comprehensive evaluation. Simply looking at a paralyzed face and proclaiming it "Bell's palsy" is not keeping with the current standards of care.

## REFERENCE

1. Sataloff RT and Sataloff JB. Embryology and Anomalies of the Facial Nerve, 2nd Edition. New Delhi, India: Jaypee Brothers; 2014.

# 23

# Squamous cell carcinoma of the temporal bone

LEONA J. TU AND ROBERT THAYER SATALOFF

The estimated incidence of temporal bone (TB) malignancy by the National Cancer Institute is 0.8–6 cases per million population per year (1, 2). They comprise < 0.2% of all head and neck malignancies (3). Squamous cell carcinoma (SCCA) represents the majority of these cases (4–6). SCCA, a rare neoplasm with an overall aggressive nature and poor prognosis, is estimated to comprise 90% of all primary malignant tumors originating in the TB (7–9). Kuhel et al. (10) described the sites of origin for TB SCCA: auricle (60%–70%), the external auditory canal (EAC) (20%–30%), and the middle ear (10%). There is a report of isolated SCCA *in situ* of the tympanic membrane (11). SCCA can also affect the TB secondarily, most commonly originating from the periauricular skin, auricular skin, parotid gland, and skull base (3, 11). The advanced nature of lesions frequently makes it harder to assess the site of origin. Most studies have reported a median age of 60–69 years at time of diagnosis (3, 5, 10, 12, 13). However, the population developing middle ear malignancy appears to be ~10 years younger (14).

While there have been conflicting data of multiple studies on the sex distribution of SCCA of TB, it appears that the distribution is slightly greater in men than in women, with a 3:2 ratio (1–18).

Definitive information about the treatment and prognosis of SCCA of the TB is not easy to obtain due to a multitude of factors: the rarity of this malignancy, the lack of an accepted staging system (prior to 1990), and the wide variety of individualized treatments. Also, many authors include tumors of multiple histology in their reports of treatment outcomes, which further complicates the issue.

## ETIOLOGY

Various etiologic factors have been associated with SCCA.

For SCCA of the auricle, sun exposure has been implicated as the most common cause. Bendl and Graham (19) found strong correlation (82%)

between the actinic or solar damage to the epidermis of the auricle and the development of SCCA. Shiffman (20) has noted the infrequency of auricular SCCA in women with long hair, and Chen and Dehner (17) found no association between SCCA of EAC with prior actinic changes of the epidermis. Some authors continue to believe that sun exposure may play some role. However, they emphasize that other factors such as genetic susceptibility contribute to SCCA malignancy after exposure to ultraviolet light (21). Individuals who are immunosuppressed also face an increased risk of developing SCCA (22).

The middle ear is sheltered from the carcinogenic effect of the sun. Thus, investigators have been concentrating on other etiologies. In 1908, Whitehead described long-standing chronic otitis media as a possible cause of SCCA. Wagenfeld et al. (23) found a history of previous otitis media in 64% of SCCA of TB patients, and many studies list chronic otorrhea as the most common presenting symptom of SCCA of the TB (10, 13). It is possible that the presence of continuous inflammation induces increased proliferation and increases the risk of malignant transformation in the surrounding tissue. For example, pseudoepitheliomatous hyperplasia (HP) is a benign skin lesion that is associated with chronic inflammations caused by various infectious agents, autoimmune skin diseases, burns, or even prolonged exposure to irritants (UV light, allergens, alcohol, chlorinated disinfectants, etc.). It bares striking resemblance to SCCA (24–26). There are several reported cases of over-treatment as a result of such histological similarity. Furthermore, Gacek et al. (24) have presented a case of HP conversion into an invasive SCCA after a 6-year symptom-free interval. HP could be an intermediate step in the continuum of the SCCA disease process. Yet, the rarity of the SCCA of the TB does not correlate with the abundant prevalence of chronic otits. Hence, it is most likely that additional factors have to be present in order to promote malignant transformation. Viral causes have been implicated. Jin et al. (27) reported high prevalence of HPV in middle ear carcinoma associated with chronic otitis media. Tsai et al. (28) identified HPV genotypes 16 and 18, and Hongo et al. (29) estimated that high-risk HPV are implicated in 3.8% of cases. The pathogenesis is postulated to be similar to that of other malignancies involving HPV, specifically by inactivation of tumor suppressors, upregulation of growth factor receptors, and uninhibited telomerase activity (13, 30). Some believe that chronic otorrhea is more likely a result than a cause of SCCA of the ear. The growth of the tumor may result in secondary infection of the middle ear via eustachian tube and EAC.

Cholesteatoma has been suggested as a causative agent of SCCA by causing localized chronic inflammation (13). Occasionally, it is present with carcinoma in the middle ear (13). However, Michaels and Wells (1980) have reviewed the TBs of 28 patients with SCCA of the middle ear (31); none of these patients had concomitant cholesteatomas. However, from 1951 to 2021, there have been six reported cases of cholesteatoma-associated TB SCCA, with four cases identifying a history of cholesteatoma and two cases presenting with concurrent cholesteatoma (32). Further research is needed to elucidate the relationship between cholesteatoma and SCCA.

In 1952, Aub et al. (33) and later in 1965 Beal et al. (34) identified radiation as a possible etiology for SCCA of the middle ear and mastoid. They noted that a significant percentage of the employees of clock and watch factories developed TB malignancy. During the 1940s, the clock industry utilized radium-containing paint to give the numerals attractive nightglow. In order to apply this paint accurately, workers would moisten the brushes with their tongue and lick the radioactive substance throughout the day. Tumor induction may have been caused by radon gas trapped in the mastoid air cell system or from the radon deposits in the cortex of the TB.

Lim et al. evaluated patients with malignant tumors of the TB. They found 7 out of 18 patients (39%) had previous history of radiation therapy (XRT) for nasopharyngeal carcinoma. Notably, five out of seven patients had SCCA. The presentation from the time of exposure averaged 13 years (35). Other authors have reported similar findings associated with >5000 cGy of radiation. Ionizing radiation is currently reported as a widely accepted risk factor, with a rate 1000x greater than the general population (32). In one study of nasopharyngeal cancer patients who received radiation treatment, the incidence of SCCA of the EAC was found to be 0.13% (36). Unfortunately, radiation-induced malignancies appear to be more aggressive and therapy-resistant than sporadic tumors

(35, 37, 38). It appears that regional postradiation changes may alter local immunity as chronic ear infections are common after radiotherapy to nasopharynx (35, 39). The authors used the criteria for diagnosis of radiation-induced malignancy proposed by Cahan et al. (40). The patient must have a history of radiation, the second neoplasm must arise in the irradiated field, and a latent period of at least 5 years must have elapsed between the radiation exposure and the development of the second neoplasm. Further, there must be histologic and roentgenographic evidence of the preexisting condition in addition to microscopic proof of a tumor; the second tumor must be a different histologic type from that previously irradiated in order to eliminate the possibility of recurrence of the original tumor.

Interestingly, unlike other head and neck cancers, tobacco and alcohol use do not appear to be a risk factor for developing primary TB SCCA (41, 42).

Local malignancies from the sites adjacent to TB may extend into its structures. These sites include the parotid gland, tympano-mandibular joint (TMJ), EAC, preauricular skin, and nasopharynx. Gidley et al. found that SCCA from the periauricular skin and parotid gland were more common than primary TB SCCA (43). The TB may also be infiltrated by metastatic tumors arising from the breast, lung, kidney, stomach, larynx, prostate, thyroid, and other organs. It is important to note the site of origin of SCCA, as prognosis varies depending on the location. Gidley et al. showed that patients with SCCA of the EAC had higher overall survival rates compared to those with TB SCCA originating from auricular, periauricular, and parotid gland sites (43).

## CLINICAL CHARACTERISTICS

Most patients present with the diagnosis of SCCA of the TB in the sixth decade, with slightly greater incidence in men compared to women (44). However, the disease is usually asymptomatic early in its course, so most patients present at an advanced stage.

Unfortunately, clinical presentation is non-specific. Kuhel et al. (10) evaluated 442 patients and identified otorrhea (61%), otalgia (51%), and EAC mass (37%) as the most common presenting symptoms. Gillespie et al. noted hearing loss as presenting symptom, although less commonly than the previously identified symptoms (45). In the report by Kenyon et al. (13), evaluation of 19 patients revealed three patients with persistent otorrhea present for at least 30 years. Many authors have found long-standing otorrhea, of ~20 years, to be common (13, 46, 47). They also noted changes in both the quality and quantity of discharge prior to patients' presentation with tumor. The amount of discharge increased, became malodorous, and occasionally bloody. Otalgia is also common and noted to become worse weeks prior to the diagnosis; it is usually described as dull and deep seated, most likely as a result of bony invasion. Presence of trismus may indicate TMJ involvement.

The majority of patients have polyps or granulation tissue within the EAC. Even though the pathology specimen can be obtained easily on an outpatient basis, the pathology findings can be misleading. Sometimes these tumors may remain asymptomatic until they become quite large. Neoplasms involving the middle ear may cause a sensation of fullness and conductive hearing loss. According to several reports, up to 50% of patients may have hearing loss of various patterns (2, 9, 48). Invasion of the otic capsule is uncommon due to the resistance of enchondral layers; yet, once the neoplasm involves the inner ear, sensorineural hearing loss and vertigo are common.

The presence of facial nerve involvement indicates more advanced disease and significantly decreases survival (2, 9, 15, 34, 49, 50). The degree of facial nerve involvement also plays a prognostic role. The treatment failure rate for patients with mild paresis has been reported as 34%, moderate paresis is 50%, and complete paralysis is 62% (RT Sataloff and JE Medina, personal communication). Other signs of advanced disease include cervical lymph node metastasis and other neuropathies (4, 5, 16, 48, 49, 51).

## DIAGNOSTIC CHALLENGE

Extremely low incidence, high frequency of ear infections, and absence of specific symptoms make the malignancy difficult to recognize. Other factors may contribute to the challenge.

One diagnostic dilemma is malignant otitis externa. The clinical presentation of the TB osteomyelitis closely resembles the presentation of TB carcinoma. Both occur in the elderly and, with regard to clinical and radiologic examination, SCCA can be indistinguishable from malignant otitis externa. Although SCCA of the TB is painful, malignant otitis externa is uniquely characterized by an acute onset of severe, recalcitrant, disabling pain. Several case reports described the simultaneous presentation of SCCA and osteomyelitis (52, 53). It is possible that the presence of necrotic or neoplastic cells may be responsible for superinfection. This highlights the importance of histological evaluation.

Another dilemma arises when one encounters pseudoepitheliomatous HP. It is a benign lesion that mimics the clinical and histologic presentation of epithelial malignancy of the EAC. It usually is associated with aural fullness but not otalgia or bloody otorrhea. If discharge is present, it is usually of recent onset. Once the diagnosis of HP is made, it is imperative that a patient be followed long-term for early detection of possible malignant transformation. Gacek et al. (24) reviewed TB specimens retrospectively diagnosed with SCCA. They found several cases of devastating misdiagnosis with resultant over-treatment. As a result, they proposed criteria for biopsy and close cooperation between the surgeon and the pathologist.

Rarity of the disease and its nonspecific presentation requires a high level of suspicion on the part of the otorhinolaryngologist. Most of the time, it is the prolonged symptomatology unresponsive to treatment that prompts further investigation; thus, the diagnosis often is delayed from 1 month to 4 years (17, 23, 54), with an average of 13 months (55). The red flags should be history of persistent aural discharge associated with change in its quality and/or quantity, development or increase in otalgia, carnial nerve (CN) VII paralysis, aural or mastoid polyp, and vertigo. If complete resolution does not occur after 2–3 weeks of vigorous medical therapy, it might be advisable to offer biopsy as surveillance for TB malignancy. Multiple authors have cautioned against reliance on a single biopsy results. They recommended strongly obtaining multiple deep biopsies including a cuff of normal tissue, even if general anesthesia or CT guidance is required. Inadequate biopsy may show only extensive inflammation and lead to delayed or missed diagnosis (17, 24, 56, 57).

## RADIOLOGY

From the earlier discussion, it is clear that the diagnosis of SCCA of TB is extremely difficult if attempted by clinical presentation alone. Chronic discharge and the frequent presence of the EAC mass preclude accurate evaluation of the canal and TM. The rarity of tumors and limited physical examination make it extremely difficult to estimate the extent of the disease. In 1983, Olsen et al. (57) evaluated the validity of CT scan in comparison to mastoid X-rays and tomography and reported its accuracy in predicting the extent of tumor. In 1990, Arriaga et al. heavily based their EAC malignancy staging system on the findings of the CT scan. In 1991, they conducted a study comparing 12 anatomical sites correlating the histopathalogic findings of the SCCA with preoperative CT scans of the TBs of 13 patients. In 94 out of 96 instances, the pathology found on histopathalogic slides coincided with pathology found on the preoperative CT scan. This confirmed the findings of other investigators that high-resolution, thin-section CT scan is the best modality for evaluating the extent of bone involvement by tumor (58, 59). As a result, they concluded that high-resolution CT (HRCT) scan provides "a consistent framework to evaluate efficacy of treatment techniques" (58). They also realized the limitations of the HRCT in distinguishing tumor from soft tissue inflammation or edema. General findings of poorly demarcated infiltrative mass, obliterated facial planes, or loss of normal fat density are highly suggestive of malignancy.

The assessment of tumor invasion into soft tissue and along fascial planes, perineural spread, and CNS infiltration is accomplished best with MRI (60, 61). Noncontrast T1-weighted images can be used to evaluate tumor invasion of bone marrow by the replacement of normal hyperintense fatty signal. The administration of contrast media may enhance the signal of the tumor. MRI with contrast is now the study of choice for evaluation of the skull base, especially the common sites of invasion: the petroclinoid fissure and foramen lacerum. Loss of smooth contour of the cortical bone indicates bone destruction. MRA may accurately determine involvement of the major vessels, although invasive angiogram is preferable in many cases.

Despite the great sensitivity of radiologic studies, intraoperative evaluation is of undisputed importance. Multiple authors recognized the limitations of current radiography. Arriaga et al., while utilizing HRCT for the design of a staging system, reported the limitations of HRCT in differentiation of tumor from soft tissue inflammation, tumor extension along fissures, and tumor progression without bone erosion (58). Spector has described perioperative findings of tumor extensions along various nerves, bones, and vascular and fascial planes that were not apparent on clinical and radiologic evaluations (62). He found the facial nerve canal to be the most common conduit for intracranial tumor extension.

Leonetti et al. concentrated on the evaluation of advanced disease (stages T3 and T4 by Pittsburgh classification). They found a fairly good correlation between preoperative radiographic and intraoperative findings for anterior and inferior tumor extensions. However, according to them, radiographic preoperative staging underestimated a significant number of patients with tumor extension to the medial, posterior, superior, and petrous carotid canal. As a result, patients were under-staged and did poorly after surgery due to high local recurrence rate (59, 62, 63). Wagenfeld et al. (23) commented "It appears that assessing the resectability of these tumors involves a significant amount of guesswork." In conclusion, Leonetti et al. (59) proposed the use of a combination of CT scan and MRI to optimize radiologic tumor mapping. Moffat et al. (21) reported a poor correlation between the extent of intracranial involvement and CT and MRI studies.

In 1998, Moharir et al. presented a computer technique of three-dimensional reconstruction based on the fusion of images from two-dimensional CT and MR. Combining the two modalities permits accurate depiction of the bone, soft tissue, blood vessels, and cartilage in one image. Several manipulations were achieved by this technology: 360° rotation in any axis, size adjustment, edge detection and transparencies capabilities, and control of color and light intensity. The ability to control the light intensity, color, and transparency of each structure allows the evaluation of the exact relationship of the tumor to the skull base. The segmented slices measure the tumor volume and planar dimensions. The three-dimensional modality offers preoperative planning, intraoperative guidance, tumor surveillance, reconstruction design, XRT field formulation, and medical education. If it proves to be as accurate as it is suggested, multiple limitations of current diagnostic modalities for SCCA of the TB will be overcome (64).

## CLASSIFICATION

For any type of cancer, it is imperative to have a system that evaluates the extent of the tumor and, based on that, accurately predicts the amount of surgery needed as well as the associated survival. The rarity of SCCA of the TB has for years hampered the formulation of an accurate classification system. Adequate analysis of the results has been difficult due to the lack of sufficient data from any single institution (65). This fact is reflected in the absence of a staging system accepted by the International Union Against Cancer or the American Joint Committee on Cancer. Many authors expressed frustration with the inability to interpret and compare the reports. Because survival is determined largely by the tumor's extent, an accurate and unanimously accepted classification system for SCCA of the TB might facilitate the exchange of clinical data in a comparable form.

One of the earliest mentions of classification was proposed <30 years ago (15). Since then, multiple authors have proposed various staging systems: Goodwin and Jesse, Stell and McCormic, Shih and Crabtree, Kinney, Spector, Pensak et al., Manolidis et al., etc. (66). Unfortunately, they were often based primarily on clinical examinations, included various histologic types of cancers, and lacked specifics for the site of tumor extension. The behavior of various types of tumors varies considerably, and the limited clinical examination of the TB is well known. Kinney and Wood (2) found that in 60% of patients, the tympanic membrane could not be observed. The presence of so many classification systems highlights the absence of uniform agreement.

In 1990, Arriaga et al. proposed a Pittsburgh staging system specific for SCCA lesions of the external auditory meatus (58). This staging system relies heavily on preoperative findings of the CT scan of the TB. They offered treatment plans for each stage and found statistically different survival rates for each tumor stage. In their later work, they describe the close correlation between histopathology of surgical specimens and preoperative CT scans (67). Several authors have used the Pittsburgh staging system and found it reproducible for both SCCA and non-SCCA tumors (8, 9, 66, 68). In 2000, Moody et al. (66) noted the significance of facial nerve paralysis as bony invasion and recommended the modification of the Pittsburgh system by upgrading a tumor stage in the presence of facial nerve paralysis. In 2002, Breau et al. (69) offered a modification for classification of early-stage lesions based on the site of the lesion within the EAC. From in-depth review, this modification appears more cumbersome than useful. Currently, the modified Pittsburgh classification system is most widely accepted due to its increased objectivity based on radiologic evaluation. Since its development, several studies have confirmed its correlation with prognosis (70–73).

## MANAGEMENT

Rarity of the disease poses challenges not only with development of a uniform classification system but also with management strategies. Despite technological advances, skull base surgery continues to be very complex. It requires cooperative efforts between a patient and an extensive team of professionals. The goal of management is to be curative; yet, due to the nature of the TB, the complete excision of the tumor, whether piecemeal or *En bloc*, is often difficult once the tumor extends beyond the EAC. Adjuvant XRT appears to play a considerable role in increasing survival, but for advanced lesions, it does not appear curative as a single modality. Chemotherapy use has been reported. It is usually offered as a palliative therapy but has not yet been shown to improve rates of survival. Nevertheless, all efforts must be made to control such devastating disease.

## SURGICAL TREATMENT

Ideally, the tumor classification system should reflect the pattern of tumor infiltration and dictate the amount of resection necessary for the best

Table 23.1 Modified Pittsburgh staging system

| | |
|---|---|
| T1 | Tumor limited to the EAC without bony erosion *or* evidence of soft tissue involvement |
| T2 | Tumor limited to the EAC with partial thickness bony erosion *or* evidence of limited (< 0.5 cm) soft tissue involvement |
| T3 | Tumor eroding the osseous EAC (full thickness) *and* limited (< 0.5 cm) soft tissue involvement or tumor involving the middle ear or mastoid |
| T4 | Tumor eroding the cochlea, petrous apex, medial wall of the middle ear, carotid canal, jugular foramen, or dura *or* with extensive soft tissue involvement (> 0.5 cm), such as involvement of TMJ or styloid process or evidence of facial paresis |
| N status | Involvement of lymph nodes is a poor prognostic finding and automatically places the patient in a higher category (i.e., stage III [T1, N1] or stage IV [T2, T3, and T4, N1] disease) |
| M status | Distant metastasis indicates a very poor prognosis and automatically places a patient in the stage IV category |

*Note:* In the rest of the discussion, all tumors will be staged according to the modified Pittsburgh classification system, unless otherwise specified.

treatment. For example, *En bloc* resection of the EAC (sleeve resection) is indicated for T1 tumors, lateral temporal bone resection (LTBR) is for tumors limited to the EAC, and subtotal temporal bone resection (STBR) or total temporal bone resection (TTBR) is for advanced tumors (74).

## SLEEVE RESECTION

Sleeve resection is designed to treat selected T1 lesions of the EAC. It involves the circumferential removal of all skin and the lateral cartilaginous portion of the canal of the EAC (**Figure 23.1**). The intact tympanic membrane and intact bony canal are the limits of resection (**Figure 23.2**). Many have cautioned against the use of these procedures due to high recurrence rate of the disease (75, 76). The term "sleeve resection" has been applied to various procedures described in the literature; thus, readers must

be cautioned to evaluate the extent of the procedure upon encountering its description (5, 50).

## LATERAL TEMPORAL BONE RESECTION

This procedure was summarized by Crabtree et al. (5). It is the workhorse for surgical management of most of the lesions confined to the EAC without middle ear involvement (intact tympanic membrane). LTBR is *en bloc* removal of the entire EAC (bony and cartilaginous), tympanic membrane, malleus, and incus. The middle ear cavity, stapes, and facial nerve are the boundaries of the resection (**Figures 23.1** and **23.2**). It is frequently accompanied by superficial parotidectomy and suprahyoid neck dissection. If a lesion extends anteriorly and is confirmed by frozen sections, resection of TMJ and condyle may be added.

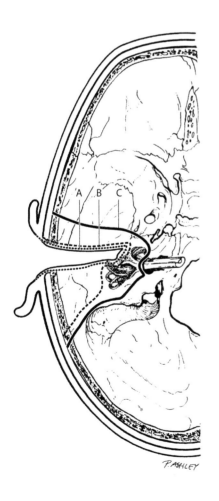

Figure 23.1 *Axial view*: (A) Dotted lines outline the extent of sleeve resection. It involves the circumferential removal of all skin and the lateral cartilaginous portion of the canal of the EAC. The intact tympanic membrane and intact bony canal are the limits of resection. (B) Dashed lines outline the extent of LTBR. It is *En bloc* removal of the entire EAC (bony and cartilaginous), tympanic membrane, malleus, and incus. The middle ear cavity, stapes, and facial nerve are the boundaries of the resection. (C) Solid lines outline the extent of partial or total TB resection. Unlike TTBR, STBR preserves the medial one-third of the petrous apex, carotid artery, and the contents of jugular foramen. The labyrinth, cochlea, facial nerve, zygoma, and mandibular condyle are sacrificed. *Abbreviations*: EAC, external auditory canal; LTBR, lateral temporal bone resection; STBR, subtotal temporal bone resection; TB, temporal bone; TTBR, total temporal bone resection.

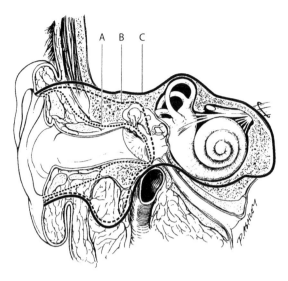

Figure 23.2 *Coronal view*: (A) Dotted lines outline the extent of sleeve resection. It involves the circumferential removal of all skin and the lateral cartilaginous portion of the canal of the EAC. The intact tympanic membrane and intact bony canal are the limits of resection. (B) Dashed lines outline the extent of LTBR. It is *En bloc* removal of the entire EAC (bony and cartilaginous), tympanic membrane, malleus, and incus. The middle ear cavity, stapes, and facial nerve are the boundaries of the resection. (C) Solid lines outline the extent of partial or total TB resection. Unlike TTBR, STBR preserves the medial one-third of the petrous apex, carotid artery, and the contents of jugular foramen. The labyrinth, cochlea, facial nerve, zygoma, and mandibular condyle are sacrificed. *Abbreviations*: EAC, External auditory canal; LTBR, Lateral temporal bone resection; STBR, Subtotal temporal bone resection; TB, Temporal bone; TTBR, Total temporal bone resection.

A long modified preauricular/parotid incision extending to the anterior neck is used to gain access to the TB, parotid gland, and cervical structures. Postauricular connection is made to include posterior nodes. When a tumor lies deep in the EAC, the majority of the peripheral auricle is preserved. The cartilage of the tragus and a portion of concha are included with the specimen. If the tumor is present in the region of the concha, the entire auricle must be sacrificed. A canal wall-down radical mastoidectomy with facial recess

exposure is performed. Incudo-stapedial joint is sectioned to prevent damage to stapes during removal of incus. The dissection continues anteriorly along the middle fossa tegmen into zygoma. The EAC is dissected of the TMJ without entering the posterior periosteum. The tympanic bone is cut below the tympanic ring, connecting TMJ with the facial recess. The bone in the hypotympanum is removed down to the area between the jugular bulb posteriorly and the carotid artery anteriorly. The styloid process is included with the specimen. The entire EAC is freed in circumferential fashion. The specimen may be left attached to the superficial lobe of the parotid gland, which is resected in continuity with the specimen. Gacek and Goodman recommend superficial parotidectomy for all *En bloc* procedures because a tumor arising in the EAC follows the path of least resistance to the preauricular soft tissue (6, 7). Total parotidectomy is performed when gross disease involves the gland. The facial nerve is preserved if there is no connection to the tumor, and the deep lobe is removed as a separate specimen. Conventional or modified neck dissection may be performed at that stage depending on the stage of disease. A frozen section of lymph node may aid the decision. The soft tissue of the remaining tragus is used to cover posterior periosteum of the TMJ.

This procedure provides tumor margins, preserves facial nerve, has little blood loss, may not require craniotomy, and may preserve serviceable conductive hearing (5, 10). Healing is completed usually by 5–6 weeks and results in a dry ear that requires no special care. Recent studies evaluating use of LTBR for T1/T2 tumors have demonstrated favorable outcomes (77, 78). Saijo et al. (79) showed that the estimated 3-year disease-free survival was 77.4% for T1 tumors and 100% for T2 tumors and that the 3-year disease-specific survival was 100% for T1/T2 tumors. In 2000, Moody et al. (66) proposed modifying LTBR by leaving the uninvolved tympanic membrane intact. In 2017, Ghavami et al. (80) proposed modifying LTBR by preserving the tympanic membrane and ossicles and reconstructing the remaining EAC with split-thickness skin graft. The goal was to preserve conductive hearing in TB SCCA patients with very limited bony canal involvement; results showed a significantly decreased mean postoperative air–bone gap (9 dB) compared to standard LTBR.

## Procedures for stage III and IV diseases

Tumors extending through the TM, arising in the middle ear or mastoid, or involving facial nerve are considered advanced because of their grave impact on the patient's prognosis. They are designated stages III or IV regardless of their size. As with other malignancies, as lesions become more advanced, the extent of surgical management becomes controversial. Various procedures have been employed to manage this disease: radical mastoidectomy, piecemeal removal of the tumor, subtotal resection of the TB, and total resection of the TB.

The general consensus is that TB cancer behaves as a local biologic process until very late in the disease. The high incidence of local recurrences and rare occurrence of distant metastasis illustrate this behavior. Because the cause of death in these patients is dominated by local recurrence, which is the highest if the tumor is not resected completely, author after author advocates an aggressive approach. In general, better survival is reported with more extensive surgery (9, 17, 65).

The extent of TB resection is the main determinant of postoperative morbidity (9, 16). Thus, it is important to identify which lesions are treated best by which procedure.

## PIECEMEAL REMOVAL OF TUMOR

Many surgeons prefer piecemeal tumor removal. Several factors have made this procedure appear to be an attractive option. Many believe that the extent of a tumor cannot be sufficiently determined by preoperative evaluation. The amount of the excised healthy tissue is considerably less than with En bloc procedures, and the close proximity of many vital structures to the TBs has made En bloc resection technically difficult and subject to significant morbidity and mortality. Thus, Kinney and Wood (2) proposed piecemeal tumor resection after initial completion of LTBR. The gross tumor is removed until tumor-free margins are confirmed. Most structures, including the internal carotid artery and uninvolved facial nerve, that otherwise would be sacrificed are preserved.

By their description, the entire parotid gland is removed and node picking is performed and submitted for frozen section to determine if there is metastatic spread. Neck dissection depends on the status of the neck nodes. If bony involvement is found, postoperative XRT is recommended.

## SUBTOTAL TEMPORAL BONE RESECTION

The very poor results obtained up to 1950 in the treatment of malignant tumors involving the TB prompted Parson and Lewis (81) to develop a more radical operation for their removal, in 1954. They reported En bloc resection of SCCA of TB in 100 patients via intracranial–extracranial approach. The overall survival rate continued to be 25%, but it signaled the return of TB resection into the therapy arsenal as a sound surgical option for advanced tumors. In the literature, one can find this procedure under different aliases, including TTBR. Unlike TTBR, STBR preserves the medial one-third of the petrous apex, carotid artery, and the contents of jugular foramen. The labyrinth, cochlea, facial nerve, zygoma, and mandibular condyle are sacrificed. Exposure is similar to LTBR. The medial resection of the petrosal ridge stops upon encountering the lateral portion of the petrosal internal carotid artery (**Figures 21.1** and **21.2**). Both the middle and posterior fossa craniotomies are necessary to obtain access. The sigmoid sinus and posterior fossa dura are exposed, and a temporal craniotomy is performed to verify that there is no intracranial tumor extension. If dura involvement is noted, the dura can be resected and grafted. The zygoma and ascending ramus of mandibular are transected and removed. The posterior infratemporal space is inspected. Total parotidectomy, facial nerve transection, and radical neck dissection are performed. The facial nerve distal stump is tagged for future anastomosis procedures. Subtemporal craniotomy is performed to isolate the internal auditory canal. It is accessed and CN VII and CN VIII are transected. The resection of the TB can then be completed. CN IX–CN XII are preserved. Several complications are associated with the procedure: frequent CSF leak, postoperative vertigo, and significant blood loss (75). Some recommend modified STBR to preserve CN VII, cochlea, and labyrinth unless they are involved with tumor.

## TEMPORAL BONE RESECTION

For extensive disease of the middle ear or involvement of the pneumatized spaces, TTBR may provide better oncologic control. In the original description of the procedure by Graham and Sataloff, the vascular and neural structures of the petrous apex are included with the resection. The goal of the procedure is *En bloc* removal of tumor without tumor transgression, providing tumor-free margins (**Figures 23.3** and **23.4**). At the initial stages, tracheotomy, ventriculoperitoneal shunt or lumbar drain, Greenfield filter, and possible intracranial bypass may be performed. The carotid artery is occluded preoperatively to assure cerebral blood flow will be adequate when the carotid artery is resected. Early in the procedure, a clip is placed on the internal carotid artery between the cavernous sinus and the origin of the opthalmic artery. This is a preventive measure to avoid an embolic event from cervical manipulation of the vasculature. Later, this maneuver permits dissection of the anterior petrous apex and carotid canal without needing to visualize the artery. Parotid gland excision, ascending ramus of the mandible resection, and neck dissections are then performed. The internal carotid artery, the jugular vein, and the cranial nerves IX–XII are resected. Pterygoid muscles are divided and left attached to the skull base. After identification, the vertebral artery is preserved. Deep cervical muscles are incised and the transverse process of C1 and/or C2 is divided if necessary for exposure. This allows medial dissection and exposure of the carotid entrance into the skull base. The mandibular division of the trigeminal nerve is identified, preserved, and traced to the foramen rotundum. A craniotomy is performed, raising a large bone flap that provides good suboccipital exposure and excellent exposure of the anterior middle fossa. The trunks and their divisions of the trigeminal nerve and carotid artery are resected and preserved. The dura of the middle fossa may be resected with the specimen. The transverse sinus is ligated. The superior petrosal sinus is occluded 0.5 cm before its entrance into the cavernous sinus. The brainstem is retracted gently to visualize the inferior petrosal sinus, jugular bulb, and foramen magnum. The anterior lateral bone cut is made through the superior petrosal sinus, the carotid canal just proximal to the cavernous sinus, and the skull base and lateral skull. This cut connects the anterior petrous apex with the neck and frees the anterior medial fossa. The eustachian tube lies inferolateral to the carotid canal. It is transected and sutured to prevent CSF leak. The final bone cuts start posteriorly to connect lateral bone with the jugular foramen. Even with this procedure, it might be impossible not to violate a tumor margin. Despite such large resection, piecemeal removal of the small amounts of residual tumor may be necessary, especially in the occipital condyle, clivus, carotid canal, or cavernous sinus. Since the original report, further modifications have been made. The clivus and the cavernous sinus have been resected in some cases; preoperative carotid artery screening with temporary balloon occlusion has been used instead of the Silverstem clamp; preoperative venous outflow evaluation has been added; and internal carotid artery and internal jugular vein sparing techniques have attempted, but resection of these structures is inevitable in most cases in the experience of this author (R.T.S.) and then (15, 46, 81–84). Sacrifice of the internal carotid artery leads to significant morbidity and the risk of mortality (24, 64, 83, 85). Unpublished data by Sobol indicates 0% 2-year survival after resection of internal carotid artery. We have not had the same experience. Moffat and Wagstaff (56) believe that even if the internal carotid artery appears to be involved, peeling the tumor off the adventitia of the arterial wall is appropriate to achieve adequate results without the neurologic sequela after carotid resection. We agree that this approach may be appropriate in the neck but do not believe it is ideal for extensive intratemporal tumor.

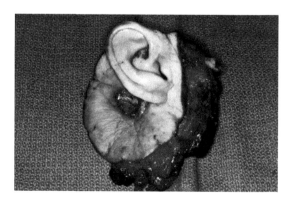

Figure 23.3 The entire TB, external auditory canal, adjacent neck tissue, and a portion of the mandible were removed. *Abbreviation*: TB, Temporal bone.

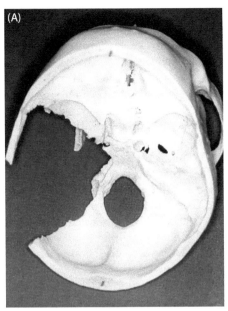 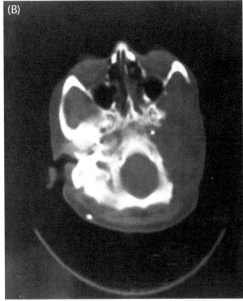

Figure 23.4  (A) Skull shows the area of bone resected. (B) A postoperative CT scan of the patient.

## COMPLICATIONS OF TEMPORAL BONE RESECTION

*Hemorrhage* of major vessels is at risk of intraoperative injury. Some authors recommend reserving 6 units of autologous whole blood prior to the surgery. Intraoperative bleeding can be reduced by hypotensive anesthesia. Acute intracranial hemorrhage is one of the most feared complications. Rapidly progressing intracranial pressure may lead to significant brain injury and possible demise in a relatively short period of time. Patients' neurologic status must be monitored closely after surgery, and, if any suspicion arises, CT scan without contrast must be obtained immediately.

*Wound infections* are not common. Preoperative XRT may increase the risk of wound infection. In this case, Pseudomonas aeruginosa is the most common causative organism and may cause flap necrosis. In the absence of CSF leak, the risk of intracranial spread of infection is low. If meningitis is suspected, CSF culture must be obtained, and IV antibiotics must be initiated until the microbiology report is available.

*CSF leak.* The main concern is risk of meningitis; thus, watertight closure is of outmost importance. Particular attention must be paid to the occlusion of the eustachian tube and adequate closure of the incision. If CSF leak develops, lumbar drains should be placed, and the patient should be monitored for signs of meningitis. In previous studies, ventriculoperitoneal shunts were required to control the leak. It is also important to avoid communication between tracheal secretions and the subcutaneous CSF leak because retrograde contamination may result in intracranial infection.

Other complications include cerebral herniation, CSF fistula, hydrocephalus, carotid artery thrombosis, and stroke.

## PATIENT SELECTION

TTBR is a formidable procedure, which commonly requires 18–24 hours and is associated often with substantial blood loss (although the author [R.T.S.] has performed one case successfully without transfusion in a Jehovah's witness). It should be performed only as a curative operation in patients who are physiologically and psychologically prepared to tolerate the procedure and a prolonged recovery. Paralysis of cranial nerves VI–XII is planned, and the patient and family must be thoroughly informed before this method is chosen. Absolute contraindications include poor health, cavernous sinus involvement, unresectable neck disease, and distant metastases (86). If the tumor encroaches upon the internal carotid artery, preoperative balloon test occlusion should be performed to determine the perfusion capacity of the contralateral side. This will help to determine whether the patient is able to tolerate the resection of the ICA or will require intracranial bypass surgery. On the basis of the ICA balloon occlusion test, Hirsch and Cheng (85) list three groups of patients based on probability of major cerebral ischemia from an acute ICA interruption. Venogram must be also performed to evaluate the venous anatomy. A unilateral dominance of the venous system is not uncommon. Significant cranial venous outflow problems may result in hydrocephalus and cerebral edema. The vein of Labbé provides the majority of venous outflow of the temporal lobe. If occluded at the entrance to the transverse sinus, severely debilitating consequences sometimes result (85). Radical neck dissection may have to be postponed or modified to prevent venous outflow problems. Sataloff et al. (84) described the transcranial sigmoid sinus balloon occlusion test in conjunction with arterial balloon occlusion to test for venous congestion.

## RECONSTRUCTION

The destructive behavior and invasive character of SCCA in the TB dictate reconstructive options. A majority of tumors arising within the EAC have a tendency for deep spread into the TB. Thus, skin loss is not a significant issue. If the lesion involves the auricle, a large soft tissue deformity may result. The goals of reconstruction include correction of functional and cosmetic defect, protection of intracranial contents, and assurance of adequate healing.

Defects from mastoidectomy or sleeve resection can be corrected by canaloplasty with split-thickness skin graft. Defect after LTBR can be corrected with tympanoplasty. It provides easy tumor surveillance of the cavity and offers potentially serviceable hearing. Fujita et al. (87) demonstrated that EAC reconstruction using rolled-up, full-thickness skin graft with tympanoplasty after LTBR can minimize hearing loss. Morita et al. (88) found that using split-thickness skin grafts can also preserve hearing as well as improve quality of life.

Unfortunately, most current treatment protocols include postoperative XRT. Once postoperative therapy is initiated, the skin or fascia graft may not provide adequate protection of bone or exposed dura, increasing the potential risk of osteoradionecrosis and fistula formation. To provide more substantial coverage, many authors recommend obliteration of the EAC with a vascularized flap. Various local and regional flaps have been used. One option is the superficial temporoparietal fascia flap. This flap is dependent on the superficial temporal artery. A temporalis muscle flap is also an excellent source of vascularized tissue in these defects (69). It is readily available in the operative field. The blood supply for this comes from anterior and posterior deep temporal arteries. Extensive dissection in the preauricular area, particularly during the resection of the ascending process of the mandible, or interruption of the external carotid artery, will compromise the viability of the flap. Gal et al., in their series, reviewed the results of seven patients with canal obliterations and two patients without and found no cases of osteoradionecrosis. They found that by rotating a temporalis muscle flap into the defect, the loss of bulk of the parotid gland and neck contents is improved easily through adequate cutaneous coverage (88). Preoperative XRT increases the risk for tissue loss and wound break down. In these patients, local rotation flaps are not recommended.

If the tumor has considerable skin involvement, the resection may result in a large soft tissue defect with exposed bone and dura. Cervical and facial rotational flaps can be used for small-to-medium-sized skin defects. They may be used also to suspend the face after resecting the facial nerve.

The defect created after STB and TTB resection is considerable (Figure 23.4). Exposure of the internal carotid artery and the high likelihood of a CSF leak generally necessitate use of either pedicled or free myocutaneous flaps, although the value of galial advancement flaps should not be underestimated. With minimal donor site morbidity, all these flaps provide excellent soft tissue bulk for cosmesis and protect bone and dura from XRT-induced damages. The pectoralis major flap is a reliable option for reconstruction of head and neck defects (90). Its use for the lateral skull base may be limited by inadequate length and undue tension exerted by gravity (89). However, recent studies have demonstrated its increasing use in lateral skull base reconstruction with promising results (91, 92). The lower island trapezius flap is a good alternative. It is based on the transverse cervical artery with a variable contribution from the dorsal scapular artery. It has several advantages: fairly good color match to the skin of the face, adequate thickness and length for surface coverage, and shorter operative time than free flaps (93, 94). Several points must be considered. The history of ipsilateral neck dissection, especially in the posterior triangle, is a relative contraindication for the use of this flap due to the uncertain status of the transverse cervical artery. The harvest of this flap requires patient placement into the lateral decubitus position. If the blood supply to the lower island trapezius flap appears to be compromised, a latissimus dorsi flap may be harvested with the patient in the same position. It is based on the thoracodorsal artery and vein (95). The benefit of the latissimus flap is its versatility. It is excellent for broad skull defects and may be used as a myofascial or myocutaneous flap. Also, if its length becomes an issue, it can be converted into a free flap (89). The rectus abdominis flap, like the latissimus, can be used as a myofascial or myocutaneous free flap. It provides excellent bulk and can cover any skull defect. Due to its remote location, a second team may harvest the flap in tandem with simultaneous TB resection. However, its use may result in ventral hernia, as it is a major support for the abdominal wall.

The radial forearm flap is a versatile flap with minimal donor site morbidity, but it lacks the bulk necessary for the obliteration of the dead space offered by other flaps. In certain instances, it can be preferable because the use of bulky flaps interferes with tumor surveillance. Also, if complete tumor resection is not assured, it may be advisable to postpone the best reconstruction option until absence of recurrence is confirmed.

There are reports that pedicled, and free flaps are associated with increased incidence of wound complications (96). Yet, if use of local tissue flaps is compromised by excessive tension, previous radiation, or other factors, one should not hesitate to use myocutaneous flaps. Emerging evidence has shown that CT perfusion and dynamic contrast-enhanced MR imaging may serve as tools for predicting wound complications after free flap reconstruction, thereby facilitating surgical planning (97).

Large cutaneous defects that include the resection of the auricle may compromise the social acceptability of the final result. With recent advances in reconstruction technology, repair of the defect should concentrate not only on the functional aspect but also prepare the site for auricular replacement. Several options for auricular replacement exist: reconstruction of the ear from autologous tissue, glued "tissue-borne" prostheses, and "implant-borne" prostheses. Granstrom et al. (98) found low aesthetic acceptability of the reconstructed ear prosthesis. The glued tissue-borne prostheses may be unacceptable due to significant movement that may occur in the reconstructed region with mandibular movement. In contrast, implant-borne prostheses maintain their position and are much better tolerated by the patient. To enhance aesthetic results, Gliklich et al. (99) utilized free flaps and camouflage techniques with osseo-integrated implant technology. They describe anchoring the implant with a bar to the remaining skull. The prosthetic auricle and bone anchoring hearing aid may be secured on the bar at the level of the contralateral ear, recreating a natural appearance. In their study, all disease-free patients were offered prosthetic rehabilitation. They reported an 89% success rate of implants in previously radiated bone. Granstrom et al. have reported 35% implant loss rate when placed in irradiated bone, but they noted that improved vascularity improves implant success, as demonstrated with hyperbaric oxygen treatment (100). Unfortunately, prostheses age with sunlight and tobacco exposure may have to be replaced every 2–3 years, prolong the rehabilitation process by several months, and require some dexterity to place. In their series, Gliklich et al. (99) found prosthetic acceptability by patients rose from 0% to 57%.

Vascular grafts and nerve grafts can be used to restore lost function. If the facial nerve is sacrificed, corneal protection and various reanimation techniques should be considered to improve both function and cosmesis.

## PROSPECTIVE

To date, there have been no treatment–control studies reported. Most of the many treatment approaches are based on individual experience. In 1994, Prasad and Janecka (65) attempted to gain perspective on the role of surgery in the management of malignant tumors of the TB. They reviewed the available literature and selected 26 publications that had comparable data. From the data analysis of 144 patients, they made the following suggestions: (a) tumors limited to EAC have a 50% overall cure rate after mastoidectomy or LTBR or STBR, (b) addition of XRT after LTBR does not appear to be advantageous, and (c) compared with mastoidectomy and LTBR, STBR improves survival once the tumor involves the middle ear. It may appear that conclusions made from such an indepth study would hold true, and indeed, multiple authors continue to use their suggestions. However, upon closer examination, one finds that for each treatment modality the patients' sample size remained small. The staging system they used was limited: tumor confined to EAC, tumor extended into the middle ear, and tumor invading petrous apex. Moreover, the XRT protocols and techniques have changed. Furthermore, multiple studies (prospective and retrospective) published since 1994 have disputed their conclusions.

One of the suggestions made by Prasad and Janecka was that, for lesions limited to EAC, there was no significant difference in 5-year survival rates between radical mastoidectomy, LTBR, and STBR (65). Other authors agree that, regardless of the treatment modality used, there is no statistical difference in the 5-year survival rates when the disease remains lateral to the tympanic membrane. Yet, much more promising cure rates ranging from 75% to 100% are reported (8, 56, 66, 101, 102).

Tumor extension in the middle ear or mastoid process mandates at least subtotal resection (103). Five-year survival rates among these patients vary from 50% to 100% (65, 66, 104). The morbidity from STBR is significant. Thus, some authors advocate piecemeal tumor removal after radical mastoidectomy, followed by high-dose postoperative XRT (2, 13, 39, 65, 105, 106). For example, Zhang et al. (107) reported the actuarial 5-year survival rate of 73% (8/11) for stage III disease and 12.5% (1/8) for stage IV disease. Nyrop and Grontved (101) applied piecemeal tumor removal for stages T3 and T4 followed by postoperative XRT. They reported 0% cure rate due to 100% local recurrence most likely related to the incomplete resection. Austin et al. compared results of procedures other than En bloc excision for stages III and IV tumors with En bloc excision and noted significantly better survival with the more aggressive approach (9). They then compared En bloc resection with and without

XRT and found better survival in the combination treatment group. Their conclusion was to proceed with En bloc excision followed by postoperative XRT. They concluded that a more radical approach with adequate margins will provide better tumor control for advanced stages. These findings were in agreement with the reports by Arena and Keen (49), Spector (62), and Dean et al. (106). Moffat and Wagstaff evaluated 15 patients with extensive T3 and T4 tumors of the TB (56). All patients had been treated previously with mastoidectomy and XRT. They criticized such treatment because of the difficulties associated with clinical and radiologic tumor surveillance of the operated site that subsequently delayed patients' presentation with recurrence. The general conclusion was that a more radical approach with adequate margins will provide better tumor control for advanced stages. This correlates with a statement by Arriaga et al., "the basic principle of surgical oncology is complete tumor extirpation" (67).

Advanced tumors extending beyond the TB require TTBR. Reported 5-year survival ranges from 12.5% to 35% with combined surgery and XRT (9, 56, 74). Despite the technical advances in neuro-otological surgery, the morbidity and the mortality rates remain high. Arriaga et al. called results of TTBR disappointing; only one patient out of five had lived past 10 months (16). He questioned the significance of pathologic margins for these resections. Gacek and Goodman believed that if the only difference between STBR and TTBR is removal of petrous apex, then there is no benefit from a procedure with significantly increased postoperative morbidity (18). However, leaving gross tumor behind almost guarantees local recurrence and demise within 12 months. Moffat and Wangstaff recognized low 5-year survival rates but advocated use of TTBR as a salvage surgery for patients with recurrence (56). They acknowledge the considerable negative impact on the patients' quality of life from recurrence of SSCA: foul otorrhea, severe intractable bone, and meningeal pain from the tumor invasion. From their experience, TTBR sparing the internal carotid artery and postoperative XRT provided palliative therapy with up to 47% 5-year survival rate.

Five-year survival rates for early carcinoma (T1 and T2) is approximately 86%; 5-year survival for T3 lesions is approximately 50%; and T4 lesions are associated with a 5-year survival rate of 41% (74).

## RADIATION THERAPY

For the first half of the 20th century, poor results associated with resection of the TB diverted physicians' attention away from the surgical approach. Treatment was concentrated mainly on the use of XRT alone or in conjunction with radical mastoidectomy. Direct beam radiotherapy or radium implants in the mastoid cavity were used extensively. Radium implants were halted because of injury to the brainstem. Overall survival of patients with middle ear SCCA after treatment in 1930–1940s was 23% (108). Some authors continue to use XRT as a sole modality. Although survival rates up to 77% have been reported with use if this modality alone, poor bone penetration, concomitant chronic infections, and constantly changing protocols (depth, site, agents, dose, frequency, techniques, etc.) have left these claims subject to skepticism and criticism. It seems that once SCCA involves the middle ear, XRT alone is curative in ~23% of cases (6, 18, 62, 108–111). In their study of long-term outcomes following TB SCCA management, Laskar et al. (112) noted that definitive XRT or chemoradiation alone was reserved for patients with unresectable tumors or had medical contraindications. They found that these patients had worse overall survival rates compared to patients who received XRT or chemoradiation in addition to surgery. The consensus is that radiation is an adjunctive therapy for SCCA of the TB.

The most common indications for XRT are large tumors, uncertain or positive margins, perineural invasion, regional adenopathy, parotid or soft-tissue extension, bony invasion, tumors involving the middle ear, mastoid, and more medial structures of the TB (9, 113).

Hashi et al. retrospectively evaluated 20 patients with SCCA of the TB. After median follow-up for 43 months, they concluded that for T1 lesions in their eight patients, 100% disease control was achieved regardless of type of therapy used, radiation alone, surgery, or combination (114). Their finding correlated with the reports of other authors (2, 9, 50, 66–68, 76, 115, 116). Patients with completely resected T1 tumors have demonstrated little benefit of postoperative XRT (117, 118). Austin et al. (9) and Moody et al. (66) noted the benefit from adjunct XRT in patients with T2 and T3 tumors. Spector (62) and Liu et al. (119) observed tumor

extension beyond the operative field despite careful intraoperative monitoring, indicating the need for control of the residual disease. Most current therapeutic recommendations call for a combination of surgery and XRT for treatment of tumors stages T2–T4.

Treatment usually starts after the wound is healed, 2–4 weeks postoperative. A tumorcidal total dose of 54–60 Gy is commonly given without serious threat of brainstem and brain injury. Spector found higher doses with deeper penetration improve significantly survival after extensive resection. He recommended boost doses to 70 Gy if margins are positive (62). Pfreundner et al. stated that only a full course of external beam radiation target (EBRT) of >66 Gy should be administered to the tumor bed of lesions extending beyond surgical margins. In their series, the tumor recurred in regions, which received <66 Gy. They hypothesize that the tumor cells at the surgical margins are hypoxic and have decreased sensitivity to radiation (74). Liu et al. caution that in order to avoid osteonecrosis, no more than 2000 rads should be given to any portion of the TB (115). The clinical target volume must take into account frequent perineural invasion (74).

There is ongoing debate whether confirmed metastatic lymph nodes should be included into the EBRT volume. Pfreundner et al. believe that the clinical target volume must take into account lymphatic drainage. They recommend incorporating an adjuvant dose of 54–60 Gy into the EBRT target volume (74). Arriaga et al. (66) point out that all of their patients who were dead from the disease died from local recurrence. Liu et al. (119) caution against intentional coverage of distal node groups, as most of the patients fail at the primary site. It is important to note that the patient population is often old and can suffer significant morbidity from high-dose radiation treatments.

To control residual or recurrent lesions, brachytherapy with intracavitary implantation of radioactive material has been used as a form of long-term irradiation (62, 74). Pfreundner et al. reported the addition of brachytherapy to external beam radiation in three patients with tumors beyond surgical margins and four patients with recurrent lesions. According to them, if the tumor is locally confined and small, brachytherapy can be used with the intent to cure (74). While uncommon, there has also been a report of a patient with T3 SCCA of the EAC successfully treated with a combination of high-dose-rate brachytherapy and EBRT. There was no evidence of disease at 15-month follow-up, but EAC stenosis and moderate conductive hearing loss were noted (120).

Several authors emphasized that postoperative XRT is not an alternative to complete resection (9, 62, 67). Nyrop and Grontved (101) confirmed findings by Goodwin and Jesse (15); an inadequately excised tumor cannot be controlled by XRT. In the experience of Wagenfeld et al. (23), treatment failure following radiotherapy was almost always within the tumor volume irradiated, suggesting that "geographic miss" was not a factor. The fact that there is a very low survival rate of patients with inoperative advanced disease despite the use of XRT furthers strengthens these conclusions (8, 9). Of course, isolated reports do exist of complete remission with postoperative external beam XRT in patients with residual tumor, but, unfortunately, they are not generally the rule (74). The hypothesis behind radiation failure is that the invading tumor reduces already low oxygen tensions of the TB. The chronic infection associated frequently with SCCA of the TB suggests the presence of hypoxic tumor cells. Thus, the reduced radiosensitivity of tumors shifts therapeutic responsibility for the patient's survival towards physical removal of the entire disease.

Complications of TB irradiation include CNS injury, osteoradionecrosis, osteomyelitis, neuropathies, delayed wound healing, and, in some instances, cochlear and vestibular damage.

## PATTERNS OF SPREAD

Understanding patterns of invasion permits accurate radiologic assessment and adequate operative planning. One must also take into account the limitations of current radiologic tests: appreciating the areas of high probability of radiologic mistakes may reduce the number of "unexpected" intraoperative findings.

SCCA arises most commonly in the cartilaginous portion of the EAC. Natural pathways provide routes of spread for small tumors. The fissures of Santorini give flexibility to the cartilage and usually are filled with connective tissue. Together with a patent foramen of Huschke, they

may permit tumor extension to the anterior soft tissues: preauricular skin, parotid gland, TMJ, or infratemporal fossa. Other points of weakness are the petrosquamous suture and the bony–cartilaginous junction. The density of the tympanic bone and the fibrous middle layer of tympanic membrane serve as barriers to tumor extension into the TB. As the tumor enlarges, it may spread in multiple directions through thin bone. Posteriorly, it can pass through the tympanomastoid suture and the retrofacial cells of Broca to involve the mastoid antrum and mastoid air cells. Medial spread through the TM permits penetration into the middle ear. Once in the middle ear, the tumor can extend into pneumotized spaces including the eustachian tube and involve the bone overlying the carotid artery. In some areas, the bone separating the eustachian tube from internal carotid artery is <1 mm thick. Involvement of the hypotympanum leads to extension into the jugular foramen. Inferior extension invades soft tissue of the neck, jugular foramen, foramen magnum, occiput, and cervical vertebrae. Cephalad extension involves the tegmen tympani or through the petrosquamous fissure, middle fossa dura, and the temporal lobe (58, 59). Posterior spread can lead to invasion of the sigmoid sinus and the posterior fossa. The fallopian canal is the most common site of deep skull invasion (62).

Perineural pathways for tumor invasion beyond the middle ear space have been well described from evaluations of pathology specimens. The lesser petrosal nerve may serve as a route to the middle cranial fossa via the inferior tympanic canaliculus, and sympathetic fibers provide access through the roof of the tympanic cavity (121). This pattern of spread is impossible to appreciate perioperatively, making it most difficult to eradicate (122).

Rouviere (123) described the lymphatic network in EAC continuous with the network of the auricle and tympanic membrane. Three zones with different lymphatic drainage are found in the EAC. The anterior zone drains into the intraparotid and preauricular nodes. The inferior portion of the canal drains inwardly. It terminates in deep intraparotid or infraauricular nodes. And, the posterior zone drainage takes a deep course below the sternoclaidomastoid muscle to the deep upper jugular nodes (74). The lymphatic network of the middle ear and mastoid empties into the retropharyngeal and deep upper jugular lymph nodes.

Cervical lymph node metastases are more likely to occur once disease extends beyond the confines of the TB.

Nonlymphatic or hematogenous spread is usually a late event and results in deposits in the lung, bone, liver, and brain (107).

## PROGNOSTIC FACTORS

Several factors are associated with decreased survival rates. These include the local extent of the tumor, facial paralysis, positive margins, dural involvement, and lymph node metastasis. Some studies have found that advanced age (> 60–65 years old) (8, 119), multiple cranial nerve involvement, moderate-to-severe pain, and female sex may worsen prognosis (124, 125).

Local extension is one of the most important issues if not the main prognostic factor (2, 16, 17, 65, 67, 76, 125). If SCCA is limited to the EAC without middle ear or CN VII involvement, it responds equally well to any kind of treatment, be a radical mastoidectomy with XRT or *En bloc* resection. The overall control rate for tumors limited to the EAC ranges from 80% to 100% (2, 8, 45, 56, 62, 74, 76, 101). Limited extension beyond the EAC reduces the control rate to 60%–70% (16) Gacek and Goodman (18) even proposed to separate and treat the lesions lateral to the tympanic membrane and the lesions extending to the middle ear as separate entities. For these patients, survival depends on aggressive tumor removal in conjunction with postoperative XRT. Once the skull base is involved, radical TB resection with adequate margins and postoperative XRT is the best oncologically sound option. Unfortunately, even though it is technically feasible, survival rates drop dramatically to 25%–38% (74). Pensak et al. (76) defined their contraindications for tumor resection. They include invasion of cavernous sinus, the internal carotid artery, the infratemporal fossa, or the paraspinal musculature. Others do find these factors limiting, but not contraindicating (56, 84).

Facial nerve involvement is an ominous sign that has been long recognized (5). Moody et al. proposed to upgrade the SCCA lesions with evidence of facial nerve paralysis to stage IV of the Pittsburgh classification system. According to them, facial nerve paralysis can only be explained by two causes. First, the tumor invades the horizontal segment of the facial nerve within the fallopian canal. In order for this to occur, the tumor must erode through the medial wall of the middle ear. Second, the tumor affects the facial nerve at the level of the stylomastoid foramen. This is only possible when soft tissue extension is >0.5 cm (66). Both causes signal aggressive behavior of the tumor and high risk of perineural spread. Histological evaluations confirmed the role of the facial nerve as a direct pathway for the intracranial spread of various nonneurogenic neoplasms (126). Chee et al. (113) noted that tumors involving facial nerves were generally extensive and invade other vital structures of the skull base. Multiple other studies reported decreased survival rate associated with facial nerve involvement (7, 8, 85, 119, 124, 125). The degree of facial nerve involvement has been reported to modify patients' prognosis. The treatment failure rate for patients with mild paresis is 34%, moderate paresis is 50%, and complete paralysis is 62% (84, 104). These findings have not been reflected in any classification system and may need further investigation.

Positive tumor margins are one of the indicators of poor prognosis. In the series by Goodwin and Jesse (15), all 13 patients with incomplete resection of advanced SCCA had developed local recurrence despite postoperative radiotherapy. Arriaga et al. (67) noted an almost 50% decrease in survival in the patients with incomplete tumor removal. "Clear margins resulted in 9 with no disease and 2 failed treatment whereas pathologically involved margins accounted for 3 with no disease and 9 treatment failures" (16). Nyrop and Grontved quote 67% overall recurrence rate among patients with positive margins at surgery (25% in stages I and II and 100% in stages III and IV). None of the patients with T3 and T4 cancers had survived after incomplete tumor resection despite postoperative XRT (101). Other authors confirmed these findings (67, 68, 74, 114). Generally, once the tumor recurs, patients succumb to disease within an average of 12 months (56).

Other local sites of invasion such as the dura, temporal lobe, and carotid artery have been implicated as separate poor prognostic factors by several authors (16, 56, 66, 67, 74, 127). On the basis of the individual experiences, authors decide whether these factors determine a tumor's resectability. For example, Pfreundner et al. (74) and Arriaga et al.

(16) believe that extension of the disease beyond the dura renders it unresectable and incurable. Others, on the contrary, reported several patients surviving 5 years after resection of involved dura and/or brain (56, 69, 84, 128). Similarly, Moffat and Wangstaff (56) believe that often peeling the tumor off the adventitia of the arterial wall is appropriate to achieve adequate results.

Several authors have attributed nodal involvement to have a negative impact on survival (7, 62, 67, 107, 124). The majority of reports describe the incidence of regional lymph node metastases to be 5%–15% (15, 48, 56, 76). It appears that cartilage invasion by the tumor is not correlated with metastasis (17). Yet, in the presence of metastatic lymphadenopathy, bony destruction is almost always present (4, 16). The reported drop in survival ranges from 20% to 60% once the nodes are involved (16, 62). This is reflected in the Pittsburgh tumor classification system. Once metastatic lymph nodes are identified, the tumor is immediately classified at least as a stage III. The question then becomes whether neck dissection is necessary. For head and neck tumors, prophylactic neck dissection in the absence of clinically and radiologically apparent metastatic lymph nodes is recommended once the risk of occult nodal involvement is at ~20%. For SCCA of the TB, some authors argue against neck dissection. Leonetti et al. (59) reported that no patients with metastatic lymph nodes die of regional lymph node disease, but instead all disease-related mortality is from the uncontrolled disease at the original site. Arriaga et al. also noted a lack of benefit from neck dissection in 2-year survival. All of their patients who were dead of the disease died from local recurrence (16, 67). Furthermore, Moody et al. (66) reported neck dissection and/or parotidectomy to have no effect on survival for any stage of disease. In addition, Liu et al. (119) caution against intentional coverage of distal node groups during XRT, as patients fail at the primary site. Other authors suggest sending the lymph nodes collected in the vicinity of the TB dissection for frozen section and proceeding with the neck dissection if they prove to have microinvasions. They believe that if the first echelon of the lymph nodes is negative for metastasis, the morbidity from the added neck dissection is unnecessary. There is a group of surgeons who perform routine selective neck dissection on every patient. Moffat et al. recommended

supraomohyoid dissection for staging purposes, better access to the skull base, and incorporating soft tissue of the neck into the postoperative XRT field (56, 128). Moffat and Wagstaff (56) and Spector (62) reported the incidence of metastatic nodes to be 23%–29%. This finding may reflect under-staging of the disease by authors who only treat TBs. In their latest discussion, Moffat and Wagstaff (56) attributed utmost prognostic importance to the presence of metastatic lymph nodes. They believe that lymph node involvement signifies more aggressive disease, which in turn elevates the risk of local recurrence and subsequent early demise (15, 56, 62, 107). Once again, a lack of uniform information forces surgeons to use personal experiences and philosophies to design their treatment plans.

The degree of tumor differentiation has shown variable impact on survival. According to the observation by Kenyon et al. (13), patients with well-differentiated tumors developed CN VII paralysis and succumbed to the disease earlier than patients with poorly differentiated tumors. Moffat et al. (128) and Liu et al. (119) reported better survival with well-differentiated carcinoma. Arriaga et al. (16) and Chen and Dehner(17) found very little difference between the histologic differentiation and survival. As we can see, there is no consensus on this subject.

Tumor recurrence, whether it occurs after surgery or external beam XRT, indicates a poor prognosis. Most treatment failures are due to local recurrence. Arriaga et al. (16) reported the incidence of local recurrences in 14 out of 17 patients with treatment failures. They also found tumor recurrence to be responsible for all the disease-related deaths (67). Because 90% of recurrence occurs locally, it must be the result of an incomplete resection. Indeed, Spector (62) notes that most of the local recurrences resulted from unexpected tumor extensions beyond the operative area. If for some reason residual tumor is left in the field and failed to respond to postoperative XRT, the majority of the patients will present within 24 months after initial surgery. The average time of presentation is 4–7 months (8, 16, 67). Once the tumor recurs, the preponderance of patients will succumb to SCCA within 18 months from the time of the diagnosis. Moffat et al. reported an incredible 47% 5-year survival rate with salvage surgery and large doses of postoperative XRT. Despite this, they continue to insist on the aggressive first treatment protocol because it offers the greatest chance for cure (56, 128).

## QUALITY OF LIFE ISSUES

While temporal bone resection is feasible. the results of such extensive surgery can be debilitating. They can cause disfigurement, social disturbances, hearing loss, facial nerve abnormality, communication difficulties, dysphagia, etc. We as physicians concentrate on technical aspects of the procedures and determine outcome of treatment by measuring tumor response rate, disease progression, and disease-free survival. However, none of these parameters reflect patients' own perception of successful outcome. Nowadays, there is increased awareness of the need for evaluating the impact of symptoms on the patient's quality of life. Kwok et al. (129) conducted a retrospective cross-sectional study of 23 patients with history of TB resection or parotidectomy with radiotherapy. They compared physicians' perceptions of success with patients' perceptions of the treatment outcome. According to their findings, with exception of hearing testing, clinical assessments did not generally correlate well with patients' ratings. Interestingly, facial disfigurement did not cause much patient distress. Several authors had reviewed life satisfaction among head and neck patients and noted that disfigurement is generally unrelated to the quality of life. Patients tend to adapt successfully and be grateful to be alive after confronting cancer (129–135). The difficulties with communication and swallowing were the most bothersome to patients and most underestimated by physicians. Additionally, de Casso et al. (136) found that patients who suffered from TMJ dysfunction following TB resection for carcinoma experienced poor quality of life measures, specifically chronic pain and psychosocial disturbances. As patient survival improves, the therapeutic decision must incorporate quality of daily life as experienced by the patients.

Hearing loss has a particularly profound consequence on quality of life. Patients can expect maximum conductive hearing loss after LTBR or complete sensorineural hearing loss after resection of the otic capsule in STBR or TTBR. Furthermore, ototoxic effects from adjuvant chemotherapy or radiotherapy can result in sensorineural hearing loss, even if the inner ear is spared during surgery. Current management of auditory rehabilitation is use of osseointegrated hearing aids. Nader et al. (137) recommended timing of implantation at initial oncologic resection and prior to radiotherapy. Nevertheless, there remains a lack of patient-reported quality of life outcomes following implantation. The insight obtained from patients' responses will guide physicians and ancillary staff in the formulation of therapeutic and rehabilitation goals.

## CHEMOTHERAPY

In the majority of cases, the increased morbidity associated with chemotherapy renders it as the last resort treatment. As a result, it is usually given in cases of aggressive, recurrent, or unresectable disease. Previously, the small number of patients receiving chemotherapy and the advanced stages of the disease for which chemotherapy is given made it virtually impossible to define the impact of chemotherapy on survival. Arriaga et al. (16) did not find the addition of chemotherapy to enhance survival. Suzuki et al. reported five patients in whom intra-arterial (as opposed to intra-venous) chemotherapy was added to the combined surgery and XRT treatment. The superficial temporal artery or superior thyroid artery was used for vascular access. They found no tumor cells in three patients after completion of combined therapy (138–140). Knegt et al. conducted a prospective study utilizing meticulous tumor debulking followed by repeated applications of 5-fluorouracil cream and necrotectomy. They report 74% overall 5-year survival. The procedure demanded eight painful sessions of follow-up after initial surgery for dressing change, necrotectomy, and 5-fluorouracil reapplication. Patients were re-evaluated intraoperatively in 2–3 months and, if found to have residual tumor, had to repeat the entire protocol and undergo XRT. The data are hard to interpret because the authors used a limited classification system, did not describe the extent of the final debulking/necrotectomy procedure, and failed to report survival outcomes separately for each stage (141). Recent studies, however, have demonstrated the promising use of chemoradiation therapy (CRT) in treating TB SCCA. Nakagawa et al. (142) showed that preoperative CRT therapy was helpful in obtaining tumor-free margins in T3 and T4 SCCA. Takenaka et al. (143) performed a meta-analysis to evaluate CRT as definitive therapy and adjuvant therapy for T3 and T4 tumors. They found that preoperative CRT was associated with improved overall survival rate, but that postoperative CRT had no effect. They also found equivalent overall survival rates between definitive CRT and surgery with adjuvant radiotherapy. This is consistent with results from more recent studies (78, 144, 145). As more evidence of the efficacy of CRT emerges, some authors have suggested utilizing definitive CRT for stage II disease (146). Cisplatin, 5-fluorouracil, and docetaxel are usually the chemotherapy agents of choice, but there are reports of success with cetuximab, bevacizumab, and pemetrexed (147). Although none of the reports is adequate for evaluation, they reflect continued interest in the use of chemotherapy agents for treatment of SCCA of the TB.

## CONCLUSION

SCCA of the TB remains a complex, challenging, and incompletely understood disease. However, it is not hopeless. Through aggressive treatment, even rare patients with advanced disease can be cured. Nevertheless, considerably more experience is needed before optimal treatment for all stages can be established with confidence.

## ACKNOWLEDGMENT

The authors appreciate contributions to the previous edition by Dr. Mikhail Vaysberg, some of which have been retained in the current edition.

## REFERENCES

1. Horn J. Surveillance, Epidemiology and End Results Rockville, MD: National Cancer Institute; 1987.
2. Kinney SE, Wood BG. Malignancies of the external ear canal and temporal bone: Surgical techniques and results. Laryngoscope. 1987;97(2):158–64.
3. Lovin BD, Gidley PW. Squamous cell carcinoma of the temporal bone: a current review. Laryngoscope Investig Otolaryngol. 2019;4(6):684–92.
4. Conley J, Schuller DE. Malignancies of the ear. Laryngoscope. 1976;86(8):1147–63.
5. Crabtree JA, Britton BH, Pierce MK. Carcinoma of the external auditory canal. Laryngoscope. 1976;86(3):405–15.
6. Lederman M. Malignant tumours of the ear. J Laryngol Otol. 1965;79:85–119.
7. Stell PM, McCormick MS. Carcinoma of the external auditory meatus and middle ear. Prognostic factors and a suggested staging system. J Laryngol Otol. 1985;99(9):847–50.
8. Testa JR, Fukuda Y, Kowalski LP. Prognostic factors in carcinoma of the external auditory canal. Arch Otolaryngol Head Neck Surg. 1997;123(7):720–4.
9. Austin JR, Stewart KL, Fawzi N. Squamous cell carcinoma of the external auditory canal. Therapeutic prognosis based on a proposed staging system. Arch Otolaryngol Head Neck Surg. 1994;120(11):1228–32.
10. Kuhel WI, Hume CR, Selesnick SH. Cancer of the external auditory canal and temporal bone. Otolaryngol Clin North Am. 1996;29(5):827–52.
11. Higgins TS, Antonio SA. The role of facial palsy in staging squamous cell carcinoma of the temporal bone and external auditory canal: a comparative survival analysis. Otol Neurotol. 2010;31(9):1473–9.
12. Woods RSR, Naude A, O'Sullivan JB, Rawluk D, Javadpour M, Walshe P, et al. Management of temporal bone malignancy in Ireland. J Neurol Surg B Skull Base. 2020;81(6):680–5.
13. Kenyon GS, Marks PV, Scholtz CL, Dhillon R. Squamous cell carcinoma of the middle ear. A 25-year retrospective study. Ann Otol Rhinol Laryngol. 1985;94(3):273–7.
14. Lewis JS. Temporal bone resection. Review of 100 cases. Arch Otolaryngol. 1975;101(1):23–5.
15. Goodwin WJ, Jesse RH. Malignant neoplasms of the external auditory canal and temporal bone. Arch Otolaryngol. 1980;106(11):675–9.
16. Arriaga M, Hirsch BE, Kamerer DB, Myers EN. Squamous cell carcinoma of the external auditory meatus (canal). Otolaryngol Head Neck Surg. 1989;101(3):330–7.

17. Chen KT, Dehner LP. Primary tumors of the external and middle ear. I. Introduction and clinicopathologic study of squamous cell carcinoma. Arch Otolaryngol. 1978;104(5):247–52.

18. Gacek RR, Goodman M. Management of malignancy of the temporal bone. Laryngoscope. 1977;87(10 Pt 1):1622–34.

19. Bendl BG, Graham JH. New concepts on the origin of squamous cell carcinoma of the skin: Solar (senile) keratosis with squamous cell carcinoma: a clinicopathologic and histochemical study. Proceeding of the Sixth National Cancer Conference. Philadelphia: Lippincott; 1968. p. 471–88.

20. Shiffman NJ. Squamous cell carcinomas of the skin of the pinna. Can J Surg. 1975;18(3):279–83.

21. Moffat DA, Grey P, Ballagh RH, Hardy DG. Extended temporal bone resection for squamous cell carcinoma. Otolaryngol Head Neck Surg. 1997;116(6):617–23.

22. Allanson BM, Low TH, Clark JR, Gupta R. Squamous cell carcinoma of the external auditory canal and temporal bone: An update. Head Neck Pathol. 2018;12(3):407–18.

23. Wagenfeld DJ, Keane T, van Nostrand AW, Bryce DP. Primary carcinoma involving the temporal bone: Analysis of twenty-five cases. Laryngoscope. 1980;90(6 Pt 1):912–9.

24. Gacek MR, Gacek RR, Gantz B, McKenna M, Goodman M. Pseudoepitheliomatous hyperplasia versus squamous cell carcinoma of the external auditory canal. Laryngoscope. 1998;108(4 Pt 1):620–3.

25. Khan AS. Pseudoepitheliomatous hyperplasia of the external ear, middle ear, and mastoid. Laryngoscope. 1979;89(6 Pt 1):984–7.

26. Monem SA, Moffat DA, Frampton MC. Carcinoma of the ear: a case report of a possible association with chlorinated disinfectants. J Laryngol Otol. 1999;113(11):1004–7.

27. Jin YT, Tsai ST, Li C, Chang KC, Yan JJ, Chao WY, et al. Prevalence of human papillomavirus in middle ear carcinoma associated with chronic otitis media. Am J Pathol. 1997;150(4):1327–33.

28. Tsai ST, Li C, Jin YT, Chao WY, Su IJ. High prevalence of human papillomavirus types 16 and 18 in middle-ear carcinomas. Int J Cancer. 1997;71(2):208–12.

29. Hongo T, Yamamoto H, Kuga R, Komune N, Miyazaki M, Tsuchihashi NA, et al. High-risk HPV-related squamous cell carcinoma in the temporal bone: a rare but noteworthy subtype. Virchows Arch. 2023;482(3):539–50.

30. Watabe-Rudolph M, Rudolph KL, Averbeck T, Buhr T, Lenarz T, Stover T. Telomerase activity, telomere length, and apoptosis: A comparison between acquired cholesteatoma and squamous cell carcinoma. Otol Neurotol. 2002;23(5):793–8.

31. Michaels L, Wells M. Squamous cell carcinoma of the middle ear. *Clin. Otolaryngol.* 1980;4(5):235–48.

32. Yanez-Siller JC, Wentland C, Bowers K, Litofsky NS, Rivera AL. Squamous cell carcinoma of the temporal bone arising from cholesteatoma: A case report and review of the literature. J Neurol Surg Rep. 2022;83(1):e13–e18.

33. Aub JC, Evans RD, Hempelmann LH, Martland HS. The late effects of internally-deposited radioactive materials in man. Medicine. 1952;31(3):221–329.

34. Beal DD, Lindsay JR, Ward PH. Radiation-induced carcinoma of the mastoid. Arch Otolaryngol. 1965;81:9–16.

35. Lim LH, Goh YH, Chan YM, Chong VF, Low WK. Malignancy of the temporal bone and external auditory canal. Otolaryngol Head Neck Surg. 2000;122(6):882–6.

36. Lo WC, Ting LL, Ko JY, Lou PJ, Yang TL, Chang YL, et al. Malignancies of the ear in irradiated patients of nasopharyngeal carcinoma. Laryngoscope. 2008;118(12):2151–5.

37. Goh YH, Chong VF, Low WK. Temporal bone tumours in patients irradiated for nasopharyngeal neoplasm. J Laryngol Otol. 1999;113(3):222–8.

38. Ruben RJ, Thaler SU, Holzer N. Radiation induced carcinoma of the temporal bone. Laryngoscope. 1977;87(10 Pt 1):1613–21.

39. Lustig LR, Jackler RK, Lanser MJ. Radiation-induced tumors of the temporal bone. Am J Otol. 1997;18(2):230–5.

40. Cahan WG, Woodard HQ, Higinbotham NL, Stewart FW, Coley BL. Sarcoma arising in irradiated bone: report of eleven cases. 1948. Cancer. 1998;82(1):8–34.

41. McRackan TR, Fang TY, Pelosi S, Rivas A, Dietrich MS, Wanna GB, et al. Factors associated with recurrence of squamous cell carcinoma involving the temporal bone. Ann Otol Rhinol Laryngol. 2014;123(4):235–9.

42. Zheng Y, Qiu K, Fu Y, Yang W, Cheng D, Rao Y, et al. Clinical outcomes of temporal bone squamous cell carcinoma: A single-institution experience. Cancer Med. 2023;12(5):5304–11.

43. Gidley PW, Thompson CR, Roberts DB, DeMonte F, Hanna EY. The oncology of otology. Laryngoscope. 2012;122(2):393–400.

44. Lechner M, Sutton L, Murkin C, Masterson L, O'Flynn P, Wareing MJ, et al. Squamous cell cancer of the temporal bone: a review of the literature. Eur Arch Otorhinolaryngol. 2021;278(7):2225–8.

45. Gillespie MB, Francis HW, Chee N, Eisele DW. Squamous cell carcinoma of the temporal bone: a radiographic-pathologic correlation. Arch Otolaryngol Head Neck Surg. 2001;127(7):803–7.

46. Ward GE, Loch WE, Lawrence W, Jr. Radical operation for carcinoma of the external auditory canal and middle ear. Am J Surg. 1951;82(1):169–78.

47. Conley J. Cancer of the middle ear. Trans Am Otol Soc. 1965;53:189–207.

48. Hahn SS, Kim JA, Goodchild N, Constable WC. Carcinoma of the middle ear and external auditory canal. Int J Radiat Oncol Biol Phys. 1983;9(7):1003–7.

49. Arena S, Keen M. Carcinoma of the middle ear and temporal bone. Am J Otol. 1988;9(5):351–6.

50. Paaske PB, Witten J, Schwer S, Hansen HS. Results in treatment of carcinoma of the external auditory canal and middle ear. Cancer. 1987;59(1):156–60.

51. Lewis JS. Cancer of the ear. CA Cancer J Clin. 1987;37(2):78–87.

52. Mattucci KF, Setzen M, Galantich P. Necrotizing otitis externa occurring concurrently with epidermoid carcinoma. Laryngoscope. 1986;96(3):264–6.

53. Grandis JR, Hirsch BE, Yu VL. Simultaneous presentation of malignant external otitis and temporal bone cancer. Arch Otolaryngol Head Neck Surg. 1993;119(6):687–9.

54. Lewis JS. Surgical management of tumors of the middle ear and mastoid. J Laryngol Otol. 1983;97(4):299–311.

55. Madsen AR, Gundgaard MG, Hoff CM, Maare C, Holmboe P, Knap M, et al. Cancer of the external auditory canal and middle ear in Denmark from 1992 to 2001. Head Neck. 2008;30(10):1332–8.

56. Moffat DA, Wagstaff SA. Squamous cell carcinoma of the temporal bone. Curr Opin Otolaryngol Head Neck Surg. 2003;11(2):107–11.

57. Olsen KD, DeSanto LW, Forbes GS. Radiographic assessment of squamous cell carcinoma of the temporal bone. Laryngoscope. 1983;93(9):1162–7.

58. Arriaga M, Curtin H, Takahashi H, Hirsch BE, Kamerer DB. Staging proposal for external auditory meatus carcinoma based on preoperative clinical examination and computed tomography findings. Ann Otol Rhinol Laryngol. 1990;99(9 Pt 1):714–21.

59. Leonetti JP, Smith PG, Kletzker GR, Izquierdo R. Invasion patterns of advanced temporal bone malignancies. Am J Otol. 1996;17(3):438–42.

60. Baker SR, Latack JT. Magnetic resonance imaging of the head and neck. Otolaryngol Head Neck Surg. 1986;95(1):82–9.

61. Levine PA, Paling MR, Black WC, Cantrell RW. MRI vs. high-resolution CT scanning: evaluation of the anterior skull base. Otolaryngol Head Neck Surg. 1987;96(3):260–7.

62. Spector JG. Management of temporal bone carcinomas: a therapeutic analysis of two groups of patients and long-term followup. Otolaryngol Head Neck Surg. 1991;104(1):58–66.

63. Kinney SE. Squamous cell carcinoma of the external auditory canal. Am J Otol. 1989;10(2):111–6.

64. Moharir VM, Fried MP, Vernick DM, Janecka IP, Zahajsky J, Hsu L, et al. Computer-assisted three-dimensional reconstruction of head and neck tumors. Laryngoscope. 1998;108(11 Pt 1):1592–8.

65. Prasad S, Janecka IP. Efficacy of surgical treatments for squamous cell carcinoma of the temporal bone: a literature review. Otolaryngol Head Neck Surg. 1994;110(3):270–80.

66. Moody SA, Hirsch BE, Myers EN. Squamous cell carcinoma of the external auditory canal: an evaluation of a staging system. Am J Otol. 2000;21(4):582–8.

67. Arriaga M, Curtin HD, Takahashi H, Kamerer DB. The role of preoperative CT scans in staging external auditory meatus carcinoma: radiologic-pathologic correlation study. Otolaryngol Head Neck Surg. 1991;105(1):6–11.

68. Yeung P, Bridger A, Smee R, Baldwin M, Bridger GP. Malignancies of the external auditory canal and temporal bone: a review. ANZ J Surg. 2002;72(2):114–20.

69. Breau RL, Gardner EK, Dornhoffer JL. Cancer of the external auditory canal and temporal bone. Curr Oncol Rep. 2002;4(1):76–80.

70. Gidley PW, Roberts DB, Sturgis EM. Squamous cell carcinoma of the temporal bone. Laryngoscope. 2010;120(6):1144–51.

71. Bacciu A, Clemente IA, Piccirillo E, Ferrari S, Sanna M. Guidelines for treating temporal bone carcinoma based on long-term outcomes. Otol Neurotol. 2013;34(5):898–907.

72. Prasad SC, D'Orazio F, Medina M, Bacciu A, Sanna M. State of the art in temporal bone malignancies. Curr Opin Otolaryngol Head Neck Surg. 2014;22(2):154–65.

73. Zanoletti E, Marioni G, Stritoni P, Lionello M, Giacomelli L, Martini A, et al. Temporal bone squamous cell carcinoma: analyzing prognosis with univariate and multivariate models. Laryngoscope. 2014;124(5):1192–8.

74. Pfreundner L, Schwager K, Willner J, Baier K, Bratengeier K, Brunner FX, et al. Carcinoma of the external auditory canal and middle ear. Int J Radiat Oncol Biol Phys. 1999;44(4):777–88.

75. Jackson CM, Ishiyama A, Canalis RF. Malignant tumors of the temporal bones. In: Canalis RF, Lambert PR, ed The Ear: Comprehensive Otology. 52. Philadelphia, PA: Lippincott, Williams; 2000. p. 835–45.

76. Pensak ML, Gleich LL, Gluckman JL, Shumrick KA. Temporal bone carcinoma: contemporary perspectives in the skull base surgical era. Laryngoscope. 1996;106(10):1234–7.

77. Bibas AG, Ward V, Gleeson MJ. Squamous cell carcinoma of the temporal bone. J Laryngol Otol. 2008;122(11):1156–61.

78. Shinomiya H, Hasegawa S, Yamashita D, Ejima Y, Kenji Y, Otsuki N, et al. Concomitant chemoradiotherapy for advanced squamous cell carcinoma of the temporal bone. Head Neck. 2016;38 Suppl 1:E949–53.

79. Saijo K, Ueki Y, Tanaka R, Yokoyama Y, Omata J, Takahashi T, et al. Treatment outcome of external auditory canal carcinoma: The utility of lateral temporal bone resection. Front Surg. 2021;8:708245.

80. Ghavami Y, Haidar YM, Maducdoc M, Tjoa T, Moshtaghi O, Lin HW, et al. Tympanic membrane and ossicular-sparing modified lateral temporal bone resection. Otolaryngol Head Neck Surg. 2017;157(3):530–2.

81. Parsons H, Lewis JS. Subtotal resection of the temporal bone for cancer of the ear. Cancer. 1954;7(5):995–1001.

82. Campbell E, Volk BM, Burklund CW. Total resection of temporal bone for malignancy of the middle ear. Ann Surg. 1951;134(3):397–404.

83. Graham MD, Sataloff RT, Kemink JL, Wolf GT, McGillicuddy JE. Total en bloc resection of the temporal bone and carotid artery for malignant tumors of the ear and temporal bone. Laryngoscope. 1984;94(4):528–33.

84. Sataloff RT, Myers DL, Lowry LD, Spiegel JR. Total temporal bone resection for squamous cell carcinoma. Otolaryngol Head Neck Surg. 1987;96(1):4–14.

85. Hirsch BC, Chang CYJ. Carcinoma of the temporal bone. In: Myers EN, ed Operative Otolaryngology Head and Neck Surgery. Philadelphia, PA: W.B. Saunders; 1997. p. 1434–58.

86. Gidley PW, DeMonte F. Temporal bone malignancies. Neurosurg Clin N Am. 2013;24(1):97–110.

87. Fujita T, Kakigi A, Uehara N, Yokoi J, Hara M, Shinomiya H, et al. Reconstruction of the external auditory canal using full-thickness rolled-up skin graft after lateral temporal bone resection for T1 and T2 external auditory canal cancer. Auris Nasus Larynx. 2021;48(5):830–3.

88. Morita S, Nakamaru Y, Homma A, Sakashita T, Masuya M, Fukuda S. Hearing preservation after lateral temporal bone resection for early-stage external auditory canal carcinoma. Audiol Neurootol. 2014;19(6):351–7.

89. Gal TJ, Kerschner JE, Futran ND, Bartels LJ, Farrior JB, Ridley MB, et al. Reconstruction after temporal bone resection. Laryngoscope. 1998;108(4 Pt 1):476–81.

90. Baek SM, Biller HF, Krespi YP, Lawson W. The pectoralis major myocutaneous island flap for reconstruction of the head and neck. Head Neck Surg. 1979;1(4):293–300.

91. Resto VA, McKenna MJ, Deschler DG. Pectoralis major flap in composite lateral skull base defect reconstruction. Arch Otolaryngol Head Neck Surg. 2007;133(5):490–4.

92. Patel NS, Modest MC, Brobst TD, Carlson ML, Price DL, Moore EJ, et al. Surgical management of lateral skull base defects. Laryngoscope. 2016;126(8):1911–7.

93. Urken ML, Naidu RK, Lawson W, Biller HF. The lower trapezius island musculocutaneous flap revisited. Report of 45 cases and a unifying concept of the vascular supply. Arch Otolaryngol Head Neck Surg. 1991;117(5):502–11.

94. Netterville JL, Panje WR, Maves MD. The trapezius myocutaneous flap. Dependability and limitations. Arch Otolaryngol Head Neck Surg. 1987;113(3):271–81.

95. Day TA, Davis BK. Skull base reconstruction and rehabilitation. Otolaryngol Clin North Am. 2001;34(6):1241–57, xi.

96. Neligan PC, Mulholland S, Irish J, Gullane PJ, Boyd JB, Gentili F, et al. Flap selection in cranial base reconstruction. Plast Reconstr Surg. 1996;98(7):1159–66; discussion 67–8.

97. Ota Y, Moore AG, Spector ME, Casper K, Stucken C, Malloy K, et al. Prediction of wound failure in patients with head and neck cancer treated with free flap reconstruction: utility of CT perfusion and MR perfusion in the early postoperative period. AJNR Am J Neuroradiol. 2022;43(4):585–91.

98. Granstrom G, Bergstrom K, Tjellstrom A. The bone-anchored hearing aid and bone-anchored epithesis for congenital ear malformations. Otolaryngol Head Neck Surg. 1993;109(1):46–53.

99. Gliklich RE, Rounds MF, Cheney ML, Varvares MA. Combining free flap reconstruction and craniofacial prosthetic technique for orbit, scalp, and temporal defects. Laryngoscope. 1998;108(4 Pt 1):482–7.

100. Granstrom G, Tjellstrom A, Albrektsson T. Postimplantation irradiation for head and neck cancer treatment. Int J Oral Maxillofac Implants. 1993;8(5):495–501.

101. Nyrop M, Grontved A. Cancer of the external auditory canal. Arch Otolaryngol Head Neck Surg. 2002;128(7):834–7.

102. Chi FL, Gu FM, Dai CF, Chen B, Li HW. Survival outcomes in surgical treatment of 72 cases of squamous cell carcinoma of the temporal bone. Otol Neurotol. 2011;32(4):665–9.

103. Neely JG, Forrester M. Anatomic considerations of the medial cuts in the subtotal temporal bone resection. Otolaryngol Head Neck Surg. 1982;90(5):641–5.

104. Medina JE, Park AO, Neely JG, Britton BH. Lateral temporal bone resections. Am J Surg. 1990;160(4):427–33.

105. Chao CK, Sheen TS, Shau WY, Ting LL, Hsu MM. Treatment, outcomes, and prognostic factors of ear cancer. J Formos Med Assoc. 1999;98(5):314–8.

106. Dean NR, White HN, Carter DS, Desmond RA, Carroll WR, McGrew BM, et al. Outcomes following temporal bone resection. Laryngoscope. 2010;120(8):1516–22.

107. Zhang B, Tu G, Xu G, Tang P, Hu Y. Squamous cell carcinoma of temporal bone: reported on 33 patients. Head Neck. 1999;21(5):461–6.

108. Figi FH, BE. Malignant tumors of the middle ear and mastoid process. Arch Otolaryngol 1943;37:149–68.

109. Arthur K. Radiotherapy in carcinoma of the middle ear and auditory canal. J Laryngol Otol. 1976;90(8):753–62.

110. Million RR, Cassisi NJ. Management of Head and Neck Cancer. A Multidisciplinary Approach. Philadelphia, PA: Lippincott; 1984.

111. Boland J, Paterson R. Cancer of the middle ear and external auditory meatus. J Laryngol Otol. 1955;69(7):468–78.

112. Laskar SG, Sinha S, Pai P, Nair D, Budrukkar A, Swain M, et al. Definitive and adjuvant radiation therapy for external auditory canal and temporal bone squamous cell carcinomas: Long term outcomes. Radiother Oncol. 2022;170:151–8.

113. Chee G, Mok P, Sim R. Squamous cell carcinoma of the temporal bone: diagnosis, treatment and prognosis. Singapore Med J. 2000;41(9):441–6, 51.

114. Hashi N, Shirato H, Omatsu T, Kagei K, Nishioka T, Hashimoto S, et al. The role of radiotherapy in treating squamous cell carcinoma of the external auditory canal, especially in early stages of disease. Radiother Oncol. 2000;56(2):221–5.

115. Wang CC. Radiation therapy in the management of carcinoma of the external auditory canal, middle ear, or mastoid. Radiology. 1975;116(3):713–5.

116. Shih L, Crabtree JA. Carcinoma of the external auditory canal: an update. Laryngoscope. 1990;100(11):1215–8.

117. Kunst H, Lavieille JP, Marres H. Squamous cell carcinoma of the temporal bone: results and management. Otol Neurotol. 2008;29(4):549–52.

118. Ogawa K, Nakamura K, Hatano K, Uno T, Fuwa N, Itami J, et al. Treatment and prognosis of squamous cell carcinoma of the external auditory canal and middle ear: a multi-institutional retrospective review of 87 patients. Int J Radiat Oncol Biol Phys. 2007;68(5):1326–34.

119. Liu FF, Keane TJ, Davidson J. Primary carcinoma involving the petrous temporal bone. Head Neck. 1993;15(1):39–43.

120. Dumago MP, Yu KKL, Jacomina LE, Yap ET, Jainar CJE, Bojador MR, et al. Technical details and clinical outcomes after high-dose-rate intracavitary brachytherapy for squamous cell carcinoma of external auditory canal and external beam radiotherapy for nodal coverage: a case report. J Contemp Brachytherapy. 2023;15(1):75–80.

121. Miller D. Cancer of the external auditory meatus. Laryngoscope. 1955;65(6):448–61.

122. Soo KC, Carter RL, O'Brien CJ, Barr L, Bliss JM, Shaw HJ. Prognostic implications of perineural spread in squamous carcinomas of the head and neck. Laryngoscope. 1986;96(10):1145–8.

123. Rouviere H. Anatomie des Lymphatiques de l'Homme. Paris: Masson et cie; 1932.

124. Birzgalis AR, Keith AO, Farrington WT. Radiotherapy in the treatment of middle ear and mastoid carcinoma. Clin Otolaryngol Allied Sci. 1992;17(2):113–6.

125. Manolidis S, Pappas D, Jr., Von Doersten P, Jackson CG, Glasscock ME, 3rd. Temporal bone and lateral skull base malignancy: experience and results with 81 patients. Am J Otol. 1998;19(6 Suppl):S1–15.

126. Selesnick SH, Burt BM. Regional spread of nonneurogenic tumors to the skull base via the facial nerve. Otol Neurotol. 2003;24(2):326–33.

127. Komune N, Miyazaki M, Sato K, Sagiyama K, Hiwatashi A, Hongo T, et al. Prognostic impact of tumor extension in patients with advanced temporal bone squamous cell carcinoma. Front Oncol. 2020;10:1229.

128. Moffat DA, De la Cruz A. Squamous cell carcinoma. Tumors of the Ear and Temporal Bone. Philadelphia, PA: Lippincott, Williams; 2000. p. 63–7.

129. Kwok HC, Morton RP, Chaplin JM, McIvor NP, Sillars HA. Quality of life after parotid and temporal bone surgery for cancer. Laryngoscope. 2002;112(5):820–33.

130. Morton RP. Evolution of quality of life assessment in head and neck cancer. J Laryngol Otol. 1995;109(11):1029–35.

131. Morton RP, Witterick IJ. Rationale and development of a quality-of-life instrument for head-and-neck cancer patients. Am J Otolaryngol. 1995;16(5):284–93.

132. Dropkin MJ, Malgady RG, Scott DW, Oberst MT, Strong EW. Scaling of disfigurement and dysfunction in postoperative head and neck patients. Head Neck Surg. 1983;6(1):559–70.

133. Long SA, D'Antonio LL, Robinson EB, Zimmerman G, Petti G, Chonkich G. Factors related to quality of life and functional status in 50 patients with head and neck cancer. Laryngoscope. 1996;106 (9 Pt 1):1084–8.

134. Kreitler S, Chaitchik S, Rapoport Y, Kreitler H, Algor R. Life satisfaction and health in cancer patients, orthopedic patients and healthy individuals. Soc Sci Med. 1993;36(4):547–56.

135. Katz MR, Irish JC, Devins GM, Rodin GM, Gullane PJ. Reliability and validity of an observer-rated disfigurement scale for head and neck cancer patients. Head Neck. 2000;22(2):132–41.

136. de Casso C, Kwhaja S, Davies S, Al-Ani Z, Saeed SR, Homer JJ. Effect of temporal bone resection on temporomandibular joint function: a quality of life study. Otolaryngol Head Neck Surg. 2010;142(1):85–9.

137. Nader ME, Beadle BM, Roberts DB, Gidley PW. Outcomes and complications of osseointegrated hearing aids in irradiated temporal bones. Laryngoscope. 2016;126(5):1187–92.

138. Harker GJ, Stephens FO. Comparison of intra-arterial versus intravenous 5-fluoroura-cil administration on epidermal squamous cell carcinoma in sheep. Eur J Cancer. 1992;28A(8–9):1437–41.

139. Suzuki K, Takahashi M, Ito Y, Tsuge I, Motai H, Takeichi Y, et al. Bilateral middle ear squamous cell carcinoma and clinical review of an additional 5 cases of middle ear carcinomas. Auris Nasus Larynx. 1999;26(1):33–8.

140. Itoh YK, Motai H. Evaluation on effective-ness of multi-drug combined intra-arterial chemotherapy as a neoadjuvant chemo-therapy in the head and neck region. J Jpn Soc Cancer Ther 1994;29:411.

141. Knegt PP, Ah-See KW, Meeuwis CA, van der Velden LA, Kerrebijn JD, De Boer MF. Squamous carcinoma of the external auditory canal: a different approach. Clin Otolaryngol Allied Sci. 2002;27(3):183–7.

142. Nakagawa T, Kumamoto Y, Natori Y, Shiratsuchi H, Toh S, Kakazu Y, et al. Squamous cell carcinoma of the external audi-tory canal and middle ear: an operation com-bined with preoperative chemoradiotherapy and a free surgical margin. Otol Neurotol. 2006;27(2):242–8; discussion 9.

143. Takenaka Y, Cho H, Nakahara S, Yamamoto Y, Yasui T, Inohara H. Chemoradiation therapy for squamous cell carcinoma of the external auditory canal: a meta-analysis. Head Neck. 2015;37(7):1073–80.

144. Nagano T, Yoshimura RI, Kojima M, Nakagawa K, Toda K. Outcomes of radio-therapy in advanced external auditory canal cancer. J Radiat Res. 2019;60(3):380–6.

145. Shiga K, Katagiri K, Saitoh D, Ogawa T, Higashi K, Ariga H. Long-term outcomes of patients with squamous cell carcinoma of the temporal bone after concomitant chemoradiotherapy. J Neurol Surg B Skull Base. 2018;79(Suppl 4):S316–S21.

146. Kitani Y, Kubota A, Furukawa M, Sato K, Nakayama Y, Nonaka T, et al. Primary defini-tive radiotherapy with or without chemo-therapy for squamous cell carcinoma of the temporal bone. Eur Arch Otorhinolaryngol. 2016;273(5):1293–8.

147. Zhong S, Zuo W. Treatment strategies for malignancies of the external audi-tory canal. Curr Treat Options Oncol. 2022;23(1):43–53.

# 24

# Sarcomas of the temporal bone

BRIAN A. NEFF AND ROBERT THAYER SATALOFF

A variety of benign and malignant lesions of the temporal bone have been described (**Table 24.1**) (1), but sarcomas that involve the temporal bone are rare. The literature contains scattered small series, case reports, and literature reviews of temporal bone sarcomas; however, most have too few cases to scientifically determine a superior treatment approach. However, most studies provide an opinion on how to handle these rare and aggressive tumors. A few definitions are important to allow proper interpretation of these scientific reports. For the purposes of this chapter, radical surgery is defined as total tumor removal with sacrifice of a vital structure, such as a nerve or artery. *En bloc* resection refers to surgery, usually radical, designed to circumscribe and remove the entire tumor without violating the tumor margins. Complete or wide surgical excision refers to surgery that attempts to obtain clear margins but does not necessarily imply radical surgery or avoidance of tumor transgression. In fact, tumor is often removed piecemeal during such procedures. Subtotal resection implies that gross residual disease remains after surgery. Examples of subtotal excision include surgical debulking and biopsy.

## RHABDOMYOSARCOMA

## DEMOGRAPHICS

Rhabdomyosarcoma (RMS) accounts for 8%–20% of all sarcomas. It is also the most common sarcoma in children. The head and neck are the most common site, accounting for 30%–50% of cases. Two-thirds of head and neck RMSs are embryonal, with a mean age of presentation between 4 and 8 years of age. The most common head and neck subsite is the orbit. The temporal bone is a much rarer location. The Armed Forces Institute of Pathology (AFIP) found that only 6.9% of all RMS of the head and neck occur in the temporal bone. Yet, RMS is currently the most common sarcoma diagnosed in the temporal bone (2). Naufel (3) found 64 cases of temporal bone RMS reported in the literature over a 100-year span ending in 1973. Numerous other cases have been described since that review (4–11). The temporal bone is considered a parameningeal subsite of the head and neck. Other parameningeal sites include the nasopharynx, nasal cavity, paranasal sinuses, infratemporal fossa, and pterygopalatine fossa (12). RMSs that affect these

DOI: 10.1201/b23379-24

areas are frequently grouped together in order to obtain sufficient numbers to make any study statistically significant. Additionally, these parameningeal sites are grouped since they are the most likely tumor areas to exhibit intracranial spread. However, such groupings make it difficult to glean information about temporal bone neoplasms specifically.

## PATHOLOGY

The World Health Organization (WHO) 2020 classification now recognizes four major histologic variants of RMS: embryonal (ERMS), alveolar (ARMS), and spindle cell/sclerosing (SSRMS). Pleomorphic RMS (anaplastic), the fourth subtype of RMS in the WHO system, is not recognized in children,

Table 24.1 Temporal bone neoplasms (1)

*Primary temporal bone tumors*

- Benign
- Meningioma
- Paraganglioma
- Neurofibroma
- Schwannoma
- Adenomas
- Eccrine cylindroma
- Pleomorphic adenoma
- Mesenchymal
- Chondroma
- Chondroblastoma
- Chondromyxoid fibroma
- Hemangiomas
- Lipoma
- Myxoma
- Fibroosseous tumors
- Fibrous dysplasia
- Ossifying fibroma
- Osteoblastoma
- Osteoma
- Giant cell granuloma
- Teratoma
- Dysontogenic
- Choristoma
- Glioma
- Chordoma

- Malignant
- Epidermal
- Squamous cell carcinoma
- Verrucous carcinoma
- Basal cell carcinoma
- Mucoepidermoid carcinoma
- Mesenchymal
- Rhabdomyosarcoma
- Chondrosarcoma
- Osteosarcoma
- Liposarcoma
- Angiosarcoma
- Undifferentiated pleomorphic sarcoma
- Ewing's sarcoma
- Malignant peripheral nerve sheath tumor
- Leiomyosarcoma
- Fibrosarcoma
- Adenocarcinomas
- Adenoid cystic
- Sebaceous cell
- Papillary cystadenocarcinoma
- Ceruminous adenocarcinoma
- Melanoma
- Plasmacytoma

*Metastatic tumors*

- Prostate, GI, renal cell, lung, breast
- Lymphoma, leukemia (chloroma)
- Multiple myeloma

*Contiguous tumor invasion*

- Meningioma
- Schwannoma
- Neurofibroma
- Gliomas
- Parotid neoplasms

- Pituitary neoplasms
- Craniopharyngioma
- Chordoma
- Nasopharyngeal carcinoma

although it is a more common subtype in adults (13). Although the histologic appearance is distinct for the different RMS subtypes, all of them arise from a similar primitive myoblast or mesenchymal stem cell (4). The embryonal subtype has an overall histologic pattern that has been likened to that of normal embryologic muscle arrested at 3–10 weeks of gestation. It is composed of small spindle-shaped cells mixed with rhabdomyoblasts, which are small, oval, eosinophilic cells. These cells are arranged in a background consisting of a loose myxoid matrix and may have a botryoid appearance (**Figure 24.1**). The alveolar histology consists of more rounded tumor cells arranged in ill-defined nests or alveolar spaces separated by fibrous strands (**Figures 24.2** and **24.3**). Some pathologists have required the presence of skeletal muscle cross-striations to make the light microscopic diagnosis of RMS; however, insistence on them will lead to underdiagnosing these lesions (5). Immunohistochemical (IHC) staining has shown that a large number of RMSs do not contain these striations. Furthermore, IHC analysis aids in the diagnosis of RMS and helps determine subtype. ERMS has a generally more favorable prognosis and is myogenin, MyoD, and desmin positive, with strong nuclear HMGA2 staining with relatively weaker AP2beta staining. ARMS has a generally poorer prognosis and stains positive for myogenin, MyoD, and desmin and has strong diffuse nuclear AP2beta staining, with weak to absent HMGA2

staining. SSRMS has a more variable prognosis and has weak to absent myogenin staining, positive desmin, and strong nuclear MyoD1 staining (13).

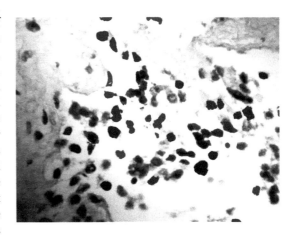

Figure 24.2 Rhabdomyosarcoma, alveolar 40× (400 magnification). Alveolar rhabdomyosarcomas are high-grade sarcomas composed of small, oval cells growing in nests or clusters separated by delicate fibrous septa. Non-cohesive cells are seen in the center of the nests while the periphery is characterized by the lepidic attachment of tumor cells simulating the morphology of pulmonary air spaces.

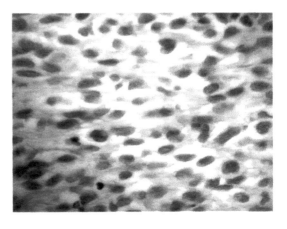

Figure 24.3 Rhabdomyosarcoma, undifferentiated 40× (400 magnification). The undifferentiated subtype shows no specific features. The growth pattern is closely packed and may be fascicular. Cells may have a moderate amount of cytoplasm and are typically larger than a mature lymphocyte. Nuclei tend to the large end of the spectrum and contain finely granular chromatin and prominent nucleoli.

Figure 24.1 Rhabdomyosarcoma, embryonal 40× (400 magnification). Embryonal rhabdomyosarcomas are composed of small, oval to elongated cells arranged in loosely cohesive sheets. The cells can have varying amounts of eosinophilic cytoplasm that displace the nuclei.

## CLINICAL PRESENTATION/ DIAGNOSTIC WORK-UP

One of the most common early presentations of RMS can mimic otitis media or acute mastoiditis. This is true for all age groups, but it is especially true in children. Many series demonstrate an average delay of up to 7 weeks from the time of initial patient presentation until definitive diagnosis (6). The presence of acute onset otalgia, acute facial nerve palsy, and an opaque tympanic membrane has often led to the early false diagnosis of acute otitis media. Patients have been treated with prolonged courses of antibiotic therapy which delayed diagnosis. Additionally, there have also been reports of incidental aural polyps being found and biopsied at the time of tympanostomy tube placement, with biopsy results revealing RMS. In this setting, otorrhea, aural granulation, or aural polyps are frequently overlooked as harbingers of a growing RMS (7, 8, 14). When reviewing the presentation of all patients with RMS of the middle ear and mastoid, they presented with the following findings: 54% had a polyp in the external auditory canal, 40% developed otorrhea, 30% of patients exhibited bloody otorrhea or frank bleeding, and conductive hearing loss and facial nerve paresis occurred 14% of the time (8). Histologic studies have shown that RMSs of the middle ear usually spread along the path of least resistance; additionally, they can demonstrate early invasion and destruction of the facial nerve in the fallopian canal, thus causing facial paresis. From that point, they can extend to the internal auditory canal and meninges (5). Virtually any cranial nerve may become involved with the tumor once it has spread to an intracranial location. Around 35% of patients with middle ear RMS develop meningeal spread which has a high mortality (9). Additionally, tumor spread can occur through the jugular fossa to cause a jugular foramen syndrome, also called Vernet's syndrome. This syndrome is caused by compression and subsequent paralysis of cranial nerves IX, X, and XI. In turn, the patient will usually manifest symptoms of hoarseness and dysphagia (due to paralysis of the palate, vocal fold, and superior pharyngeal constrictor).

Around 25% of RMSs can arise in the area of the eustachian tube with extension to the petrous apex. These masses present differently from the more lateral lesions involving the mastoid and middle ear. Frontal headaches, retro-orbital pain, and diplopia from abducens nerve palsy are common. This clinical picture mimics petrous apicitis. Aural symptoms and facial nerve paresis are usually absent until late in the disease process. These lesions usually exhibit signs of intracranial spread earlier in the disease course. Common areas of spread include Meckel's cave and the carotid canal which can cause facial paresthesias and Horner's syndrome, respectively (5).

A history of otitis media in a child unresponsive to antibiotics, with a polyp in the external auditory canal, should raise the suspicion of tumor until biopsy proves otherwise. If cranial neuropathies are present, imaging is indicated as well as biopsy of any mass present on physical exam or radiograph. If the diagnosis of RMS is made at biopsy, work-up should include a computed tomography (CT) of the temporal bones if it has not already been obtained. If there is evidence of extensive soft tissue extension to the infratemporal fossa, other extracranial areas, or intracranially, a magnetic resonance imaging (MRI) is needed. If meningeal spread is questioned, most oncologists will perform a lumbar puncture for cytology as well as a bone marrow biopsy. Around 14% of parameningeal RMSs in the early Intergroup Rhabdomyosarcoma Study (IRS) had evidence of distant metastasis at the time of presentation. The most common site was the lungs, with other frequently involved areas including skeletal bone and liver (8). Consequently, the metastatic work-up should include a CT of the chest and abdomen, liver function tests, and wholebody 18-fluorodeoxyglucose (18-FDG)-positron emission tomography (PET) scan.

## HISTORICAL TREATMENT

Early case reports and series prior to current multimodality therapy used surgical excision of varying degrees with radiation therapy or chemotherapy in some cases. Most surgical resections were not complete. Jaffe et al. (15) reported no 2-year survivors among 40 patients who underwent resection of their temporal bone RMS. Deutsch and Felder reported similar, poor survival statistics with only five survivors out of 78 patients at 31–54 months follow-up. These patients had their temporal bone RMSs treated by combinations of surgical excision, radiation, and chemotherapy (10). It was because of these dismal statistics that in 1972, the Intergroup Rhabdomyosarcoma Study Group (IRSG) was formed with the primary goal of performing large, randomized trials designed to try to improve survival rates with initial treatments. Since 2000, the Children's Oncology Group (COG) has taken over study oversight and direction. These groups evaluated treatment protocols for all body sites for patients <21 years of age. They have completed and published numerous large prospective trials to evaluate the efficacy of newer radiation regimens and chemotherapy agents in the treatment of RMS. These studies have developed treatment protocols using the multimodality approach of surgery, radiation therapy, and chemotherapy to almost triple the cure rate and survival in the last 30 years (16). The North American-based COG and European protocols are probably the most widely accepted treatment approaches for eradicating RMS of all sites, including the temporal bone. They are, however, not without flaws that make surgical decision-making more difficult.

# TREATMENT

The Clinical Oncology Group (COnG) RMS committee categorizes patients according to their tumor stage, completeness of resection following surgery (postsurgical pathologic grouping), and risk categories. The COnG modified Tumor, Node, Metastasis (TNM) pretreatment staging system (**Table 24.2**) stages RMSs by the location of the primary site, tumor size, the presence or absence of lymph node metastasis, and the presence or absence of distant metastatic disease (17). RMS of the orbit and non-parameningeal head and neck sites are stage I independent of their size or lymph node status. RMSs of the parameningeal head and neck sites are stage II if they are ≤5 cm and have no regional or distant metastatic disease. Parameningeal sites include tumors of the nasopharynx, nasal cavity, middle ear, mastoid, temporal bone, paranasal sinuses, pterygopalatine fossa, and infratemporal fossa. These same sites are also termed unfavorable primary sites by the COnG system. These same parameningeal tumors are upstaged to stage III if neck lymph nodes are present or if the tumor is >5 cm. All head and neck lesions with distant metastatic disease are stage IV (17).

Table 24.2  Clinical Oncology Group (COnG) rhabdomyosarcoma (RMS) modified Tumor Node Metastasis (TNM) pretreatment staging system (previously the IRSG Staging) (17)

| Stage | Site | T | Size | Lymph node | Metastasis |
|---|---|---|---|---|---|
| I | Head and neck (excluding parameningeal sites) Orbit, biliary tract/liver, and genitourinary (excluding prostate/bladder) | T1/T2 | a or b | $N_0$, $N_1$, or $N_x$ | M0– |
| II | Cranial parameningeal, prostate/bladder, extremity, other (retroperitoneum, trunk, etc.; excludes biliary/liver) | T1/T2 | A | $N_0$, $N_x$ | M0– |
| III | Cranial parameningeal, prostate/bladder, extremity, Other (retroperitoneum, trunk, etc.; excludes biliary/liver) | T1/T2 | A | $N_1$ | M0– |
| | | T1/T2 | B | $N_0$, $N_1$, or $N_x$ | M0– |
| IV | Any site | T1/T2 | a or b | $N_0$, $N_1$, or $N_x$ | M1 |

*Note:* Tumor: T1: Confined to anatomic site of origin; T2: Extension and/or fixation to surrounding tissue; a: ≤5 cm in size diameter; b: >5 cm in size diameter. Regional nodes: $N_0$: Regional nodes not clinically involved; $N_1$: Regional nodes clinically involved as defined as (a) >1 cm by CT or MRI or (b) [18]FDG avid; $N_x$: Clinical status of regional nodes unknown (especially sites that preclude lymph node evaluation. Metastases: M0: No distant metastases; M1: Distant metastases present: (includes positive CSF, pleural fluid, abdominal fluid cytology, or carcinomatosis of pleural/abdominal/CNS surfaces).

*Abbreviation:* FDG, Fluorodeoxyglucose.

The Clinical Group Classification System pathologic grouping (**Table 24.3**) classifies patients according to the completeness of their surgical resection and, thus, the amount of residual disease present. Group 1 contains patients whose lesions were completely resected with microscopically negative margins and no regional nodal disease, which, for temporal bone tumors, would mean no facial or neck lymph node involvement. Group 2 contains patients with complete tumor resection (all visible tumor removed) with residual microscopic disease along with the nodal basin status noted in **Table 24.3**. Group 3 includes patients with gross residual disease after subtotal surgical resection or biopsy. Lastly, group 4 encompasses patients who had distant metastatic disease or positive CSF cytology or CNS imaging consistent with CNS carcinomatosis at the time of their presentation (17).

The COnG system finally assigns a risk category to each patient depending on their stage and postsurgical pathology group. Patients were separated into low-, intermediate-, and high-risk categories which were then used to determine event-free survival (**Table 24.4**). Recent advances in molecular staging has incorporated the *FOXO1* fusion gene status in the risk stratification. The presence of a *FOXO1* fusion refers to one of two chromosomal translocations—t(2;13) resulting in fusion of *PAX3* to *FOXO1* or t(1;13) resulting in fusion of *PAX7* to *FOXO1*. The *FOXO1* fusion status is a better prognostic classifier than histologic subtype, such as alveolar vs. embryonal, and it has now replaced histology in the COnG risk stratification for RMS. Approximately 80% of tumors that are morphologically alveolar subtype carry a *FOXO1* fusion, whereas more than 95% of tumors that are morphologically embryonal have no *FOXO1* fusion, and it is now understood that the presence or absence of the *FOXO1* fusion gene drives the clinical behavior of RMS. Only distant metastatic status surpassed *FOXO1* fusion status as a poor prognostic predictor (18, 19).

The higher the risk category, the poorer the disease-free survival and EFS for the patient. In more recent COG trials, patients with low-risk RMS comprise over a quarter of all patients with RMS and carry an excellent prognosis with a 4-year EFS of approximately 90%. Patients with intermediate-risk RMS represent the most heterogeneous risk group with 5-year EFS rates between 50% and 75% and comprise more than half of newly diagnosed patients with RMS. Lastly, patients with high-risk RMS comprise approximately 15% of all patients with RMSs but represent the most challenging to treat, with generally poor outcomes. Patients younger than 10 years of age with high-risk RMS had 3-year EFS ranging from 60% to 64%. In contrast, the 3-year EFS for high-risk RMS patients older than 10 years was 32%–48% (18). This risk schema can be applied to temporal bone RMS. Low-risk temporal bone lesions are stage II tumors if ≤5 cm, without face/neck lymphadenopathy. Additionally, low-risk patients need to be in the group 1 postsurgical pathology grouping, and consequently, the temporal bone RMSs must be completely excised with negative margins. All remaining lesions are intermediate-risk tumors except for those presenting as stage IV with metastatic disease. Patients with stage IV RMS are placed in the high-risk category.

It can be seen from the COnG system that the patient risk category and survival are dependent not only on the location and extent of disease but also on the completeness of surgical resection. Therefore, theoretically, the patient's prognostic group and future treatment depend on the aggressiveness of the surgeon. As previously mentioned, the only way that a temporal bone lesion can be low risk is if it demonstrated localized disease of ≤5 cm and was resected completely at the time of initial surgery (**Table 24.4**) (16, 18, 19). This scenario was extremely uncommon in any of the IRSG or COG trials. With the evolving field of cranial base surgery, removal of previously unresectable lesions is now possible. How then should one decide how aggressive to be when resecting a temporal bone RMS? There are no definitive answers since there is a paucity of these lesions, making it nearly impossible to design a significant, randomized, prospective study to address this question. The COG and European Cooperative Sarcoma group have emphasized retaining form/function for quality of life in other areas such as the orbit. For now, common sense conclusions are all that can guide cranial base surgeons and attempts to preserve functioning cranial nerves and neurovascular structures, such as the carotid artery, are probably prudent even when risking microscopic or small amounts of gross residual disease. Radical resection should only be attempted if they include non-functional cranial nerves or occluded vascular structures until future studies show a survival

Table 24.3 Clinical Group Classification System (former IRSG Postsurgical Pathology Group) (16, 17)

| | |
|---|---|
| Group 1 | Local disease, gross total (complete) resection; microscopic negative margins; no regional nodal disease |
| Group 2 | Localized disease, grossly resected with microscopic residual disease or regional disease, grossly resected with or without microscopic residual disease |
| | a. Localized disease, grossly resected tumor with microscopic residual disease; regional nodes not involved |
| | b. Regional disease with involved nodes completely resected with no microscopic residual (including most distal node histologically negative) |
| | c. Regional disease with involved nodes, grossly resected with evidence of microscopic residual and/or histologic positive distal node) |
| Group 3 | Localized local or regional disease |
| | Biopsy only or incomplete resection with gross residual tumor |
| Group 4 | Distant metastasis present at initial patient presentation |
| | Includes positive CSF, pleural or abdominal fluid cytology, or presence of tumor implants on pleural, abdominal, or CNS surfaces. |
| | Regional lymph nodes are not considered distant metastasis. |

Abbreviation: IRSG, Intergroup Rhabdomyosarcoma Study Group.

benefit in routinely sacrificing these important structures, when functional. *En bloc* resection is usually not possible for most cases that require subtotal or total temporal bone resection, so by default, margin assessment becomes difficult or impossible. With this extent of disease, it is probably most accurate to assume microscopic positive margins even if they cannot be definitively demonstrated (20). Future studies should also consider redefining the staging system for parameningeal sites or attempt to evaluate the temporal bone and other parameningeal sites as a distinct subset of patients in order to assess whether modern techniques of skull base tumor resection will improve survival over patients undergoing lesser aggressive

subtotal resection of the tumor mass, which the author does not routinely advocate.

With the significant expansion of chemotherapy and molecularly targeted agents, it is not possible to completely cover numerous treatment regimens that are available. All of the staging systems, risk stratifications, and primary tumor sites have led to innumerous combination therapy studies; therefore, current optimal treatment should involve a team led by an oncologist with expertise in treating RMS. Low-risk groups tend to be treated with 24–48 weeks of vincristine and dactinomycin (VA regimen) or vincristine, dactinomycin, and cyclophosphamide (VAC regimen) with some sites and stages receiving radiation

Table 24.4 Children's Oncology Group rhabdomyosarcoma risk stratification (18, 19)

| Risk group | COG mod TNM stage | Clinical group class | Age | Fusion status (FOXO1) |
|---|---|---|---|---|
| Low | 1 | I, II, III (orbit only) | Any | − |
| | 2 | I, II | Any | − |
| Intermediate | 1 | III (non-orbit) | Any | − |
| | 1, 2, 3 | I, II, III | Any | + |
| | 2, 3 | III | Any | − |
| | 3 | I, II | Any | − |
| | 4 | IV | < 10 years | − |
| High | 4 | IV | ≥ 10 years | − |
| | 4 | IV | Any | + |

Abbreviation: TNM, Tumor node metastasis.

treatments of 36–50.4 Gy. There are also attempts to select very-low-risk groups that may be candidates for de-escalation therapy in ongoing and future trials. Intermediate risk groups seem to be treated with similar VA or VAC chemotherapy and radiation regimens, but many studies are showing benefit of molecular targeted therapies such as irinotecan and temsirolimus (mechanistic Target of Rapamycin [mTOR] inhibitor). In the intermediate risk group, some studies are also showing benefit of low-dose maintenance therapy with cyclophosphamide and/or vinorelbine for 24 weeks after primary chemotherapy completion. The optimal timing to deliver radiation treatment continues to evolve, and treatment dosages also vary similar to low-risk disease from 36 to 50.4 Gy. The current recommendations are for radiation treatment to commence after four cycles (12 weeks) of chemotherapy, even for patients with parameningeal involvement (18, 21) High-risk RMS are usually enrolled in treatment studies that attempt to maximize dose intensity, incorporating all known active agents (vincristine, doxorubicin, cyclophosphamide, ifosfamide/etoposide, and VAC) into an interval compressed, intensified backbone. These studies are also trying to evaluate promising novel agents (irinotecan, temozolomide, or cixutumumab) for various time intervals. (18). Additionally, for the high-risk group, whose treatment outcomes have not improved much over the years, antibodies and immunotherapy drugs are being incorporated into promising current and future treatment trials (22) Radiation treatment is even more highly variable in this group which can often include patients with distant metastasis. Radiation treatment is given to the primary site with doses up to 59.4 Gy, usually after 16–20 weeks of initial chemotherapy. Guidelines are defined by the site and clinical group. Whole-lung radiation therapy to 15 Gy is indicated for patients with lung metastases. Focal radiation therapy is also recommended for bone metastases, when possible. (21).

Some physicians have tried to look at the controversial question of how aggressive of a resection should be attempted for temporal bone RMS. Prasad et al. (23) treated 14 RMS patients with complete skull base resection followed by postoperative chemotherapy. Radiation therapy was utilized for close or microscopically positive margins. They noted a 2-year survival of 42%. Healy

et al. (24) reported nine patients with infratemporal fossa RMS treated with chemotherapy followed by complete radical resection using microsurgical techniques. With this radical approach, they reported a 44% long-term survival. Both studies failed to include a less radical surgical or nonsurgical chemoradiotherapy arm. The poor 2-year survivals could easily be explained by the fact that these radically resected lesions were, on average, more advanced than those who were treated in the IRSG studies. Additionally, the tumors were in locations that carry a worse prognosis than many of the cases in the IRSG studies. Consequently, the authors were unable to delineate any positive or negative effects that aggressive surgical resection may have.

The RMS trial physicians have discouraged aggressive surgery of the skull base in children. They make this statement based on the excellent response that they have seen with chemotherapy and radiation therapy in the COG and older IRS trials and on their desire to avoid the morbidity associated with resection of cranial nerves. Raney et al. (25) reported the IRS I trial results in which there were 24 temporal bone RMSs. All were treated with surgical biopsy followed by chemotherapy and radiation therapy. They reported an improved 5-year survival of 46% when compared to previous retrospective studies that used a variety of surgical approaches as the main treatment option. Consequently, it was concluded that surgical resection should be done only if it does not require extensive reconstruction or sacrifice of neurovascular and other functional structures; therefore, subtotal resection or biopsy of temporal bone lesions was deemed the appropriate initial surgical management (25). Again, the fault of this study is that they failed to ask whether their improved survival rate could have been even better if complete resection had been combined with their chemoradiation protocols. They also do not clearly defend their position that functional concerns seem to supersede the oncologic principle that any malignancy should be removed entirely. Surgical debulking is not appropriate in squamous cell neoplasms of the head and neck and possibly is detrimental to survival in the treatment of sarcomas. Unfortunately, the subsequent IRS II–IV studies have not examined temporal bone tumors as an isolated group. In addition to the above controversies, the IRS protocols created significant morbidity in the children treated with high-dose radiation therapy. Frequent episodes of xerostomia, osteoradionecrosis, and asymmetric growth disorders of the craniofacial skeleton were reported (16).

## CHONDROSARCOMA

## EMBRYOLOGY

There are a few different theories proposed as to how chondrosarcomas develop in the temporal bone. The bones of the skull base mature predominantly by endochondral ossification while the bones of the skull vault develop primarily by intramembranous ossification (26). The areas of the petro-occipital, spheno-occipital, and sphenopetrosal synchondroses, as well as a large part of the petrous portion of the temporal bone, are sites in the mature skull that underwent endochondral development (27). It is hypothesized that islands of residual endochondral cartilage may be present in these areas and that chondrosarcoma develops from these chondrocytes (28, 29). Alternatively, it is suggested that chondrosarcomas may arise from pluripotent mesenchymal cells involved in the embryogenesis of the skull base and temporal bone. Lastly, metaplasia of mature fibroblasts has been implicated as an inciting mechanism in the development of chondrosarcomas (28, 29).

## DEMOGRAPHICS

Chondrosarcomas account for 0.1% of all head and neck tumors and ~6% of all skull base lesions (30). The most common skull base site varies between differing studies, with common sites of involvement including the petrous apex, middle cranial fossa, clivus, temporo-occipital junction, sphenoethmoid complex, and anterior cranial fossa (29, 31, 32). The mean age at presentation is the fourth and fifth decades of life, with most studies not showing a sex predilection (28, 32, 33). Primary chondrosarcoma develops *de novo* in normal bone. Most temporal bone chondrosarcomas arise in this manner. Rarely, there are secondary chondrosarcomas which arise from preexisting cartilaginous tumors or abnormalities. Chondrosarcoma has been reported in association with Paget's disease, Maffucci syndrome, osteocartilaginous exostoses, Ollier's disease, and osteochondromas (34, 35).

## PATHOLOGY

There have been several subtypes of chondrosarcomas proposed. The conventional subtype consists of hyaline, myxoid, or a combination of these components. The hyaline component has been described as neoplastic chondrocytes residing within lacunar spaces surrounded by a hyaline matrix. The myxoid component features areas of chondrocytes that are surrounded by a frothy mucinous matrix (28, 32) (**Figure 24.4**). Mesenchymal and undifferentiated subtypes are rare histologies that reveal a more anaplastic appearance, and these lesions usually present with aggressive, advanced disease. The clear cell subtype (malignant chondroblastoma) is extremely rare with only a few cases reported in the head and neck (30, 36).

Chondrosarcomas have been placed into three categories based on cellularity and nuclear atypia. Rosenberg reviewed 200 cases of skull base chondrosarcoma and found that 50.5% of tumors were grade 1 (well differentiated), 21% were grade 2 (moderately differentiated), 28.5% were a mixture of grades 1 and 2, and 0% were grade 3 (poorly differentiated) tumors (32) (**Table 24.5**). This grading system is important since it corresponds to prognosis based on tumor biology, distinct from its location or stage of presentation. Evans et al. (37) reported on chondrosarcomas from all body sites and found a correlation between survival and histologic grade. Five-year survival for chondrosarcomas of grades I, II, and III is 90, 81, and 43%, respectively. Koch et al. (30) reported additional factors that bode a poorer prognosis which included advanced stage, metastatic disease, and mesenchymal or pure myxoid tumors. Others have stated that location (unresectable location) and dedifferentiated subtypes also bear a poorer prognosis (31, 36, 38). The differential diagnosis for chondrosarcomas of the temporal bone and skull base includes chordoma, chondroid chordoma, osteosarcoma, meningioma, enchondroma, and glomus jugulare (24, 25). Most of these can be distinguished with a thorough history and physical as well as imaging studies. However, most radiologists agree that chordoma, chondroid chordoma, and chondrosarcoma are difficult to distinguish reliably by MRI and CT scan (34). Histologic differentiation is often difficult as well. Chordomas differ from chondrosarcomas in that they contain an abundance of cells with bubbly eosinophilic cytoplasm called physaliphorous cells. Chondroid chordomas contain features of both chondrosarcoma and chordoma. They contain neoplastic chondrocytes along with physaliphorous cells which are present but much rarer than in chordomas (26, 29). Frequently, analysis by an IHC panel of antibodies is needed for definitive diagnosis. Typically, chordomas stain positive for cytokeratin, epithelial membrane antigen, S-100 protein, and vimentin (VIM). Conversely, chondrosarcomas stain positive for VIM and S-100 and negative for cytokeratin and epithelial membrane antigen (28, 32, 39). Wojno et al. (39) were able to demonstrate both staining patterns within a single tumor, and hence, they helped distinguish these masses as chondroid chordomas.

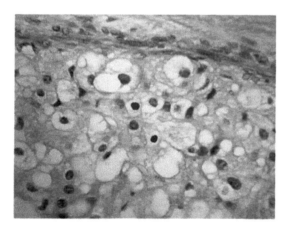

**Figure 24.4** Chondrosarcoma (400 magnification). This conventional chondrosarcoma consists of neoplastic cells within lacunar spaces embedded in a hyaline matrix. Nuclei are large, sometimes binucleate, and have prominent nucleoli. Mitotic figures are rare in low-grade tumors and are readily identified in high-grade lesions.

## CLINICAL PRESENTATION

Several clinical presentations have been reported for chondrosarcoma of the skull base. The symptoms correlate with the anatomic site of destruction or compression. Initial complaints may include hearing loss, pulsatile tinnitus, vertigo/unsteadiness, aural fullness, and headache. Multiple cranial

neuropathies are common and present as diplopia, facial pain, paresthesias, hemifacial spasm, facial paresis, dysphagia, hoarseness, shoulder weakness, and hemi-tongue weakness and atrophy. A comprehensive neurotologic work-up is indicated when temporal bone lesions are suspected. The work-up includes pure tone and speech audiometry, CT of the temporal bones and brain, MRI/MRA, as well as any other tests that are indicated clinically (27, 31). Chondrosarcomas generally arise from the petroclival synchondrosis, although 28% may originate more centrally from the clivus (32). CT often demonstrates areas of tumor calcification (40). Chondrosarcomas are generally hypo- to isointense with T1-weighted MRI, hyperintense on T2-weighted MRI, and heterogeneous enhancement with gadolinium enhancement (41). Although not universally adopted, a recent staging system for temporal bone and skull base chondrosarcoma has been proposed (42).

**Table 24.5** Petroclival chondrosarcoma staging system

| | |
|---|---|
| Stage 1 | Tumor size <2 cm |
| | Limited to bone |
| Stage 2 | Tumor size 2–4 cm |
| | Limited to bone or evidence of middle or posterior fossa extension |
| Stage 3 | Tumor size >4 cm, or > 270 degree encasement of internal carotid artery |
| Stage 4 | Any tumor size with spinal seeding, lymph node metastasis, and distant metastasis; any histologic grade 3 tumor |

*Source:* Reference [42].

## TREATMENT

Treatment approaches have evolved throughout the years and include combinations of surgical debulking, complete surgical excision, radiation, and chemotherapy. Although most studies report a treatment bias, the paucity of patients with chondrosarcoma of the temporal bone makes it impossible to perform prospective trials that could lead to definitive treatment conclusions. Anecdotal protocols are common and will be reviewed here. Due to a concern that surgical debulking violates tumor boundaries and oncologic principles, the concept of total *En bloc* resection with total gross removal of disease has been suggested as the preferred surgical procedure when removing chondrosarcoma of the skull base and temporal bone. Others have reported aggressive subtotal or near total resection with preservation of critical anatomy such as cranial nerves, carotid artery, or cavernous sinus and its contents (42). A few authors have reported small surgical series with successful outcomes. Kveton et al. (31) reported the House clinic's experience of five cases of skull base chondrosarcoma involving the temporal bone. They conveyed their preference for total *En bloc* resection and stated that they were successful in removing petrous apex lesions via an infratemporal fossa approach in most cases. Similarly, Charabi et al. (43) completely resected a temporal bone chondrosarcoma with jugular foramen extension through an infratemporal fossa approach. Al-Mefty et al. (44) described a combined infratemporal and posterior fossa approach for total removal of two temporal bone chondrosarcomas with posterior fossa extension. Additionally, Watters and Brookes (27) reported eight cases of petrous temporal bone chondrosarcoma and concurred that total *En bloc* resection was ideal. Siedman et al. (29) reviewed 31 cases of chondrosarcomas of the temporal bone, but they did not report a clear treatment protocol. However, the authors did suggest that optimal treatment would include complete surgical excision followed by radiation (29). Lastly, Carlson et al. reported on 55 cases of successfully treated petroclival chondrosarcomas with the goal of gross total resection, but the majority received aggressive subtotal or near total resection with adjuvant proton beam radiation therapy to preserve critical neurovascular structures (42).

Radiation treatment for chondrosarcomas used to be considered futile. Harwood et al. reported on chondrosarcomas that occurred at multiple body sites and found that conventional external beam radiation of 5000 rads (cGy) over 4–5 weeks locally controlled 50% of 31 cases. Complete remission was seen in three of these cases after 15 years of follow-up. They stated that earlier claims that chondrosarcomas were radio-resistant failed to consider that clinical regression of tumor after radiation treatment was slow. Additionally, the radiographic appearance of bone involved with the lesion never completely returns to normal after radiation therapy despite prolonged evidence of clinical remission. Both these factors may have falsely led earlier investigators to claim treatment failures in patients who may have been treated successfully (38). Several recent series have reported on the advantage of proton beam radiation in the treatment of skull base chondrosarcomas. With this modality, very large radiation doses are deliverable to the mass while achieving a rapid reduction in dose outside the defined target volume (45). Rosenberg et al. (32) reported the largest series to date of skull base chondrosarcomas which included temporal bone lesions. They reported treating 200 patients with proton beam therapy of 64.2–79.6 Gy equivalents in 38 fractions. All patients had been treated previously with surgical procedures ranging from biopsy to total excision. They report the most successful 5- and 10-year local control rates of 99% and 98%, respectively, as well as 5- and 10-year survival rates of 99% and 98%, respectively. Their mean follow-up was reported as 65 months. Austin-Seymour et al. (46) reported on 28 patients with low-grade chondrosarcoma of the skull base treated with 69 Gy equivalents of proton beam therapy in 31–41 fractions. Their results were not as favorable as Rosenburg's results and demonstrated 5-year local control and survival rates of 82% and 76%, respectively. However, they failed to separate chondrosarcomas from chordomas when reporting these group figures, and this may have impacted negatively upon their 5-year statistics. They concluded that surgery followed by proton beam radiation was the treatment of choice for chondrosarcoma and chordoma of the skull base. Coltrera et al. (28) reported 13 cases of temporal bone chondrosarcoma. They generalized that proton beam therapy was the preferred radiation modality and that conventional external beam radiation has yielded poor results. However, they did not comment on radiation dosage, success of treatment in their series, or the specific role of surgery.

Stereotactic radiosurgery has also been described in the treatment of chondrosarcoma of the skull base (28). Radiosurgery combines the accuracy of stereotactic guidance with high-dose, single-session irradiation. There is steep radiation fall-off outside the image-defined tumor margin. Hence, the tumor gets a tumoricidal dosage while the surrounding brain and neural structure receive tolerable levels of radiation, usually without serious side effect. Muthukumar et al. (47) treated six cases of chondrosarcoma of the skull base with

24–40 Gy to the tumor while the tumor margins received 12–20 Gy. Tumor volume was the limiting factor for this treatment modality. They limited treatment to those with masses <3 cm diameter and 10.3 cm³ of volume. They showed improvement in over half of their patients but did not separately group their chondrosarcoma lesions from their patients with chordomas when reporting results (47). Debus et al. (33) used fractionated stereotactic radiotherapy to treat eight chondrosarcomas of the skull base. A linear accelerator was used with the head immobilized in a stereotactic frame to deliver 64.9 Gy to the tumor center. The advantage of fractionated delivery is that it allows treatment of larger tumor volumes than previous single-session radiosurgery approaches. All patients had undergone previous resection of their lesions, and when combined with stereotactic radiation, 100% 5-year local control and survival rates were achieved. They did acknowledge that they had a small number of patients, and consequently, they cautioned that fractionated proton beam therapy was still the standard for postoperative radiation therapy.

There is no agreement as to when and if chemotherapy should be utilized in the treatment of skull base chondrosarcoma. Several reports state that chemotherapy is not effective in head, neck, and skull base chondrosarcomas, and therefore, it should not be utilized (35). Conversely, Finn et al. (36) stated that multi-agent chemotherapy protocols used to treat other soft tissue sarcomas may be useful in treating chondrosarcomas with a high probability of aggressive local spread or metastasis. Included were grade II or III conventional chondrosarcoma, mesenchymal chondrosarcomas, and undifferentiated chondrosarcomas. Chemotherapy may also offer palliation for chondrosarcomas that are unresectable. Koch et al. (30) concurred that advanced, high-grade lesions and mesenchymal subtypes may benefit from multi-agent chemotherapy.

## OSTEOSARCOMA

## DEMOGRAPHICS

Osteogenic sarcoma or osteosarcoma is a highly aggressive malignant tumor that usually presents in the metaphysis of long bones. The majority of

cases occur between the ages of 10 and 30 years with the median age of 28. There are ~7400 new cases and 4200 deaths from osteosarcoma occurring annually in the United States. Approximately 10% of cases occur in the head and neck, and this accounts for ~900 new cases per year (48, 49). In a review of the world literature, Sataloff et al. (50) found 19 reported cases of osteosarcoma involving the temporal bone, with the largest series reporting three cases. At least nine additional cases have been reported for a total of at least 28 cases (49–53). The total number of primary temporal bone cases is difficult to ascertain because some series include patients with maxilla or mandibular primary lesions extending to involve the skull base. No matter the total number, skull base and temporal bone osteosarcomas are very rare tumors. Almost every bone of the skull has been involved as a primary site; however, the mandible was clearly the most common primary location in the head and neck (48, 54, 55).

## PATHOLOGY

Osteosarcoma is thought to arise from immature bone-forming cells or through neoplastic differentiation of other immature mesenchymal cells into osteoblasts. Histologically, a tumor is considered to be an osteosarcoma if it demonstrates malignant spindle cells producing osteoid in various stromal backgrounds (**Figure 24.5**). Subtypes are based on the predominant characteristic of the cells and stroma and include osteoblastic, chondroblastic, broblastic, small cell, and telangiectatic types (54, 56).

Additionally, tumors are graded with regard to the degree of histologic differentiation with grade 1 being well differentiated and grade 4 being poorly differentiated (54). Ninety-five per cent of extragnathic craniofacial osteosarcomas present with an aggressive histology of grade 3 or 4; however, many authors are not able to clearly correlate a high-grade histology with poorer survival (48, 52, 56). There are a few commonly named factors that have been reported as significant in the development of osteosarcoma: previous radiation therapy, a history of hereditary retinoblastoma, fibrous dysplasia, and Paget's disease (48, 56). Three cases of osteosarcoma of the temporal bone have been reported to arise in areas of previous radiation treatment. One of these occurred in a patient previously treated with 66 Gy for nasopharyngeal carcinoma (50, 51). Patients with retinoblastoma have a 500 times increased risk of developing an osteosarcoma during their lifetime, independent of previous radiation treatment to their primary site. Both retinoblastoma and osteosarcoma patients have shown specific deletions in the long arm of chromosome 13, and a retinoblastoma gene that has been implicated in the development of both retinoblastoma and osteosarcoma has been reported (48). Approximately, 1% of patients with head and neck fibrous dysplasia will eventually develop osteosarcoma; however, these patients do not appear to have a poorer prognosis than patients with *de novo* osteosarcoma (48). On the other hand, patients who develop osteosarcoma in an area of Paget's disease seem to develop an aggressive form of the lesion with a reported 5-year survival of 2% (57).

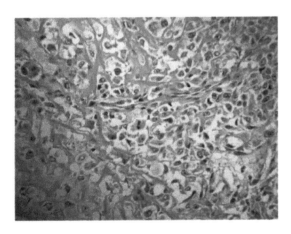

Figure 24.5 Osteosarcoma (200 magnification). The production of osteoid defines an intramedullary tumor as osteosarcoma. This definition holds regardless of histologic pattern. Cell size and shape can vary widely. Nuclei are typical large, pleomorphic, and contain one or more prominent nucleoli. The chromatin pattern is usually coarse and clumped.

## CLINICAL PRESENTATION/ DIAGNOSTIC WORK-UP

In most studies of head and neck osteosarcoma, the most common presentation is pain and swelling over the area of bone containing the lesion (49). In their review of 19 patients with temporal bone

osteosarcoma, Sataloff et al. (50) demonstrate that the most common presenting symptoms or signs were a mass in the temporal fossa, mastoid, or external ear canal in 84%, facial paralysis in 47% (9/19), conductive hearing loss in 37% (7/19), otalgia in 32% (6/19), bloody or purulent otorrhea in 16% (3/19), and other cranial nerve deficits in 16% (3/19) (50). As with other skull base and temporal bone malignancies, symptoms caused by cranial nerve deficits are determined by the site of tumor involvement.

Work-up for temporal bone and skull base osteosarcoma again starts with a CT of temporal bones and brain. On CT scan, skull base osteosarcoma displays osteolysis and osteoblastic bone destruction, or a mixture, as well as an irregular tumor margin and tumor calcifications. MRI for temporal bone osteosarcoma is complementary to CT, and tumors are isointense on the T1-weighted images, hypointense on the T2-weighted images, and tumors demonstrate intense contrast enhancement (53). The only significant associated clinical laboratory finding is an elevated alkaline phosphatase, which is nonspecific and not always present (49, 56). Regional metastasis to lymph nodes are very rare in osteosarcoma, but distant metastatic disease has been reported in 17–51% of head and neck lesions. The overwhelming majority of metastases are to the lungs, with less frequent sites including the liver, bone, and brain (48, 56). Routine metastatic work-up should include a chest CT, as well as liver function tests, bone scans, or whole-body FDG-PET scan. Poor prognostic factors include osteosarcoma in association with Paget's disease, as well as site of lesion, positive surgical margins, and metastatic disease at presentation (48, 54). Nora et al. (52) showed that head and neck osteosarcomas of the extragnathic bones had a much poorer 5-year survival of 10% than those that involved the mandible and maxilla whose 5-year survival approached 40%.

## TREATMENT

Again, very few cases of osteosarcoma of the temporal bone have been reported in the English literature since 1910 (49–52, 58). Over that time, treatment has widely varied, and follow-up was inconsistent or not reported in nearly one-third of the cases. Consequently, treatment protocols for temporal bone osteosarcoma have to be extrapolated from series reporting osteosarcomas located in the head, neck, and other body sites. The two largest head and neck series were reported by Garrington et al. at the AFIP, and Caron et al. at Memorial Sloan Kettering Cancer Center. They looked at 56 and 43 patients, respectively, and concluded that radical resection was the treatment of choice, with 5-year survivals of 35% and 23.3%, respectively. However, both these studies failed to distribute patients equally into alternative therapy treatment arms with very small numbers receiving radiation, chemotherapy, or combinations of the two (47, 48). Kassir et al. (54) performed a meta-analysis of 173 patients in 23 different reports and found an overall 5-year survival for head and neck osteosarcoma of 37%. They found that patients with negative surgical margins did the best and stated that radiation and chemotherapy still had an unproven role in the adjuvant treatment of osteosarcoma. However, they did admit that their retrospective analysis lent significant bias to their results since chemotherapy and radiation were used mainly in more advanced or unresectable lesions (54). More recently, Guo reported on 19 cases of osteosarcoma involving the skull base and advocated for attempted gross total surgical resection followed by planned postoperative radiation and chemotherapy treatment. They also performed a literature review showing a 37.8% 5-year survival for patients with osteosarcoma involving skull base subsites (53).

Several studies have shown that adjuvant radiation improves local control and survival. Chambers and Mahoney (59) reported a higher 5-year survival of 73% when they used high-dose preoperative radiation followed by wide surgical resection for osteosarcomas of all body sites. Additionally, Mark et al. (48) obtained better results with wide surgical excision of head and neck osteosarcomas followed by postoperative radiation and chemotherapy, but they did not compare results to surgery alone. There have been no prospective trials to evaluate chemotherapy efficacy in head and neck or temporal bone osteosarcomas. There have been a few prospective, randomized studies showing a survival benefit when utilizing chemotherapy to treat osteosarcoma of the extremities. Link et al. (60) enrolled 114 patients with extremity osteosarcomas and

showed that 2-year disease-free survival was 56% in the surgery plus chemotherapy arm vs. 18% in the surgery alone group. Eibler et al. (61) randomized 59 patients with a surgery arm alone vs. surgery with adjuvant multi-agent chemotherapy. Patients received four, 6-week cycles of chemotherapy postoperatively. Two-year disease-free and overall survivals were 55% and 80% in the adjuvant chemotherapy arm vs. 20% and 48% in the surgery alone group, respectively. For temporal bone lesions, ideally the patient should receive *En bloc* excision followed by 55–69 Gy of postoperative radiation therapy. However, Castro et al. (62) have shown some benefit in treating with heavy charged particle irradiation to deliver 66 gray equivalents to a more defined tumor target. Early success with chondrosarcomas and osteosarcomas may make this the radiation modality of choice for most skull base and temporal bone sarcomas. Chemotherapy can also be given concurrently with the postoperative radiation. Most recent reports including Sataloff et al. (50) and Sharma et al. (49) support the radical resection of temporal bone osteosarcoma with the use of adjuvant radiation and chemotherapy.

## UNDIFFERENTIATED PLEOMORPHIC SARCOMA

## DEMOGRAPHICS

Undifferentiated pleomorphic sarcoma, formerly known as malignant fibrous histiocytoma, has undergone many nomenclature and definition changes over the years, making it difficult to follow outcome and treatment studies over time. The category is a pathological redefinition into a more well-defined sarcoma type. Initially, this category drew from a pool of lesions that had been misdiagnosed as high-grade fibrosarcomas, liposarcomas, pleomorphic RMSs, and undifferentiated sarcomas. The tumor is a fairly common sarcoma in adults and arises most frequently in the extremities, pelvis, and retroperitoneum; however, it is a rare tumor of the head and neck. Rarely, undifferentiated pleomorphic sarcoma also can affect bone, but it is extremely rare in skull bones with only 17 reported cases in the English literature (63). There are three reported cases of undifferentiated pleomorphic sarcoma that involve the temporal bone (63–65). It is also possible that the number of undifferentiated pleomorphic sarcoma cases has been underestimated. Many of Naufel's (3) 89 cases of undifferentiated sarcomas and 17 cases of fibrosarcomas might be reclassified as undifferentiated pleomorphic sarcoma if examined by today's pathologic criteria. None of the studies clearly summarized the clinical presentation of these temporal bone undifferentiated pleomorphic sarcomas, but there is no reason to believe that they would differ greatly from other sarcoma histologies. Work-up includes a thorough head and neck exam, cranial nerve exam, and CT and MRI imaging of the primary tumor as a starting point. FDG-PET and chest/abdominal imaging with CT or MRI can be utilized for metastatic evaluation.

## PATHOLOGY

The microscopic appearance of undifferentiated pleomorphic sarcoma includes rounded histiocytic cells mixed with spindle broblastic cells in a matted pattern (**Figure 24.6**). There are various subtypes based on microscopic characteristics which include the angiomatoid, inflammatory, and pleomorphic subtypes. It is thought that undifferentiated pleomorphic sarcoma arises from a primitive mesenchymal cell which has the ability to form both broblastic and histiocytic elements. IHC staining is positive for CD 68 which is a histiocyte stain. It is negative for S-100 and EMA (53, 55).

## PROGNOSIS

Head and neck undifferentiated pleomorphic sarcoma has an average age at presentation of ~43 years, with a slight predilection for males (56%). Male sex and increasing age were independently found to be associated with a poorer prognosis. Additionally, tumors arising from or extending into bone showed a more aggressive clinical course and a poorer prognosis than those restricted to soft tissues. Tumors > 3 cm were also shown to do more poorly than smaller primary tumors. The metastatic rate was 32% for head and neck undifferentiated pleomorphic sarcoma, and these patients had a poorer survival (63, 64). The lung was by far the most common metastatic site with brain, bone, liver, and regional neck lymph node metastases also reported. Regional neck metastasis was seen in 15% of patients; however, neck dissection is not suggested in the absence of clinically positive nodes (63, 64).

## TREATMENT

Raney et al. treated seven children with undifferentiated pleomorphic sarcoma of which three had head and neck lesions. The treatment protocol closely mirrored the IRS protocols used for treating RMS in children. They stated that every child should have as complete a resection as possible; however, all of the head and neck lesions were simply biopsied with no attempt at complete surgical resection. Biopsy was then followed by multi-agent chemotherapy for 2 years. If initial surgical therapy left gross or microscopic disease, 40–50 Gy was delivered to the tumor over 5–6 weeks. Even with this aggressive treatment, three of seven children died of distant metastatic disease (65). Nakayama et al. (63) suggested that radical resection of head and neck undifferentiated pleomorphic sarcoma with involved bone was appropriate. They reported a total temporal bone resection with facial nerve sacrifice as an example of their treatment philosophy. They suggested that postoperative chemoradiation would also be beneficial. Their patient was alive without disease at 18 months. The same authors also reviewed several small series containing 15 other cases of undifferentiated pleomorphic sarcoma involving bones of the skull and reported a 34%–50% 5-year survival. In their review of 87 cases of head and neck undifferentiated pleomorphic sarcoma, Blitzer et al. stated that wide surgical resection was the treatment of choice. They also advocated chemotherapy of some type, using doxorubicin since this agent seemed to provide the best partial tumor regression. Radiotherapy was not effective in their series; however, they did support its use with chemotherapy in the inoperable patient or as palliation in those patients with distant metastatic disease. They reported a 45% mortality rate in their own 11 patients but were unable to give 5-year survival statistics for the 87 reviewed cases due to incomplete and variable follow-up (64).

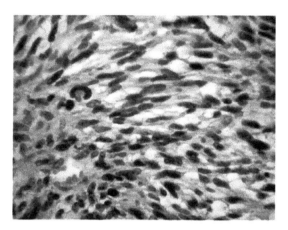

Figure 24.6 Undifferentiated pleomorphic sarcoma (400 magnification). Undifferentiated pleomorphic sarcoma can show any number of different morphologic patterns, but all consist of varying proportions of myofibroblasts, histiocytoid cells, and fibroblasts. Typically, the cells are arranged in random bundles with an intersecting fascicular pattern.

## FIBROSARCOMA

## DEMOGRAPHICS

Fibrosarcoma used to be the most commonly diagnosed head and neck sarcoma, but the frequency has dropped with more rigid histologic criteria and the development of new pathologic categories. In reviews of previous fibrosarcomas, up to one-half would be regrouped into other diagnoses (2, 66). There are numerous lesions to be considered in the differential diagnosis of fibrosarcoma-like or spindle cell tumors including such benign processes as fibromatosis, fibromas, nodular fasciitis, and malignant sarcomas such as undifferentiated pleomorphic sarcoma (malignant fibrous histiocytoma), RMS, liposarcoma, monophasic synovial sarcoma, and malignant peripheral nerve sheath tumor (MPNST; neurogenic sarcoma). Some authors have reported that fibrosarcomas account for 5%–10% of sarcomas, with 10%–20% of these occurring in the head and neck (2). Fibrosarcomas commonly affect the 40- to 70-year age range with the average age being 44 years old. Like osteosarcoma, fibrosarcoma is common in areas of previous tissue injury. Up to 10% of all fibrosarcoma

patients have a history of distant radiation therapy, 4% have a history of trauma to the site, and 0.8% have a history of thermal injury to the site. The soft tissue of the neck was the most common site involved with fibrosarcoma, and the soft tissue of the face and scalp followed closely in frequency (66). In a review of the literature, 17 cases of fibrosarcoma were found to involve the temporal bone. Temporal bone fibrosarcoma will also likely become a much rarer diagnosis due to the more current, stringent histologic criteria (3, 67, 68). History, physical, and radiologic evaluations should mirror other skull base sarcomas.

## PATHOLOGY/PROGNOSIS

Fibrosarcoma is composed of spindle-shaped fibroblasts arranged in intersecting fascicles that give rise to a "herringbone pattern" (**Figure 24.7**). This is very similar to neurogenic sarcoma which will be discussed briefly later. Immunohistochemistry is not diagnostic for fibrosarcoma, but it is helpful in excluding lesions in its pathologic differential. Pathologists designate these tumors as grade 1 (well differentiated) to 4 (poorly differentiated). Most tumors usually present with a grade 2 or 3 histology (2, 66).

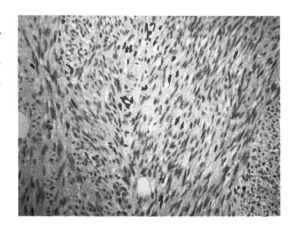

Figure 24.7 Fibrosarcoma (100 magnification). Fibrosarcomas are composed of slender spindle-shaped cells oriented in interweaving bundles. This interlacing arrangement gives rise to the term herring-bone pattern and is associated with lower grade tumors. Nuclear pleomorphism is minimal.

Similar to other sarcomas, higher grades appear to correlate with increased local recurrences, increased metastatic rate, and decreased overall survival. Additional poor prognostic factors include tumors > 5 cm, presence of metastatic disease, and incomplete surgical resection. Metastatic disease from head and neck fibrosarcoma occurs in 19% of cases (66, 69).

## TREATMENT

Frankenthaler et al. (66) reviewed 118 cases of head and neck fibrosarcoma at MD Anderson. They supported wide local excision but were unable to obtain negative margins in 47% of their cases. If the surgical margins were microscopically positive or questionable, then 60 Gy of radiation therapy was given postoperatively over 6 weeks. Up to nine courses of multi-agent chemotherapy, consisting of doxorubicin-based regimens, were given preoperatively when the biopsy showed either grade 3 or 4 lesions or for an unresectable tumor. Unresectable sarcomas were debulked surgically after induction chemotherapy, and then they were treated with radiation therapy. They reported a 63% 5-year overall survival with this approach. Freedman et al. (70) employed a bi-treatment approach. Their primary goal was obtaining wide surgical margins followed by postoperative radiation in cases when there were high-grade lesions, close margins, or microscopically positive margins. They reported a 5-year survival of 68%. Conley et al. (69) reported using surgery and postoperative radiation in his treatment approach, but he stated that radical *en bloc* resection should definitely be used for more aggressive, poorly differentiated lesions since radical resection was their only chance for survival. Extrapolating these treatment philosophies to temporal bone lesions, total "radical" resection of skull base lesions seems appropriate, when possible, with postoperative radiation and possibly induction chemotherapy in high-grade lesions.

## EWING'S SARCOMA

## DEMOGRAPHICS

Ewing's sarcoma represents 6%–9% of primary malignant bone tumors and is encountered most commonly in the long bones, pelvis, ribs, or vertebrae (71, 72).

During the early IRS trials, pathologists discovered that there was a distinct subgroup of extra-osseous tumors that could be distinguished from undifferentiated RMS. They termed this group as extra-osseous Ewing's sarcoma. Consequently, future IRS trials excluded these from their study treatment groups (4, 25). This extra-skeletal form is extremely rare in the head and neck. Ewing's sarcoma that involves the facial bones and skull is also extremely rare, accounting for < 1% of all reported Ewing's sarcomas. The most common head and neck site affected is the mandible. Approximately 50 cases of Ewing's sarcoma of the skull or skull base have been reported in the literature. Most Ewing's sarcomas of the skull arise in the convexities of the calvarium; however, a handful have been reported in the temporal bone (73, 74). The literature reports nine lesions involving the temporal bone, of which most arise from the squamous portion of the temporal bone. Additionally, there are reports of five cases of petrous apex Ewing's sarcoma and three cases involving the mastoid portion of the temporal bone. The average patient age of those affected with head and neck Ewing's sarcoma was 14.5 years old, and the age range for those with temporal bone tumors was from 3 to 19 years of age (3, 72, 74–76).

## PATHOLOGY

Grossly, Ewing's sarcomas are firm, rubbery vascular masses arising from bone. Microscopically, these lesions consist of small, blue, round cells arranged in sheets with a few pseudorosettes present (**Figure 24.8**). Additionally, there are glycogen granules in the cytoplasm of these cells after periodic acid–Schiff staining; however, this is also seen in ERMS. The histologic differential for a cranial Ewing's sarcoma includes neuroectodermal tumor, RMS, metastatic neuroblastoma, and lymphoma. IHC staining is important in helping to distinguish among these lesions. Ewing's sarcoma is positive for CD 99, VIM, and MIC-2 which is a specific marker for Ewing's sarcoma. These lesions are negative for the skeletal marker, desmin, as well as the neural markers S100 and chromogranin and the lymphoma markers such as leukocyte common antigen, CD20, and CD3 (74–76).

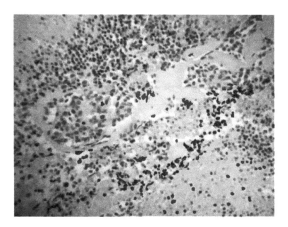

Figure 24.8 Ewing's sarcoma (200 magnification). Tumors cells are arranged in sheets and lobules with broad areas of necrosis. Individual cells have a small amount of amphophilic cytoplasm and contain well-defined, oval nuclei with finely dispersed chromatin and small nucleoli. Intracellular glycogen can be demonstrated by PAS stain.

## CLINICAL PRESENTATION AND WORK-UP

Patients presenting complaints differ depending upon the anatomic site within the temporal bone affected by the tumor. A mass arising from the squamous portion of the temporal bone will present as temporal scalp swelling and pain. Additionally, headache and signs of increased intracranial pressure such as vomiting, and papilledema can be present. These latter symptoms will be more prominent with large intracranial extensions of tumor causing midline shift of the cerebrum. In the middle ear, Ewing's sarcoma will present with otalgia, facial nerve paresis, conductive hearing loss, and multiple cranial neuropathies (71, 77). Work-up includes CT and MRI of the temporal bones and brain and other neurotological studies as indicated based on symptoms and signs. Ewing's sarcoma will appear isodense to bone with enhancement after IV dye administration, and extensive bone erosion and destruction are usually present (73). A technetium-99 bone scan will show increased uptake at the primary site as well as any metastatic sites; however, metastatic disease is extremely uncommon in Ewing's sarcoma of the skull (71). A skeletal survey, in addition to the bone scan, is obtained to further evaluate for a non–head and neck Ewing's sarcoma primary that may have metastasized to the skull. Bilateral bone marrow biopsies are also done in select patient work-ups. More current metastatic surveys with whole-body FDG-PET or PET-CT scans are good alternative options to older plain films and bone scans. Hadfield et al. (74) reported that metastatic Ewing's sarcoma to the skull and skull base is much more common than a primary Ewing's sarcoma of the skull base. A 24-hour urine should be collected for VMA in order to exclude a metastatic neuroblastoma from the differential diagnosis. Osteosarcoma may also be in the radiologic differential of Ewing's sarcoma; however, biopsy clearly differentiates these two lesions. MRI has a limited role in the evaluation of these tumors due to poor delineation of bony detail (75).

## TREATMENT

Desai et al. (75) reported 14 patients with primary Ewing's sarcoma of the cranium. They supported *En bloc* excision of each tumor; however, they did not report any cases involving the temporal bone. Surgical treatment was then followed by the round cell chemotherapy protocol (RCT II). It consisted of two alternating cycles of iodipamide and etoposide with vincristine, doxorubicin, and cyclophosphamide. At 8–9 weeks after starting chemotherapy, 40–50 Gy of radiation was delivered to the primary site. Six courses of maintenance chemotherapy were given after the radiation was complete. They were able to achieve a 57% 5-year survival with this protocol. Multiple other small series report that optimal treatment would include complete excision followed by chemoradiation. There were no reported cases in any series where radical skull base surgery was utilized to eradicate tumor from the middle ear cleft, mastoid, or petrous apex. The authors advocating radical removal of lesions were mainly basing their opinions on wide local excision of calvarium lesions which are easier to remove without functional deficits (75–77). Horowitz et al. (78) supported a different treatment approach. They suggested that multi-agent chemotherapy, such as RCT II, should be the initial treatment after biopsy-proven diagnosis. This would be followed by surgical debulking of as much disease as possible without sacrificing vital structures. Lastly, postoperative chemoradiation would be given to treat the residual disease. The goal of this treatment approach was to reduce surgical morbidity while achieving the same survival as those series that utilized wide local excision as a primary treatment.

## MALIGNANT PERIPHERAL NERVE SHEATH TUMOR

### DEMOGRAPHICS

A brief review of definitions will hopefully help clarify this rare head and neck sarcoma. A neurofibroma is a benign peripheral nerve mass composed of perineural cells, fibroblasts, neurites, and Schwann cells. The nerve fibers are essentially engulfed in this un-encapsulated mass, and, therefore, the nerve is not separable from the tumor during surgery. Neurofibromas are usually multiple with 22%–40% occurring in the head and neck. Additionally, neurofibromas are the tumor associated with von Recklinghausen's disease or neurofibromatosis type 1 (NF1), which originates from a genetic abnormality on chromosome 17. This is not to be confused with neurofibromatosis-related schwannomatosis, or the older term neurofibromatosis type 2 (NF2), which is manifested as multiple or bilateral vestibular schwannomas which are a different entity from a neurofibroma. Schwannomas arise from Schwann cells on the surface of their nerve of origin. The chromosomal lesion in neurofibromatosis-related schwannomatosis is found on chromosome 22 instead of 17 (79).

MPNSTs are the malignant counterpart of neurofibroma. MPNST has been previously called by multiple names including neurogenic sarcoma, neurofibrosarcoma, and malignant schwannoma. All of these names have fallen out of favor, but the last two are currently discouraged because they can lead to incorrect inferences as to the origin of this tumor (79). In the early years of light microscopy, many pathologists found it very difficult to distinguish, histologically, between fibrosarcoma and MPNST. The only reliable way to clearly identify MPNST was its gross pathologic origin from a nerve or by a surgeon's report that the mass arose from a nerve. They then called the variant neurofibrosarcoma (80). Recently, however, IHC stains have made the distinction more clearly, and consequently, it has been determined that neurofibrosarcomas are not true fibrosarcomas. Malignant schwannoma is also discouraged because Enzinger stated that schwannomas have almost no malignant potential, except in a few very rare cases; however, this point is debatable (79). MPNSTs arise almost exclusively from preexisting neurofibromas, but very rarely they may arise *de novo*. A few studies disagree about

which is more common; additionally, the frequency of these malignancies arising in the setting of NF1 remains controversial. Literature reports of MPNST arising in patients with NF1 range from 5% to 50%. The most common areas affected by MPNST are the trunk and extremities. Head and neck MPSNT accounts for 6–17% of cases, and the neck is the most common area, with the brachial plexus and vagus nerve as the most common sites (80, 81).

### HISTOLOGY

MPSNT is very similar to fibrosarcoma. MPSNT contains microscopic fields composed of spindle-shaped cells arranged in interlacing fascicles in a herringbone pattern (**Figure 24.9**). Occasionally, there may be a clue that some neurogenic features are present, but diagnosis really relies upon immunohistochemistry. MPSNT stains heavily for S-100 antigen (a neural marker which is not seen in fibrosarcoma.) It also stains for myelin basic protein and leu 7 which are not as specific. Pathologically, MPSNT also appears quite similar to amelanotic melanoma, but melanoma stains positive for HMB-45, whereas MPSNT does not (79, 80).

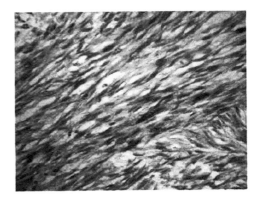

Figure 24.9 Malignant peripheral nerve sheath tumor (MPNST, 400 magnification). MPNSTs are composed of tightly packed spindle cells arranged in interlacing bundles. Cell nuclei are large and can be pleomorphic. Often, there is a suggestion of nuclear palisading. Higher grade tumors are associated with increasing cellularity, nuclear atypia, and mitoses.

### CLINICAL PRESENTATION

MPNST of the temporal bone is an extremely rare lesion. Naufel in 1973 reviewed the world literature and found three MPNST (neurogenic sarcomas) in case reports that arose from cranial nerve VII (3, 82, 83). The masses were found on the mastoid segment of the facial nerve, and none arose from an existing lesion per the authors report. Clinical presentation was similar to other middle ear sarcomas with symptoms which included preauricular or mastoid swelling or mass, polyps in the external auditory canal, otorrhea, conductive hearing loss, and facial nerve paralysis (82, 83). Since then, there have been isolated case reports of MPNST arising within the temporal bone or extending to include the temporal bone, confirming the pathologies rareness (81, 84)

## TREATMENT

Treatment strategies need to be adapted from larger series of MPNSTs arising from other body sites. Hutcherson et al. (80) reviewed seven patients with head and neck MPNST. The patients varied widely in surgical treatment, and they also received various treatments of either radiation therapy, chemotherapy, or both. However, they concluded that wide surgical excision is the mainstay of treatment with postoperative radiation being helpful in local control and prevention of local recurrences. They had a 43% 5-year survival in this series. D'Agostino et al. (85) studied 24 cases of which six were located in the head and neck region. Again, no specific protocol was evaluated; however, they felt that wide surgical excision was the only effective treatment. They did not believe radiation conferred any survival advantage. Greager et al. (81) reported 17 patients with head and neck MPNST. They found that wide local excision with resection of the involved neurovascular structures were the mainstay of treatment. They did not find adjuvant radiation or chemotherapy to be helpful but admitted that their experience with these techniques was limited and their role needed further study. Hellquist and Lundgren (79) and Goepfert et al. (86) both retrospectively reviewed small series of patients with head and neck MPNST and found radical surgery plus 60 Gy radiation afforded the best survival. Greager et al. (81) reported 2-, 5-, and 10-year overall survivals of 65%, 47%, and 29%, respectively. A poor prognosis was also reported in patients with associated von Recklinghausen's disease (NF1) which may be due to a more aggressive lesion. Other negative prognostic indicators included presence of metastatic disease which occurs in up to 47% of head and neck MPNST, tumors >5 cm in size, and possibly tumor grade; however, histologic differentiation did not always correlate well with survival (80, 81).

## ANGIOSARCOMA

Angiosarcoma is a malignant vascular tumor most commonly arising in the skin and soft tissue of the scalp in elderly men (**Figure 24.10**). They are aggressive tumors that tend to recur locally and metastasize early despite early treatment. Most give a history of a several-month period of an enlarging purple skin lesion with pain, edema, and intermittent bleeding (87). There have been five case reports of angiosarcoma arising from the petrous portion of the temporal bone (88–90). Naufel and Mark et al. have reported nine patients with "ear" involvement by an angiosarcoma, but neither author delineated whether these lesions arose from the middle ear and mastoid or whether they primarily involved the skin of the pinna or external auditory canal. The latter is more likely the case since nearly all of these tumors arise in the subcutaneous tissues (3, 87). Linthicum and Schwartzman (91) provided a pathology slide demonstrating an angiosarcoma adjacent to the stapes footplate; however, clinical presentation and treatment were not reported. Treatment is aimed at wide surgical excision, which is not always possible in the skull base, followed by 50–60 Gy of postoperative radiation. Adjuvant chemotherapy is not standard therapy but may be useful for advanced tumors. Most head and neck series reported 5-year survivals of 10%–41% (87, 92).

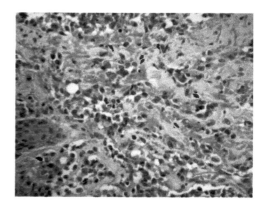

Figure 24.10 Angiosarcoma (400 magnification). These vasoformative tumors are composed of malignant endothelial cells that arrange themselves in complex anastomosing channels. The cellular nuclei are plump and tend to heap-up and project into the lumens. Mitoses are common, and extravasated red cells are seen in the stroma.

## LIPOSARCOMAS

Liposarcomas are composed of malignant lipoblasts situated in a loose stroma (**Figure 24.11**). The head and neck are involved in only 2%–6% of cases. The myxoid subtype was the most common subtype reported in the head and neck. The tumor arises *de novo*, not from benign lipomas. Statistics of 5-year survival depend on the histologic subtype. Well-differentiated myxoid liposarcomas have a 5-year survival of 75%–100%. The more poorly differentiated tumors such as the round and pleomorphic subtypes have 5-year survivals of 6%–27% (2). In Naufel's (3) review, he reported one case involving the temporal bone which was reported in the German literature. They did not suggest any general treatment approaches; however, combination therapy consisting of surgery, radiation, and chemotherapy would probably be most effective.

## LEIOMYOSARCOMA

Leiomyosarcoma is a malignant tumor of smooth muscle origin (**Figure 24.12**). In the head and neck, smooth muscle is scarce and is located in the walls of blood vessels and arrector pili musculature of skin. IHC staining is positive for smooth muscle-specific actin. The most common head and neck site is the sinonasal tract. Zbaren and Ruchti (93) reported one case involving the middle ear which was deemed unresectable and was treated unsuccessfully with chemotherapy. They recommended surgical excision, followed by postoperative radiation and chemotherapy. Prognosis is poor, with 1-year survival reported at 50% for tumors of the sinonasal tract.

## CONCLUSION

In conclusion, sarcomas of the temporal bone are rare. With the exception of RMS, there is very little literature that gives a clear picture of how to optimally treat these lesions. Using broad generalizations, RMS is the only temporal bone sarcoma where combined surgery, chemotherapy, and radiation therapy are commonly accepted as the primary treatment modalities, with non-radical surgery being the role for the surgeon. However, this has not been proven definitively to be the best approach. Other non-RMS sarcomas are usually treated with wide and/or radical surgical resection with varying protocols utilizing pre- and postoperative radiation and chemotherapy. Proton beam radiation has been used increasingly to treat chondrosarcomas and osteosarcomas of the temporal bone and skull base, with encouraging results. Further research and wider application may confirm this as a good radiation modality for all skull base sarcomas. As with most head and neck malignancies, true leaps in survivorship await treatments aimed at correcting the underlying molecular and genetic origins of these tumors.

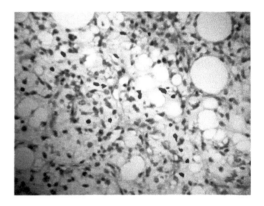

Figure 24.11 Liposarcoma (200 magnification). Malignant lipoblasts are the hallmark of this lesion. They appear as vacuolated cells with eccentrically displaced nuclei, resembling altered adipose tissue. Cell nuclei are large, variably pleomorphic, and may appear in the form of rings or florets.

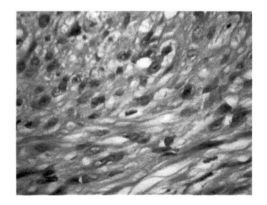

Figure 24.12 Leiomyosarcoma (200 magnification). Leiomyosarcomas consist of intersecting bundles of spindle-shaped smooth cells. Nuclei are cigar-shaped and have blunt ends. The neoplastic cells contain a moderate degree of eosinophilic cytoplasm that appears fibrillar in the longitudinal axis. When cut on end, tumor cells appear to have perinuclear halos.

# REFERENCES

1. Marsh M, Coker N, Jenkins H. Temporal bone neoplasms and lateral cranial base surgery. In: Cummings C, ed. Otolaryngology Head and Neck Surgery. 3rd ed. St. Louis, MO: Mosby, 1996:3245–3281.
2. Kyriakos K, Batsakis JG, eds. Tumors of the Head and Neck. 3rd ed. Baltimore, MD: Williams & Wilkins, 1987.
3. Naufel PM. Primary sarcomas of the temporal bone. Arch Otolaryngol 1973; 98:44–50.
4. Newton WA, Gehan EA, Webber BL et al. Classification of rhabdomyosarcomas and related sarcomas. Cancer 1995; 76(6):1073–1085.
5. Canalis RF, Gussen R. Temporal bone findings in rhabdomyosarcoma with predominantly petrous involvement. Arch Otolaryngol 1980; 106:290–293.
6. Anderson GJ, Tom LWC, Womer RB et al. Rhabdomyosarcoma of the head and neck in children. Arch Otolaryngol Head Neck Surg 1990; 116:428–431.
7. Goepfert H, Cangir A, Lindberg R et al. Rhabdomyosarcoma of the temporal bone. Is surgical resection necessary? Arch Otolaryngol 1979; 105:310–313.
8. Wiatrak BJ, Pensak ML. Rhabdomyosarcoma of the ear and temporal bone. Laryngoscope 1989; 99:1188–1192.
9. Tefft M, Fernandez C, Donaldson M et al. Incidence of meningeal involvement by rhabdomyosarcoma of the head and neck in children. A report of the intergroup rhabdomyosarcoma study. Cancer 1978; 42:253–258.
10. Deutsch M, Felder H. Rhabdomyosarcoma of the ear-mastoid. Laryngoscope 1974; 84:586–592.
11. Schouwenburg PF, Kupperman D, Bakker FP et al. New combined treatment of surgery, radiotherapy, and reconstruction in head and neck rhabdomyosarcoma in children: The AMORE Protocol. Head Neck 1998; 20:282–283.
12. Daya H, Chan HSL, Sirkin W et al. Pediatric rhabdomyosarcoma of the head and neck. Is there a place for surgical management? Arch Otolaryngol Head Neck Surg 2000; 126:468–472.
13. Rudzinski ER, Kelsey A, Vokuhl C, et. Al Pathology of childhood rhabdomyosarcoma: A consensus opinion document from the Children's Oncology Group, European Pediatric Soft Tissue Sarcoma Study Group, and the Cooperative Weichteilsarkom Studiengruppe. Pediatr Blood Cancer 2021; 68: e28798.
14. El-Gothamy B, Fujita S, Hayden RC. Rhabdomyosarcoma—a temporal bone report. Arch Otolaryngol 1973; 98:106–110.
15. Jaffe BF, Fox JF, Batsakis JG. Rhabdomyosarcoma of the middle ear and mastoid. Cancer 1971; 27(1):29–37.
16. Baker KS, Anderson JR, Link MP et al. Benefit of intensified therapy for patients with local or regional embryonal rhabdomyosarcoma: Results from the Intergroup Rhabdomyosarcoma Study IV. J Clin Oncol 2000; 18(12):2427–2434.
17. Crane JN, Xue W, Qumseya A, et al. Clinical group and modified TNM stage for rhabdomyosarcoma: A review from the Children's Oncology Group. Pediatr Blood Cancer 2022; 69: e29644.
18. Haduong JH, Heske CM, Allen-Rhoades W, et al. An update on rhabdomyosarcoma risk stratification and the rationale for current and future Children's Oncology Group clinical trials. Pediatr Blood Cancer 2022; 69: e29511.
19. Hibbitts E, Chi YY, Hawkins DS, et al. Refinement of risk stratification for childhood rhabdomyosarcoma using FOXO1 fusion status in addition to established clinical outcome predictors: a report from the Children's Oncology Group. Cancer Med 2019;8(14):6437–6448.
20. Gluth MB. Rhabdomyosarcoma and other pediatric temporal bone malignancies. Otolaryngol Clin N Am 2015; 48: 375–390.
21. Yechieli RL, Mandeville HC, Hiniker SM, et al. Rhabdomyosarcoma. Pediatr Blood Cancer 2021; 68(Suppl. 2): e28254.
22. Hosoi H. Current status of treatment for pediatric rhabdomyosarcoma in the USA and Japan. Pediatr Int 2016; 58: 81–87.
23. Prasad S, Snyderman C, Janecka IP et al. Role for surgical resection of parameningeal rhabdomyosarcoma in childhood. In: Proceedings of the 1994 Joint

Annual Meeting of the German and North American Skull Base Society. New York: Thieme; 1994:8.

24. Healy GB, McGill TJI, Janecka I. The surgical management of sarcomas of the head and neck in children. Proceedings of the 4th International Conference on Head and Neck Cancer. Madison, WI: Omni Press, 1996:379–384.

25. Raney RB, Lawrence W, Maurer HM et al. Rhabdomyosarcoma of the ear in childhood. A report from the Intergroup Rhabdomyosarcoma Study I. Cancer 1983; 51(12):2356–2361.

26. Lau DPC, Wharton SB, Antoun NM et al. Chondrosarcoma of the petrous apex. Dilemmas in diagnosis and treatment. J Laryngol Otol 1997; 111:368–371.

27. Watters GWR, Brookes GB. Chondrosarcoma of the temporal bone. Clin Otolaryngol 1995; 20:53–58.

28. Coltrera MD, Googe PB, Harrist TJ et al. Chondrosarcoma of the temporal bone. Diagnosis and treatment of 13 cases and review of the literature. Cancer 1986; 58:2689–2696.

29. Siedman MD, Nichols RD, Raju UB et al. Extracranial skull base chondrosarcoma. Ear Nose Throat J 1989; 68:626–632.

30. Koch BB, Karnell LH, Hoffman HT et al. National Cancer Database Report on chondrosarcoma of the head and neck. Head Neck 2000; 22:408–425.

31. Kveton JF, Brackmann DE, Glasscock ME et al. Chondrosarcoma of the skull base. Otolaryngol Head Neck Surg 1986; 94:23–31.

32. Rosenberg AE, Nielson GP, Keel SB et al. Chondrosarcoma of the base of the skull: a clinicopathologic study of 200 cases with emphasis on its distinction from chordoma. Am J Surg Pathol 1999; 23:1370–1378.

33. Debus J, Schulz-Ertner D, Schad L et al. Stereotactic fractionated radiotherapy for chordomas and chondrosarcomas of the skull base. Int J Radiat Oncol Biol Phys 2000; 47:591–596.

34. Brown E, Hug EB, Weber AL. Chondrosarcoma of the skull base. Neuroimaging Clin North Am 1994; 4:529–541.

35. Burkey BB, Hoffman HT, Baker SR et al. Chondrosarcoma of the head and neck. Laryngoscope 1990; 100:1301–1305.

36. Finn DG, Goepfert H, Batsakis JG. Chondrosarcoma of the head and neck. Laryngoscope 1984; 94:1539–1544.

37. Evans HL, Ayala AG, Romsdahl MM. Prognostic factors in chondrosarcoma of bone: A clinicopathologic analysis with emphasis on histologic grading. Cancer 1977; 40:818–831.

38. Harwood AR, Krajbich JI, Fornasier VL. Radiotherapy of chondrosarcoma of bone. Cancer 1980; 45:2769–2777.

39. Wojno KJ, Hruban RH, Garin-Chesa P et al. Chondroid chordomas and low-grade chondrosarcomas of the craniospinal axis: An immunohistochemical analysis of 17 cases. Am J Surg Path 1992; 16:1144–1152.

40. Grossman RI, Davis KR. Cranial computed tomographic appearance of chondrosarcoma of the base of the skull. Radiology 1981;141:403–408.

41. Meyers SP, Hirsch WL Jr, Curtin HD, et al. Chondrosarcomas of the skull base: MR imaging features. Radiology 1992;184:103–108.

42. Carlson ML, O'Connell BP, Breen JT, et al. Petroclival chondrosarcoma: A multicenter review of 55 cases and new staging system. Otol Neurotol 2016; 37: 940–950.

43. Charabi S, Engel P, Bonding P. Myxoid tumours in the temporal bone. J Laryngol Otol 1989; 103:1206–1209.

44. Al-Mefty O, Fox JL, Rifai A et al. A combined infratemporal and posterior fossa approach for the removal of giant glomus tumors and chondrosarcomas. Surg Neurol 1987; 28:423–431.

45. Suit HD, Goitein M, Munzenrider J et al. Definitive radiation therapy for chordoma and chondrosarcoma of base of skull and cervical spine. J Neurosurg 1982; 56:377–385.

46. Austin-Seymour M, Munzenrider J, Goitein M et al. Fractionated proton radiation therapy of chordoma and low-grade chondrosarcoma of the base of the skull. J Neurosurg 1989; 70:13–17.

47. Muthukumar N, Kondziolka D, Lunsford LD et al. Stereotactic radiosurgery for chordoma and chondrosarcoma: Further experiences. Int J Radiat Oncol Biol Phys 1998; 41:387–392.

48. Mark RJ, Sercarz JA, Tran L et al. Osteogenic sarcoma of the head and neck. The UCLA experience. Arch Otolaryngol Head Neck Surg 1991; 117:761–766.

49. Sharma SC, Handa KK, Panda N et al. Osteogenic sarcoma of the temporal bone. Am J Otolaryngol 1997; 18(3):220–223.

50. Sataloff RT, Myers DL, Spiegal JR et al. Total temporal bone resection for osteogenic sarcoma. Ear Nose Throat J 1998; 67:626–627, 630–632, 634.

51. Goh YH, Chong VFH, Low WK. Temporal bone tumours in patients irradiated for nasopharyngeal neoplasm. J Laryngol Otol 1999; 113:222–228.

52. Nora FE, Unni KK, Pritchard DJ et al. Osteosarcoma of extragnathic craniofacial bones. Mayo Clin Proc 1983; 58:268–272.

53. Guo Z, Hu K, Bing Z, et al. Osteosarcoma of the skull base: An analysis of 19 cases and literature review. J Clin Neuroscience 2017; 44: 133–142.

54. Kassir RR, Rassekh H, Kinsella JB et al. Osteosarcoma of the head and neck: Meta-analysis of nonrandomized studies. Laryngoscope 1997; 107:56–61.

55. Hazarika P, Nayak DR, Sahota JS et al. Osteogenic sarcoma of sphenoid bone: An extended lateral skull base approach. J Laryngol Otol 1995; 109:1101–1104.

56. Garrington GE, Scofield HH, Cornyn J et al. Osteosarcoma of the jaws. Analysis of 56 cases. Cancer 1967; 20(3):377–391.

57. Odell PF. Head and neck sarcomas: a review. J Otolaryngol 1996; 25(1):7–13.

58. Caron AS, Hadju SI, Strong EW. Osteogenic sarcoma of the facial and cranial bones: a review of forty-three cases. Am J Surg 1971; 122:719–725.

59. Chambers RG, Mahoney WD. Osteogenic sarcoma of the mandible: Current management. Am Surg 1970; 36:463–471.

60. Link M, Goorin A, Miser A et al. The role of adjuvant chemotherapy in the treatment of osteosarcoma of the extremities: Preliminary results of the multi-institutional osteosarcoma study. Proc Am Soc Clin Oncol 1985; 4:237.

61. Eibler F, Giuliano J, Eckardt J et al. Adjuvant chemotherapy for osteosarcoma: A randomized prospective trial. J Clin Oncol 1987; 5(1):216.

62. Castro JR, Linstadt DE, Bahary JP et al. Experience in charged particle irradiation of tumors of the skull base: 1977–1992. Int J Radiat Oncol Biol Phys 1994; 29(4):647–655.

63. Nakayama K, Nemoto Y, Inoue Y et al. Malignant fibrous histiocytoma of the temporal bone with endocranial extension. AJNR Am J Neuroradiol 1997; 18:331–334.

64. Blitzer A, Lawson W, Zak FG et al. Clinical–pathological determinants in prognosis of fibrous histiocytomas of head and neck. Laryngoscope 1981; 91:2053–2069.

65. Raney RB, Allen A, O'Neill J et al. Malignant fibrous histiocytoma of soft tissue in childhood. Cancer 1986; 57:2198–2201.

66. Frankenthaler R, Ayala AG, Hartwick RW et al. Fibrosarcoma of the head and neck. Laryngoscope 1990; 100(8):799–802.

67. Pope EM. Fibrosarcoma of dura, middle fossa, radical mastoid operation. Case report. Laryngoscope 1931; 41:555–556.

68. Apte NK. Fibrosarcoma of the temporal bone. J Laryngol Otol 1965; 79(12):1101–1103.

69. Conley J, Stout AP, Healey WV. Clinicopathologic analysis of eighty-four patients with an original diagnosis of fibrosarcoma of the head and neck. Am J Surg 1967; 114:564–569.

70. Freedman AM, Reiman HM, Woods JE. Soft-tissue sarcomas of the head and neck. Am J Surg 1989; 158(4):367–372.

71. Fitzer PM, Steffey WR. Brain and bone scans in primary Ewing's sarcoma of the petrous bone. J Neurosurg 1976; 44:608–612.

72. Davidson MJC. Ewing's sarcoma of the temporal bone. A case report. Oral Surg Oral Med Oral Pathol 1991; 72:534–536.

73. Desai K, Goel A, Nadkarni TD. Primary petrous bone Ewing's sarcoma. Br J Neurosurg 2000; 14(2):143–145.

74. Hadfield MG, Luo VY, Williams RL et al. Ewing's sarcoma of the skull in an infant. A case report and review. Pediatr Neurosurg 1996; 25:100–104.

75. Desai KI, Nadkarni TD, Goel A et al. Primary Ewing's sarcoma of the cranium. Neurosurgery 2000; 46(1):62–69.

76. Wantanabe H, Tsubokawa T, Katayama Y et al. Primary Ewing's sarcoma of the temporal bone. Surg Neurol 1992; 37:54–58.

77. Sharma RR, Netalkar A, Lad SD. Primary Ewing's sarcoma of the greater wing of the sphenoid bone. Br J Neurosurg 2000; 14(1):53–57.

78. Horowitz ME, Malawer MM, Woo SY et al. Ewing's sarcoma family of tumors: Ewing's sarcoma of bone and soft tissue and the peripheral neuroectodermal tumors. In: Pizzo PA, Poplock DG, eds. Principles and Practice of Pediatric Oncology. 3rd ed. Philadelphia, PA: Lippincott-Raven Publishers, 1997:831–863.

79. Hellquist HB, Lundgren J. Neurogenic sarcoma of the sinonasal tract. J Laryngol Otol 1991; 105:186–190.

80. Hutcherson RW, Jenkins HA, Canalis RF et al. Neurogenic sarcoma of the head and neck. Arch Otolaryngol 1979; 105:267–270.

81. Greager JA, Reichard KW, Campana JP et al. Malignant schwannoma of the head and neck. Am J Surg 1992; 163:440–442.

82. Kettel K. Intratemporal sarcoma of the facial nerve. Arch Otolaryngol 1950; 52:778–781.

83. Guttman MR, Simon MU. Neurofibrosarcoma of the facial nerve involving the tympanomastoid. Arch Otolaryngol 1951; 54:162–166.

84. Chen A, Wang T, Xu X. Giant malignant peripheral nerve sheath tumor of the head and neck: A case report and literature review. Ear Nose Throat J 2021; 100(5 Suppl): 624S–628S.

85. D'Agostino AN, Soule EH, Miller RH. Primary malignant neoplasms of nerve (malignant neurolemmomas) in patients without manifestations of multiple neurofibromatosis (von Recklinghausen's disease). Cancer 1963; 16:1003–1014.

86. Goepfert H, Lindberg RD, Sinkovics JG. Soft-tissue sarcoma of the head and neck after puberty. Arch Otolaryngol 1977; 103(6):365–368.

87. Mark RJ, Tran LM, Sercarz J et al. Angiosarcoma of the head and neck. The UCLA experience 1955 through 1990. Arch Otolaryngol Head Neck Surg 1993; 119:973–978.

88. Kinkade JM. Angiosarcoma of the petrous portion of the temporal bone. Ann Otol Rhinol Laryngol 1948; 57:235–240.

89. Bernstock JD, Shafaat O, Hardigan A, et al. Angiosarcoma of the temporal bone: Case report and review of the literature. World Neurosurg 2019; 130: 351–357.

90. Chen JX, Kozin ED, O'Malley J, et al. Otopathology in angiosarcoma of the temporal bone. Laryngoscope 2018; 129: 737–742.

91. Linthicum FH, Schwartzman JA. An Atlas of Micropathology of the Temporal Bone. San Diego, CA: Singular Publishing Group, Inc., 1994:78–79.

92. Aust MR, Olsen KD, Lewis JE et al. Angiosarcomas of the head and neck: Clinical and pathological characteristics. Ann Otol Rhinol Laryngol 1997; 106:943–951.

93. Zbaren P, Ruchti C. Leiomyosarcoma of the middle ear and temporal bone. Ann Otol Rhinol Laryngol 1994; 103:537–541.

# Hearing in dogs

D. CAROLINE COILE

The domestic dog serves in a variety of roles, including sentry, patrol, herding, hunting, and guide dog functions, all of which require acute hearing for optimal performance. Many of these roles involve exposure to loud noises, placing dogs at risk for noise-induced hearing loss. In addition, some kenneling and even veterinary practices may expose them to high noise levels that would cause hearing deficits in humans. Yet little research has been done in this area, and in fact, there's still insufficient data about hearing in normal dogs and the extent to which it may differ across breeds or with physical differences—and possibly, the extent to which some features might put dogs at greater or lesser risk for noise-induced hearing loss. Without this knowledge, dogs may be subjected to noise levels that could adversely affect their hearing and thus ability to work or even live a normal life.

A popular subject of early research in comparative hearing, the dog eventually fell from favor as a research subject, in part because of its lack of uniformity. Yet, it is exactly this diversity that makes the dog a particularly intriguing subject in which to examine the influence of for example head size and pinna configuration on hearing within the same species. In addition, the presence of hereditary (particularly pigment-related) deafness in dogs has both basic and applied implications. Despite such a wealth of incentives, a paucity of information about canine hearing exists.

## INTERAURAL DISTANCE AND HIGH-FREQUENCY DETECTION

As a rule of thumb, smaller species of land mammals can hear higher frequencies compared with the frequencies larger species can hear; this difference has been conjectured to be an adaptation for sound localization in smaller animals. The wider the ears are separated, the easier it is to use differences in arrival time of sounds to either ear as a localization cue. Sound shadowing from the animal's own head provides another important localization cue; the smaller the sound waves are in comparison to the head width, the greater this effect. This means that an animal with a narrower head must be able to perceive higher frequency sound in order to use this cue. The trend toward higher frequency hearing in smaller animals could be an adaptation enabling the animal to use high-frequency sound for localization cues despite its small head size. These interspecies observations might suggest that dogs with small or narrow heads should have either poorer sound

DOI: 10.1201/b23379-25

localization or better high-frequency hearing than dogs with larger, wider heads. Most working dogs are of necessity larger breeds with wider heads. Although there are no comparison studies between breeds in sound localization ability, in a comparison of the hearing thresholds of four dogs representing four breeds (Chihuahua, Dachshund, Poodle, and Saint Bernard) of different sizes, no differences in high- or low-frequency hearing were found. All had maximal sensitivity at ~8000 Hz, with a high frequency cut-off ~41,000–47,000 Hz—a far smaller difference than would be predicted by the variation in head size. When compared with other species of comparable sizes, small dogs have a slightly better ability to hear high frequencies, and large dogs have a much better ability to hear high frequencies, than would be expected on the basis of their size (1). Note, however, that an unpublished study did find a more substantial relationship between interaural distance and maximum high-frequency hearing in dogs, with dogs with more narrow heads hearing frequencies up to 60,000 Hz (2).

Rodent vocalizations can be of a higher frequency (for example, mice around 40,000 Hz) than humans can detect but are easily detected by dogs. Rodent and insect ultrasonic deterrents emit frequencies above the hearing range of humans, typically ranging from 25,000 to 65,000 kHz. Manufacturers claim that dogs and cats also cannot hear the high frequencies emitted by these devices—but they can. Dogs can hear frequencies as high as ~47,000 or even 60,000 Hz, and cats can hear even higher frequencies, up to ~85,000 Hz (3). They are thus subjected to a barrage of high-frequency sound emitted from many of these devices.

It is unknown the extent to which constant exposure to high-frequency ultrasounds might affect hearing. It could conceivably interfere with the work of search and rescue dogs or patrol dogs that may need to detect low-amplitude sounds. And constant exposure could lead to noise-induced hearing loss or to stress. Ultrasonic pest deterrents should be removed from areas in which dogs spend extended times or in which they are expected to perform tasks based on auditory detection. Other household devices, such as televisions, audio systems, and motion detectors can also emit ultrasounds that dogs may hear. High-intensity (120 dB) ultrasonic sweeps of 5000–55,000 Hz have

been reported to repel most dogs (4). Research is needed to determine the extent of chronic ultrasound exposure any effects on dog hearing and well-being.

## PINNA CONFIGURATION

Dog pinnae vary greatly in design, but no data exist on how their configuration affects hearing. The most popular police and military dog breeds, the German Shepherd Dog and Belgian Malinois (and other Belgian Shepherd breeds), have pricked ears. The only popular military breed that doesn't, the Doberman Pinscher, has drop ears that are traditionally cropped. The most popular guide and service dogs tend to be retrievers, Poodles, and their mixes, all with drop ears. Gun dog breeds all have drop ears. While it's intuitive that prick ears would be more sensitive than drop ears, nobody knows if it's actually true, or to what extent, and if that difference is enough to select for that trait in working dogs or against it in dogs subjected to gunshot noise. Nor is it known if hanging ears confer a protection against noise-induced hearing loss. It's also not known if hearing protective gear might work better for one configuration than another.

As if the natural variation in pinna conformation was not enough, humans have cropped dogs' ears for centuries. The reason was often originated with function but remained due to style. One intriguing functional reason was the belief it increased hearing ability in dogs with otherwise hanging ears.

A hanging ear flap cannot function in the same manner as an erect ear. The erect ear can swivel to direct its opening toward a sound source. Its configuration directs the sound waves into the ear canal and, additionally, amplifies them slightly. In cats, the pinna produces up to 28-dB amplification of sounds (especially high-frequency sounds) emitted within the pinna's optimal axis of reception directly in front of its cup (5). The naturally erect dog ear probably has a comparable amplification ability that is not available to dogs with other ear configurations.

The hanging pinna also imposes a barrier between the sound waves and the ear canal, which could conceivably dampen sounds. Despite the rich array of dog ears waiting to be tested, only one study has addressed the effects of pinna configuration on hearing thresholds. In a comparison of four dogs, one of which had erect pinnae, and three of which had hanging pinnae, no significant differences in high- or low-frequency hearing were detected. When one dog with hanging ears was retested with its pinnae taped over its head, no differences in its low-frequency thresholds and only minor differences (> 3 dB) in its high-frequency threshold were found (1). Taping the dog's ear back does not give the pinna the same acoustic powers that a normally erect pinna has; however, neither does ear cropping. A cropped ear is missing a good portion of the natural bell shape that a naturally erect ear has; it is thus questionable that cropping ears affords any worthwhile gain in auditory sensitivity.

The pinna does play a large role in sound localization, especially in discriminating front vs. back and high vs. low sources (6). The asymmetry of the entire pinna, coupled with the various folds within it, transforms sound waves differently depending upon the angle at which they impinge upon the pinna, providing further cues for sound localization. Dogs with hanging ears may thus be compromised compared to erect-eared dogs at locating the source of a sound in the high vs. low dimension or front vs. back dimension but should not be compromised at left vs. right localization. A mobile pinna would seem to be an asset in localization, but the movement of the pinna is too slow to aid in localization of brief sounds. In a study of 10 dogs, the minimum audible angle varied from 1.3 degrees to 13.2 degrees, depending on the individual, but no clear relationship was found between localization ability and ear or head shape (7).

The pinna funnels the sound waves into the auditory meatus, which differs from the human canal because it initially travels downward and then turns abruptly inward. The horizontal section can be difficult to treat in cases of otitis externa. Some breeds have hair growing within or at the entrance to the canal, which could influence hearing. Chronic otitis externa can sometimes result in impaction or occlusion of the ear canal and, ultimately, ossification of the canal, all circumstances that can cause conductive deafness. Surgical procedures can often re-establish hearing in such dogs (8).

The influence of pinna configuration is another area needing research for both basic science and practical reasons, both to optimize hearing for the task at hand and to protect hearing if needed.

## MIDDLE EAR

Differences in the size of the tympanic membrane between species have long been thought to affect auditory response properties. The single study to examine this in dogs found the area of the tympanic membrane varied from 30 $mm^2$ in the Chihuahua to 55 $mm^2$ in the Saint Bernard (1). Despite this large difference, no differences in hearing ability between these breeds were documented.

The tympanic membrane can rupture due to chronic ear disease or trauma. Working dogs exposed to explosive shocks can have ruptured tympanic membranes in one or both ears. The forces at which this occur appear to be similar for dogs and humans, that is, about 194 dB for humans and 192 dB for dogs. For static pressure exposure, the levels are 198 dB for humans and 194 dB for dogs (9). Dogs with ruptured membranes can still hear but at a compromised level. Vibration of the tympanic membrane causes a lever-like action of the ossicles of the middle ear; this, combined with the concentration of energy onto the tiny oval window, results in an increase in sound pressure level that approximately counteracts the loss of energy that would otherwise occur when going from the air-filled middle ear to the fluid-filled cochlea. The dog's malleus is relatively larger compared to the human malleus, increasing its leverage and thus amplification. Decreased articulation of the ossicles may contribute to hearing loss in older dogs (presbycusis) but is probably a comparatively minor factor.

The stapedius and tensor tympani muscles are attached to the ossicles and serve to stiffen the tympanic membrane and retract the stapes from its normal position in the oval window in response to loud noise. These actions decrease the sound amplitude by as much as 30 dB in humans and probably at least that much in dogs. This acoustic reflex, which has a threshold of 70–110 dB in dogs at frequencies of 1000 and 2000 Hz (10), protects the ear from damage from continued loud noise, though it cannot protect it from sudden loud noise or from continued extreme loud noise. This study found that removing the tensor tympani tendon had no effect on the acoustic reflex. No other studies examining the efficiency of the acoustic reflex in dogs exist despite its importance in preserving hearing in working dogs.

## NOISE-INDUCED HEARING LOSS

A paucity of research on noise-induced hearing loss exists for dogs, although it is much needed. Many canine occupations expose dogs to sudden or continuous loud noises that could impact their ability to do their jobs. Many other situations expose them to noise levels that could impact their ability to communicate with people.

Dogs housed in kennels are often subjected to prolonged noise levels over 100 dB with peaks of 120 dB from barking (11), a situation compounded by the lack of acoustic insulation in most kennel buildings. In one study comparing hearing thresholds of 14 dogs housed in a kennel for 9 months, the dogs had a threshold at least 10 dB higher afterward (12). This could prove problematic to shelter dogs, military dogs, boarding dogs, or commercial breeding dogs housed in kennels or even to dogs at daycare establishments. Noise-abatement design in kennel buildings should be a consideration that could improve dog and human welfare (13).

Some researchers speculate that the level of noise acceptable as being safe for people is too intense for dogs by about 20 dB (so, a limit of 50 dB averaged through the day) because dogs have more sensitive hearing, especially at high frequencies, which are more vulnerable to noise-induced hearing loss (14).

Police, military, and hunting dogs may be exposed to repeated gunfire sound. A study comparing 40 German Shorthaired Pointers immediately following a day hunting alongside gunfire (143 dB) found they experienced a substantial decline in amplitude values in brainstem auditory-evoked response (BAER) records obtained with a click stimulus (15).

Military dogs subjected to loud helicopter sounds have displayed hearing loss of up to 50 dB after even brief flights (16). Dogs shipped by air are often subjected to high noise levels by airline personnel who place dogs along with baggage on the tarmac next to jet engines. Dogs employed as airline bomb or contraband detectors may have to work around jet engines but can be trained to wear ear protection. Police dogs on patrol at rock concerts can also be subjected to high noise levels. Dogs competing in certain dog sports, such as flyball, are subjected to high noise from barking for hours at a time.

Dogs undergoing veterinary procedures or experimental procedures may be subjected to loud MRI noise without benefit of ear protection as would be afforded to humans. MRI noise can reach 130 dB and has been shown to significantly reduce frequency-specific cochlear function in dogs (17).

Several products have been introduced for hearing protection in dogs. Some of these are aimed at the military or police dog segment whereas others are aimed at muffling sounds for noise-reactive dogs in the home. Although exact noise reduction has not been quantified, anecdotal reports support their effectiveness.

It's as yet unclear the extent of noise-induced hearing loss in dogs compared to humans, but in a review of dog vs. human hearing, the authors point out that

> as dogs hear better in higher frequency range and higher frequencies are most often affected by loud noises, in general noise induced hearing loss could be more easily induced, and possibly more severe, in dogs compared with humans, although empirical data are missing (18).

Many dogs' jobs or roles as companions depend on good hearing, and many situations put them at risk of noise-induced hearing loss. This is an area in which research is needed, both to elucidate the extent of hearing loss and to establish guidelines for diminishing hearing loss, including noise abatement and otoprotective gear and drugs.

## INNER EAR

Movement of the ossicles transmits vibrations to the cochlea via the oval window, causing movement of the cochlear fluid and basilar membrane. Within the cochlea, the organ of Corti contains hair cells, each of which has many stereocilia that extend to and are embedded in another membrane, the tectorial membrane. Movement of cochlear fluid produces movement of the basilar membrane upon which the hair cell stereocilia of the organ of Corti are embedded; because the tectorial membrane remains stationary, a shearing force upon the hair cells is created. It is this shearing force that results in a nerve impulse from the hair cell. With repeated or sustained exposure to loud noise, the hair cells become damaged or disarranged, resulting in hearing loss.

Hair cells can also be damaged by certain drugs, many of which are routinely prescribed in veterinary practice. The most common of these ototoxic drugs are the aminoglycoside antibiotics, which include the frequently prescribed gentamicin and neomycin (19). Routine administration of these drugs seldom causes loss of hearing, but prolonged systemic administration, or topical administration in dogs with ruptured tympanic membranes, can result in irreversible hearing loss.

Hereditary deafness is known in many breeds of dogs, with the best known being the Dalmatian. Affected Dalmatians are born with normal auditory structure, but soon after birth, the stria vascularis (the vascular bed of the cochlear duct) degenerates. The cochlear duct in turn collapses and the hair cells degenerate so that these dogs are deaf by ~1 month of age (20). In some other breeds, deafness results from degeneration of hair cells without any circulatory involvement (21).

In dogs with normal hearing and hair cells, the hair cells send their signals to the brain by way of the auditory nerve fibers that leave the organ of Corti via the spiral ganglion. Acquired hearing loss in old dogs is often associated with loss of cells in the spiral ganglion (22). This structure also degenerates in the deaf Dalmatian, possibly secondarily to the loss of hair cells. Normal auditory nerve fibers leave the ear and travel to the brain, with most entering the brainstem, where they make contact with cells in the cochlear nucleus.

Because the auditory signals must travel by way of the brainstem, recordings of the electrical activity of the brainstem in response to auditory stimuli can indicate whether a dog's ear is functioning normally. The most widespread and useful test of hearing in dogs is the BAER.

In dogs with normal hearing, the signals travel from the brainstem to several other structures of the brain, including the superior olivary complex, lateral lemniscus, inferior colliculus, and medial geniculate nucleus, all of which process the auditory information before sending it on, until it ultimately arrives in the auditory cortex. In the absence of auditory stimulation, the auditory cortex will deteriorate, an observation that led some early researchers to ascribe the hereditary deafness in the Dalmatian to brain abnormalities. These abnormalities are secondary to the initial cochlear losses, however, and do not suggest that deaf Dalmatians have abnormal brains. In fact, deafness in dogs due to brain abnormalities is rare, and in such cases usually is the least of the dog's problems.

## PIGMENT-RELATED DEAFNESS

The most common cause of deafness in young dogs is hereditary pigment-related deafness such as that associated with genes responsible for lack of pigmentation in the coat, iris, and other body parts. The most prominent of these genes are the merle (M) and extreme piebald ($s^w$) alleles.

In merle dogs, the presence of one M allele results in the merle coat coloration (a patchwork of dark and light coat such as that often seen in the Catahoula Leopard Dog and Australian Shepherd). The merle coat color is governed by a short interspersed nuclear element (SINE) insertion in the silver locus protein homolog (SILV; also called premelanosome protein [PMEL17]) gene. Having a single *M* allele raises the chance of being deaf, although the chance of an *Mm* merle being bilaterally deaf is still less than 1%. The presence of two *M* genes, however, greatly increases the chance of deafness, depending on what breed it's in. For example, in one study, about 10% of *MM* Catahoula Leopard Dogs, about 56% of *MM* Australian Shepherds, and about 85% of all other *MM* dogs studied were deaf in both ears (23).

In extreme piebald dogs, the presence of two $s^w$ alleles results in a predominantly white dog with spots (such as the pattern seen in Dalmatians and English Setters). The gene responsible for extreme white, called *Melanocyte-Inducing Transcription Factor (MITF)*, has been assumed by many to also cause deafness, with all extreme-white dogs in a breed equally at risk, but with random expression of deafness, somewhat similar to how spots are randomly expressed. But despite many attempts to uncover the genetic basis of this type of deafness, no DNA study has been able to positively identify a genetic cause—not even *MITF*.

However, a risk haplotype that consists of a combinations of genes near the *MITF* gene has been identified that is associated with deafness in Dalmatians (24). All Dalmatians have the *MITF* gene, but three possible haplotypes at another nearby location then affect hearing. So extreme-white is a necessary but insufficient cause of deafness. Dalmatians with one of the three haplotypes were at greater risk of deafness than those with the other possible types.

Looking at Dalmatians from Australia, and validating with Dalmatians from the UK and US, these University of Sydney researchers found 62% of bilaterally dogs were homozygous for the risk haplotype, while 30% of bilaterally deaf and 45% of hearing dogs carried one copy of the risk haplotype. Dalmatians that were homozygous for the risk haplotype were 10 times more likely to be bilaterally deaf compared to those that carried one or no copies of the risk haplotype. They were also more likely to be unilaterally deaf. The risk haplotype's incomplete penetrance could be due to interactions with genes at as yet undiscovered locations. It's possible that a similar association may be found in other breeds with deafness associated with white, particularly white Boxers and Australian Cattle Dogs. The varying frequency of the haplotype from breed to breed could explain why deafness is more common in some extreme-white spotted breeds than in others.

This association with coat color is more than just coincidental; animals with alleles that result not only in absence of coat pigmentation but also in missing pigment on other body structures may be lacking normal pigment on internal body structures. For example, normal blood vessels have pigment-producing cells (melanocytes) within them; it is likely that blood vessels missing melanocytes do not develop normally. Melanocytes in the stria vascularis seem to be suppressed by the action of the merle or extreme piebald genes. The melanocytes may be responsible for maintaining potassium levels in endocochlear fluid, as well as for the maintenance of the cochlear duct (25, 26). In addition, pigment molecules are thought to play a role in guiding some neural connections during development; abnormal connections are seen

in association with some other alleles resulting in reduced pigment such as those in the albino series (27). Not all white dogs are the result of such alleles; those with the greatest likelihood of having deafness associated with white or merle coloration seem to be those in whom coat color is often associated with absence of normal ocular pigment.

## OTHER DEAFNESS

Not all non-noise-induced deafness in dogs is pigment related. Deafness in Doberman Pinschers, for instance, results from primary degeneration of the cochlear hair cells (without vascular involvement) and is not associated with merle or piebald genes. This type of deafness, which also affects the sense of balance, is caused by a single recessive allele (21). Many other breeds have hereditary deafness caused by breed-related mutations.

In addition, age-related hearing loss is extremely common in dogs. No research exists on whether it varies by breed (some breeds age faster than others) or prior noise exposure, although the latter at least seems probable. Age-related hearing loss, which occurs starting around 8–10 years (28), can cut short the working life of some dogs, and also is corelated with future canine cognitive disorder, which can cut short the enjoyable companion life of some dogs (29).

Dogs suspected of or at risk of being deaf can have a BAER test performed at most veterinary teaching hospitals and several specialty clinics (30). Preliminary screening tests can be conducted in the home or veterinary clinic, but the results may not be very accurate. Saying a word to which the dog normally responds when the dog's attention is elsewhere and when the dog cannot see the person speaking is a simple preliminary test. Ringing a bell or sounding a novel stimulus from behind the dog should result in either the dog's attention (as evidenced by head turning and ear twitching) or a startle reaction. Dogs that are panting will characteristically stop panting momentarily in order to listen, so this can be used as a tentative sign of hearing. Testers must be careful that no wind currents from clapping hands or vibrations through the floor reach the dog and that the dog cannot see the tester out of the corner of its eye (bearing in mind that dogs have a greater peripheral field of vision than humans) or cannot see the tester's shadow or reflection. Other dogs that could provide cues by their response should be removed from the area. Dogs habituate to auditory stimuli rapidly; repeating the test will often result in lack of responsiveness. These tests can generally detect a dog that is bilaterally deaf. A dog with unilateral deafness will still respond to words and sounds in a manner almost indistinguishable from a dog with normal hearing. It will swivel both pinnae in response to a sound, even though one pinna may be leading to a totally deaf ear. A dog with unilateral hearing loss may have some difficulty in localizing sounds in the left vs. right dimension, but this can be difficult to test without more sophisticated techniques.

Good hearing is essential in most working dogs. Unilaterally deaf dogs make excellent companions, and their owners often are never aware that the dog has any loss of hearing. Bilaterally deaf dogs present a more challenging, and controversial, situation. These dogs are at greater risk of being killed or injured in an accident because they cannot hear their owner's calls or cannot hear approaching danger. They may be more likely to snap because they can be easily startled by the sudden appearance of a dog or person. They can be difficult to train because special ways of first having the dog watch the owner must be taught, and then visual or tactile signals must be used. Owners who do not realize their dog is deaf too often conclude it is stupid or stubborn and may abuse or abandon it. Many people have raised deaf dogs successfully, however. They use hand signals, flashlights, vibrating collars, and even other dogs to help them communicate with their deaf pets. Nonetheless, living with a totally deaf dog presents hardships not encountered when living with a dog that can hear. Owners of deaf dogs can find advice through several sources (31).

# REFERENCES

1. Heffner HE. Hearing in large and small dogs: absolute thresholds and size of the tympanic membrane. Behav Neurosci 1983; 97:310–318.
2. McMahon, DH. Investigating the relationship between the frequency ranges a dog can hear compared to its head size. Unpublished BSc (Hons) thesis, University of Lincoln. 2015. Cited in Barber, et al.
3. Heffner RS, Heffner HE. Hearing range of the domestic cat. Hear Res 1985; 19:85–88.
4. Blackshaw JK, Cook GE, Harding P, Day C, Bates W, Rose J, Bramham D. Aversive responses of dogs to ultrasonic, sonic and flashing light units. Appl Anim Behav Sci 1990; 25:1–8.
5. Phillips DP, Calford B, Pettigrew JD, Aitkin LM, Semple MN. Directionality of sound pressure transformation at the cat's pinna. Hear Res 1982; 8:13–28.
6. Heffner RS, Koay G, Heffner HE. Sound localization in chinchillas III: effect of pinna removal. Hear Res 1996; 99:13–21.
7. Guérineau C, Lõoke M, Broseghini A, Dehesh G, Mongillo P, Marinelli L. Sound localization ability in dogs. Vet Sci 2022; 9:619.
8. Krahwinkel DJ, Pardo AD, Sims MH, Bubb WJ. Effect of total ablation of the external auditory meatus and bulla osteotomy on auditory function in dogs. J Am Vet Med Assoc 1993; 202:949–952.
9. Richmond DR, Fletcher ER, Yelverton JT, Phillips YY. Physical correlates of eardrum rupture. Ann Otol Rhinol Laryngol Suppl 1989; 98 (5, Suppl.): 35–41.
10. Sims MH, Weigel JP, Moore RE. Effect of tenotomy of the tensor tympani muscle on the acoustic reflex in dogs. Am J Vet Res 1986; 47:1022–1031.
11. Sales G, Hubrect R, Peyvandi A, Milligan S, Shield B. Noise in dog kenneling: Is barking a welfare problem for dogs? Appl Anim Behav Sci 1997; 52, 321–329.
12. Scheifele P, Martin D, Clark JG, Kemper D, Wells J. Effect of kennel noise on hearing in dogs. Am J Vet Res 2012; 73: 482–489.
13. Coppola CL, Enns MR, Grandin T. Noise in the animal shelter environment: Building design and the effects of daily noise exposure. J Appl Anim Welf Sci 2006; 9: 1–7.
14. Mak SL, Au SL, Tang WF, Li CH, Lee CC, Chiu WH. A Study on Hearing Hazards and sound measurement for Dogs. *2022 IEEE International Symposium on Product Compliance Engineering – Asia (ISPCE-ASIA)*, Guangzhou, Guangdong Province, China, 2022; 1–4.
15. Sirin Ö, Sirin Y Beşalti, Ö. Does acoustic trauma occur in pointers due to firearm noise? A prospective study on 50

hunting dogs. Ankara Universitesi Veteriner Fakultesi Dergisi. 2018; 65, 365–372. 10.1501/Vetfak_0000002869.

16. Scheifele P, Martin D, Clark JG, Kemper D, Wells J. Effect of kennel noise on hearing in dogs. Am J Vet Res 2012; 73: 482–489.

17. Venn RE, McBrearty AR, McKeegan D, Penderis J. The effect of magnetic resonance imaging noise on cochlear function in dogs. Vet J 2014; 202:141–145.

18. Barber AL, Wilkinson, A, Montealegre-Z F, Ratcliffe VF, Guo K, Mills DS. A comparison of hearing and auditory functioning between dogs and humans. Comp Cogn Behav Rev 2020; 15: 45–94.

19. Strain GM, Clark LA, Wahl JM, Turner AE, Murphy KE. Prevalence of deafness in dogs heterozygous or homozygous for the merle allele. J Vet Intern Med 2009; 23: 282–286. 10.1111/j.1939-1676.2008.0257.x

20. Oishi N, Talaska AE, Schacht J. Ototoxicity in dogs and cats. Vet Clin North Am Small Anim Pract 2012; 42:1259–1271.

21. Wilkes MK, Palmer AC. Congenital deafness and vestibular deficit in the doberman. J Small Anim Pract 1992; 33:218–224.

22. Knowles K, Blauch B, Leipold H, Cash W, Hewitt J. Reduction of spiral ganglion neurons in the aging canine with hearing loss. J Vet Med 1989; 36:188–199.

23. Strain GM, Clark LA, Wahl JM, Turner AE, Murphy KE. Prevalence of deafness in dogs heterozygous or homozygous for the merle allele. J Vet Internal Med 2009; 23: 282–286.

24. Haase B, Willet CE, Chew T, Samaha G, Child G, Wade CN. De-novo and genome-wide meta-analyses identify a risk haplotype for congenital sensorineural deafness in Dalmatian dogs. Sci Rep 2022; 12:15439.

25. Steel KP, Barkway C. Another role for melanocytes: their importance for normal stria vascularis development in the mammalian inner ear. Development 1989; 107:453–463.

26. Cable J, Huszar D, Jaenisch R, Steel KP. Effects of mutations at the W locus (c-kit) on inner ear pigmentation and function in the mouse. Pigment Cell Res 1994; 7: 17–32.

27. Witcop CJ, Jay B, Creel D, Guillery RW. Optic and otic neurological abnormalities in oculocutaneous and ocular albinism. In: Cotlier, Maumenee, Berman, eds. Genetic Eye Diseases: Retinitis Pigmentosa and Other Inherited Eye Disorders. Proceedings of the International Symposium on Genetics and Ophthalmology. New York, NY: Alan R. Liss, 1981.

28. Ter Haar G, Venker-van Haagen AJ, Van Den Brom WE, Van Sluijs FJ, Smoorenburg GF. Effects of aging on brainstem responses to toneburst auditory stimuli: A cross-sectional and longitudinal study in dogs. J Vet Internal Med 2008; 22: 937–945.

29. Fefer G, Khan MZ, Panek WK, Case B, Gruen ME, Olby NJ. Relationship between hearing, cognitive function, and quality of life in aging companion dogs. J Vet Internal Med 2022; 36:1708–1718.

30. Strain G. Deafness in dogs and cats. BAER Test Sites. In: Deafness in Dogs and Cats. Available from https://www.lsu.edu/deafness/deaf.htm

31. Cope-Becker S. Living With a Deaf Dog: A Book of Advice, Facts and Experiences about Canine Deafness. Cincinnati: Cope-Becker S, 1997.

# 26

# Implications of nutraceutical modulation of glutathione with cystine and cysteine in general health and otology

KATHERINE MULLEN, THOMAS A. KWYER (DECEASED),
AND ROBERT THAYER SATALOFF

## INTRODUCTION

As knowledge regarding the ear has advanced, it has become clear that otologic abnormalities are similar to conditions elsewhere in the body. For example, presbycusis is but one manifestation of aging. Similarly, autoimmune inner ear disease (AIED) has much in common with other autoimmune disorders such as rheumatoid arthritis, psoriasis, and thyroiditis. Like all other body systems, ear function is dependent on efficient operation of biochemical pathways that provide essential nutrients to cells.

Investigation of nutraceutical use in otologic patients is in its infancy; however, glutathione (GSH) modulation appears to be beneficial in conditions such as otitis media and AIED. Oxidative stress might contribute to the pathogenesis of otologic conditions such as otitis media, presbycusis,

and noise-induced hearing loss. Due to the small body of literature regarding nutraceutical supplementation in otologic patients, the first part of the chapter will focus on the role of GSH in human immunodeficiency virus (HIV)/acquired immunodeficiency syndrome (AIDS). GSH modulation in HIV/AIDS has been investigated extensively, and presentation of the pathogenesis of this condition allows for a nuanced discussion of oxidative stress and the application of GSH as an antioxidant in the immune system.

Maintenance of the neuronal networks connecting the vestibulocochlear apparatus to the brain is essential for hearing. A brief discussion of neurodegenerative disorders outlines GSH modulation in nerves, which is of potential value to the otologist, as GSH modulation might show benefit in sensorineural hearing loss. A brief discussion of GSH and its role in aging are included since presbycusis is a manifestation of aging.

DOI: 10.1201/b23379-26

Nutraceutical materials are discussed briefly to give readers a sense of their evidenced-based use in medicine. The chapter concludes with an in-depth discussion of the state of nutraceutical use in otologic patients. This discussion serves to support the adjunctive use of nutraceuticals in this population and to highlight the limits of the current body of literature regarding nutraceuticals in otologic patients.

## GLUTATHIONE: AN INTRACELLULAR ANTIOXIDANT

## GLUTATHIONE

Numerous seemingly unrelated diseases such as HIV/AIDS, amyotrophic lateral sclerosis (ALS), cataract pathogenesis, Alzheimer's disease, rheumatoid arthritis, and autoimmune thyroiditis are unified by the unique properties of GSH as an antioxidant.[1] GSH is a tripeptide of L-glutamate, glycine, and L-cysteine, a sulfur-containing amino acid that is the rate-limiting substrate in GSH synthesis. GSH is a powerful antioxidant because of its ability to donate protons and reduce disulfide bonds, which can occur spontaneously with GSH alone or with GSH-dependent enzymes. Cysteine alone also can donate protons and reduce disulfide bonds, which makes it another antioxidant of interest. Essential functions of the immune system (such as antigen presentation), reversal of cataract formation, and repair of denatured enzymes are dependent on the availability of GSH to reduce disulfide bonds.

## GLUTATHIONE ENZYMES

GSH is synthesized in a two-step enzymatic reaction that requires adenosine triphosphate (ATP). The rate-limiting step is catalyzed by the first enzyme in the reaction, γ-glutamate cysteine ligase (γ-GCL), which joins glutamate and cysteine to form γ-glutamylcysteine. The second step of the reaction is catalyzed by GSH synthetase which attaches glycine to γ-glutamylcysteine to form γ-L-Glutamyl-L-cysteine. GSH exerts a feedback inhibition on γ-GCL that safeguards against the overproduction of intracellular GSH.

Excess GSH also stimulates γ-glutamyl transpeptidase (GTT), the enzyme that modulates the first step in GSH breakdown back into its component amino acids. The highest density of GTT is found on the outside of cells that have a secretory or absorptive function.[2] The extracellular location of GTT prevents intracellular GSH breakdown; however, the breakdown of GSH by GTT allows for the redistribution of its component amino acids, particularly cysteine, to cells that are deficient in cysteine or GSH.[2] In this way, GSH functions as the "storage" molecule for cysteine and as such the GSH level is a good measure of the efficiency of cysteine absorption and availability. However, GSH has functions beyond the storage of cysteine.

GSH functions as an important intracellular antioxidant, particularly in the mitochondria in which it reduces reactive oxygen species (ROS) produced during cellular metabolism.[3] GSH-Px is an enzyme that functions to defend cells against ROS as it reduces hydrogen peroxide and lipid peroxide (LPO). The glutathione-S-transferase (GST) family of enzymes works in tandem with the P450 cytochrome system of the liver to detoxify many organic toxins. GSH is a potent antioxidant because of its ability to donate free electrons to reduced oxidizing molecules in the cell. Once oxidized, reduced GSH is regenerated by glutathione reductase (GSSG).

Beyond ROS management, GSH reduces and returns ascorbate (vitamin C) and α-tocopherol (vitamin E) back to their bioactive reduced forms.[4] GSH participates in a number of other well-documented metabolic reactions, including DNA synthesis and repair, protein synthesis, prostaglandin synthesis, amino acid transport, metabolism of toxins and carcinogens, enzyme activation, and enhancement of immune system function.[5]

## GLUTATHIONE AND THE IMMUNE SYSTEM

## GLUTATHIONE AND ANTIGEN PRESENTATION

Macrophages and dendritic cells are antigen-presenting cells (APCs) that function as the first responders of the innate immune response, processing antigens for presentation to cells of the cellular and adaptive immune systems. GSH levels in APCs determine how antigens are processed and which cytokines (signaling molecules) are produced. Cytokine production can direct the immune system to generate a cellular immune response (adequate GSH associated, T helper type-1 [Th1] cytokine response; deficient GSH associated, T helper type-2 [Th2] cytokine response) or a humoral immune response.[6]

When APCs encounter an antigen, GSH is used to split the antigenic protein–protein disulfide bonds to form protein–GSH disulfide bonds. The formation of protein GSH disulfide bonds are required for antigenic protein unfolding, and GSH depletion impedes the APC's ability to process antigens into protein fragments in antigens with disulfide bonds.[7]

GSH has roles in both the cellular and adaptive immune systems and is necessary for the generation of a cellular immune response and humoral immune system regulation. Adequate GSH levels lead to effective antigen unfolding followed by the release of Th1-specific cytokines that mediate lymphocyte activation and enhance the cellular immune response. It has been shown that intracellular redox status influences Th type-17 (Th17) and T-regulatory (T reg) cell differentiation with increased T reg cell differentiation in prooxidant environments.[8] Repletion of cells with N-acetyl cysteine (NAC) has restored Th17 cell generation in cell lines affected by ROS damaged.[9,10] GSH also has been shown to regulate B cell confinement in germinal centers which is necessary for maintenance of the normal organization of the adaptive immune system in secondary lymphoid organs.[11]

## ADEQUATE GLUTATHIONE LEVEL FAVORS LYMPHOCYTE-MEDIATED CELLULAR IMMUNITY

In cell culture, cellular vs. humoral immune determination occurs in the first few hours of APC/antigen interaction.[7] The immune response generated is specialized and optimized to eradicate the type of infection against which it is activated. Effector T helper (Th) cell (CD4+) differentiation is coordinated by the complex interaction between the cytokine milieu, costimulatory molecules, and the antigen presented by macrophages or dendritic cells. CD4+ T cells differentiate into three main types, Th1, Th2, and Th17. A Th1 response is generated in response to infections with bacteria, fungi, protozoa, and viruses[12,13] and is involved in activating macrophages and inducing inflammation. A Th2 response is generated in response to helminth and parasite infections and environmental allergens and is involved in antibody production and allergic responses.[12] Th17 cells are generated in response to extracellular pathogens such as invasive candida and are involved in neutrophil activation and tissue inflammation.[14] While not included as a T-cell subset involved in inflammation and thus not extensively discussed here, T regs are a distinct population of T cells that are identified by FoxP3 positivity and modulate immune responses.[15] The immune system generally functions optimally when the cellular immune response is activated, especially as it can eradicate a wider range of pathogens and assist in activation of the humoral immune system. GSH is required to maintain this cellular immune response. In addition, mitochondrial ROS alter T-cell metabolism after activation by an antigen to promote T-cell proliferation during the effector phase of an immune response, serving as an indirect link between GSH and T-cell function.[16]

## LYMPHOCYTES AND MACROPHAGES DIFFER IN THEIR PREFERENCE FOR CYSTEINE OR CYSTINE

Lymphocytes are known to preferentially absorb cysteine.[17] Macrophages regulate intracellular GSH levels of lymphocytes by preferentially consuming cystine, two cysteine molecules connected by a disulfide bond, for intracellular GSH synthesis, and then releasing cysteine at a variable and regulated rate for lymphocyte absorption.[17] This has a significant effect on lymphocyte proliferation.[18]

Therefore, macrophages regulate the immunological response by making cysteine available to lymphocytes on an "as-needed" basis. For this reason, cystine supplementation feeds all of the cells of the immune system starting with the macrophages and then, through controlled release, to lymphocytes.

On the other hand, cysteine supplementation is not as effective for macrophage GSH production.

Because macrophage GSH is the optimal source of the cysteine secreted by macrophages to lymphocytes, providing cysteine instead of cystine reduces the ability of the macrophage to deliver cysteine to the lymphocytes optimally.

## LYMPHOCYTE PROLIFERATION AND CYTOKINE SELECTION

Hamilos also reports that GSH levels play a major role, "Lymphocyte proliferation in response to mitogenic lectins is directly dependent upon glutathione availability. Thus, proliferation can be enhanced by providing lymphocytes with excess GSH, and strongly inhibited by limiting the quantity of intracellular GSH available during the mitogenic stimulation."[18] Lymphocyte proliferation has been the standard method used to document a material to be immune-enhancing.

Cytokines are the cell-signaling molecules that direct the immune differentiation of lymphocytes during the effector phase of an immune response. The production of interleukin-2 (IL-2), IL-12, and interferon-gamma (IFN-γ) promotes the differentiation of T cells into Th1 cells, which in turn secrete IL-2 and IFN- γ. Thus, IL-2 and IFN-γ are referred to as Th1 cytokines. The availability of IL-4 stimulates the differentiation of Th2 cells, which in turn secrete IL-4, IL5, IL-10, and IL-13. IL-4 and IL13 stimulate antibody production, especially class-switching to IgE production, aiding in helminth eradication, and causing allergic responses. Thus, a "Th2 response" is often characterized by IL-4 and IL-10 production and up-regulation of various antibody responses.[6]

Many disease states have been associated with GSH deficiency[4-7,19-29], but none is more clearly related to immune deficiency and low GSH than HIV/AIDS. Peterson concludes, "GSH depletion in APC populations may play a key role in exacerbating HIV and other infectious diseases in which Th2 predominance is an important aspect of the disease pathology."[6]

Immune deficiency in AIDS is strongly associated with GSH deficiency. Increasing the intracellular GSH level would be expected to enhance the cellular response of the immune system and have a favorable impact on immune deficiency states, such as the progression of HIV infection to AIDS. Survival rates in AIDS give insight into the effect of GSH on the progression of HIV to AIDS and the important impact of GSH on survival. Lymphocyte proliferation and cytokine profiles are two immune responses that are potentially modulated by GSH and, thus, may explain the association between immune deficiency and GSH deficiency and will be further explored further in this chapter.

The fundamental biochemical properties of GSH disulfide bond reduction and proton donation underlie the clinically proven benefit of cystine supplementation that provides a reliable, safe, and predictable source of GSH for individuals with HIV[30] and probably extend to patients with neurodegenerative diseases.[31]

## GLUTATHIONE AND HIV/AIDS PATHOGENESIS

## GLUTATHIONE DEFICIENCY IN HIV/AIDS AND SURVIVAL

GSH deficiency is recognized to influence four important components of the immune response, namely antigen processing[6], lymphocyte proliferation[18], cytokine selection[6,20], and lymphocyte apoptosis (programmed cell death).[32] Clinical observations support the concept that GSH deficiency may play a role in HIV/AIDS, which is the prototypic immune deficiency state, and other autoimmune diseases. When GSH levels are maintained or augmented, improvements in HIV/AIDS clinical outcomes have been documented.[32]

Rodriguez found HIV-infected children to be deficient in GSH, compared with healthy controls.[22] Furthermore, it was found that increasing CD4+ T-cell counts were associated with higher average GSH concentration and that viral load was inversely related to GSH concentration; however, no association was found between clinical disease progression and average GSH concentrations.[22] In other words, the observations by Rodriguez showed that low GSH concentrations are associated with low CD4+T-cell counts and higher viral loads.

Herzenberg has reported that the GSH level in white blood cells was a *determinant factor* in the survival of AIDS patients.[21] A $p < 0.0001$ level of statistical significance was documented using Kaplan–Meier and logistic regression analyses to evaluate survival data from all HIV+ patients as well as from those with a CD4+ T-cell count <200/μL.

The 3-year survival rates in this study were as follows:

Survival in all HIV+: GSB > 0.91 = 90%
Survival in all HIV+: GSB < 0.91 = 32%
When CD4+ < 200/μL: GSB > 1.05 = 87%
When CD4+ < 200/μL: GSB < 1.05 = 17%
(GSB = GSH-S-bimane, a fluorescent form of GSH)

Immune deficiency is associated with GSH deficiency, and as such increasing the intracellular GSH level is likely to enhance the cellular response capacity of the immune system. The role of GSH in HIV/AIDS disease progression is still under investigation, and Levin suggested that GSH helps to prevent accelerated aging noted by decreased muscle strength and exercise capacity and increased muscle breakdown and fat accumulation in HIV patients.[33] The randomized controlled trial found that supplementation with NAC plus glycine reversed several markers for accelerated aging in HIV patients.[33] Although the exact mechanism of the effect of GSH on cellular metabolism and the immune systems is still under investigation, it is evident that it helps to modulate disease progression.

## PATHOGENESIS OF IMMUNE DEFICIENCY IN HIV/AIDS: CYTOKINE SHIFT

Historically, HIV/AIDS pathogenesis has been described by a shift in cytokine predominance within the Th1 vs. Th2 paradigm. Clerici described a shift in cytokines within this dichotomy and noted that in HIV-seropositive patients with delayed or absent disease progression, a type 1 cytokine milieu predominated over type 2 cytokine production.[20] A type 2 cytokine predominance was noted in patients with progressive disease, and a shift between type 1 and type 2 cytokines may indicate the rate of decline of CD4+ T cells, time to AIDS diagnosis, and time to death.[20] Other studies have further supported the predominance of pro-inflammatory cytokines and cytokine imbalance in HIV disease progression, suggesting cytokine shift/imbalance as a potential mechanism of immune deregulation, especially by affecting T-cell survival and function, during HIV pathogenesis.[34,35]

Since the establishment of the Th1 vs. Th2 paradigm, the role of Th17 cells and T reg cells has been established in HIV/AIDS pathogenesis. It has been noted that HIV infection is associated with increased IL-17 production, a proinflammatory cytokine, in Th17 cells.[36] Jiao et al. reported that T reg cell populations were decreased in patients with disease progression.[37] T reg cells were found to be maintained at high levels in the peripheral blood mononuclear cells (PBMCs) of patients with HIV type-1 who maintain normal CD4+ T-cell counts and are not treated with any form of antiretroviral therapy.[38] These results indicated that HIV progression results from a complex change in T-cell populations and the cytokine environment. Further research is needed to understand the interplay between these components and to determine how GSH status affects the relationships between all of these elements.

## PATHOGENESIS OF IMMUNE DEFICIENCY IN HIV/AIDS: APOPTOSIS

According to Clerici, shifts in cytokines lead to CD4+ T-cell loss.[20] Antigen stimulation (viral exposure) of lymphocytes of HIV-seropositive individuals in the presence of abnormally low concentrations of type 1 cytokines (IL-2, IL-12, and IFN-γ) and/or of abnormally elevated concentrations of type 2 cytokines (IL-4 and IL-10) can result in the induction of antigen-induced cell death (AICD)[20] or more recently termed as activation-induced cell death.

In a review, Cummins and Badley suggest that there are four main mechanisms for cell death in HIV infection: decreased production, increased destruction via direct cytotoxicity of virally infected cells, apoptosis of effected cells or bystander cells (nearby cells uninfected with HIV), and immune cell redistribution.[39] Apoptosis is one of these mechanisms and is not inherently pathologic. Conceptually, programmed cell death represents the reciprocal of monoclonal expansion. As such, it is an integral part of the contraction mechanism of the immune system. However, T cells that have been repeatedly stimulated with a specific antigen (such as HIV) undergo apoptosis more rapidly than normal, which is why this process is also known as AICD.[24] In AIDS, with sustained stimulation of T cells, AICD may account for much of the CD4+ T-cell loss. Fas and Fas-ligand (FasL) engagement is a mechanism of AICD of CD4+ T cells during HIV progression, and elevated levels of Fas and FasL are observed in people living with HIV infection and correlated with disease progression.[40,41] In addition, it has been shown that programed death 1 (PD1) receptor is expressed at the highest level on the surface of exhausted T cells in HIV and that engagement of PD1 with its ligand leads to a dysregulated state in T cells.[40] Day et al. also found that up-regulation of the PD 1 receptor correlates positively with viral load and inversely correlates with CD4+ T-cell count.[42]

As HIV infection is associated with persistent or recurrent viral replication throughout the course of the disease, the accelerated apoptosis of T cells observed in HIV reflects the intensification of normal AICD occurring in response to the HIV-1 virus as the persistent and recurrent stimulus.[23] Apoptotic susceptibility is affected by the number of antigenic exposures; the more the exposures, the more rapidly apoptosis is initiated. Started with the engagement of either Fas-FasL or PD1-PD1L on the cell surface, the intracellular reactions that initiate apoptosis are modulated by cell-signaling molecules such as GSH and B-cell lymphoma factor 2 (Bcl-2).

## APOPTOSIS, GLUTATHIONE, AND Bcl-2

Bcl-2 is an oncoprotein that is expressed during times of cellular stress, such as infection, inflammation, and disease. It is one of a large group of cell-signaling proteins that are referred to as heat shock proteins. The Bcl-2 family of proteins regulates T cell's susceptibility to apoptosis.[23]

Under normal circumstances, over-expression of Bcl-2 has been shown to inhibit some of the common initiators of apoptosis in HIV/AIDS and other inflammatory states including anti-Fas and tumor necrosis factor-alpha (TNF-α)-mediated apoptosis.[25] One of the determinant factors in this response is the intracellular level of GSH.

Depletion of GSH caused cells to over-express Bcl-2 and to become sensitized to and succumb to apoptotic induction.[32] On the other hand, in cells with adequate levels of GSH, Bcl-2 over-expression led to relocalization of GSH into the nucleus, thereby altering nuclear redox status and blocking caspase activity, as well as other nuclear initiators of apoptosis.

GSH depletion also is linked to disruption of the mitochondrial transmembrane potential ($\Delta\Psi m$), considered an early step in apoptosis.[26] The mitochondrial transmembrane potential disruption is followed by hyper-production of ROS with disruption of $Ca^{2+}$ homeostasis.

When there is a sufficient quantity of GSH, Bcl-2 maintains the $\Delta\Psi m$ by enhancing proton efflux from mitochondria, even in the presence of $\Delta\Psi m$-loss-inducing stimuli such as $Ca^{2+}$, $H_2O_2$, and *tert*-butyl hydroperoxide.[27] The proton donor function of GSH appears to provide the necessary proton for the proton efflux regulating effect of Bcl-2. The action of Bcl-2 prevents apoptotic mitochondrial dysfunction when GSH levels are adequate. This would explain the pivotal role GSH plays in Bcl-2 anti-apoptosis.

## MECHANISM OF CD4+ CELL INVASION IN HIV/AIDS: CELL SURFACE ANTIGEN EXPRESSION

Sprietsma has reported that as AIDS progresses, the immune response moves to a Th2-dominant state.[28] Research has shown that HIV multiplies almost exclusively in Th2 cells and rarely, if ever, in Th1 cells.[29,43] The Th2 cytokine, IL-4, promotes the production of the cell surface antigen CXCR4 which allows the more virulent strains of HIV to infect CD4+ T cells.[44] BLTR is a high-affinity receptor for leukotriene B4 and, like CXCR4, is another CD4+ T-cell surface co-receptor that preferentially admits the more aggressive HIV-1 virus into the cells.[45]

Sufficient intake of essential nutrients[28] (cysteine, methionine, arginine, vitamins A, B, C, and E, zinc, and selenium) maintains the Th1 influence on the immune system, thereby inhibiting the proliferation of viruses such as HIV: This is accomplished by inactivating the HIV protease and downregulating the number of BLTR receptors.

Amino acids such as cysteine, methionine, and arginine are among the most commonly deficient essential nutrients in typical diets. Consequently, supplementation with a source of these amino acids, especially cysteine, is necessary to produce the regulator molecules: GSH, metallothionein, and nitric oxide. Adequate quantities of these three regulatory molecules promote the production of Th1 cytokines and reduce the expression of the cell surface antigens associated with HIV-1 entrance into CD4+ T cells and progression of HIV to AIDS.

Sprietsma further points out that immune activities under Th1 control can offer protection against a broad range of other clinical conditions such as viral infections and autoimmune diseases (diabetes, rheumatoid arthritis, Crohn's disease, and others). Thus, HIV/AIDS is only one of many medical conditions affected by cytokine selection.[28]

Therefore, it should be no surprise that HIV/AIDS is not the only clinical condition favorably affected by cysteine supplementation.[30] Published reports of (1) a case report of pulmonary function improvement in COPD,[46] (2) a study in hepatitis B,[47] (3) a compilation of case reports in urogenital cancer patients,[48] (4) a study of systemic lupus erythematosus,[49] and (5) and a randomized controlled clinical trial in patient with COVID-19 infection[50] expand the knowledge base found in the peer-reviewed medical literature regarding the impact of cysteine supplementation.

The common denominators in these reports appear to be the promise of essential nutrients and the cell-signaling molecules that these nutrients are synthesized into, especially cysteine and GSH. Consistent with this view are other reports in the GSH research literature strongly suggesting that many medical conditions are affected, and even controlled, by the GSH level and redox status of cells. This links the actions of GSH to the common underlying mechanism of oxidative stress. Oxidative stress has been implicated in a number of diseases, but the research literature is particularly convincing in its association with neurodegenerative diseases, especially Parkinson's disease.

## A SUMMARY OF THE EFFECTS OF GLUTATHIONE AND CYSTEINE

The Th1 vs. Th2 axis used to describe the immunologic role of T cells in the pathogenesis of HIV/AIDS serves as a foundation to describe the role that GSH and cellular redox status play in this condition. However, since publication of the previous edition of this chapter in Sataloff, R.T. and Sataloff, J., *Hearing Loss, 4th Edition*,[51] the immunology community has made exciting advances in understanding the role of Th17 cells and T reg cells. The role of Th17 cells and T reg cells in HIV/AIDS has been established, and advances have been made that improve understanding of apoptosis in HIV/AIDs through the PD1 receptor. The full body of literature that encompasses the current understanding of HIV/AIDS pathogenesis is well beyond the scope of this chapter; however, a discussion was included to show how GSH and cysteine modulation affects disease pathogenesis in the prototypic immune deficiency state.

From the discussion above, readers should note that GSH is an essential antioxidant and plays a pivotal role in offsetting both physiologic and pathologic oxidative stress. GSH maintenance and/or augmentation regulates many basic immune functions such as optimization of antigen processing, maximization of lymphocyte proliferation and antibody synthesis, maintenance of Th1 cytokine production (IFN-γ, IL-2, and IL-12), and reduction of lymphocyte loss due to disease-initiated apoptosis. GSH is a requirement in a wide array of metabolic reactions that are pivotal to many cellular functions that are summarized in **Table 26.1**. These functions are likely to have a significant impact on a number of disease states and health-related conditions.

Table 26.1  Functions of GSH

- Functions as the central reservoir for cysteine
- Protects against disease-initiated apoptosis
- Optimizes immune function
- Maximizes interferon-γ
- Up-regulates IL-2
- Assists DNA synthesis
- Renews enzyme activation
- Contributes to protein synthesis
- Supports amino acid transport
- Prevents oxidative cell damage (antioxidation)
- Metabolizes toxins and carcinogens (detoxification)

This discussion paired with the next topic presented (GSH modulation in neurodegenerative diseases) serves as a foundation for a broader discussion regarding nutraceutical use in otology because otologic conditions can have components of both immune system dysregulation and neurodegeneration in their pathogenesis.

## NEURODEGENERATIVE DISORDERS AND GLUTATHIONE

## NEURODEGENERATIVE DISORDERS: GLUTATHIONE PREVENTION OF NEURONAL DEATH

During periods of oxidative stress, GSH is an important protector of mitochondrial function.[52] Dopaminergic neurons are very sensitive to changes in the internal oxidant buffering capacity of the cell, and reductions in GSH levels can lead to disruption of calcium homeostasis and cell death.[53] Therefore, GSH protects human neural cells from dopamine-induced apoptosis.[54] Notably, dopamine treatment during GSH depletion is documented to produce defects in psychomotor behavior in a laboratory animal model.[55]

Oxidative stress has been implicated in various neurodegenerative disorders and may be a common mechanism underlying various forms of cell death including excitotoxicity, apoptosis, and necrosis. Bains and Shaw hypothesized that diminished GSH plays a role in ALS, Parkinson's disease, and Alzheimer's disease.[31] GSH modulation may prove to be beneficial in spinal cord injury,[56] multiple sclerosis,[57] and stroke.[58,59] As cysteine supplementation increases GSH, it may hold promise as a method to modulate neurodegenerative diseases.

## GLUTATHIONE, DOPAMINE, AND GLUTAMATE: ROLES IN PARKINSON'S DISEASE

GSH is utilized by the granular storage system of dopamine in PC12 pheochromocytoma cells, and it is likely that GSH protects susceptible parts of the granular transport system against (possibly dopamine-induced) oxidative damage.[60] In PC12 and C6 glial cell lines, glutamate toxicity causes oxidative stress and GSH depletion by reducing cystine uptake which results in apoptotic cell death.[61,62] These mechanisms are implicated in the pathogenesis of Parkinson's disease.

The suggested pathogenesis of Parkinson's disease suggests a key role for GSH in glutamate excitotoxicity. Strategies designed to maintain GSH levels protect against glutamate toxicity and prevent dopamine-induced cell death—this results in enhanced neuronal survival.[63,64]

Astrocytes play a vital neuroprotective role that includes expression of antioxidant enzymes, synthesis of GSH, recycling of vitamin C, as well as transport and metabolism of glucose that yields reducing equivalents for antioxidant regeneration and lactate for neuronal metabolism.[65] Many of these functions require GSH or cystine. Astrocytes, like macrophages, prefer cystine and glutamate for GSH synthesis,[6,66,67] whereas cysteine and glutamine are preferred by neurons. These differential preferences allow astrocytes to regulate neuronal GSH.[68] It has been shown that astrocyte mediation of enhanced neuronal survival is abolished by GSH deficiency.[68] Wei et. al found that astrocyte dopamine receptor, DRD2, induces GSH synthesis and that decreased dopamine release causes GSH depletion and oxidative stress in astrocytes leading to disease progression in Parkinson's disease.[69]

## GLUTATHIONE-MEDIATED REVERSAL OF AGE-RELATED EVENTS: EVIDENCE FOR BIOCHEMICAL REJUVENATION

Senescent changes lead to either reduced response capacity, such as reduced immunological response, or to progressive degeneration, as exemplified by cataract formation. The age-dependent decline in the ability of T cells to mount a proliferative response is due to an age-related defect in signal transduction.[70] Proliferation of aged T cells, which is typically 10%–30% of the level of young controls, was enhanced almost 10-fold by increasing GSH and reached levels of young controls.[70]

GSH-dependent reversal of cataract has been reported[71] and results in improved transparency of the lens. A two-step GSH reduction of disulfide bonds occurs. First, GSH nonenzymatically forms protein–GSH disulfide bonds from lens protein–protein disulfide bonds; then the GSH-dependent enzyme thioltransferase (TTase) reduces the protein–GSH disulfide bond to a protein sulfhydryl bond that unfolds the crystalline protein of the lens,[72] as TTase is found in the human lens.[73] Reversing age-related GSH loss in the lens through GSH enhancement holds great promise for cataract patients.[74] TTase also has been shown to reactivate metabolically important enzymes that have been oxidized such as pyruvate kinase, phosphofructokinase, and GST.[72] This may hold promise for patients with diabetes.

Research on life extension has identified endogenous free radical reactions as a major cause of aging and "possibly the only one."[75] The higher intracellular GSH levels found in food-restricted experimental animals has been exposed as the explanation of the life-prolonging effect of food restriction treatment.[76] As GSH is the major endogenous antioxidant, its preservation and enhancement is central to anti-aging and rejuvenating strategies.

## NUTRACEUTICALS AND CLINICAL OUTCOMES

### INCREASING INTRACELLULAR GLUTATHIONE WITH CYSTEINE AND CYSTEINE PRO-DRUGS

A number of strategies have been tried to increase GSH. Most approaches use pharmacological doses of GSH or a form of the rate-limiting substrate, cysteine. Administering GSH by oral, intravenous, intratracheal, and intraperitoneal routes has been tried with no sustained increase in tissue GSH.[77,78] GSH is digested if taken orally, has a short half-life if delivered intravenously, and does not significantly increase liver or lymphocyte GSH if given intratracheally or intraperitoneally. Esterified GSH compounds have increased GSH in a few tissues[79] but have limited value in clinical applications due to harmful and potentially toxic metabolic products.[80]

Providing cysteine or methionine directly is associated with substantial toxicity.[81] Cysteine is metabolized readily,[78] and methionine can be converted to cysteine in the liver, but this requires energy. Also, the conversion process could increase an intermediate metabolite, homocysteine. If it is not fully metabolized, increased levels of homocysteine lead to homocystinuria, and elevated homocysteine appears to be associated with atherosclerotic vascular disease.

NAC has been used for treatment of AIDS to increase GSH.[6,19,82–87] However, NAC has only 10% bioavailability when given orally and is associated with substantial side effects (rashes and severe gastro-intestinal upset) at therapeutic doses of ≥ 4 g/day.[21] Anaphylactic reactions have been reported.[88]

Even at more moderate pharmacological doses, cysteine pro-drugs, such as NAC, are associated with mobilization of heavy metals across the placenta[89–91] and blood–brain barrier,[92–96] as well as into liver, kidney,[86] and astrocytes.[97] Though this may prove useful for some interventional applications, it also may limit its usefulness as a daily source of cysteine for GSH enhancement. Various forms of cysteine, including NAC, cause excitotoxin release in certain areas of the brain such as the hippocampus, a primary location of neurodegeneration in Alzheimer's disease. Excitotoxin release has been documented with various forms of cysteine; however, excitotoxin release does not occur with cystine

supplementation.[98] This may limit the application of cysteine in neurodegenerative conditions because excitotoxin release is thought to be implicated in the pathogenesis of these conditions.[99]

### CYSTINE IS THE OPTIMAL FORM OF CYSTEINE FOR INTRACELLULAR GLUTATHIONE SYNTHESIS

Cystine has been shown to be the cysteine precursor of choice in macrophages[16] and astroglial cells.[66,67] Macrophages and astroglial cells then provide cysteine to lymphocytes and neurons in a highly regulated fashion. The increase in the GSH levels in astrocytes is substantially greater with cystine than with any other cysteine source.[66] Therefore, cystine represents the optimal form of cysteine for GSH production in the antigen-presenting macrophage and the neuron-protecting astroglial cell.

One way to avoid the drawbacks of using pharmacological doses of cysteine pro-drugs is to use an *undenatured* source of complete amino acids that contain a high concentration of cystine, such as Immunocal® (Immunotec Research Ltd., Montreal, Quebec, Canada). Immunocal® administration effectively enhances GSH production,[100] and the GSH produced by this method benefits patients suffering from AIDS with wasting syndrome.[30] The bioactivity and effectiveness of Immunocal® appear to depend on the *undenatured* amino acids in protein derived whey. The undenatured amino acids preserve the disulfide bond in cystine which allows a high concentration of cystine to be made available to the liver. This is not a property found in commercial whey proteins.

A full discussion of this topic is beyond the scope of this chapter. Interested readers can find a more comprehensive discussion in a text edited by Montagnier, Olivier, and Pasquier.[101]

### IMMUNONUTRIENTS AND CLINICAL OUTCOMES

Supplementation with immune-enhancing formulas has been found to improve immune response and efficiency in a number of clinical studies.[102] Immune efficiency has a profound effect on resistance to infection, need for antibiotic therapy, and length of stay in the hospital. IMPACT (Novartis Nutrition, Bern, Switzerland) and Immun-Aid (McGaw, Irvine, CA)

Table 26.2 Summary of meta-analysis outcomes of immunonutrient enteral feeds

| Outcomes | Patient group | Treatment number | Control number | Treatment effect (95% CI) | p-value |
|---|---|---|---|---|---|
| Infection rate | All | 437 | 425 | 0.60 (0.42, 0.86) | 0.005 |
| | Surg. | 224 | 223 | 0.48 (0.28, 0.83) | 0.01 |
| Length of stay (days) | All | 631 | 642 | −2.9 (−4.4, −1.4) | 0.0002 |
| | Surg. | 273 | 280 | −2.3 (−4.0, −0.6) | 0.007 |
| | Med. | 133 | 125 | −9.7 (−17.1, −2.3) | 0.01 |
| Ventilator days | All | 357 | 369 | −2.6 (−5.1, −0.6) | 0.04 |
| | Tr. | 95 | 101 | −4.0, (−7.5, −0.6) | 0.02 |

*Abbreviations:* CI, Confidence interval; Surg., Surgical; Med., Medical; Tr., Trauma.

are two immune-enhancing nutrients that have been fully documented to be safe and effective in many peer-reviewed medical journals, as well as a large (1482 patients), well-controlled, meta-analysis (**Table 26.2**).[102] Of note, Immunocal® has been shown to have a significant effect on clinical conditions associated with serious disease states—pulmonary functions in COPD,[47] wasting syndrome in HIV/AIDS,[30] and liver function in hepatitis B.[48]

One study using Immun-Aid in patients with severe abdominal trauma has documented the dramatic benefit of immune-enhancing nutrients on a number of clinical outcomes in seriously ill patients in the ICU setting.[103] This study compares patients fed either an immune-enhancing (Immun-Aid) or an isonitrogenous, isocaloric diet with a control of no diet.

As demonstrated by this study (**Table 26.3**), antibiotic usage is not the only outcome statistic affected. Significant reduction in length of treatment is noted in this study, as well. All of the findings were found to be statistically significant except hospital charges. This is only one of the 12 studies complied in a 1482 patient meta-analysis.[102]

In a meta-analysis, IMPACT (10 studies) or Immun-Aid (two studies) were given to critically ill patients.[102] Dramatically improved outcome statistics were documented including a 40% decreased rate of infection ($p = 0.005$) and reduced hospital stay of 2.3 days ($p = 0.007$) in surgical patients and 2.9 days ($p = 0.0002$) in all patients; however, no statistically significant reduction in ICU length of stay was found.

Table 26.3 How an immune-enhancing diet affects outcome parameters in severe abdominal trauma

| Antibiotic use and hospital stay | IED (16) | ISO (17) | Significant value | Control (19) |
|---|---|---|---|---|
| Antibiotic use (days ± SEM) Prophylactic | 3.8 ± 0.9 | 2.7 ± 0.5 | NS | 4.2 ± 0.7 |
| Empiric | 1.4 ± 0.8 | 2.6 ± 1.1 | NS | 0.7 ± 0.5 |
| Therapeutic | 2.8 ± 1.6 | 7.1 ± 1.7 | $p = 0.02$ | 17.4 ± 4.6 |
| Hospital stay (days ± SEM) Total | 18.3 ± 2.8 | 32.6 ± 6.6 | $p = 0.03$ | 34.9 ± 6.0 |
| In ICU | 5.8 ± 1.8 | 9.5 ± 2.3 | $p = 0.10$ | 15.7 ± 4.9 |
| On ventilator | 2.4 ± 1.3 | 5.4 ± 2.0 | $p = 0.09$ | 9.0 ± 4.2 |
| Hospital charges | $80,515 ± 21,528 | $110,599 ± 19,132 | NS | $141,049 ± 34,396 |

*Source:* Adapted from Kudsk et al.[103]

*Abbreviations:* ICU, Intensive care unit; IED, Immune-enhancing diet; ISO, Isonitrogenous, isocaloric diet; NS, Not significant; SEM, Standard error of the mean.

## ADVANTAGES AND LIMITATIONS OF NUTRACEUTICALS

An early example of nutraceutical modulation is the use of Vitamin C in scurvy. Nutraceutical treatment in the context of scurvy has been accepted widely. However, the benefit of nutraceutical modulation in prostate cancer was a historically surprising application that allowed for a deeper understanding of the pathogenesis of prostate cancer. Antioxidants that are either rejuvenated by GSH or are integral to GSH-dependent enzymes appear to play a role in mitigating against carcinogenesis in the prostate.[104] The generation of a prooxidant environment also has been associated with the promotion of prostate cancer.[105] Interestingly, a study showed that physiological levels of androgens decrease GSH content in human prostate cells,[105] which suggests that GSH reduction is consistent with the prooxidant mechanism for prostate cancer.

The advantage of nutraceutical applications in the disease states discussed above is that the body has a well-developed and wide array of enzymes to metabolize them. In the case of the GSH system, these enzymes synthesize, breakdown, mobilize, and revitalize GSH and its precursor amino acids. Since the body has a system to regulate GSH's use and metabolism, the possibility of adverse effects and overdose from GSH administration is reduced drastically. These features are particularly important because increasing the concentration of GSH precursors is central to increasing the synthesis of GSH itself.

Quantifying and standardizing bioactivity is one of the most challenging aspects in the clinical application of nutraceuticals. These products are frequently promoted as, "good for you," but there is little information on how much of a nutraceutical is needed to produce a proven effect. This has given rise to the "more is better" theory, which has inspired a number of food fads that have damaged the credibility of nutraceutical and functional foods use in the medical community.

Vitamin C is a good example of the discourse surrounding the optimal dose of a nutraceutical in clinical practice. High-dose vitamin C was ardently promoted by Dr. Linus Pauling, an early proponent of nutraceutical therapies, while other physicians were concerned about Vitamin C overdose. Over the years, this debate has waned to obscurity due to the lack of reported side effects. The concern of overdose with many nutraceuticals is negligible; however, physicians should consult the specific nutrient in question because some do cause toxicity with high doses and prolonged use (i.e. vitamin A).

Although nutraceuticals are generally safe, effective for promoting health, and benefit a variety of conditions, manufacturers and distributors of nutraceuticals are prohibited from claiming to diagnose, treat, cure, or prevent any disease. This stipulation, enforced by the FDA, has made it difficult to report outcomes of research in plain language, thereby limiting clinicians' and patients' awareness and understanding of the potential benefits these products.

Another limiting factor to wider recognition and broader application of nutraceuticals in health care is the pharmacologic model for developing drugs with a specific action and target. Emphasis on this model has precluded consideration and focus on development of broad-spectrum, universal agents that mediate a wide array of cellular functions to improve health status and fight disease. Despite these limitations, nutraceutical application with immune-enhancing formulations such as Immunocal® (Immunotec Research Ltd., Montreal, Quebec, Canada), Immun-Aid (McGaw, Irvine, CA), and IMPACT (Novartis Nutrition, Bern, Switzerland) have shown benefit in several disease states. It is hoped that continued exploration of nutraceuticals via randomized controlled trials will clarify the benefit of adjunctive treatment with these nutrients and that evidenced-based guidelines will be developed to help guide physicians in their use.

## NUTRACEUTICAL SUPPLEMENTATION IN OTOLOGY

### INTRODUCTION

There is a limited body of research investigating the use of nutraceuticals in otologic patients. A systematic review in 2016 synthesized the literature on GSH levels and oxidative stress in otolaryngologic patients, specifically addressing the following otologic conditions: otitis media with effusion, chronic otitis media (COM), COM and cholesteatoma, tympanic membrane sclerosis, and

Ménière's disease.[106] Although the chapter initially outlines the benefit of GSH in the immunomodulation of HIV/AIDs, a wider discussion of the current literature of nutraceuticals in otologic patients is included below. The benefit of antioxidant use, alone or in conjunction with the current gold standard of medical treatment, has been investigated most extensively in otitis media and presbycusis; so, the nutraceutical research surrounding these two disease states will be highlighted.

## OTITIS MEDIA

Otitis media with effusion is an ideal disease in which to study oxidative stress in human ears because effusion fluid can be removed from patients for study during routine procedures. Testa et al. studied LPO concentrations in effusion fluid from pediatric patients who presented with otitis media with effusion, flat tympanograms, and conductive hearing loss and found that the LPO concentration values were comparable to other chronic disease states.[107] The authors chose to measure LPO as a marker of oxidative stress because when antioxidant systems are overwhelmed, a pro-oxidative state is formed in which free radicals can cause damage to cell membranes, producing LPOs. The authors concluded that the higher LPO values determined that free radical oxidation occurs in otitis media with effusion.

Advances in evidenced-based antioxidant treatment in otologic conditions have been stymied by the challenge of studying the effect of an antioxidant on tissue samples in humans; as such, most of the literature exploring the use of antioxidants in otitis media relies on animal models. However, one randomized controlled trial showed the benefit of GSH supplementation in patients with otitis media with effusion.[108] Testa et al. followed patients for 3 months who had otitis media with effusion who had hearing loss and flat tympanograms, documented unresponsiveness to antibiotics and steroids, and were treated with either saline nasal spray (control group) or 600mg of GSH in a nasal aerosol (treatment group).[108] At the conclusion of the study, 66% of children treated with GSH showed improvement in the gross appearance of the tympanic membrane, tympanometry, and audiometry as compared to 8% of children in the control group.[108] The authors concluded that the results showed both a potential role for GSH

in the treatment of otitis media with effusion and that the inflammation observed in this condition is due in part to oxidative stress.[108]

Animal models allow for the analysis of both serologic markers of inflammation and histologic examination of middle ear epithelial tissue. In a study evaluating the anti-inflammatory and antioxidant properties of alpha-lipoic acid in acute otitis media (AOM), researchers noted that the experimental group treated with alpha-lipoic acid and penicillin G had well-preserved epithelial integrity, appearing the same as in the control group in whom AOM was not induced.[109] Serologic evaluation also showed that the alpha-lipoic acid and penicillin G group had superior superoxide dismutase (SOD) and GSH levels, markers of antioxidant capability, when compared to experimental groups treated with alpha-lipoic acid, penicillin G, and saline.[109] Another study investigated the use of selenium in AOM and found that rats treated with selenium for 10 days had increased GSH-Px and SOD levels when compared to the control group that was treated just with saline; however, only the increase in GSH-Px reached the level of statistical significance.[110] These results suggest that selenium supplementation for 10 days could potentially augment GSH-Px and SOD levels in acute inflammation. Aladag et al. showed a significant increase in GSH-Px and SOD activity when investigating the role of vitamin A as a supplemental treatment with ampicillin–sulbactam; researchers noted that epithelial integrity was better in rats receiving antibiotics and vitamin A when compared to rats that were receiving only antibiotics.[111] These animal models show promise for continued investigation of the role of antioxidants in AOM. More research is necessary to determine whether antioxidant use affects hearing loss, AOM infections per year, length of antibiotic use, and other clinically relevant variables. Despite the lack of evidenced-based algorithms for the use of the antioxidants mentioned in the discussion above, it is likely that these antioxidants can be used in AOM infection with little likelihood of adverse events from administration.

## PRESBYCUSIS

Oxidative stress inherent to the biochemical process of aging has been implicated as part of the pathophysiology of presbycusis. Coling et al. studied GSH-Px activity in Fischer 344 rats (an animal model for presbycusis) and found that GSH-Px activity was increased in the spiral ligament and stria vascularis and was age-related.[112] The authors postulated that the increase in GSH-Px activity stemmed from an age-related decrease in GSH, causing tissues to be exposed to greater amounts of free radicals. The role that GSH-Px activity and the GSH:GSSG ratio play in the development of presbycusis was elucidated in a case–control study in which patients with presbycusis had increased activity of erythrocyte GSH-Px and a decreased GSH:GSSG ratio with an odds ratio of 135:1 when compared to healthy controls.[113] However, the confidence interval for the odds ratio was very wide; so, although this relationship may exist, the magnitude of the relationship is unknown.

The role of oxidative stress in presbycusis is supported further by genetic studies. GSTM1 and GSTT1 are two genes in a family of genes associated with GST. Angeli et al. found that subjects with deletions in the alleles for GST were more likely to have a high-frequency, steeply sloping audiogram pattern[114]; the association between this pattern of hearing loss and the increased susceptibility of cochlear hair cells may be an indication that the basal turn of the cochlea is particularly sensitive to oxidative stress. The elevated risk of presbycusis with GSTT1 deletions was supported further by a study by Karimian et al., which also showed an increased risk of presbycusis with GSTMI deletion.[115] A comprehensive review of the genetic literature with respect to presbycusis is outside the scope of this chapter, but interested readers are encouraged to consult current papers.

Several animal model studies support the involvement of oxidative stress in the pathogenesis of presbycusis. A study using mice that were homozygous for a loss of function mutation for the gamma-glutamyl transferase 1 gene found that supplementation with N-acetyl-L-cysteine (L-NAC) prevented hearing deficits and inner hair cell loss; interestingly, when the L-NAC supplementation was stopped, hearing deficits and inner hair cell loss were noted.[116] However, Davis et al. found no difference between auditory brainstem response and histopathology in C57BL/6J mice (a mouse strain for studying age-related hearing loss) that received L-NAC in their drinking water.[117] The difference in hearing preservation between the two studies may be due to the mouse models used. It is possible that the benefit of

L-NAC supplementation is most pronounced when gamma-glutamyl transferase enzyme activity is lost completely and that L-NAC provides no appreciable benefit when enzyme activity is normal. Another study in C57BL/6J mice showed that mice supplemented with an antioxidant mixture comprised of L-cysteine-glutathione, mixed disulfide, ribose-cystine, NW-nitro-L-arginine methyl ester, vitamin B12, folate, and ascorbic acid had decreased threshold shifts with ABR from baseline when compared to the control group.[118] The antioxidant mixture was chosen because each nutraceutical targets a site in the oxidative pathway. In aggregate, the mixture is beneficial for decreased threshold shifts; however, the specific benefit of each antioxidant cannot be determined from this study.

The possibility of modifying the speed and severity of age-related hearing loss is compelling. The studies discussed above support the role that oxidative stress plays in presbycusis. Further genetic research has the potential to advance knowledge regarding the pathophysiology of presbycusis and identify specific molecular risk factors that contribute to its development. More research is necessary to support evidenced-based use of antioxidants in hearing preservation, but there is hope that nutraceutical use can benefit hearing in the aging population.

## AUTOIMMUNE INNER EAR DISEASE

The pathophysiology of AIED is poorly understood, and the treatment of the disease often comprises a non-focal "shotgun" method using immunosuppressive medications such as corticosteroids and cytotoxic drugs. A more targeted approach to treatment is desired. However, broad immunosuppression is the gold standard treatment, and no other regimen has demonstrated equal or superior efficacy. Immunomodulation of AIED with nutraceuticals might provide a beneficial adjunctive treatment to the management of AIED. Pathak et al. found that NAC abrogated approximately 60% of lipopolysaccharide (LPS)-mediated TNF-α release in the PBMC smears of patients with AIED and in the PBMC smears of control patients.[119] Svrakic et al. found that AIED patients with high levels of TNF-α had increased steroid sensitivity[120]; so, it can be suggested that NAC supplementation in AIED patients may help to act as an effective adjunctive treatment in patients who respond well to steroids. These studies suggest that antioxidant supplementation may benefit AIED patients; however, more research is necessary to determine whether patients benefit clinically from nutraceutical supplementation.

## VERTIGO

There is a growing body of literature regarding nutraceutical use in benign paroxysmal positional vertigo (BPPV): the most common cause of peripheral vertigo.[121] Low vitamin D status has been implicated in the pathogenesis of BPPV, and a meta-analysis found that patients with recurrent BPPV attacks had lower levels of vitamin D when compared with BPPV patients who did not experience BPPV recurrence.[122] However, the authors found an insignificant reduction in vitamin D levels in BPPV patients when compared with healthy controls.[122] This suggests that vitamin D status may play a role in disease severity. A meta-analysis found approximately a 63% reduction in the recurrence of BPPV attacks in patients who were supplemented with vitamin D.[123] The authors suggested that vitamin D may be used as a secondary prevention agent in this patient population.[123] The reduction in BPPV recurrence was supported further by another meta-analysis that found a 59% reduction in BPPV recurrence with vitamin D supplementation.[124] A randomized controlled trial evaluated LICA® (Difass International, Coriano [RN], Italy), a nutritional supplement comprised of alpha-lipoic acid, L-carnosine, zinc, and vitamins B and D3 in preventing BPPV recurrences, and found that only patients who had insufficient or deficient vitamin D levels had a statistically significant reduction in BPPV attacks.[125] So, it is difficult to determine whether the change in relapse events in vitamin D-deficient patients is due to supplementation with LICA® or supplementation with just vitamin D.

The role of oxidative stress in vertigo has been investigated in several preliminary studies that have determined that patients with vertigo have higher markers of oxidative stress.[126–128] However, the exact role of oxidants in the pathogenesis of vertigo has not been determined. More targeted studies are necessary to determine whether nutraceutical supplementation might be beneficial in the treatment of central and peripheral vertigo.

## NOISE-INDUCED HEARING LOSS

Why do some people develop noise-induced hearing loss, while others, who abuse their ears equally, fail to develop impairment in their hearing? Various factors at the cellular level determine an individual's response to noise-induced temporary threshold shifts, and, like all other cells in the body, cells in the cochlea and auditory pathways depend upon biochemical antioxidant mechanisms to manage free-radical generation. Since the cells of the cochlea are susceptible to free radical damage, one might hypothesize that supplementation with nutraceuticals could have a positive impact on primary or secondary prevention of noise-induced hearing loss. However, research has yielded few clinically relevant findings. A systematic review reported that NAC, methionine, acetyl-L-carnitine, and resveratrol supplementation in animal models had an otoprotective effect.[129] Of the antioxidants listed in the review, NAC was the only one studied in humans, with mixed results.[129] Several meta-analyses investigating the role of genetic polymorphisms in antioxidant genes have revealed non-significant generalizable relationships between the investigated polymorphism and noise-induced hearing loss.[130–132] Studying nutraceutical use in industrial environments is challenging; however, research in this setting is recommended to investigate whether nutraceuticals are otoprotective.

## OTOLOGIC SURGERY

Even in the hands of the most experienced surgeon, outcomes following otologic surgery are not invariably perfect. Perforations occur following a small percentage of tympanoplasties, some stapedectomies result in sensorineural hearing loss (sometimes mild and restricted to high frequencies, but sometimes profound), and sometimes even straightforward mastoidectomy can result in unexpected tinnitus, hearing loss, and vertigo. A randomized controlled trial investigated the role of NAC in protecting high-frequency hearing in patients undergoing stapedotomy and found that the administration of NAC 1 hour before surgery did not have an effect on the hearing thresholds of patients 1 year after surgery.[133] Research investigating surgical outcomes with respect to nutraceutical supplementation is needed before a definitive opinion can be issued on the benefit of nutraceuticals in otologic surgery patients.

## CONCLUSION

GSH has been shown to regulate basic immune functions, which may prove beneficial to patients with a broad spectrum of immune-related conditions. It may also play a beneficial role in various neurodegenerative diseases. A growing body of literature supports the use of nutraceuticals in otologic patients, with the use of vitamin D in BPPV and GSH in otitis media showing promising results. For nutraceuticals to become evidence-based adjunctive therapies in otologic conditions, randomized controlled clinical trials are needed in conditions for which research is limited to animal models. The authors of this chapter look forward to advances in the application of nutraceuticals to otologic patients.

## ACKNOWLEDGMENT

Thanks to Youngjin Cho for her contributions to the discussion of the immune system and HIV/AIDS pathogenesis, and thanks to Gustavo Bounous for his contributions to the previous edition of this chapter first published in Sataloff, R.T. and Sataloff, J., *Hearing Loss, Fourth Edition*.[51]

## REFERENCES

1. Perricone C, De Carolis C, Perricone R. Glutathione: a key player in autoimmunity. Autoimmun Rev 2009; 8(8):697–701.
2. Meister A, Anderson ME. Glutathione. Annu Rev Biochem 1983; 52:711–760.
3. Fernández-Checa JC, Kaplowitz N, García-Ruiz C, et al. GSH transport in mitochondria: defense against TNF-induced oxidative stress and alcohol-induced defect. Am J Physiol 1997; 273(1 Pt 1):G7–G17.
4. Meister A. The antioxidant effects of glutathione and ascorbic acid. In: Pasquier C et al., eds. Oxidative Stress, Cell Activation and Viral Infection. Molecular and Cell Biology Updates. Bäsel, Switzerland: Birkhäuser Basal; 1994:101–111.
5. Lomaestro BM, Malone M. Glutathione in health and disease: pharmacotherapeutic issues. Ann Pharmacother 1995; 29:1263–1273.
6. Peterson JD, Herzenberg LA, Vasquez K, Waltenbaugh C. Glutathione levels in antigen-presenting cells modulate Th1 versus Th2 response patterns. Proc Natl Acad Sci U S A 1998; 95(6):3071–3076.
7. Short S, Merkel BJ, Caffrey R, McCoy KL. Defective antigen processing correlates with a low level of intracellular glutathione. Eur J Immunol 1996; 26(12):3015–3020.
8. Liang J, Ziegler JD, Jahraus B, et al. Piperlongumine acts as an immunosuppressant by exerting prooxidative effects in human T cells resulting in diminished $T_H17$ but enhanced $T_{reg}$ differentiation. Front Immunol 2020; 11:1172.
9. Fu G, Xu Q, Qiu Y, et al. Suppression of Th17 cell differentiation by misshapen/NIK-related kinase MINK1. J Exp Med 2017; 214(5):1453–1469.
10. Gerriets VA, Kishton RJ, Nichols AG, et al. Metabolic programming and PDHK1 control CD4+ T cell subsets and inflammation. J Clin Invest 2015; 125(1):194–207.
11. Lu E, Wolfreys FD, Muppidi JR, Xu Y, Cyster JG. S-Geranylgeranyl-L-glutathione is a ligand for human B cell-confinement receptor P2RY8. Nature 2019; 567(7747):244–248.
12. Romagnani S. Lymphokine production by human T cells in disease states. Annu Rev Immunol 1994; 12:227–257.
13. Zhang T, Kawakami K, Qureshi MH, Okamura H, Kurimoto M, Saito A. Interleukin-12 (IL-12) and IL-18 synergistically induce the fungicidal activity of murine peritoneal exudate cells against Cryptococcus neoformans through production of γ interferon by natural killer cells. Infect Immun 1997; 65:3594–3599.
14. Kaiko GE, Horvat JC, Beagley KW, Hansbro PM. Immunological decision-making: how does the immune system decide to mount a helper T-cell response? Immunology 2008; 123(3):326–338.
15. Vignali DA, Collison LW, Workman CJ. How regulatory T cells work. Nat Rev Immunol 2008; 8(7):523–532.
16. Franchina DG, Dostert C, Brenner D. Reactive oxygen species: involvement in T cell signaling and metabolism. Trends Immunol 2018; 39(6):489–502.

17. Gmunder H, Eck HP, Benninghoff B, Roth S, Dröge W. Macrophages regulate intracellular glutathione levels of lymphocytes. Evidence for an immunoregulatory role of cysteine. Cell Immunol 1990; 129:32–46.

18. Hamilos D. Lymphocyte proliferation in glutathione-depleted lymphocytes: direct relationship between glutathione availability and the proliferative response. Immunopharmacology 1989; 18(3):223–235.

19. Dröge W, Holm E. Role of cysteine and glutathione in HIV infection and other diseases associated with muscle wasting and immunological dysfunction. FASEB J 1997; 11(13):1077–1089.

20. Clerici M. Type 1 and type 2 cytokines in HIV infection—a possible role in apoptosis and disease progression. Ann Med 1997; 29(3):185–188.

21. Herzenberg LA. Glutathione deficiency is associated with impaired survival in HIV disease. Proc Natl Acad Sei USA 1997; 94(5):1967–1972.

22. Rodriguez JF. Plasma glutathione concentrations in children infected with human immunodeficiency virus. Pediatr Infect Dis J 1998; 17(3):236–241.

23. Oyaizu N, Pahwa S. Role of apoptosis in HIV disease pathogenesis. J Clin Immunol 1995; 15:217–231.

24. Ucker DS, Aswell JD, Nickas G. Activation-driven T cell death. 1: requirements for de novo transcription and translation and association of genome fragmentation. J Immunol 1989; 143:3461–3469.

25. Itoh N, Tsujimoto Y, Nagata S. Effect of bcl-2 on Fas antigen mediated cell death. J Immunol 1993; 151:621–627.

26. Macho A, Hirsch T, Marzo I, et al. Glutathione depletion is an early and calcium elevation is a late event of thymocyte apoptosis. J Immunol 1997; 158:4612–4619.

27. Shimizu S, Eguchi Y, Kami ike W, et al. Bcl-2 prevents apoptotic mitochondrial dysfunction by regulating proton flux. Proc Natl Acad Sei USA 1998; 95:1455–1459.

28. Sprietsma IE. Modem diets and diseases: NO-zinc balance. Under Th1, zinc and nitrogen monoxide (NO) collectively protect against viruses, AIDS, autoimmunity, diabetes, allergies, asthma, infectious diseases, atherosclerosis and cancer. Med Hypotheses 1999; 53(1):6–16.

29. Mosmann TR. Cytokine patterns during the progression to AIDS. Science 1994; 265:193–194.

30. Bounous G, Baruchel S, Falutz J, Gold P. Whey protein as a food supplement in HIV-seropositive individuals. Clin Invest Med 1993; 16:204–209.

31. Bains IS, Shaw CA. Neurodegenerative disorders in humans: the role of glutathione in oxidative stress-mediated neuronal death. Brain Res Brain Res Rev 1997; 25(3):335–358.

32. Voehringer DW. Bcl-2 expression causes redistribution of glutathione to the nucleus. Proc Natl Acad Sei USA 1998; 95(6):2956–2960.

33. Sekhar RV, Hsu J, Suliburk J, et al. Reversing Accelerated Aging in HIV patients: Metabolic and Mitochondrial Mechanisms. Paper presented at: Conference on Retroviruses and Opportunistic Infections; March 4–7, 2018; Boston, MA.

34. French MA, Cozzi-Lepri A, Arduino RC, et al. Plasma levels of cytokines and chemokines and the risk of mortality in HIV-infected individuals: a case-control analysis nested in a large clinical trial. AIDS 2015; 29(7):847–851.

35. Osuji FN, Onyenekwe CC, Ahaneku JE, Ukibe NR. The effects of highly active antiretroviral therapy on the serum levels of pro-inflammatory and anti-inflammatory cytokines in HIV infected subjects. J Biomed Sci 2018; 25(1):88.

36. Maek-A-Nantawat W, Buranapraditkun S, Klaewsongkram J, Ruxrungtham K. Increased interleukin-17 production both in helper T cell subset Th17 and CD4-negative T cells in human immunodeficiency virus infection (published correction appears in Viral Immunol. 2007 Summer;20(2):328. Ruxrungthum, Kiat [corrected to Ruxrungtham, Kiat]). Viral Immunol 2007; 20(1):66–75.

37. Jiao Y, Fu J, Xing S, et al. The decrease of regulatory T cells correlates with excessive activation and apoptosis of CD8+ T cells in HIV-1-infected typical progressors, but not in long-term non-progressors. Immunology 2009; 128(1 Suppl):e366–e375.

38. Chase AJ, Yang HC, Zhang H, Blankson JN, Siliciano RF. Preservation of FoxP3+ regulatory T cells in the peripheral blood of human immunodeficiency virus type 1-infected elite suppressors correlates with low CD4+ T-cell activation. J Virol 2008; 82(17):8307–8315.

39. Cummins NW, Badley AD. Mechanisms of HIV-associated lymphocyte apoptosis: 2010. Cell Death Dis 2010; 1(11):e99. Published 2010 Nov 11.

40. Hosaka N, Oyaizu N, Kaplan MH, Yagita H, Pahwa S. Membrane and soluble forms of Fas (CD95) and Fas ligand in peripheral blood mononuclear cells and in plasma from human immunodeficiency virus-infected persons. J Infect Dis 1998; 178(4):1030–1039.

41. Ghare SS, Chilton PM, Rao AV, et al. Epigenetic mechanisms underlying HIV-infection induced susceptibility of CD4+ T cells to enhanced activation-induced FasL expression and cell death. J Acquir Immune Defic Syndr 2021; 86(1):128–137.

42. Day CL, Kaufmann DE, Kiepiela P, et al. PD-1 expression on HIV-specific T cells is associated with T-cell exhaustion and disease progression. Nature 2006; 443(7109):350–354.

43. Maggi E, Mazzetti M, Ravina A et al. Ability of HIV to promote a Th1 to Th0 shift and to replicate preferentially in Th2 and Th0 cells. Science 1994; 265:244–248.

44. Valentin A, Lu W, Rosati M et al. Dual effect of interleukin 4 on HIV-1 expression: implications for viral phenotypic switch and disease progression. Proc Natl Acad Sei USA 1998; 95:11880–11885.

45. Owman C, Garzino-Demo A, Cocchi F, Popovic M, Sabirsh A, Gallo RC. The leukotriene B4 receptor functions as a novel type of coreceptor mediating entry of primary HIV-1 isolates into CD4-positive cells. Proc Natl Acad Sci U S A 1998; 95:9530–9534.

46. Lothian B, Grey V, Kimoff R, Lands L. Treatment of obstructive airway disease with a cysteine donor protein supplement: a case study. Chest 2000; 117(3):914–916.

47. Watanabe A, Okada K, Shimizu Y, et al. Nutritional therapy of chronic hepatitis by whey protein (non-heated). J Med 2000; 31(5–6):283–302.

48. Bounous G. Whey protein concentrate (WPC) and glutathione modulation in cancer treatment. Anticancer Res 2000; 20(6C):4785–4792.

49. Lai ZW, Hanczko R, Bonilla E, et al. N-acetylcysteine reduces disease activity by blocking mammalian target of rapamycin in T cells from systemic lupus erythematosus patients: a randomized, double-blind, placebo-controlled trial. Arthritis Rheum 2012; 64(9):2937–2946.

50. Rahimi A, Samimagham HR, Azad MH, Hooshyar D, Arabi M, KazemiJahromi M. The efficacy of N-Acetylcysteine in severe COVID-19 patients: a structured summary of a study protocol for a randomised controlled trial. Trials 2021; 22(1):271. Published 2021 Apr 12.

51. Kwyer TA, Bounous G, Sataloff RT. Implications of nutraceutical modulation of glutathione with cystine and cysteine in general health and otology. In: Hearing Loss. 4th ed. Boca Raton, FL: Taylor & Francis; 2005:603–633.

52. Zeevalk GD, Bernard LP, Nicklas WJ. Role of oxidative stress and the glutathione system in loss of dopamine neurons due to impairment of energy metabolism. J Neurochem 1998; 70(4): 1421–1430.

53. Jurma OP, Hom DG, Andersen JK. Decreased glutathione results in calcium-mediated cell death in PC12. Free Radic Biol Med 1997; 23(7):1055–1066.

54. Gabby M, Tauber M, Porat S, Simantov R. Selective role of glutathione in protecting human neuronal cells from dopamine-induced apoptosis. Neuropharmacology 1996; 35(5):571–578.

55. Shukitt-Hale B, Denisova NA, Strain JG, Joseph JA. Psychomotor effects of dopamine infusion under decreased glutathione conditions. Free Radic Biol Med 1997; 23(3):412–418.

56. Lucas JH, Wheeler DG, Emery DG, Mallery SR. The endogenous antioxidant glutathione as a factor in the survival of physically injured mammalian spinal cord neurons. J Neuropathol Exp Neurol 1998; 57(10):937–954.

57. Singh I, Pahan K, Khan M, Singh AK. Cytokine-mediated induction of ceramide production is redox-sensitive. Implications to proinflammatory cytokine-mediated apoptosis in demyelinating diseases. J Biol Chern 1998; 273(32):20354–20362.

58. Weisbrot-Lefkowitz M, Reuhl K, Perry B, Chan PH, Inouye M, Mirochnitchenko O. Overexpression of human glutathione peroxidase protects transgenic mice against focal cerebral ischemia/reperfusion damage. Brain Res Mol Brain Res 1998; 53(1–2):333–338.

59. Skaper SD, Ancona B, Facet L, Franceschini D, Giusti P. Melatonin prevents the delayed death of hippocampal neurons induced by enhanced excitatory neurotransmission and the nitridergic pathway. FASEB J 1998; 12(9):725–731.

60. Drukarch B, Jongenelen CA, Schepens E, Langeveld CH, Stoof JC. Glutathione is involved in the granular storage of dopamine in rat PC12 pheochromocytoma cells: implications for the pathogenesis of Parkinson's disease. J Neurosci 1996; 16(19):6038–6045.

61. Froissard P, Monrocq H, Duval D. Role of glutathione metabolism in the glutamate-induced programmed cell death of neuronal-like PC12 cells. Eur J Pharmacol 1997; 326(1):93–99.

62. Mawatari K, Yasui Y, Sugitani K, Takadera T, Kato S. Reactive oxygen species involved in the glutamate toxicity of C6 glioma cells via xc antiporter system. Neuroscience 1996; 73(1):201–208.

63. Offen D, Ziv I, Stemin H, Melamed E, Hochman A. Prevention of dopamine-induced cell death by thiol antioxidants: possible implications for treatment of Parkinson's disease. Exp Neurol 1996; 141(l):32–39.

64. Nakamura K, Wang W, Kang UJ. The role of glutathione in dopaminergic neuronal survival. J Neurochem 1997; 69(5):1850–1858.

65. Wilson JX. Antioxidant defense of the brain: a role for astrocytes. Can J Physiol Pharmacol 1997; 75:1149–1163.

66. Kranich O, Dringen R, Sandberg M, Hamprecht B. Utilization of cysteine and cysteine precursors for the synthesis of glutathione in astroglial cultures: preference for cystine. Glia 1998; 22(1):11–18.

67. Kranich O, Hamprecht B, Dringen R. Different preferences in the utilization of amino acids for glutathione synthesis in cultured neurons and astroglial cells derived from rat brain. Neurosci Lett 1996; 219(3):211–214.

68. Drukarch B, Schepens E, Jongenelen CA, Stoof JC, Langeveld CH. Astrocyte-mediated enhancement of neuronal survival is abolished by glutathione deficiency. Brain Res 1997; 770(1–2):123–130.

69. Wei Y, Lu M, Mei M, et al. Pyridoxine induces glutathione synthesis via PKM2-mediated Nrf2 transactivation and confers neuroprotection. Nat Commun 2020; 11(1):941.

70. Weber GF, Mirza NM, Yunis EJ, Dubey D, Cantor H. Localization and treatment of an oxidation-sensitive defect within the TCR-coupled signaling pathway that is associated with normal and premature immunologic aging. Growth Dev Aging 1997; 61(3–4):191–207.

71. Wang G-M, Raghavachari N, Lou MF. Relationship of protein-glutathione mixed disulfide and thioltransferase in $H_2O_2$-induced cataract in cultured pig lens. Exp Eye Res 1997; 64:693–700.

72. Gravina SA, Mieyal JJ. Thioltransferase is a specific glutathionyl mixed disulfide oxidoreductase. Biochemistry 1993; 32:3368–3376.

73. Raghavachari N, Lou MF. Evidence for the presence of thioltransferase in the lens. Exp Eye Res 1996; 63:433–441.

74. Takemoto L. Increase in the intramolecular disulfide bonding of alpha-A crystallin during aging of the human lens. Exp Eye Res 1996; 63(5):585–590.

75. Harman D. Extending functional life span. Exp Gerontol 1998; 33(1–2):95–112.

76. Armeni R, Pieri C, Marra M, Saccucci F, Principato G. Studies on the life prolonging effect of food restriction: glutathione levels and glyoxalase enzymes in rat liver. Meeh Ageing Dev 1998; 101(1–2):101–110.

77. Witschi A, Reddy S, Stofer B, Lauterburg BH. The systemic availability of oral glutathione. Europ J Clin Pharmacol 1992; 43:667–669.

78. Bray TM, Taylor CO. Enhancement of tissue glutathione for antioxidant and immune functions in malnutrition. Biochem Pharmacol 1994; 47:2113–2123.

79. Puri RN, Meister A. Transport of glutathione as γ-glutamylcysteinylglycyl ester, into liver and kidney. Proc Natl Acad Sei USA 1983; 80:5258–5260.

80. Anderson ME, Powrie F, Puri RN, Meister A. Glutathione monoethyl ester: preparation, uptake by tissues, and conversion to glutathione. Arch Biochem Biophys 1985; 239:538–548.

81. Birnbaum SM, Winitz M, Greenstein JP. Quantitative nutritional studies with water-soluble, chemically defined diets. III. Individual amino acids as sources of "non-essential" nitrogen. Arch Biochem Biophys 1957; 72:428–436.

82. Dröge W, Gross A, Hack V, et al. Role of cysteine and glutathione in HIV infection and cancer cachexia: therapeutic intervention with N-acetylcysteine. Adv Pharmacol 1997; 38:581–600.

83. Gross A, Hack V, Stahl-Hennig C, Dröge W. Elevated hepatic γ-glutamylcysteine synthetase activity and abnormal sulfate levels in liver and muscle tissue may explain abnormal cysteine and glutathione levels in SIV-infected rhesus macaques. AIDS Res Hum Retroviruses 1996; 12(17):1639–1641.

84. Kinscherf R, Fischbach T, Mihm S, et al. Effect of glutathione depletion and oral N-acetyl-cysteine treatment on CD4+ and CD8+ cells. FASEB J 1994; 8(6):448–451.

85. Staal FJT, Roederer M, Herzenberg LA, Herzenberg LA. Intracellular thiols regulate activation of nuclear factor kB and transcription of human immunodeficiency virus. Proc Natl Acad Sci U S A 1990; 87:9943–9947.

86. Roederer M, Staal FJT, Raju PA, Ela SW, Herzenberg LA, Herzenberg LA. Cytokine-stimulated human immunodeficiency virus replication is inhibited by N-acetyl-L-cysteine. Proc Natl Acad Sci U S A 1990; 87:4884–4888.

87. Kalebic T, Kinter A, Poli G, Anderson ME, Meister A, Fauci AS. Suppression of human immunodeficiency virus expression in chronically infected monocytic cells by glutathione, glutathione ester, and N-acetylcysteine. Proc Natl Acad Sci U S A 1991; 88:986–990.

88. Mant TGK, Tempowski JH, Volans GN, Talbot JCC. Adverse reactions to acetylcysteine and effects of overdose. Br Med J 1984; 289:217–219.

89. Kajiwara Y, Yasutake A, Adachi T, Hirayama K. Methylmercury transport across the placenta via neutral amino acid carrier. Arch Toxicol 1996; 70:310–314.

90. Aschner M, Clarkson TW. Mercury 203 distribution in pregnant and nonpregnant rats following systemic infusions with thiol-containing amino acids. Teratology 1987; 36:321–328.

91. Aschner M, Clarkson TW. Distribution of mercury 203 in pregnant rats and their fetuses following systemic infusions with thiol-containing amino acids and glutathione during late gestation. Teratology 1988; 38:145–155.

92. Aschner M, Clarkson TW. Methyl mercury uptake across bovine brain capillary endothelial cells in vitro: the role of amino acids. Pharmacol Toxicol 1989; 64:293–297.

93. Mokrzan EM, Kerper LE, Ballatori N, Clarkson TW. Methylmercury-thiol uptake into cultured brain capillary endothelial cells on amino acid system L. J Pharmacol Exp Ther 1995; 272:1277–1284.

94. Aschner M, Clarkson TW. Uptake of methylmercury in the rat brain: effects of amino acids. Brain Res 1988; 462:31–39.

95. Kerper LE, Ballatori N, Clarkson TW. Methylmercury transport across the blood-brain barrier by an amino acid carrier. Am J Physiol 1992; 262:R761–R765.

96. Aschner M. Brain, kidney and liver 203 Hg-methyl mercury uptakes in the rat: relationship to the neutral amino acid carrier. Pharmacol Toxicol 1989; 65:17–20.

97. Aschner M, Eberle NB, Goderie S, Kimelberg HK. Methylmercury uptake in rat primary astrocyte cultures: the role of the neutral amino acid transport system. Brain Res 1990; 521:221–228.

98. Abbas AK, Jardemark K, Lehmann A, Weber SG, Sandberg M. Bicarbonate-sensitive cysteine induced elevation of extracellular aspartate and glutamate in rat hippocampus in vitro. Neurochem Int 1997; 30:253–259.

99. Blaylock RL. Excitotoxins: The Taste that Kills. Santa Fe, NM: Health Press, 1997.

100. Bounous G, Batist G, Gold P. Immuno-enhancing property of dietary whey protein in mice: role of glutathione. Clin Invest Med 1989; 12:154–161.

101. Baruchel S, Viau G, Olivier R, Bounous G, Wainberg M. Nutriceutical modulation of glutathione with a humanized native milk serum protein isolate, Immunocal™: application in AIDS and cancer. In: Montagnier L, Oliver R, Pasquier C, eds. Oxidative Stress in Cancer, AIDS, and Neurodegenerative Diseases, New York, NY: Marcel Dekker, 1997.

102. Beale RJ, Bryg DJ, Bihari DJ. Immunonutrition in the critically ill: a systematic review of clinical outcome. Crit Care Med 1999; 27(12):2799–2805.

103. Kudsk KA, Minard G, Croce MA, et al. A randomized trial of isonitrogenous enteral diets after severe trauma. Ann Surg 1996; 224(4):531–543.

104. Fleshner NE, Kucuk O. Antioxidant dietary supplements: rationale and current status as chemopreventive agents for prostate cancer. Urology 2001; 57(4, suppl 1):90–94.

105. Ripple MO, Henry W, Rago R, Wilding G. Prooxidant-antioxidant shift induced by androgen treatment of human prostate carcinoma cells. J Nat Cancer Inst 1997; 89:40–48.

106. Asher BF, Guilford FT. Oxidative stress and low glutathione in common ear, nose, and throat conditions: a systematic review. Altern Ther Health Med 2016; 22(5):44–50.

107. Testa D, Guerra G, Marcuccio G, Landolfo PG, Motta G. Oxidative stress in chronic otitis media with effusion. Acta Otolaryngol 2012; 132(8):834–837.

108. Testa B, Testa D, Mesolella M, D'Errico G, Tricarico D, Motta G. Management of chronic otitis media with effusion: the role of glutathione. Laryngoscope 2001; 111(8):1486–1489.

109. Tatar A, Korkmaz M, Yayla M, et al. Anti-inflammatory and anti-oxidative effects of alpha-lipoic acid in experimentally induced acute otitis media. J Laryngol Otol 2016; 130(7):616–623.

110. Aydoğan F, Taştan E, Aydın E, et al. Antioxidant role of selenium in rats with experimental acute otitis media. Indian J Otolaryngol Head Neck Surg 2013; 65(Suppl 3):541–547.

111. Aladag I, Guven M, Eyibilen A, Sahin S, Köseoglu D. Efficacy of vitamin A in experimentally induced acute otitis media. Int J Pediatr Otorhinolaryngol 2007; 71(4):623–628.

112. Coling D, Chen S, Chi LH, Jamesdaniel S, Henderson D. Age-related changes in antioxidant enzymes related to hydrogen peroxide metabolism in rat inner ear. Neurosci Lett 2009; 464(1):22–25.

113. Hasansulama W, Madiadipoera T, Sunarjati S, Garna H. Glutathione peroxide and glutathione to disulfide glutathione ratio in presbycusis: a case-control study. Med Arch 2022; 76(3):209–214.

114. Angeli SI, Bared A, Ouyang X, Du LL, Yan D, Zhong Liu X. Audioprofiles and antioxidant enzyme genotypes in presbycusis. Laryngoscope 2012; 122(11):2539–2542.

115. Karimian M, Behjati M, Barati E, Ehteram T, Karimian A. CYP1A1 and GSTs common gene variations and presbycusis risk: a genetic association analysis and a bioinformatics approach. Environ Sci Pollut Res Int 2020; 27(34):42600–42610.

116. Ding D, Jiang H, Chen GD, et al. N-acetylcysteine prevents age-related hearing loss and the progressive loss of inner hair cells in γ-glutamyl transferase 1 deficient mice. Aging 2016; 8(4):730–750.

117. Davis RR, Kuo MW, Stanton SG, Canlon B, Krieg E, Alagramam KN. N-Acetyl L-cysteine does not protect against premature age-related hearing loss in C57BL/6J mice: a pilot study. Hear Res 2007; 226(1–2):203–208.

118. Heman-Ackah SE, Juhn SK, Huang TC, Wiedmann TS. A combination antioxidant therapy prevents age-related hearing loss in C57BL/6 mice. Otolaryngol Head Neck Surg 2010; 143(3):429–434.

119. Pathak S, Stern C, Vambutas A. N-Acetylcysteine attenuates tumor necrosis factor alpha levels in autoimmune inner ear disease patients. Immunol Res 2015; 63(1–3):236–245.

120. Svrakic M, Pathak S, Goldofsky E, et al. Diagnostic and prognostic utility of measuring tumor necrosis factor in the peripheral circulation of patients with immune-mediated sensorineural hearing loss. Arch Otolaryngol Head Neck Surg 2012; 138(11):1052–1058.

121. Froehling DA, Silverstein MD, Mohr DN, Beatty CW, Offord KP, Ballard DJ. Benign positional vertigo: incidence and prognosis

in a population-based study in Olmsted County, Minnesota. Mayo Clin Proc 1991;66(6):596–601.

122. AlGarni MA, Mirza AA, Althobaiti AA, Al-Nemari HH, Bakhsh LS. Association of benign paroxysmal positional vertigo with vitamin D deficiency: a systematic review and meta-analysis. Eur Arch Otorhinolaryngol 2018; 275(11): 2705–2711.

123. Jeong SH, Lee SU, Kim JS. Prevention of recurrent benign paroxysmal positional vertigo with vitamin D supplementation: a meta-analysis. J Neurol 2022; 269(2):619–626.

124. Yang Z, Li J, Zhu Z, He J, Wei X, Xie M. Effect of vitamin D supplementation on benign paroxysmal positional vertigo recurrence: a meta-analysis. Sci Prog 2021; 104(2):368504211024569.

125. Libonati GA, Leone A, Martellucci S, et al. Prevention of recurrent benign paroxysmal positional vertigo: the role of combined supplementation with vitamin D and antioxidants. Audiol Res 2022; 12(4):445–456.

126. Ozbay I, Topuz MF, Oghan F, Kocak H, Kucur C. Serum prolidase, malondialdehyde and catalase levels for the evaluation of oxidative stress in patients with peripheral vertigo. Eur Arch Otorhinolaryngol 2021; 278(10):3773–3776.

127. Li J, Wu R, Xia B, Wang X, Xue M. Serum levels of superoxide dismutases in patients with benign paroxysmal positional vertigo. Biosci Rep 2020; 40(5):BSR20193917.

128. Ohara K, Inoue Y, Sumi Y, et al. Oxidative stress and heart rate variability in patients with vertigo. Acute Med Surg 2014; 2(3):163–168.

129. Hullfish H, Roldan LP, Hoffer ME. The use of antioxidants in the prevention and treatment of noise-induced hearing loss. Otolaryngol Clin North Am 2022; 55(5):983–991.

130. Wu J, Jiang Z, Huang X, Luo Z, Peng H. Association of polymorphisms in the catalase gene with the susceptibility to noise-induced hearing loss: a meta-analysis. Am J Otolaryngol 2023; 44(2):103699.

131. Wang J, Li J, Peng K, et al. Association of the C47T polymorphism in superoxide dismutase gene 2 with noise-induced hearing loss: a meta-analysis. Braz J Otorhinolaryngol 2017; 83(1):80–87.

132. Zong S, Zeng X, Guan Y, et al. Association of Glutathione s-transferase M1 and T1 gene polymorphisms with the susceptibility to acquired sensorineural hearing loss: a systematic review and meta-analysis. Sci Rep 2019; 9(1):833.

133. Bagger-Sjöbäck D, Strömbäck K, Hakizimana P, et al. A randomised, double blind trial of N-Acetylcysteine for hearing protection during stapes surgery. PLOS ONE 2015; 10(3):e0115657.

# 27

# Tables summarizing differential diagnosis

ROBERT THAYER SATALOFF

The preceding 26 chapters discuss a great many causes of hearing loss, associated symptoms, and diagnostic distinctions. The tables in this chapter help summarize the information so that similarities and differences are apparent at a glance. While they certainly do not cover all the information presented, the tables include most of the common and important conditions discussed so far, highlighting their most important distinguishing features (**Tables 27.1–27.7**).

DOI: 10.1201/b23379-27

Table 27.1 Audiologic criteria for classifying hearing loss[a]

| | Air conduction pattern | Bone conduction pattern | Air–bone gap | Lateralization of 500-Hz fork | Recruitment | Abnormal tone decay | Discrimination |
|---|---|---|---|---|---|---|---|
| Conductive | Greater low-tone loss, except when fluid is in the ear Maximum loss is 60- to 70-dB ANSI | Normal or almost | At least 15 dB | To worse ear | Absent | Absent | Good |
| Sensory | Greater low-tone loss or high-tone dip | BC = AC | No gap | To better ear with low intensity To worse ear with high intensity | May be marked and continuous | Absent | Poor |
| Neural | Greater high-tone loss | BC = AC or BC worse than AC | No gap | To better ear | Absent | Marked tone decay in acoustic neuroma and nerve injuries | Reduced |
| Sensorineural | Greater high-tone loss or flat loss | BC = AC | No gap | To better ear | Absent or slight | Absent | Reduced |
| Functional | Flat | Usually, no BC | No gap | Vague | Absent | Variable | Usually, good or no response |
| Central | Variable or even normal threshold | BC = AC or absent BC | No gap | None | None | Undetermined | Reduced |

Table 27.1 (Continued)

| | Audiometric responses[b] | Tinnitus | Békésy tracings | Impedance audiometry | Patient's voice[b] | Other findings |
|---|---|---|---|---|---|---|
| Conductive | Vague and slow | Absent or low | Overlap of pulsed and continuous tracings | • Often abnormal and diagnostic tympanogram | Soft or normal | • No diplacusis<br>• Hears better in noisy environment |
| Sensory | Sharp | Low roar or seashell | • Pulsed tracings slightly wider at higher frequencies<br>• Little or no separation | • Normal tympanogram<br>• Metz recruitment (stapedius reflex at low intensity) | Normal | • Diplacusis<br>• Hears worse in noisy environment<br>• Lowered threshold of discomfort |
| Neural | Sharp | Hissing or ringing | Separation of tracings in acoustic neuroma | • Normal tympanogram<br>• Stapedius reflex absent or decayed | Louder | • No diplacusis<br>• Hears worse in noisy environment |
| Sensorineural | Sharp | Hissing or ringing | Slight separation of tracing | • Normal tympanogram<br>• Other test variable | Louder | • No diplacusis<br>• Hears worse in noisy environment |
| Functional | Inconsistent | Absent | Separation of tracing with poorer threshold for pulsed tone | • Normal | Normal | • No diplacusis<br>• Hears worse in noisy environment |
| Central | Slow | None | Undetermined | • Normal tympanogram<br>• Difference between ipsilateral and contralateral stapedius reflex responses | Normal | • No diplacusis<br>• Hears poorly in noise<br>• Poor integration of complex stimulus |

*Abbreviations:* AC, Air conduction; ANSI, American National Standards Institute; BC, bone conduction.

a These criteria are the usual ones, but many variations and exceptions are encountered.

b These are common findings, but there are many exceptions.

Table 27.2 Causes of conductive hearing loss with abnormal findings originating in external canal

| Diagnosis | History | Onset of hearing loss | Otoscopic findings | Tinnitus | Audiologic and impedance | Special findings |
|---|---|---|---|---|---|---|
| Congenital aplasia | • Ear deformed at birth with hearing impairment<br>• Unilateral or bilateral | Congenital | • Auricular deformity and canal closed | None | Flat hearing loss about 60–70 dB, worse if inner ear is involved | If deformity is bilateral, speech development is impaired |
| Treacher Collins syndrome | • Abnormal findings present at birth bilaterally | Congenital | • Auricular deformity and canal closed | None | Flat hearing loss about 60–70 dB | *Bilateral deformity:* slanted eyes, receding jaw and malar bones |
| Stenosis | • Ear blocked either since birth or following infection, trauma, or surgery to the ear | Congenital or slowly developing | • Eardrum not visible due to closure of canal | None | • Flat hearing loss about 60 dB<br>• Type B | • Auricle is normal, but canal is closed uniformly<br>• Usually no inflammation is present |
| Cerumen | • Ear blocked after attempting to clean canal or after chewing | Slow or sudden after attempting to clean ear canal | • Wax blocking canal and drum not visible | Rarely | • Flat loss, about 45 dB<br>• Type B | • Wax is visible, and hearing returns after wax is removed |
| Fluid in canal | • After swimming or bathing or applying medication in ear | Sudden | • Fluid in canal | Occasionally | • Mild loss with loss in higher frequencies<br>• Bone conduction normal<br>• Type B | • Eardrum normal after fluid is removed |
| External otitis | • Pain and itching in canal, aggravated by chewing or moving auricle<br>• Tenderness<br>• No pain on nose blowing | Insidious | • Canal wall inflamed and debris present<br>• Eardrum intact | None | • Flat loss, about 45 dB<br>• Type B | • Tender canal walls and surrounding areas<br>• Hearing improves with removal of debris |

Table 27.2 (Continued)

| Diagnosis | History | Onset of hearing loss | Otoscopic findings | Tinnitus | Audiologic and impedance | Special findings |
|---|---|---|---|---|---|---|
| Exostosis or osteoma | • Either constant blockage or intermittent if small opening opens and closes with wax or debris | Sudden or intermittent | • Hillocks of bony projections from canal wall or large bony occlusion | None | • Flat loss, about 45 dB<br>• Type B | • Canal closed by hillocks or mounds of bone from canal wall<br>• X-ray films: normal middle ears and external bony projections |
| Granuloma | • Fullness in ears—often painless | Slow | • Firm granulation with or without excessive bleeding<br>• Eardrum normal if visible<br>• Often no inflammation | None | • Flat loss, about 45 dB<br>• Type B | • Often no pain or inflammation<br>• Middle ear normal<br>• Occasional palpable bony defect in canal<br>• Positive biopsy |
| Cysts | • Little or no discomfort but fullness | Slow | • Soft mass in canal covered with skin | None | Flat loss, about 45 dB | Drum normal if visualized |
| Collapse of canal | • Hearing loss only during testing | Only with earphones | • Relaxed opening to external canal | None | Mild low-tone loss, sometimes apparent high-tone loss | • Patient says he hears worse with earphones |
| Foreign body | • Foreign body in ear<br>• In children, no clear history | Sudden | • Foreign body in ear | None, except live insect in ear | Mild flat loss | • Mass in ear not attached to canal wall and not covered with skin |

Table 27.3 Conductive hearing loss with abnormal findings visible in tympanic membrane and middle ear

| Diagnosis | History | Onset | Tinnitus | Audiologic findings | Otoscopic | Special findings |
|---|---|---|---|---|---|---|
| Myringitis bullosa (Blebs on drum) | • Discomfort, fullness in ear, not aggravated by swallowing or chewing and not associated with general malaise | Slow | Slight | Very mild hearing loss of about 25 or 30 dB | • Clear or hemorrhagic blebs on drum involving only outer layer | • Drum is intact and moves with air pressure through canal or nose |
| Ruptured eardrum | • Severe explosive, slap on ear, or foreign body poked into ear, with sudden pain, hearing loss, and possible bleeding and fullness | Sudden | Sometimes | • Flat loss from 40 to 60 dB, sometimes with sensorineural component<br>• Type B | • Jagged central perforation of drum with no inflammation if seen early | • Perforation in drum is jagged and not associated with infection |
| Perforated drum caused by burns | • Spark in ear from welding or exposure to fire | Sudden | None | Flat loss of about 60 dB | • Usually, complete destruction of drum with little infection | • Marked destruction of drum with history of severe pain caused by burn |
| Dry perforation in drum Anterior or central | • Previous otitis media due to adenoid hypertrophy, allergy, or eustachian tube pathology, or following secretory otitis media | Slow | None | Usually less than 40 dB and worse in lower frequencies | • Central or anterior perforation<br>• No infection and normal middle ear mucosa<br>• Edge of perforation usually smooth and regular | • Discharge usually intermittently with colds or water in ears |
| Superior (Shrapnell's area) or posterior perforation on large portion of drum | • Previous otitis media with chronic otorrhea or mastoid infection | Slow | None | • Variable from 15 to 60 dB<br>• Type B | • Posterior or superior perforation | • The amount of hearing loss depends on damage to ossicular chain and other pathology in the middle ear |

Table 27.3 (Continued)

| Diagnosis | History | Onset | Tinnitus | Audiologic findings | Otoscopic | Special findings |
|---|---|---|---|---|---|---|
| Healed perforation | • Previous ear infections | Gradual | None | • From minimal to 70-dB loss<br>• Type $A_S$ or $A_D$ or normal | • Thick scars or transparent closure in drum that looks like perforations | • Drum moves with gentle air pressure in canal or through nose<br>• Hearing loss depends on damage in middle ear |
| Hypertrophied adenoids | • Intermittent ear blocking and fullness<br>• Some mouth breathing | Gradual | None | • Maximum loss usually about 40 dB and often worse at higher frequencies<br>• Type B or C | • Clear fluid level in middle ear or thickened or retracted drum | • Large lymph tissue masses in lateral recesses of nasopharynx |
| Cleft palate | • Recurrent otitis in childhood | Gradual | None | As above | • Type B or C<br>• Opaque, thickened, or retracted drum | • Congenital malformation leads to abnormal eustachian tube function |
| Retracted drum | • Stuffiness in ears | Gradual | None | As above | • Abnormalities in nasopharynx or eustachian tube, such as allergy, adenoids, or neoplasm | • Pressure disparity in middle ears and poor eustachian-tube function |
| Serous otitis media | • Stuffiness in ears, feeling of fluid | Gradual | None | • As above<br>• Type C | • Fluid in middle ear, sometimes with evidence of inflammation and associated with upper respiratory infection | • Blocked eustachian tube and abnormal findings in nasopharynx or tubes |
| Acute otitis media | • Stuffiness, pain, and fullness in ear, sometimes fever | In several hours | None | • Maximum loss usually about 40 dB and often worse at higher frequencies | • Inflamed or bulging drum with prominent vessels<br>• Absent landmarks | • Associated with inflammation in nasopharynx and upper respiratory infection |

*(Continued)*

Table 27.3 (Continued) Conductive hearing loss with abnormal findings visible in tympanic membrane and middle ear

| Diagnosis | History | Onset | Tinnitus | Audiologic findings | Otoscopic | Special findings |
|---|---|---|---|---|---|---|
| Secretory otitis media | • Generally, without upper respiratory infection but may follow it<br>• Recurrent fullness<br>• No pain or systemic symptoms | Slowly | None | • As above<br>• Bone conduction may be slightly reduced<br>• Type B | • Fluid level or bubbles and straw-colored fluid or even gel-like mass | • Eustachian tube is patent, and condition recurs<br>• Nasal mucosa also secretory |
| Aerotitis media | • Sudden pain and fullness on descending in airplane or elevator | Sudden | None | • Mild and usually mostly in higher frequencies<br>• Type B or C | • Retracted drum with possible fluid level<br>• Hearing returns with politzerization or myringotomy | • Resolution often is spontaneous, but early myringotomy resolves hearing loss |
| Chronic otitis media Dry with ossicular damage | • Previous otitis media with prolonged otorrhea for many months before cessation<br>• No pain | Gradual | None | • Flat loss, 60–70 dB | • Large marginal perforation in drum and disruption of ossicular chain by erosion | • Usually, end of incus or crura of stapes are eroded<br>• X-ray films show sclerosis but no active infection in mastoid |
| Mucoid discharge | • Intermittent otorrhea especially following upper respiratory infection but dry in between<br>• No pain | Gradual | None | • Mild with maximum of 40 dB and mostly in lower frequency<br>• Type B | • Usually, anterior perforation | • Associated with eustachian-tube and nasopharyngeal infections<br>• Ossicular chain intact<br>• X-ray films, no mastoid involvement |
| Putrid and purulent discharge | • Persistent otorrhea with evidence of mastoid bone destruction<br>• Occasional discomfort | Gradual | None | • Flat loss up to about 60 dB | • Marginal perforation or no drum | • Degree of hearing loss depends on damage to ossicles<br>• X-ray films show chronic mastoiditis |

Table 27.3 (Continued)

| Diagnosis | History | Onset | Tinnitus | Audiologic findings | Otoscopic | Special findings |
|---|---|---|---|---|---|---|
| Putrid and purulent discharge with cholesteatoma | • As above<br>• Usually discharge | Gradual | None | • Flat loss up to about 60 dB | • Marginal perforation or no drum<br>• White cholesteatoma<br>• Debris in canal | • As above and cholesteatoma |
| Putrid and purulent discharge with cholesteatoma and erosion into semicircular canal | • As above<br>• Vertigo | Gradual | Occasional tinnitus | • Flat loss up to 60 dB | • As above<br>• Vertigo and eye deviation with pressure of air in ear canal | • As above<br>• Positive fistula test |
| Glomus jugular tumor | • Gradual stuffiness in one ear or persistent discharge | Gradual | Often hears own heartbeat | • Very mild hearing loss at first and later up to about 60 dB | • Red appearance of drum and middle ear or hemorrhage<br>• Tissue appears granulomatous | • Much bleeding in ear on manipulation, X-ray films show erosion |
| Tuberculosis | • Mild hearing loss with chronic ear infection<br>• May be associated with tuberculosis elsewhere | Gradual | None | • Minimal to 60-dB flat loss | • Granulation tissue that resists treatment<br>• Later, cervical adenopathy<br>• Multiple perforation of eardrum | • Biopsy and culture show tuberculosis (acid-fast bacilli) |
| Granuloma | • Chronic otorrhea with fullness in ear and little pain | Gradual | None | • Minimal to 60-dB flat loss | • Firm granulations that regrow after removal | • Biopsy shows specific etiology |
| Carcinoma | • As above and sometimes some pain and nodes | Gradual | None | • As above | • As above | • As above |
| Letterer–Siwe disease | • Generalized skin rash<br>• Chronic otorrhea | Gradual | None | • As above | • Bleeding and erosive granulations causing stenosis of canal | • X-ray films show bone erosion and punched-out areas in skull |

(Continued)

Table 27.3 (Continued) Conductive hearing loss with abnormal findings visible in tympanic membrane and middle ear

| Diagnosis | History | Onset | Tinnitus | Audiologic findings | Otoscopic | Special findings |
|---|---|---|---|---|---|---|
| Tympanosclerosis | • Chronic otitis media in the past | Gradual | None | • Using flat and about 60–70 dB | • Eardrum eroded or scarred and thick; deformed appearance in middle ear | • Sclerosis in mastoid bone |
| Hemotympanum | • Blow to head or ear, with pain and fullness | Sudden | Roaring | • 40–70 dB with greater loss at higher frequencies<br>• Type B | • Bloody fluid in middle ear | • No infection is present and eardrum does not move with pressure |
| Systemic diseases: measles, scarlet fever | • Acute otitis media, often followed by chronic otitis and hearing loss | Sudden | None | • 30–70 dB flat loss<br>• Type B | • Perforated drum with or without chronic otitis | • Chronic ear infection since childhood disease |
| Adhesion in middle ear | • Slight hearing loss and fullness in ear with colds | Gradual and fluctuating | None | • Up to about 35 dB or worse in lower frequencies | • Drum retracted or scarred, reflecting previous otitis media | • Hearing loss not corrected by inflation |
| Flaccid tympanic membrane | • Feeling of flutter in eardrum corrected by self-politzerization and nose blowing | Gradual and fluctuating | None | • As above<br>• Type $A_D$ | • Wrinkled and loose eardrum | • Drum is easily blown out and seems to be loose and redundant |
| Blue eardrum | • Fullness in ear | Fluctuates | None | • Up to about 45 dB and worse in higher frequencies | • Drum seems to be blue or purple and does not move | • Drum is dark blue and does not politzerize easily<br>• Normal X-ray findings in mastoid<br>• No infection |
| Simple mastoidectomy | • Ear infection followed by surgery—usually postauricularly<br>• No subsequent ear discharge | After infection | None | • Often little or no hearing loss, but sometimes up to 70 dB if ossicular chain is disrupted | • Eardrum often almost normal, or only small perforation and normal auditory canal | • Usually, postauricular scar and no progressive hearing loss |

Table 27.3 (Continued)

| Diagnosis | History | Onset | Tinnitus | Audiologic findings | Otoscopic | Special findings |
|---|---|---|---|---|---|---|
| Modified radical mastoidectomy | • Ear infection and surgery without removal of ossicles | After infection | None | • About 40-dB flat loss | • Eardrum slightly deformed and posterior canal wall taken down | • Postauricular or endaural scar and malleus are visible |
| Radical mastoidectomy | • Ear infection and surgery with removal of eardrum remnants and ossicles | After infection | None | • 70-dB flat loss | • No eardrum or ossicles visible and mastoid cavity seen through canal wall | • X-ray films show surgical defect in mastoid |
| Fenestration | • Hearing loss and surgical correction | Insidious hearing loss over years | May be low-pitched | • Variable hearing loss from 30 to 70 dB, depending on success of surgery | • Partially exenterated mastoid cavity with displaced eardrum | • Positive fistula test |
| Myringoplasty | • Hearing loss and hole in drum with surgical repair<br>• Often vein or skin was used | Mild and gradual | None | • Flat loss up to 70 dB | • Healed perforation or large, thick drum repair, landmarks may be missing | • Drum is in good position, and patient has scar at donor site |
| Tympanoplasty | • Chronic otitis and hearing loss followed by surgery for hearing and infection | Gradual | None | • About 50–70 dB | • Large middle ear may be covered with skin<br>• Ossicles may be absent, and cavity resembles radical mastoidectomy | • Varying findings, depending on type of surgery done |
| Artificial prosthesis | • Ear infection with large defect in eardrum | Gradual | None | • 50- to 70-dB flat loss | • Much of drum is absent, and patient uses artificial prosthesis that is inserted into canal to middle ear | • Patient improves hearing with prosthesis |
| Radiation therapy to nasopharynx or thyroid | • Clear fluid in ear following irradiation | Gradual | None | • 30–40 dB, with greater loss in higher frequencies | • Fluid level and pressure disparity | • X-ray treatment |

Table 27.4  Sensory hearing loss

| History | Onset of hearing loss | Otoscopic | Tinnitus | Audiologic and/or special | Diagnosis |
|---|---|---|---|---|---|
| Recurrent intermittent vertigo, nausea<br><br>Ear feels full<br>Voices sound tinny and hollow<br><br>Difficulty understanding speech | • Intermittent and then permanent | Normal | Ocean roar or hollow seashell | • Recruitment complete, continuous, and hyperrecruitment<br>• Diplacusis<br>• Poor discrimination compared with hearing loss<br>• Discrimination worse with intensity<br>• Small-amplitude (type II) Békésy tracings | • Recruitment may be complete and often hyperrecruitment<br>• Diplacusis<br>• Patient distraught<br>• Usually, unilateral — Ménière's disease with vertigo |
| Occasional mild imbalance<br>Some ear fullness<br>No noise exposure | • Insidious or sudden | Normal | Absent or high-pitched | • Marked recruitment in some patients<br>• Loss only in high frequencies in most cases | • Complete recruitment<br>• Usually, unilateral<br>• No noise exposure — Viral disease |
| Exposure to sudden noise such as gunfire or explosion | • Sudden hearing loss with tinnitus and then improves | Normal | Ringing | • Starts with 4000-Hz dip and widens if severe<br>• Sometimes permanent | Highest frequency normal unless advanced age or severe damage<br>Nonprogressive — Acoustic trauma |
| Direct blow to head | • Sudden with ringing tinnitus<br>• May be some improvement | Normal | Ringing | • 4000-Hz dip, loss in high frequencies or "dead" ear<br>• Labyrinth also may be affected | • X-ray film may reveal fracture of temporal bone<br>• Vertigo may be present — Head trauma |
| Surgery for otosclerosis<br>Sound distortion and some imbalance | • Following surgery for stapes mobilization or stapedectomy | Normal | Usually present with buzz or roar | • High-tone hearing loss—worse postoperative; discrimination reduced | • Discrimination worse postoperatively than preoperatively, even if hearing loss is impaired — Poststapedectomy |

Table 27.4 (Continued)

| History | Onset of hearing loss | Otoscopic | Tinnitus | Audiologic and/or special | Diagnosis |
|---|---|---|---|---|---|
| Daily exposure to intense noise for many months. No vertigo | • Insidious | Normal | Uncommon | • Early 4000-Hz dip or slightly broader dip | • Marked and continuous recruitment<br>• Only a little discrimination change because only high tones involved | Occupational deafness (early) |
| Slight difficulty in understanding speech | • Insidious | Normal | Occasional hissing, sometimes ringing | • High-tone drop at 8000, 6000, and 4000 Hz<br>• Mild recruitment but continuous<br>• Discrimination reduced<br>• Bilateral usually | • Age group about 50–60<br>• Bilateral hearing loss | Presbycusis |
| Taking ototoxic drugs, especially in presence of kidney infection | • Insidious or sudden | Normal | Generally high-pitched | • High-tone loss bilaterally but may progress to all frequencies | • Recruitment present<br>• Hearing loss usually associated with prolonged administration of drug | Drug ototoxicity |
| Hearing loss, with or without imbalanced | • Insidious or sudden, unilateral or bilateral | Normal | High-pitched or seashell | • Asymmetric, progressive but may be sudden and total, unilateral, or bilateral | • Recruitment common<br>• Decreased discrimination | Autoimmune, syphilis and Lyme disease |

Table 27.5 Neural hearing loss

| History | Onset of hearing loss | Otoscopic | Tinnitus | Audiologic and/or special | Diagnosis |
|---|---|---|---|---|---|
| Early unilateral high-tone hearing loss Sometimes persistent vertigo | • Insidious | Normal | Variable | • Abnormal tone-decay • Wide separation on continuous and interrupted Békésy tracings • Poor discrimination compared with hearing loss • Unilateral • Marked tone decay decreased • No response to caloric test • Spontaneous nystagmus • Erosion visible by X-ray film late in disease • Stapedius reflex decay • Abnormal BERA • Other neurological deficits | Acoustic neuroma |
| Trouble understanding some people with soft voices | • Insidious | Early atrophic eardrum; more white than normal | Occasional hissing | • Gradual high-tone hearing loss • Reduced discrimination • No abnormal tone decay • Bone conduction often worse than air conduction • Age range roughly 60–75 • Bilateral progressive deterioration of hearing • No abnormal tone decay | Presbycusis |
| Severe head injury with loss of consciousness | Sudden | Normal, or blood in canal if fracture involves middle ear | Ringing or none | • Total, usually unilateral loss of hearing from injury to auditory nerve • X-ray film may show fracture around internal auditory meatus | Skull fracture |
| Sudden hearing loss, occasionally with vertigo or pain in ear | Sudden | Normal | High-pitched | • Severe unilateral hearing loss • Other symptoms of herpes may be present | Viral |

*Abbreviation:* BERA, Brainstem evoked-response audiogram.

Table 27.6 Sensorineural hearing loss

| History | Onset of hearing loss | Otoscopic | Tinnitus | Audiologic | Special | Diagnosis |
|---|---|---|---|---|---|---|
| Difficulty in hearing and understanding speech | Insidious | Normal | Occasional | • Usually reduced hearing in all frequencies, especially in higher range; reduced discrimination | • Usually over 50<br>• Bilateral progressive hearing loss<br>• No abnormal tone decay; starts at 3000–6000 Hz<br>• Presbycusis starts at highest frequencies | Presbycusis |
| Exposure to intense noise over many months or years | Insidious | Normal | Uncommon | • Early high-tone loss (C-5 dip), later involving lower frequencies<br>• Reduced discrimination<br>• Békésy tracings depend on stage | • In working age group; bilateral<br>• Starts usually at 3000–6000 Hz and spreads: no abnormal tone decay | Noise-induced hearing loss |
| Severe head injury often with unconsciousness, subjective vertigo | Sudden | Normal or some middle ear pathology due to fracture | Hissing | • Hearing loss usually is severe but may be only high-tone dip or high-tone loss | • Fractured temporal bone with absent caloric responses<br>• Eardrum often appears to be normal<br>• No spontaneous nystagmus, except early | Head trauma |
| Ototoxic drug, usually in large doses, or a small dose in presence of kidney disease | Sudden | Normal | High-pitched | • Rapid, sometimes severe bilateral hearing loss | • Rapid and severe bilateral hearing loss, worse in high frequencies | Ototoxicity (neomycin, streptomycin kanamycin, or other ototoxic drugs) |

*(Continued)*

Table 27.6 (Continued)  Neural hearing loss

| History | Onset of hearing loss | Otoscopic | Tinnitus | Audiologic | Special | Diagnosis |
|---|---|---|---|---|---|---|
| Exposure to intense noise | Sudden hearing loss and tinnitus, followed by gradual recovery | Normal | Temporary ringing | • High-tone dip or more severe losses, mostly in high frequencies | • Except in unusual cases, recovery occurs within several days | Auditory fatigue Temporary threshold shift |
| Rh incompatibility in parents Kernicterus and speech defect in child | Congenital | Normal | None | • Descending audiogram • Nonprogressive hearing loss | • Speech defect • Sometimes other neurological deficits | Rh factor incompatibility |
| Sudden unilateral hearing loss during or following mumps | Sudden | Normal | None | • Total unilateral hearing loss | • Normal vestibular reaction | Mumps |
| Severe hearing loss after meningitis with high fever | Sudden | Normal | None | • Generally subtotal bilateral hearing loss | • Labyrinth also is involved in many cases | Meningitis |
| Sudden unilateral hearing loss with or without dizziness | Sudden | Normal | High-pitched or motorlike | • Subtotal high-tone loss, usually unilateral | • Occasionally associated with hypotension but generally no specific vascular disease | Vascular disorders or membrane ruptures May follow barotrauma |
| Child has retarded or defective speech | Congenital | Normal | None | • High-tone loss bilaterally | • Often follows maternal rubella in first trimester of pregnancy or anoxia, trauma, or jaundice at birth | In utero and birth lesions |
| Disturbing unilateral tinnitus and hearing loss | Sudden and sometimes progressive | Normal | May be hissing | • High-tone loss or subtotal loss of hearing, usually unilateral • Test for acoustic neuroma negative | • Often follows a viral infection | Auditory neuritis |

Table 27.7  Distinguishing external otitis from otitis media

|  | External otitis | Otitis media |
|---|---|---|
| History | Onset after getting water in ear or irritating auditory canal | After rhinitis or blowing nose hard or sneezing |
| Pain | In auditory canal and around meatus<br>Aggravated by moving auricle and chewing | Deep in ear<br>Aggravated by sneezing and blowing nose |
| Tenderness | Around auricle | No tenderness |
| Otoscopic | Skin of canal infected and absence of normal cerumen; eardrum not inflamed | Skin of canal not infected, but eardrum injected or bulging |
| Discharge | Debris from skin of canal | Often mucoid or mucopurulent through tympanic perforation |
| With air pressure in canal | Eardrum moves with positive pressure | Eardrum does not move well, especially if perforation is present |
| Hearing | Hearing loss disappears when canal is cleared | Hearing loss is present even with clear canal |
| With politzerization | Eardrum moves<br>If the external canal is infected and there is mucoid discharge, it is a combination of external otitis and otitis media since the mucus comes from the middle ear through a perforated eardrum | Eardrum does not move well |
| Fever | Comparatively little | Often general malaise and fever |
| Imaging | Normal mastoids and middle ears | Congestion in mastoid and middle ears |

# Appendix I: Anatomy of the ear

This book will not review anatomy of the head and neck in detail. Most anatomy relevant to otolaryngologic practice is taught in medical school. However, many medical school curricula omit detailed discussion of special sensory structures including the ear. Consequently, a more complete discussion of otologic anatomy is provided here. Understanding the ear requires not only observation of gross anatomy but also histologic study. There are two basic techniques for studying histology of the ear.

1. *Traditional temporal bone histology*: Decalcification, staining, section. Takes several months. Good for bones. Less useful for membranous structures. Unsatisfactory for studying hair cell loss.
2. *Surface preparation*: Microdissection after special staining. Excellent for non-bony structures. Takes only hours. Phase contrast microscope studies. Electron microscopy is also used to study the ear, of course.

The ear is divided into three parts differing in their gross anatomy, their histology, and their functions. The italicized items in the following outline are most important structures. A good clinician should review them mentally as he/she examines an ear in order to recognize their normal conditions and understand the implications of their pathology. Familiarity with the non-underlined structures facilitates *special and functional understanding* of the major structures.

## THE EXTERNAL EAR

1. *Auricle*: Elastic cartilage, elastic fibers in perichondrium, skin with subcutaneous layer posteriorly only, a few hairs, sebaceous glands, and very few sweat glands. The helix should meet the cranium at a level not below a line drawn straight back from the lateral canthus of the eye. The axis of the ear should not be >10° off a perpendicular line dropped from the lateral canthal line.
2. *External Auditory Meatus*: S-shaped, curving inferomedially. Lateral portion, cartilaginous. Medial portion, bony. Thin skin, generally lacking papillae, firmly attached to perichondrium and periosteum.
   a. *Cartilaginous portion*: Hairs. Extremely large sebaceous glands connected with hair follicles. Ceruminous glands are specialized coiled tubular apocrine sweat glands, surrounded by myoepithelial cells. Ducts open onto surface or into hair follicles.
   b. *Bony portion*: Small hairs and sebaceous glands on the upper wall only.

## THE MIDDLE EAR

1. Tympanic cavity
   a. *Lateral wall*: Tympanic membrane.
   b. *Medial wall*: Bony wall of the inner ear, facial nerve canal.
   c. *Posterior wall*: Connects through tympanic antrum with *mastoid air cells.*
   d. *Roof*: Tegmen tympani, *very thin bone* (also forms roof of mastoid air cells, antrum, and eustachian tube).
   e. *Floor*: Bony covering of *jugular venous bulb.*
   f. *Anterior wall*: Opening of eustachian tube, and bony covering of *internal carotid artery.*

g. *Contents*: *Ossicles*, tendons of tensor tympani and stapedius muscles, *chorda tympani nerve*, facial nerve canal.

h. Mucosa with simple squamous epithelium except there is ciliated, cuboidal, or columnar epithelium near the tympanic membrane and the auditory (eustachian) tube.

2. Tympanic membrane—The "Eardrum"
   a. *Semi-transparent*: cone-shaped, with *malleus* attached to apex.
   b. *Four layers*: Two layers of collagenous fibers and fibroblasts deficient in the anterior superior quadrant forming the flaccid Shrapnell's Membrane. Collagen fibers are radially arranged in the outer layer, circularly in the inner layer. Lined by skin laterally, by mucosa medially. Vessels and nerves reach the center of the tympanic membrane along the area of the manubrium of the malleus.

3. Ossicles
   a. *Malleus*: Attaches to tympanic membrane at the *umbo*.
   b. *Incus*: Connects the malleus and incus.
   c. *Stapes*: Fits into oval window. Held in place by fibrous annular ligament. Fixed in the disease *otosclerosis*.
   d. The ossicles are supported by ligamentous attachments to bone.

4. Mucosa of the middle ear
   There are five types of cells in the mucosa of the human middle ear, mastoid, and eustachian tube. These cells are (1) the nonciliated cell without secretory granules, (2) the nonciliated cell with secretory granules (including the goblet cell), (3) the ciliated cell, (4) the intermediate cell, and (5) the basal cell. The mastoid cavity has predominantly simple squamous or cuboidal epithelium, although ciliated cells can be found in some specimens. The posterior part of the mesotympanum and the epitympanum have tall epithelium, which is often ciliated. The promontory has secretory and nonsecretory columnar cells, occasional ciliated cells, and rarely goblet cells and glands. The middle ear mucosa has modified respiratory mucosa, and the nonciliated cell is the principal secretory cell of the middle ear. In its most active secretory phase, the nonciliated cell has the cytological characteristics of a goblet cell.

5. Auditory Tube = Eustachian Tube = Pharyngotympanic Tube
   a. One-third of the eustachian tube nearest the ear is bony. Two-thirds nearest the nasopharynx are cartilaginous. Elastic cartilage, except where bone meets cartilage (the isthmus), where there is hyaline cartilage. Cartilage runs mostly medially, but a superolateral ridge of cartilage gives a shepherd's crook appearance in cross-section. There is fat adjacent to the open portion of the cartilaginous eustachian tube.
   b. Mucous membrane, thin, low columnar ciliated in the bony part, but abundant pseudostratified ciliated tall columnar with mucous-secreting tubuloalveolar glands and goblet cells at the pharyngeal end. Tubal tonsils (lymphoid tissue) may be found at the pharyngeal end.

## THE LABYRINTH

A membranous labyrinth filled with endolymph is suspended in perilymph within a bony labyrinth. The whole inner ear is embedded in hard bone within which are large cavity called the vestibule, the spiraling cochlea, and three semi-circular canals. The inner ear has two divisions: *acoustic* (hearing) and *vestibular* (balance).

1. *Membranous labyrinth*
   a. All parts arise from a single otic vesicle of ectodermal origin. Cochlear duct and saccus endolymphaticus are derived from the saccule; semicircular ducts are derived from the utricle. Generally, squamocuboidal epithelium. All parts are interconnected. All parts are filled with endolymph.
   b. Components: Three semicircular ducts, utricle, ductus endolymphatics, saccus endolymphaticus, saccule, ductus reuniens, and the spiraling cochlear duct ending as the cecum cupulare.

2. *Vestibule*: Through the oval window, the footplate of the stapes contacts the perilymph filling most of the vestibule. The vestibule contains the utricle, the saccule, five openings for semicircular canals, the opening for the

vestibular aqueduct, the opening to the scala vestibuli of the cochlea, and the ductus reuniens leading to the cochlear duct.

   a. *Utricle*: Oblong membranous structure, five openings to the semicircular ducts and ampullae. Sensory functions at the macula. Simple squamous epithelium except around the macula. Gives off a duct medially which joins the duct from the saccule to form the endolymphatic duct.

   b. *Saccule*: Spherical. Anterior and inferior to the utricle. Contains a macula. Gives off ductus reuniens and a small duct that joins the duct from the utricle to form the endolymphatic duct.

   c. *Maculae*: Sensory structures within the utricle and saccule. Supporting cells and hair cells similar to those described under the vestibular system. Hairs embedded in gelatinous otolithic membrane which contains otoliths—3- to 5-micron stones of calcium carbonate and protein.

   d. *Ductus endolymphaticus* (endolymphatic duct) leads through the petrous portion of the temporal bone to the saccus endolymphaticus which lies between the layers of the meninges. Squamocuboidal epithelium in the duct changes to two types of tall columnar epithelium in the sac, suggesting specialization for resorption. Cellular debris is common in the sac, but not elsewhere in the labyrinth.

3. *The vestibular system*

   a. Includes utricle (position of the head and linear acceleration) and saccule (function uncertain) and semicircular ducts.

   b. *Three semicircular ducts* called superior, posterior, and horizontal (or lateral). The nonampullated ends of the superior and posterior canals join, entering the utricle as the common crus (hence, five openings into the utricle instead of six). Sensory structures of the semicircular ducts: Epithelium of the ampulla makes a transverse ridge called the *crista ampullaris*. It is covered with sensory epithelium and bounded on either end by the planum semilunatum. The hairs are embedded in the "gelatinous" cupula (no otoliths) which fits like a saddle over the crista.

   c. *Hair cells*

     i. Type I: Flask shaped; round basal nucleus surrounded by mitochondria. Mitochondria also near surface. Enclosed in a chalice-like nerve terminal.

     ii. Type II: Simple columnar. Nuclei at various levels, but usually higher than Type I. Numerous small nerve endings: granulated (efferents) and nongranulated (afferents).

     iii. Features common to both types: 40–80, stereocilia, long microvilli, probably nonmotile. One kinocilium—a modified cilium lacking a central pair of fibrils. Hairs are constricted at base, arranged in a regular hexagonal pattern on the cell surface, according to height and varying in size from 100 micron to 1 micron. The longest hairs are next to the kinocilium, which is at one side of the cell. Complicated specialized organelles differ between Types I and II. Nerve fibers leave the cells and transverse the crista becoming the nerves of the ampullae, which combine with each other and the nerves of the utricle and saccule to form the vestibular division of the eighth cranial nerve.

4. *Cochlea*: The acoustic system. Bony spiral anteromedial to the vestibule. Makes 2 and 3/4 turns around its axis, the modiolus. The curvature of the cochlea, rather than its size, is correlated with the low-frequency hearing limit in numerous mammals. Only mammals have spiral-shaped cochleae. Low-frequency hearing limit varies with the ratio of the radius of the curvature of the cochlea's base to the curvature of its apex. Ratios in different species vary from about two to about nine. The greater the ratio, the lower the frequency the animal can hear. Implications for humans remain to be clarified, but it appears likely that this information should be useful in understanding hearing problems in patients with cochlear malformations, for example, as well as other hearing variations among people.

   a. *Modiolus*: Conical pillar of porous bone containing blood vessels, nerve bundles of the cochlear division of VIII, spiral ganglia. Its base is the deep end of the internal acoustic meatus.

b. *Spiral lamina* divides the cochlear spiral into upper and lower compartments meeting at the apex as the helicotrema. Spiral lamina itself is divided into two sections.

   i. *Osseous spiral lamina* (medial, with respect to the modiolus). Carries blood vessels, myelinated nerves. Spiral limbus at its lateral lip is the site of attachment for Reissner's membrane and the area where the nerve fibers lose their myelin.

   ii. *Membranous spiral lamina* or *basilar membrane* contains the *organ of Corti.* Lateral attachment to the bony spiral is a thickening of periosteum called the spiral ligament (it is not a ligament).

c. From the area of the spiral ligament, arching up to the bony wall of the cochlea, are the spiral prominence and the *stria vascularis.* At the top of the stria, Reissner's membrane (the vestibular membrane) originates and courses diagonally down to join the spiral osseous lamina the medial border of the spiral limbus.

d. *Reissner's membrane*: Differentiated cells probably for fluid and electrolyte transport. Divides the compartment above the spiral lamina in two. The upper part communicates with the perilymphatic space of the vestibule and is called *scala vestibuli.* The lower division of the upper compartment is the *scala media.* It is filled with endolymph and connects via the ductus reuniens with the saccule. The compartment below the spiral lamina is the scala tympani, a perilymphatic space that meets the scale vestibuli at the helicotrema and leads basally to the round window (covered by the secondary tympanic membrane, hence scala tympani) and to the cochlear aqueduct, which connects the perilymphatic space with the posterior cranial fossa.

e. *Stria vascularis*: There are at least two cell types. Basal cells with few mitochondria, but numerous ascending processes which separate marginal cells. Marginal cells, with smooth convex free surface, but basally, labyrinthine infoldings of plasmalemma containing many mitochondria. Abundant capillaries throughout.

f. Spiral prominence is continuous with epithelium of stria vascularis superiorly. Inferiorly, it reflected from the wall onto the basilar membrane, forming the external spiral sulcus. Over the basilar membrane, the cells become cuboidal cells of Claudius. In parts of the basal turns, cells of Boettcher come between the basilar membrane and cells of Claudius.

g. *Organ of Corti*: The organ of hearing. Supporting cells and hair cells.

   i. *Supporting cells*: Tall, slender cells extending from basilar membrane to free surface. Upper surfaces are in contact with each other forming, with the upper surfaces of hair cells, the reticular lamina (reticular membrane). Pillar cells form the inner tunnel, through which nerves cross to the outer hair cells. Hensen's cells, Deiters cells, and the outer row of outer hair cells form the outer tunnel or space of Nuel. The arch formed by the pillars overlies the zona arcuata of the basilar membrane. Laterally, the membrane continues as the zona pectinata containing "auditory strings." Inner phalangeal cells support inner hair cells and some nerve fibers. Deiters cells support outer hair cells, enclosing the nerve endings around the base of the hair cells, and giving off finger-like processes which surface about three cells away to join the reticular lamina. Border cells are also supporting cells.

   ii. Hair cells: *Inner hair cells* form a single row and resemble vestibular Type I cells, somewhat. Similar hairs. No kinocilium, but basal body persists. Hairs arranged in a W-pattern. Mitochondria under the terminal web and at the base of the cells. Granular and nongranular nerve endings on base of cell. Inner hair cells receive 90–95% of all nerve endings. *Outer hair cells* generally form three rows, but may be five rows near basal end. Highly specialized. Nerve endings as on inner hair cells. No kinocilium. More rows of hairs, and they are long toward the periphery and short in the center of the cells. Dense lipid-like inclusions, convoluted granular endoplasmic reticulum, and some mitochondria below terminal web. Mitochondria at base and alongside parallel to plasmalemma. Outer hair cells receive only 5%–10% of nerve endings.

iii. Sound amplification occurs in the inner ear as well as through the mechanical mechanisms of the outer and middle ears. There are two theories as to how the outer hair cells amplify sound as they transform sound into electrical signals. The stereociliary motility theory posits that amplification occurs because of vibrations of bundles of cilia extending from the outer hair cells. The somatic motility theory suggests that the signal is amplified by a protein called prestin embedded in the hair cell membrane and powered by voltage within the membrane that is produced by mechanical sound vibrations.

h. Spiral limbus is the inner edge of scala media. Overhangs inner spiral sulcus. Auditory teeth of Huschke (collagenous fibers). Uniformly spaced between teeth on upper margin are interdental cells which secrete the tectorial membrane.

i. *Tectorial membrane*: Highly organized protein, fibrous, cellular structure. Overlies hairs like a cuticle. Hair marks detectable.

j. Nerves

i. Direct myelinated acoustic fibers radiate from spiral ganglia bipolar cells to nearest part of Corti's organ. Spiral fibers are thicker and fewer than direct. Spiral fibers go radially toward organ of Corti but turn and follow a spiral course. Inner spiral bundle, spiral tunnel bundle, and outer spiral bundle.

ii. The simple processes from the spiral ganglion cells synapse in the cochlear nucleus. Axons from the cochlear nucleus cross the midline in the dorsal and intermediate acoustic striae and the trapezoid body. Trapezoid body fibers continue to the superior olivary nucleus which receive ipsilateral and contralateral cochlear input. Cochlear and superior olivary axons ascend in the lateral lemniscus. Some synapse in the nuclei of the lateral lemniscus and cross through Crobst's commissure. Lateral lemniscus fibers eventually synapse in the inferior colliculus. Inferior colliculus axons course to the medial geniculate nucleus of the thalamus. Thalamic cells project homolaterally to the primary auditory cortex in the superior temporal gyrus (Brodmann's area 41 and 42).

k. *Blood vessels of the cochlea*

i. Vestibulocochlear artery is the lowest part of first cochlear turn.

ii. Cochlear artery proper penetrates modiolus. Its branches spiral to apex as the spiral tract. Supplies spiral ganglia and inner parts of the basilar membrane in arcades in the tympanic cover layer under the inner tunnel and the limbus. Stria vascularis and spiral ligament vessels do not communicate with vessels of the basilar membrane.

iii. Vein distribution does not follow arterial distribution. Most of the veins traverse the scale tympani.

iv. *Rationale*: Arteries are in the wall of the scala vestibuli and in the modiolus. Veins are in the scala tympanic. This distribution provides optimum damping of pulsations, protecting the ear from the sound of its own blood supply.

# Appendix II: Otopathology

This appendix is not intended to be complete. It was designed to summarize the scope of otopathology and to serve as an aid for organizing further study of the field.

Most of these notes are in brief, outline form. However, certain diseases have been discussed in some detail. They have been selected either for their special interest because of their incidence or because of difficulty finding information about them in standard reference sources. In particular, an extensive discussion of diseases of the external ear is included here because it is generally not well covered in many standard texts.

## CONGENITAL DISEASES OF THE EAR

This topic is so broad and interesting that even a modestly thorough discussion of it would more than double the size of this outline. Therefore, because it is such a specialized area, the topic is merely sketched to suggest its scope and present a few of the most common and relevant lesions. The reader is encouraged to consult other literature.

1. *Embryology of the ear (in brief)*
   a. A series of six tubercles located around the margins of the first pharyngeal or mandibular cleft develop into the auricle, and the cleft becomes the external auditory meatus.
   b. The middle ear is derived from the first and second branchial arches, for the most part. The malleus and incus are from the first branchial arch (Meckel's cartilage), from which the mandible is also derived.
   c. Most of the stapes, except for the vestibular wall of the footplate, is derived from the second branchial arch (Reichert's cartilage) as is the tympanic portion of the facial canal.
   d. The vestibular aspect of the footplate is from a differentiation of the otocyst called the lamina stapedialis which is at first continuous with the rest of the otic capsule but later differentiates into the annular ligament.
      i. Otic vesicles in the ectoderm form as invaginations of the otic placodes.
      ii. The otic vesicles or otocysts develop into a ventral component which gives rise to the saccule and the cochlear duct, and a dorsal part which forms the utricle, semicircular canals, and the endolymphatic duct.
      iii. These comprise the membranous labyrinth. They are imbedded in mesenchyme which develops into the bony labyrinth.

2. *Malformations of the external and middle ear*: External and middle ear deformities may occur separately, but often they are associated.
   a. *Primarily outer ear*: Aplasia (also middle ear, often), absence of part of an ear, asymmetry of the ears, polyotia, microtia, macrotia, Macacus ear (helix points up), Satyr ear (helix is pointed and retains the Darwinian tubercle), abnormal protrusion, drooping roll or dog ear, malposition or malrotation, adhesions, atresia of membranous or osseous canal, cleft lobule, fistula auris (defective closure of the first branchial cleft), supernumerary auricle, Darwinian tubercle (local thickening on the upper posterior border of the helix).

b. Middle ear anomalies, continued. In addition to the preceding list, note there can be complete agenesis of the middle ear.

   i. Important ossicular malformations include congenital fixation of the stapes (failure of differentiation of the lamina stapedialis), ossicular absence, and monopolar stapes.

   ii. Middle ear anomalies with unknown etiology, without associated anomalies, include entities such as abnormally positioned facial nerve, ossicular abnormalities, mal-positioned carotid artery, congenital absence of the oval of round window, persistent stapedial artery, internal carotid artery aneurysm, high jugular bulb, and congenital absence of the stapedial muscle and tendon. Middle ear anomalies with unknown etiology but with associated **anomalies** include some ossicular malformations, congenital cholesteatoma (associated with branchial arch anomalies), and anomalies associated with Trisomy 18, Trisomy 13, and Trisomy 15.

   iii. There are numerous middle ear anomalies of genetic origin. Some have no associated anomalies such as otosclerosis.

c. Middle ear anomalies may be associated with branchial arch anomalies and others.

   i. With branchial arch anomalies
     A. Atresia auris congenita
     B. Cleft palate, micrognathia, and glossoptosis
     C. Mandibulofacial dysostosis
     D. Mixed hearing loss, low-set malformed ear, and mental retardation

   ii. With skeletal anomalies
     A. Active phalosyndactylia
     B. Brevicollis
     C. Craniofacial dysostosis
     D. Craniometaphyseal dysplasia
     E. Dominant proximal Symphalangus and hearing loss
     F. Knuckle pads, leukonychia, and deafness
     G. Oral-facial-digital Syndrome 11
     H. Osteitis deformans
     I. Osteogenesis imperfecta
     J. Osteopetrosis
     K. Otopalatodigital syndrome

   iii. With cardiac anomalies
     A. Congenital heart disease, deafness, and skeletal malformation

   iv. With renal anomalies
     A. Recessive renal, genital, and middle ear anomalies

   v. With connective tissue anomalies
     A. Achondroplasia
     B. Hurler's syndrome

   vi. With ophthalmologic anomalies
     A. Congenital facial diplegia
     B. Duane's retraction syndrome

   vii. And with other abnormalities
     A. Chemodectoma of middle ear
     B. Histiocytosis
      *Note*: Inner ear anomalies can also be associated with prenatal infection (congenital syphilis and congenital rubella syndrome) and iatrogenic ototoxicity (thalidomide).

d. *Middle ear anomalies without associated anomalies.*

   i. Aberrant facial nerve
   ii. Anomalies of ossicles
   iii. Anomalous internal carotid artery in middle ear
   iv. Congenital absence of oval window
   v. Congenital absence of round window
   vi. Congenital absence of stapedial muscle and tendon
   vii. High jugular bulb
   viii. Internal carotid artery aneurysm
   ix. Persistent stapedial artery

e. *Middle ear anomalies with other associated anomalies.*

   i. With branchial arch anomalies
     A. Congenital cholesteatoma of middle ear
     B. Ossicular malformations

   ii. With chromosomal abnormalities
     A. Gonadal aplasia
     B. Trisomy 13–15 syndrome
     C. Trisomy 18 syndrome

f. *Anomalies of the inner ear.*

   i. Five recognized groups:
     A. (1) *Michel*: Complete absence of the inner ear.

B. (2) *Bing-Siebenmann*: Osseous labyrinth is normal, basilar membrane is deformed, as are the organ of Corti and the spiral ganglion and some of the membranous vestibular labyrinth.

C. (3) *Mondini*: Cochlea flattened from base to apex; lack of interscalar septum between middle and endolymphatic duct is dilated. Organ of Corti atrophic in some areas. Spiral ganglion may have reduced numbers of cells. Semicircular canals are usually normal.

D. (4) *Scheibe*: Most common; osseous labyrinth normal. Reissner's membrane distended. Saccule may be dilated. Organ of Corti, stria vascularis, and macula of the saccule are somewhat atrophic. Spiral ganglion is lacking.

E. (5) Michel and Mondini are present before birth; Bing-Siebenmann and Scheibe may occur after birth. *Note*: See below for Mondini–Alexander types.

g. Hereditary sensorineural deafness (see Chapter 13 and other topics below in this Appendix).

3. Other congenital disease
   a. *Congenital cholesteatoma*:
      i. Originates from epidermis.
      ii. Rests deposited in the temporal bone during development.
      iii. Detected by damage to facial nerve or ossicles.
      iv. Smooth, pearl-like surface, grossly and histologically like acquired cholesteatoma see acquired middle ear diseases.
   b. *Congenital cysts and tumors*: In addition to preauricular cysts and fistula, may see dermoid, hemangioma and lymphangioma, in the external ear.
   c. *Mondini–Alexander type*: Anomalies of cochlear and vestibular divisions. Varying degrees of aplasia, usually incomplete spiral lamina. Dysplastic cochlear duct. Often anomalies of semicircular canals. Otic capsule boney abnormalities.

d. Manifestations of retrocochlear disease (see other literature and Chapter 10 in this book).

e. *Otosclerosis*: Hereditary, but not truly congenital.

f. *Acquired congenital deafness*: Thalidomide, chloroquine, other drugs, Rubella, encephalitis especially due to chicken pox virus, erythroblastosis fetalis, anoxia, hypoxia, and prematurity.

4. Diseases with middle ear anomalies
5. Dominant hereditary sensorineural deafness
   a. Hereditary sensorineural hearing loss without associated abnormalities.
6. Hearing loss and inborn errors of metabolism
   a. Schaeffer's syndrome, Treacher Collins (TC) syndrome, and Waardenburg's syndrome
7. Hearing loss in renal abnormalities
   a. Alport syndrome and Herrmann's syndrome
   b. Muckle–Wells syndrome
8. Hearing loss and ectodermal abnormality
   a. von Recklinghausen's disease
9. Hearing loss and degenerative neurological disease
   a. Huntington's chorea
10. Recessive hereditary sensorineural hearing loss.
    a. Hereditary recessive sensorineural hearing loss without associated abnormality.
    b. Recessive hereditary hearing loss and inborn errors of metabolism.
    c. Albinism and hearing loss, Hurler's syndrome; Morquio's disease, onychodystrophy, Tay–Sachs disease, and Wilson's disease.
11. Hearing loss and degenerative neurological disease
    a. Friedreich's ataxia, Schilder's disease, and Unverricht's epilepsy
12. Hearing loss and heart disease
    a. Jervell's and Lange–Nielsen syndrome
    b. Lewis's syndrome
13. Hearing loss in endocrine disease
    a. Pendred's syndrome
14. Hearing loss and ophthalmologic disease
    a. Alström's syndrome
    b. Cokayne's syndrome
    c. Norrie's disease
    d. Usher's syndrome

## ACQUIRED DISEASES OF THE EAR

*External ear*

1. Diseases of unknown etiology
   a. *Malfunction of skin glands*
      i. *Seborrheic dermatitis*: Erythematous, greasy, scaly eruption which flakes. Usually associated with seborrhea of scalp. Frequent secondary changes imposed by excoriations: crusting, inflamed, and weeping. May be difficult to distinguish from contact dermatitis and streptococcal dermatitis.
      ii. *Diffuse external otitis*: discussed under Gram-negative organisms.
      iii. *Asteatosis*: Dry ear. Deficiency of sebaceous secretion. May be iatrogenic. May occur with eczema or ichthyosis and seen frequently in old age.
      iv. Infantile eczema
         A. *Infantile intertrigo*:
            - Small children.
            - Lobule and post-auricular sulcus.
            - Bilateral and symmetrical.
            - Erythematous and scaly with vesicular or vesico-pustular border.
            - Itching.
            - Secondary infection.
            - Psoriasis often underlying. If due to Candida, more pinkish and glazed and more extensive.
         B. *Infantile dermatitis*:
            - Irritation without involvement of the auricle of other exposed skin (although skin may be involved at times).
            - No edema or adenopathy.
            - Itching.
            - Dry crusted debris at the entrance of the auditory canal.
            - Soft, pale yellowish, moist fetid secretion fills the canal.
            - Cultures often show corynebacterium diphtheriae.

      v. *Membranous external otitis*:
         A. Rare.
         B. Meatal skin swollen, gray, and wrinkled.
         C. May be seropurulent discharge, marked discomfort.
         D. After 5–7 days, fibrinous membrane can separate as a complete cast of the meatus.
         E. Improves in 2–3 days, no consistent flora.
      vi. *Chronic idiopathic myringitis*:
         A. Usually myringitis is a manifestation of disease of the meatus, middle ear, or mastoid.
         B. Persistent changes may include chronic infection, superficial ulceration, or low-grade suppuration, all limited to the tympanic membrane (TM).
         C. Cultures often show micrococci and Gram-negative organisms such as *Aerobacter*.
      vii. *Hyperceruminosis*: Usually apparent "wax formers" do not extrude wax easily because of anatomy of the meatus. May be due to rapid cerumen formation.
   b. *Miscellaneous*
      i. *Lupus erythematosus*:
         A. *Chronic discoid*:
            - Erythematous, circumscribed lesions with firm adherent scale.
            - Pigmentation and atrophy.
            - Ear is frequently involved, especially the lobule and concha.
         B. *Systemic*: Diagnosis in usual manner.
      ii. *Psoriasis*: Superficial, pink lesions, with mica-like scale. Usually also on scalp, elbows, knees, and nails. Not as greasy as seborrhea and there is a greater tendency to form circumscribed plaques.
      iii. *Lichen planus*: Annular and linear patches of flat, lilac-colored, angulated papules. Dry and shiny. Scale. Trunk and flexor surfaces of the extremities. Mucous membranes in 25%.
      iv. *Pemphigus*: Lethal. Large flaccid bullae from noninflamed bases on the skin and mucous membranes. Occasionally seen on the ears.

2. Infections
  a. *Bacteria*
    i. Gram positive
      A. *Furunculosis*: Hair infection. *Staphylococcus*.
      B. *Impetigo*: *Staphylococcus* (*Staph.*), *Streptococcus* (*Strep.*), or both.
      C. *Pyoderma*: Deep, boggy, frequently follow trauma. Usually, (*Staph.*).
      D. *Ecthyma*: Infrequent in ear. Inflammatory. May lead to scarring and stenosis of canal. Mixed flora.
      E. *Cellulitis*: Lymphangitis and adenopathy. Usually (*Strep.*) or (*Staph.*).
      F. *Erysipelas*: Hemolytic strep, occasionally staph pain, fever, anorexia. Warm, tender, smooth, elevated tense shining, red, indurated appearance with sharp line of demarcation. Rapid extension. May be vesicles and bullae.
    ii. Gram negative
      A. *Diffuse otitis externa*: Swimmer's ear; hot, humid weather.
        – *Preinflammatory stage*:
          . Initiated by swimming, diving, trauma.
          . Edema of stratum corneum interferes with formation of lipid cover.
          . Absence of wax.
          . Dry skin.
          . Itching.
        – *Acute inflammatory stage*:
          (i) *Mild*:
            . Pain on manipulation.
            . Edema, redness, odorless secretion, or exfoliated debris.
            . Some luster of drum.
          (ii) *Moderate*:
            . Lumen partially occluded.
            . Moderate periauricular edema without adenopathy, obliteration of canal, gray or green seropurulent secretions, and exfoliated debris.
            . Small pustules appear.
          . Infecting organism in all of the above is usually Gram negative but may be fungal.
        – Chronic *inflammatory stage*:
          . Thickening of the skin.
          . Dry, adherent debris.
          . Secretion may be present, gray-brown, or greenish with a fetid odor.
          . Usually Gram negative, rarely fungal.
      B. *Hemorrhagic or Bullous external otitis*: No preceding URI. Sudden onset of severe pain. Later bloody discharge, without pain. Hemorrhagic bullae on meatal wall. TM is normal.
      C. *Otitis externa granulosis*: Skin raw and coated with scanty, creamy pus, and granulations. Peculiar stalk nature of the granulations. Usually antecedent neglected otitis externa.
      D. *Perichondritis*: May follow infection, trauma including surgery and temperature. Auricular cartilage becomes warm, soft, reddish, and thickened. Pus between the cartilage and perichondrium interferes with nourishment. Deformity is a common sequel. Cauliflower ear.
    iii. Acid fast
      A. *Tuberculosis* (*TB*): Lupus vulgaris, apple jelly nodules. Less common: TB of skin; TB of subcutaneous tissues.
      B. *Leprosy*: Auricle becomes infiltrated, nodular, and enlarged.
  b. *Fungi and yeasts*
    i. Saprophytic
      A. Aspergillaceae, Mucoraceae, yeast-like fungi, dermatophytes, Actinomycetaceae and miscellaneous fungi
        – Chronic or recurrent.
        – Tropical climates.
        – Itching and fullness, and there may be pain, deafness, and tinnitus in severe cases.

- Moist cerumen with exfoliated scales, sheets of epithelium.
- Canal may be line with structure like those on culture media.
  B. *Aspergillus niger*: Skin of osseous meatus and TM covered velvety gray membrane with black spots.
  ii. Pathogenic
     A. *Superficial*: Candida albicans and others.
     B. *Deep*: Blastomycosis, actinomycosis, and sporotrichosis. Should be thought of with granulomatous lesion of the canal.
  c. *Virus*
     i. *Bullous myringitis*: Associated with URI. Acute vesicular or hemorrhagic bullae of the TM and adjacent canal. Sudden severe pain, relieved by rupturing blebs.
     ii. *Herpes simplex*: Vesicles usually also on lips.
     iii. *Herpes zoster*: Unilateral. Tense vesicles following course of cutaneous nerve.
     iv. *Molluscum contagiosum*: Usually children. One or more small, circumscribed raised, waxy nodules with central umbilication.
     v. *Variola and varicella*: Pustular vesicles as elsewhere.
  d. *Protozoa*
     i. *Syphilis*: Primary, secondary, and tertiary.
     ii. *Yaws*: Treponema pertenue. Clinically resembles syphilis, although not as serious. Indigenous to tropics.
  e. *Animal parasites*
     i. *Pediculosis*: Edematous, red papules, may have central punctate from proboscis. Sometimes vesicles and bullae.
     ii. *Scabies*: Itching, excoriated papules, and burrows. Ear lesions usually in children. Acarus scabiei.
3. Neurogenic eruptions
  a. *Simple pruritus*: Predominantly middle-aged women, tense, hyperactive. No gross lesions. Must rule out contact dermatitis, diabetes, jaundice, nephritis, bloody dyscrasias and dry skin, as well as other causes.

  b. *Neurodermatitis*
     i. *Localized*: Lichen chronicus simplex, excoriated, scaly, dry patches, more sharply circumscribed than in seborrhea. Neck, eyelids, antecubital, and popliteal areas, and ankles.
     ii. *Disseminated*: Lesions as above, but wider distribution. Frequently psychogenic. Rule out atopic dermatitis.
  c. Neurotic excoriations
  d. *Artifact dermatitis (malingering)*: Do not follow natural forms. Are usually discrete, inflamed, crusted, and ulcerated; different geometric appearances.
4. Allergic dermatoses
  a. *Contact dermatitis*: Suspect ear medicines, cosmetics, hair spray, eyeglass temples (nickel), telephone receivers, perfumes, and earrings.
  b. *Atopic dermatitis*: Associated with dermatitis of eyelids, face, neck, popliteal, and cubital fossae. History of other allergic disease such as asthma and hay fever. Family history common.
  c. *Drug eruptions*: Any morphological form. Usually, other parts of body also affected.
  d. *Infectious eczematoid dermatitis*: Adjacent focus of infection discharges and sensitizes skin leading to this condition.
  e. *Physical allergy*: Exposure to cold, heat, pressure, ultraviolet (UV) rays, or visible rays may result in urticaria or erythema. Mechanism may be a true antigen antibody reaction against protein altered by the physical agent, or it may actually be another mechanism of response to trauma.
5. Traumatic lesions
  a. *Contusions and lacerations*
     i. Traumatic
     ii. *Chondrodermatitis nodularis chronica helicis*: Harmless, common in telephonists, soldiers, nuns, and physicians. Hard, small immovable nodule surrounded by a hyperemic abscessed area on the helix.
  b. Surgical incisions
  c. *Hemorrhages*
     i. *Hematoma*: Between cartilage and perichondrium secondary to trauma;

may result in cauliflower. Hemorrhages into skin of canal may occur secondary to base of skull and osseous meatus fracture.

  ii. *Vesicles and bullae*: Follow manipulation.

d. Burns

e. *Frostbite*: Common site.

f. *Radiation injury*

  i. UV

  ii. *Roentgen rays*: Auricle is said to be able to tolerate up to 600 R.

g. *Chemical*: Acids and alkalis. Medicines used in excessive strengths.

6. Senile changes

a. Thinning of the epidermis, loss of elasticity, freckling and dryness, and pruritus. Keratoses.

b. Indolent ulcer, usually in one ear. Mild discomfort and pain, slight discharge, and foul odor. Granulations in circumscribed area of osseous canal. Exposed bone in midst of ulcer. Differentiate from malignancy.

7. Vitamin dyscrasias

a. *Vitamin A*: Dry skin, scaly small follicular papules.

b. *Vitamin B*: Pellagra occasionally involving ears.

c. *Vitamin C*: Scurvy with subsequent acanthosis and hyperkeratosis.

8. Endocrine dyscrasias

a. *Hypothyroidism*: Pale, sallow, greasy skin varying to cold, thick dry, and scaly skin.

b. *Hyperthyroidism*: Warm, moist thin, and translucent skin.

c. *Addison's disease*: Soft and bronzed skin, pigmentation associated with pigmentation elsewhere.

9. *Foreign bodies*: Vegetable, animal, and mineral.

10. Otalgia (see other literature)

11. Tumors

a. *Benign cysts*

  i. *Pseudocysts*: Fluid in tissue space without epithelial lining.

  ii. *Sebaceous cyst*: Common around the auricle, especially in the post-auricular crease.

  iii. *Preauricular cysts*: See congenital diseases.

  iv. *Incisional cyst or epidermal implantation cyst*: Due to implantation of squamous epithelium into subcutaneous tissue. Secretions are from sweat or sebaceous glands implanted.

  v. *Dermoid cyst*: See congenital diseases.

b. *Benign tumors*

  i. See congenital diseases.

  ii. *Papilloma*: Rare in the external canal and even less common on the auricle.

  iii. Keratosis obturans or cholesteatoma of the external auditory meatus is rare. Desquamating squamous epithelial mass is found deep in the canal. Frequently associated with bronchiectasis and sinusitis. Cause unknown. Pain. Sometimes deafness and otorrhea.

  iv. Osteoma or hyperostosis

    A. *Exostosis*:

      – Most common tumor of the external canal.

      – Much more common in males.

      – Usually, bilateral.

      – Most common in saltwater swimmers.

      – Covered by skin.

      – Attached by broad base to osseous canal.

      – Usually, asymptomatic.

    B. *Osteoma*:

      – Single cancellous osteoma is relatively rare.

      – Hearing loss and discomfort common.

      – Will continue to grow.

  v. *Adenoma*: Rare; glandular. Originate from sebaceous glands in the outer part of the canal. Small, soft, and painless.

  vi. *Ceruminoma (Hidradenoma, sweat gland tumor)*: Uncommon. Smooth, polypoid swelling. Local recurrence and malignant change are common.

  vii. *Chondrodermatitis nodularis chronica helicis*: Discussed earlier.

  viii. *Chondroma*: Rare lesion of the auricle, usually associated with trauma. Enchondromas are cartilaginous spicules in the external canal which continue to grow.

    ix. *Lipoma*: Extremely rare on the ear.

    x. *Fibroma*: Very rare. Two types: soft and hard.

    xi. *Keloid*: Connective tissue hypertrophy, scar-like tumor. Commonly on lobule secondary to earring.

    xii. *Xanthoma*: Not a true neoplasm but may resemble one. Diseases associated with a disturbance in cholesterol metabolism.

    xiii. *Myoma*: Striated muscle, extrinsic muscles of the ear. Smooth muscle, arrectores pilorum, or muscular coats of vessels. Extremely rare.

    xiv. *Mixed salivary gland tumors*: Rare. Moveable masses tightly related to overlying skin. Ectodermal origin.

    xv. *Melanoma*: Fairly common. Usually intradermal (common mole).

c. *Malignant tumors*

    i. Incidence

      A. Approximately 90% of all skin cancers occur in the head and neck, and 6% of all skin cancers occur on the ear.

      B. The majority are on the helix and antihelix.

      C. Squamous cell is most common, then basal cell. Approximately 80%–85% of aural cancers involve the auricle, 10%–15% involve the canal, and 5%–10% involve the middle ear.

    ii. Malignant tumors of the auricle

      A. *Squamous cell carcinoma*: Grows slowly, metastasizes late. Small lesions on the helix or antihelix have excellent prognosis. Near the cartilaginous canal, much poorer.

      B. *Endothelioma*: Perivascular origin, much slower than Epi.

      C. *Basal cell*: Men more than women. Fifth or sixth decade. Locally malignant, but slow growing and does not usually metastasize. Rodent ulcer.

      D. Cylindroma, adenocarcinoma, sarcoma, and malignant melanoma are rare on the auricle, but do occur.

    iii. Malignant tumors of the external auditory canal

Serious disease. Pain, otorrhea, bleeding, fullness, and decreased hearing may all be symptoms. Urgent to diagnosis early.

    A. *Squamous cell*:
- 70% of all canal malignancies.
- First nodes are usually pretragal.
- Distant metastases are rare.
- Death is from local extension.

    B. *Basal cell*: Rarer than on auricle, but prognosis worse because of late discovery and invasion of bone and middle ear.

    C. *Adenocarcinoma*:
- Least common.
- Arises from sweat or sebaceous glands.

    D. *Cylindroma and adenoid cystic epithelium*:
- Not common.
- It is an adenocarcinoma arising from the ceruminous glands.
- Fifth decade of life.
- Slow growth.
- Pain becomes extremely severe.
- Bony destruction.
- Yellow firm, smooth masses in the canal.
- Distant metastasis late to pulmonary cervical nodes and kidneys.

    E. *Sarcoma*:
- Mesoblastic origin.
- Extremely rare, but in the ear, one sees chondrosarcoma, fibrosarcoma, osteosarcoma, lymphosarcoma, rhabdomyosarcoma, leiomyosarcoma, and undifferentiated cylindrical cell type sarcoma.
- Prognosis relates to site and differentiation, but they metastasize early, and the outlook is usually not good.

    F. *Malignant melanoma*:
- Extremely rare.
- Prognosis is guarded as elsewhere with this lesion.

iv. Addition to diseases of the auditory canal
   A. *Stenosis of ear canal*:
      – Traumatic, postoperative, or congenital.
      – Collapse of ear canal.

# DISEASES OF THE TYMPANIC MEMBRANE

1. Many of the diseases of the external ear may involve the drum. See preceding discussion.
2. *Infection of middle ear reflected in the drum.*
   a. *Acute suppurative otitis media*
      i. Pain, fullness, and congestion of vessels.
      ii. Hyperemia, exudation, suppuration following rupture.
      iii. Resolution with desquamation, closer of perforation.
   b. *Acute viral otitis media*
      i. Minimal findings, associated with blocked eustachian tube.
      ii. *Bullous myringitis*:
         A. Severe pain without fever or hearing loss.
         B. Epidemics.
         C. Multiple blebs in drum and canal.
   c. *Acute necrotizing otitis media*
      i. Bacterial, usually beta-hemolytic strep.
      ii. Areas of poorest blood supply (kidney-shaped center of the pars tensa) affected first.
      iii. True necrosis.
   d. Tuberculous otitis media usually secondary to primary TB spread through eustachian tube. Cloudy exudate, continued drainage. Pain is rare.
   e. *Non-TB chronic otitis media*:
      i. Can result from persistent perforation, bone destruction, inflammation, cholesterol, granuloma, cholesteatoma, allergy, and dermatitis.
      ii. When behavior or response to treatment is atypical, must consider chloroma, lupus, malignant otitis externa, or granulomatosis disease such as Wegener's of histiocytosis X.

3. *Tympanosclerosis*:
   a. Benign; result of repeated infection.
   b. Not invasive. Tunica propria of the mucous membrane of the middle ear and TM becomes edematous and infiltrated with inflammatory cells during acute infections.
   c. Repeated recurrence leads to invasion by fibroblasts and organization of tunica propria into thick collagenous connective tissue.
   d. Hyaline degeneration results in smooth, white, slightly raised areas of dense tissue.
   e. Calcification may occur. In middle ear, ossicles may be fixed.
   f. Chalky, white patches are seen in the TM.
4. *Traumatic perforations*: Compression; instrumentation; burns or caustic agents; blasts 90% heal spontaneously, usually within a month.
5. *Chronic granular myringitis*: Itching, otorrhea, and hearing loss. Replacement of the squamous layer by proliferating granulation tissue. Rare.
6. *Keratosis obturans*: Ear canal cholesteatoma. See external auditory canal discussion.
7. *Chronic adhesive otitis media*: Late sequel of chronic otitis media, middle layers of drum destroyed.
8. *TM in chronic otitis media*: Destruction of drum, partial (fibrous layers), or complete. Retraction perforation, cholesteatoma.

# DISEASES OF EUSTACHIAN TUBE

See other standard otolaryngologic literature.

# DISEASES OF THE FACIAL NERVE

Bell's palsy, facial palsy (inflammatory, traumatic, and herpetic), and Ramsey–Hunt syndrome. Facial nerve tic, hemifacial spasm, and facial nerve neuroma.

# DISEASES OF THE MIDDLE EAR

1. Middle ear effusions
   a. *Etiologies*:
      i. Adenoid hypertrophy, cleft palate, barotrauma, and tumors (especially unilateral effusion in adult).

ii. High incidence of nasopharyngeal carcinoma (especially in Cantonese), inflammation and antibiotics, allergy, iatrogenic (inadequate antibiotic therapy, radiation therapy, trauma especially to the torus during adenoidectomy), other causes (viral, immune, etc.).

b. *Classification of middle ear fluids*: Serous, mucoid, bloody, and purulent.

c. *Symptoms*: Plugged up feeling, conductive hearing loss, autophony, often pain, often history of URI.

d. *Findings*: Opaque or amber drum, creamy colored drum, retraction (or bulging) of drum, fluid level or bubbles, and blue drum.

e. *Sequelae*: Atrophic TM, ossicular erosion, tympanosclerosis, cholesterol granuloma and gland formation, chronic otitis media, and cholesteatoma.

2. Acute otitis media and mastoiditis

a. *Types*

i. *Acute bacterial*:

A. Usually, acute middle ear infection.

B. *Haemophilus influenzae* (rare in patients > 5 years old), *pneumococci*, and β-*hemolytic streptococci* are most common.

C. *Staphylococcus aureus* occasionally; also, pseudomonas aeruginosa.

D. Self-limited diseases.

E. Bulging drum. About 1%–5% will become chronic and may erode bone and lead to extradural or perisinus abscess or a subperiosteal abscess, leptomeningitis, sigmoid sinus thrombophlebitis, brain abscess, suppurative labyrinthitis, petrositis, or facial nerve palsy.

ii. *Acute necrotic otitis media*:

A. Chiefly in children severely ill with exanthem or other systemic infection.

B. Rare.

C. Usually β-*hemolytic streptococci*.

D. Necrosis or localized gangrene.

E. Virulent because of impaired host resistance.

F. Requires treatment.

iii. *Acute viral myringitis*: Normal hearing and absence of significant fever.

b. *Malignant otitis externa*:

i. In diabetics, granuloma rises from floor of external.

ii. Canal at bony cartilaginous junction.

iii. Pain out of proportion.

iv. Poor response to prescription.

v. Not a cancer.

vi. *Pseudomonas aeruginosa*.

vii. Severe destruction of middle ear and temporal bone.

viii. Gangrene, may lead to facial paralysis, death.

3. Chronic otitis media and mastoiditis

a. *Types*: Allergic secretory; suppurative, benign mucosal type; tubercular; suppurative with osteitis or osteomyelitis; suppurative with cholesteatoma.

b. *Bacteriology*: Usually (in order) *S. aureus* (32%), *Bacterium proteus, Pseudomonas pyocyanea, S. aureus* penicillin resistant, mixed, *E. coli, Streptococcus pyogenes, St. viridans*, and pneumoniae (5%). No growth in 10.6%.

c. *Location*: Chronic infection in ciliated columnar areas is usually confined to the mucosa. In flat pavement epithelium of the attic and antrum, it is in association with erosion of bone and requires more vigorous attention.

d. *Tubotympanic disease*: Permanent perforation syndrome; persistent tubotympanic mucosal infection.

e. *Attic and antrum disease*

i. Occlusion of the attic floor by a chronic process limited to the anterior and posterior tympanic isthmuses.

ii. *Cholesteatoma*: Congenital—see congenital disease.

A. *Primarily acquired*: Squamous epithelial cyst that arises in the pars flaccida and gradually invades the epitympanum, aditus, and middle ear. Possibly an extension of rete pegs into unresolved mesenchyme in early life. Origin not visible by otoscopy. Conductive hearing loss due to immobility of destruction of ossicles. Wall (matrix) produces enzymes that result in absorption of bone (not proven). Thin layer of squamous epithelium forms the wall of the cyst. Center consists of desquamated keratinizing epithelium which undergoes degeneration. Cholesterol accumulates, giving rise to misnomer. Is really an epithelioma, or keratoma. Secondary acquired—repeated infections destroy fibrous layer of drum, usually in posterior superior quadrant. Perforations from disease. Negative pressure in ear that led to infection encourages invagination of squamous tissue when perforation heals. Negative pressure causes drum to retract in posterior superior quadrant, and desquamation of the squamous epithelium fills the retraction pocket. Histology the same as primary acquired. Another theory suggests that the secondary type results directly from metaplasia of the middle ear mucosa provoked by infection. Symptoms—foul, mild otorrhea, hearing loss variable, bleeding, earache, dizziness, and headache suggestive of intracranial extension.

f. *Late middle ear sequelae*
    i. Adhesive otitis media
   ii. Tympanosclerosis
  iii. *Cholesterol granuloma*: Stasis with mucosal edema, exudation, and hemorrhage, usually blood vessels to the ossicles and along the facial canal. Blue drum. Breakdown of red cells releases cholesterol crystals which act as foreign bodies and stimulate granulation tissue. Mucosa often undergoes metaplasia becoming ciliated secretory throughout the middle ear and mastoid. Granulation tissue walls off preexisting effusion producing cysts containing cholesterol crystals. Cholesterol clefts also in granulation tissue. Macrophages, round cells, and foreign body giant cells around clefts. Fibroblasts may invade and obliterate entire middle ear space.

g. Complications of suppurative otitis media and mastoiditis facial paralysis, labyrinthitis, suppurative labyrinthitis, petrositis (Gradenigo's syndrome), meningitis, lateral sinus thrombophlebitis, extradural abscess, subdural abscess, brain abscess, and otitis hydrocephalus.

4. Postsurgical pathology: Not covered in this discussion.

5. Temporal bone fractures: Not covered.

6. Granulomas and other diseases of the ear and temporal bone
   a. Tuberculous otitis media
   b. *Syphilis*: Any syphilitic lesions (gummas, etc.) may occur in the middle or inner ears. There is a syndrome of sudden deafness associated with late congenital syphilis in children or in later years. Pathology includes marked ectasia of the cochlear duct. Corti's organ may be absent, may be bone or connective tissue in the scala media. There is some evidence that this syndrome may be reversible if the diagnosis is made rapidly. Hearing loss in ~35% of all lues cases, incidence higher in women.
   c. Polyps of various types
   d. *Histiocytosis X*
      i. Acute disseminated histiocytosis (Letterer–Siwe disease) before age of 2. Lesions in soft tissue and bone.
     ii. Chronic disseminated histiocytosis (Hand–Schuller–Christian disease). Children and young adults. Bone. Soft tissue. Juvenile xanthogranuloma is benign histiocytosis disease that may be isolated or occur in association with histiocytosis X.
    iii. Eosinophilic granuloma:
         A. Benign chronic disease.
         B. One or several bony lesions.
         C. May arise in soft tissue.
            – Temporal bone lesion in histiocytosis X expands and presents as a granuloma in the external canal and may erode the mastoid cortex, tegmen, dura, labyrinth, lateral sinus, and zygoma.
            – Secondary infection is common. Sheet-like layers of histiocytes. Occasional lymphocytes, plasma cells, and multinucleated giant cells.

e. *Wegener's Granulomatosis*:
   i. Uncommon in the ear.
   ii. Usually white male adults.
   iii. Nasal sinus or ear symptoms.
   iv. Appears severely ill out of proportion to usual nose or ear disease.
   v. Fever, facial paralysis common.
   vi. Tissue resembles closely periarteritis nodosa.
   vii. Nonspecific granuloma with many round cells and some giant cells.
   viii. Round cells are typically perivascular.
7. Tumors of the middle ear
   a. *Glomus jugulare*:
      i. Glomus bodies (solid masses of epitheloid cells) exist normally along the course of Arnold's and Jacobson's nerves and in the adventitia of the jugular bulb.
      ii. Nerves from IX and blood supply through the tympanic branch of the ascending pharyngeal artery.
      iii. Tumors enlarge concentrically.
      iv. Five times more common in women.
      v. Familial disposition.
      vi. Ten percent are multicentric.
      vii. Histopathology shows large epitheloid cells with abundant acidophilic cytoplasm, often vacuolated.
      viii. Nuclei are small and nonhyperchromatic without mitotic figures, small alveolar.
         Patterns separated by fibrous septa containing vessels. In some cases, cordlike deposition. Two kinds:c
         1. *Glomus tympanicum*: From Jacobson's nerve. Slow.
         2. *Glomus jugulare*: From jugular bulb. Sometimes very rapid spread to adjacent and intracranial structures. The are nonchromaffin paragangliomas.
   b. *Aquamous cell*: Intractable external otitis, bleeding paralysis of facial nerve, severe pain especially at night. Prognosis is poor.
   c. *Fibrosarcoma*: Transitory paralysis of the facial nerve in attacks; prolonged pain.
   d. *Neurofibroma*: Can occur on any of the nerve structures.
   e. *Giant cell tumor*: Rare in the middle ear. Usually, in long bones or temporomandibular joint (TMJ) but does occur in ear.

f. *Osteoma*: Relatively rare. Damage by expansion.
g. *Rhabdomyosarcoma*: Most common temporal bone tumor in children < 6 years. Painless otorrhea or bleeding. Prognosis poor. Four types:
   1. *Pleomorphic*: Dense cellularity of spindle-shaped cells, Multiple nuclei. Striations.
   2. *Alveolar*: Connective tissue septa. Closely applied to the inner aspect of the trabecular longitudinal and cross striations.
   3. *Embryonal*: Abundant eosinophilic cytoplasm. Long, tiny cells with bipolar processes. Enlarged around their single nuclei. Cross-striations in some.
   4. *"Tadpole cells" Botryoid*: Gross description. Rest under mucous membrane. Histology-like embryonal type.
h. *Salivary gland choristoma*: Rare. Histologically normal salivary tissue on the middle ear cleft. It is usually associated with facial and ossicular chain congenital anomalies. Tumor usually covered by pseudostratified columnar epithelium.
i. *Metastatic tumors*: In order of frequency— Mammary cancer. Renal cell cancer and bronchogenic cancer. Melanoma also reported.
j. *Tumors invading from adjacent structures*: Meningioma, gliomas, neurilemmoma, cylindroma, dermoid cyst, and tumors of the nasopharynx.
8. *Otosclerosis: Extensive literature readily available, so only a brief discussion here*
   a. *Incidence*: About 10% of the population.
      i. Females: Males are about 2:1;
      ii. *Hereditary*: Usually second-, third-, and fourth-decade presentation with conductive hearing loss.
      iii. Tinnitus often present.
      iv. Pregnancy accelerates clinical findings.
   b. Lesion may occur anywhere in the capsule, but symptoms only if stapes is fixed or if cochlea (especially the stria vascularis region) or vestibule is involved.
   c. *Two types:*
      i. *Otospongiotic*:
         A. Active

B. Multinucleated osteoclasts and osteoblasts enlarged marrow spaces.

C. No osteoclastic activity occurs in the normal otic capsule bone.

   ii. *Otosclerotic*

     A. Inactive

     B. Narrower marrow spaces with osteoblast on the walls. (Endochondral and endosteal layers.)

d. Conductive, sensorineural, or mixed loss may develop.

9. Other Labyrinth Capsule Lesions (with generalized disease)

  a. *Paget's disease*:

    i. Polyostotic or monostotic.

    ii. Often familial.

    iii. Continuous resorption and regeneration of bone.

    iv. Deformities of the normal structures.

    v. Stapes fixation less frequent than in Otosclerosis.

  b. *Osteogenisis imperfecta*: Congenita and tarda.

  c. *Late congenital syphilis*:

    i. Often a Ménière's-like syndrome.

    ii. Positive Hennebert's sign (positive fistula test with intact drum, especially with negative pressure).

    iii. Often negative or equivocal serology with negative spinal fluid serology and positive FTA.

  d. Radium-induced necrosis and carcinoma

  e. Histiocytosis X.

# DISEASES OF THE INNER EAR

This set of notes outline only a few of the major ailments of the inner ear which are especially common and/or especially exciting in terms of future advancement in managing otologic disease.

1. Diseases of the labyrinth

  a. Non-genetic sensorineural deafness in children—See other literature.

  b. *Sudden deafness*:

    i. Etiology unclear but several factors appear related in some cases:

     A. Virus, vascular, noise (special case), and pressure changes.

    B. *Symptoms*: Deafness, tinnitus, and vertigo.

    C. About one-third return to normal, one-third return partially, and one-third remain totally deaf, see Chapter 11.

  c. *Functional deafness*: Diagnosed by special audiometric tests.

  d. *Presbycusis*:

    i. Old-age deafness.

    ii. High frequencies.

    iii. Discrimination difficulties.

    iv. *According to Schuknecht, four types*:

     A. (1) Sensory (2) Neural (3) Metabolic (4) and Mechanical.

     B. Recruitment and diplacusis may be present.

  e. *Noise-induced hearing loss*: Exposure to blasts, gunfire, or other loud noises or chronic unprotected exposure to > 90 dBA daily is likely to lead to bilateral, symmetrical hearing and diplacusis may be present. A major problem in American industry.

  f. *Ototoxic drugs*:

    i. *Partial list*: Streptomycin, dihydro-streptomycin, neomycin, gentamicin, cisplatin, chloramphenicol, kanamycin, vancomycin, polymyxin B, ethacrynic acid, furosemide, salicylates, quinine, nitrogen mustard, tetanus antitoxin, and thalidomide.

    ii. *Chemicals*: Carbon monoxide, mercury, tobacco, gold, lead, arsenic, aniline dyes, and alcohol.

  g. *Labyrinthitis*: Toxic, epidemic, viral, circumscribed labyrinthitis paralabyrinthitis, labyrinthitis fistula, and perilabyrinthitis), serous labyrinthitis, suppurative (commonly hematogenic), and labyrinthine ossification.

  h. *Tinnitus*: Etiology unknown. Relation of character to lesion unreliable. Occurs with a great many lesions, see Chapter 18.

  i. *Vertigo*: Tabes dorsalis, pellagra, pernicious anemia, cerebral anoxemia, postural hypotension, paroxysmal atrial fibrillation, aortic stenosis, Adams–Stokes disease, metabolic disturbances, epilepsy, meningitis, encephalitis, syphilis, and head injury all produce non-rotational dizziness, *not true vertigo*, see Chapter 19.

- *Vertigo*: Sensation of motion.
  - *Ménière's syndrome*: Paroxysmal attacks of spinning vertigo lasting hours and accompanied by perceptive hearing loss, frequently fluctuating, usually more severe in one ear and with tinnitus and usually with a feeling of fullness. Audiogram is usually flat. Calorics are usually depressed bilaterally. Path: Endolymphatic hydrops.
  - *Postural vertigo*: Cupulolithiasis syndrome, labyrinthine circumscribed labyrinthitis, serous labyrinthitis, Lermoyez's syndrome, otosclerosis inner ear syndrome, vestibular neuronitis, and secondary endolymphatic hydrops.
2. *Disorders of the central auditory nervous system*: Brainstem, temporal lobe, and other CNS lesions
3. Otologic manifestations of retrocochlear disease
   a. Congenital diseases
   b. *Infectious*: Meningitis, Ramsay Hunt's syndrome, encephalomyelitis, neurosyphilis, and brain abscess
   c. *Neoplasms*
      i. *Childhood*: Glioma, medulloblastoma, astrocytoma, and ependymoma.
      ii. *Adult*: Subtentorial have especially definitive auditory and vestibular signs. Angle tumors may be meningioma, glioma, cholesteatoma, cyst, granuloma, metastatic, or aneurysm, but neuroma is most common.
         A. *Acoustic neuroma*:
            - More than half of all tumors of the cerebellopontine angle.
            - 9% of all intracranial tumors.
            - Usually 30- to 40-year group.
            - Usual site is Scarpa's ganglion.
            - Bilateral in cases of von Recklinghausen's disease.
            - Early symptoms are tinnitus, hearing loss, and dizziness and often a feeling of fullness.
            - Later, weakness of other nerves.
            - Sensorineural loss, poor discrimination, usually no recruitment or diplacusis, but tone decay present.
            - Usually visible on X-ray.
   d. *Vascular lesions*: Hypotension, hypertension, vertebrobasilar artery insufficiency, thrombosis of the posterior–inferior cerebellar artery, and thrombosis of the internal auditory artery
   e. *Traumatic lesions*: Cervical vertigo and skull fracture
   f. *Metabolic and drug induced*: Hormonal effects, hypervitaminosis D or Vitamin B1 def, nicotinic acid def (nystagmus in 20%), and numerous drugs
   g. *Demyelination and degenerative disease*: Multiple sclerosis, diffuse sclerosis, subacute combined degeneration, syringobulbia and syringomyelia, olivocerebellar atrophy, and Friedreich's ataxia
   h. *Idiopathic disorders*: Vestibular neuronitis and epilepsy
   i. Psychogenic disorders

## MISCELLANEOUS ADDITIONS

Tumors not mentioned that occur in the temporal bone are Ewing's sarcoma, angiosarcoma, osteogenic sarcoma, and others.

# Appendix III: Otosclerosis, Paget's disease, and osteogenesis imperfecta involving the ear

Otosclerosis, Paget's disease, and osteogenesis imperfecta may present similar clinical pictures as far as their otologic manifestations are concerned. Consequently, some older literature suggests that they may be related or, in fact, that otosclerosis is actually one of the other two diseases. It now appears clear that these three diseases are distinct entities with some clinical similarities, but quite distinct histopathologic features. There are other diseases not covered in this short discussion whose presentation and pathology allows them to be confused with the diseases discussed. The basic features of these diseases are outlined in brief.

## OTOSCLEROSIS

I. *Incidence*: About 10% of the population. Females:Males are ~2:1. Hereditary, probably autosomal dominant. Presentation after puberty, usually in second, third, or fourth decade. Pregnancy accelerates clinical picture.

II. Presentation usually with conductive hearing loss. Tinnitus often present. Lesions may occur anywhere in the human otic capsule, but symptoms occur only if stapes is fixed or if cochlear (especially in area of stria vascularis) is involved, or the area of the vestibule.

III. Two types of otosclerosis can be found: (1) *Otospongiotic-active*: Multinucleated osteoclasts and osteoblasts, enlarged marrow spaces. No osteoclastic activity occurs in the normal otic capsule. (2) *Otosclerotic-inactive*:

Narrower marrow spaces with osteoblasts on the walls.

IV. Conductive, sensorineural, or mixed hearing loss.

## PAGET'S DISEASE

I. *Incidence*: Less common than otosclerosis, but there are more subclinical than apparent cases, so the disease is more common than it appears to be. Males:Females are 4:1. Hereditary, probably autosomal dominant previously considered sex-linked recessive. Usually presents after fourth decade.

II. Often found incidentally on X-ray. When clinical, usually presents with enlarged skull. Often, progressive mixed hearing loss (interestingly, Paget's original case was hard of hearing). Skull, spine, pelvis, femur, and tibia are most often involved. May be polyostotic or monostotic. When temporal bone is involved, lesions may involve otic capsule, bone of the tympanic cavity, and occasionally the ossicles themselves.

III. The otic capsule lesions tend to involve the vascular periosteum and spare the endosteal layer and membranous labyrinth except in advanced lesions. The ossicles are usually fixed by impingement by deformed bone and spurs from their surrounding structures. The ossicles themselves may be involved and may be fixed by increased mass or, rarely, actual ankylosis. The external auditory canal may be stenosed, as by the internal canal (leading to pressure on the eighth nerve). Alkaline phosphatase is elevated. Blood is shunted to the lesions. About 1% progress to osteogenic sarcoma.

IV. Conductive, sensorineural, or mixed hearing loss.

## OSTEOGENESIS IMPERFECTA

I. *Incidence*: 1 in 25,000 births. No sex predilection. Autosomal dominant. A few reports of autosomal recessive families. Variable expressivity. Two types.

II. Osteogenesis imperfecta congenita is usually severe. Multiple fractures *in utero* or at birth. Still-born or low survival.

Osteogenesis imperfecta tarda is seen at later age. Relatively painless fractures with minor trauma. Long bones with slender shafts and abrupt widening near epiphyses. Small structure. Pectus excavatum and kyphoscoliosis are common. Hyperextensible joints and ligaments. Odontogenesis imperfecta, blue sclera. Hearing loss clinically identical to otosclerosis. Usually begins after puberty. Thirty-five percent have hearing loss by age 40 and 50% by age 60. More sensorineural incidence than in otosclerosis. May have bony lesion in footplate or atrophy of crura. Middle ear mucosa is hyperemic, and stapes is fixed due to thick, friable bone. Some authors report bone similar to otosclerotic lesion in some cases. The two diseases have been known to co-exist. Van der Hoeve–de Kleyn syndrome: blue sclera, bone fragility, and hearing loss.

III. Abnormalities of collagen fibers at the reticular stage. Calcium and phosphorus content are low, but enzyme activity is normal. Bone matrix is immature with large numbers of osteoblasts, but no apparent osteoblastic activity.

IV. Conductive, sensorineural, or mixed loss.

# Appendix IV: Neurofibromatosis

Von Recklinghausen's disease (1882) occurs in three forms (overlap of forms also occurs).

1. Central forms, known as neurofibromatosis-II (NF-II)
   a. Multiple intracranial and intraspinal tumors
   b. Bilateral acoustic schwannomas
2. Peripheral form (NF-I) (Today, only NF-I is referred to as von Recklinghausen's disease)
   a. Café au lait spots
3. Visceral form

## NF-II

1. First report of bilateral acoustic tumors was by Wishart in 1882 and Knoblauch.
2. In 1940, Turner reported a family with bilateral acoustic tumors transmitted through generations.
3. No gross difference in appearance between unilateral and bilateral acoustic schwannomas. However, in NF-II, there may be multiple schwannomas involving an individual nerve, or involving numerous nerves, as well as multiple meningiomas. Schwannomas and meningiomas may be present in the same surgical specimen and indistinguishable grossly.

   Microscopically, NF-II schwannomas are histologically identical to sporadic acute unilateral acoustic schwannomas. In some cases, they may show an intermediate pattern between meningioma and schwannoma (the cells of schwannomas and meningiomas originate from the neural crest). These schwannomas are different, however, from neurofibromas.

4. *Recurrence*
   a. Tumor behavior can be different from unilateral acoustic schwannomas (old data).
   b. NF-II tumors may be more invasive and may infiltrate the cochlear nerve. This infiltration may be responsible for low success rate with tumor debulking.
   c. No real evidence that recurrence rate is higher, although there is a risk of new tumor on adjacent or residual cranial nerve. Tumor recurrence or recurrence has been reported infrequently, and usually after suboccipital/retrosigmoid approach, and these probably represent residual tumor.
5. Overall acoustic neuroma recurrence rate is ~0.5%. True recurrence rate with NF-II is unknown but appears to be higher. The average time interval from removal to recurrence overall is ~10 years. Growth rate of recurrences range between 0.79 and 5.2 mm per year. Recurrence is most likely to occur in large tumor.
6. NF-II effect primarily brain and spinal cord, although there may be other tumors.
7. NF-II afflicts 1 in 35,000 or 40,000 individuals, but NF-1, which is usually diagnosed in infancy, does not become apparent in early adulthood or later.
   a. Accepted average tumor growth rate is 2.8 mm per year. House believes in one postop MRI at 5 years, at which time recurrent tumor would be 1.5 cm.
   b. NIH consensus conference diagnostic criteria for NF-II.
   c. Bilateral eighth nerve masses on MRI or CT.
   d. First-degree of relative with NF-II and either a unilateral eighth nerve tumor

or two of the following: Neurofibroma, meningioma, glioma, schwannoma, or posterior subcapsular lenticular opacity.

8. *Hearing preservation surgery usually is indicated*
   a. Growth pattern is unpredictable.
   b. Surgery is the mainstay of treatment, although radiation and chemotherapy have been used.
   c. Old concepts noted above have been abandoned, and hearing preservation is tried with all tumors less than ~2 cm. If hearing is lost on the first side, second tumor is observed until hearing begins to deteriorate. If hearing is preserved, second tumor is removed with attempted hearing preservation.
   d. If cochlear nerve can be preserved, cochlear implantation can be performed.

9. *Hearing preservation—Factors that influence*:
   a. Serviceable hearing 50 dB, 50% discrimination.
   b. Success in NF-II for saving hearing is the same as that in acoustic neuromas in general, 67%.
   c. Tumor located more medially in the internal auditory canal may be more favorable for middle fossa approach for hearing preservation and may be less adherent to the cochlear nerve.
   d. Reduced caloric may indicate superior compartment tumor and be more favorable.
   e. Good preoperative brainstem evoked response audiometry morphology may be more favorable.

4. Penetrance is 100%, but expression is variable.
5. About 50% of NF-II cases are new mutations.
6. Heterogeneous expression between families; there are two clinical subtypes of NF-II.
   a. *Gardner's subtype* (Milder form)
      i. Onset of symptoms, usually hearing loss from bilateral vestibular schwannomas.
      ii. Few or other associated brain or spinal cord tumors.
      iii. Main age of onset is 27 years, only 12% have meningiomas.
   b. *Wishart's subtype* (Severe form)
      i. Multiple intracranial and spinal tumors.
      ii. Developed at an early age with rapid progression of signs and symptoms.
      iii. Average age of presentation 17.4 years, > 70% with meningiomas.
   c. *Third subtype, called the Lee/Abbott subtype*
      i. Childhood cataracts and early death due to cranial and spinal meningiomas and schwannomas.
      ii. Average age of presentation 14 years, > 70% incidence of meningiomas.

## SCREENING

1. Molecular testing peripheral blood sample.
2. Screening by MRI.
3. Screening should be performed early (under age 8) for at-risk family members, and gene carrier should be screened yearly.

## GENETICS

1. Autosomal dominant.
2. Deletion on the long arm of chromosome 22.
3. The NF-II is a tumor suppressor gene that is inactivated in NF-II tumors. The DNA sequence and protein product on which it acts had been determined.

# Index

T - #0257 - 160425 - C158 - 254/178/29 - PB - 9781032567594 - Gloss Lamination